Essentials of Clinical Geriatrics

Essentials of Clinical Geriatrics

Edited by Roger Simpson

hayle
medical

New York

Hayle Medical,
750 Third Avenue, 9th Floor,
New York, NY 10017, USA

Visit us on the World Wide Web at:
www.haylemedical.com

ISBN: 978-1-63241-495-3

Cataloging-in-Publication Data

Essentials of clinical geriatrics / edited by Roger Simpson.
    p. cm.
Includes bibliographical references and index.
ISBN 978-1-63241-495-3
1. Geriatrics. 2. Older people--Diseases. 3. Older people--Health and hygiene.
I. Simpson, Roger.
RC952 .E87 2018
618.97--dc23

Table of Contents

Permissions

List of Contributors

Index

Preface

This book aims to highlight the current researches and provides a platform to further the scope of innovations in this area. This book is a product of the combined efforts of many researchers and scientists, after going through thorough studies and analysis from different parts of the world. The objective of this book is to provide the readers with the latest information of the field.

Geriatric medicine focuses on the prevention and treatment of diseases found in older people. Some of these diseases are atherosclerosis, dementia, osteoporosis, orthogeriatrics, Parkinson's disease, etc. Geriatrics is rapidly evolving as people are becoming more aware to medical problems related to aging. This book is a compilation of chapters that discuss the most vital concepts and emerging trends in the field of geriatrics. Students, researchers, experts, medical practitioners and all associated with geriatrics and gerontology will benefit alike from this book.

I would like to express my sincere thanks to the authors for their dedicated efforts in the completion of this book. I acknowledge the efforts of the publisher for providing constant support. Lastly, I would like to thank my family for their support in all academic endeavors.

Editor

Isolation of a Stable Subpopulation of Mobilized Dental Pulp Stem Cells (MDPSCs) with High Proliferation, Migration, and Regeneration Potential Is Independent of Age

Hiroshi Horibe[1,2❾], Masashi Murakami[1❾], Koichiro Iohara[1], Yuki Hayashi[1,3], Norio Takeuchi[1,4], Yoshifumi Takei[5], Kenichi Kurita[2], Misako Nakashima[1]*

1 Department of Dental Regenerative Medicine, Center of Advanced Medicine for Dental and Oral Diseases, National Center for Geriatrics and Gerontology, Research Institute, Morioka, Obu, Aichi, Japan, 2 Department of Oral and Maxillofacial Surgery, School of Dentistry, Aichi-gakuin University, Nagoya, Aichi, Japan, 3 Department of Pediatric Dentistry, School of Dentistry, Aichi-gakuin University, Nagoya, Aichi, Japan, 4 Department of Endodontics, School of Dentistry, Aichi-g akuin University, Nagoya, Aichi, Japan, 5 Department of Biochemistry and Division of Disease Models, Center for Neurological Diseases and Cancer, Nagoya University Graduate School of Medicine, Nagoya, Aichi, Japan

Abstract

Insights into the understanding of the influence of the age of MSCs on their cellular responses and regenerative potential are critical for stem cell therapy in the clinic. We have isolated dental pulp stem cells (DPSCs) subsets based on their migratory response to granulocyte-colony stimulating factor (G-CSF) (MDPSCs) from young and aged donors. The aged MDPSCs were efficiently enriched in stem cells, expressing high levels of trophic factors with high proliferation, migration and anti-apoptotic effects compared to young MDPSCs. In contrast, significant differences in those properties were detected between aged and young colony-derived DPSCs. Unlike DPSCs, MDPSCs showed a small age-dependent increase in senescence-associated β-galactosidase (SA-β-gal) production and senescence markers including p16, p21, Interleukin (IL)-1β, -6, -8, and Groα in long-term culture. There was no difference between aged and young MDPSCs in telomerase activity. The regenerative potential of aged MDPSCs was similar to that of young MDPSCs in an ischemic hindlimb model and an ectopic tooth root model. These results demonstrated that the stem cell properties and the high regenerative potential of MDPSCs are independent of age, demonstrating an immense utility for clinical applications by autologous cell transplantation in dental pulp regeneration and ischemic diseases.

Editor: Irina Kerkis, Instituto Butantan, Brazil

Funding: The work was supported by Research Grant for Longevity Sciences (23-10) from the Ministry of Health, Labour and Welfare to MN. The funders had no role in study design, data collection and analysis, decision to publish, or preparation of the manuscript.

Competing Interests: The authors have declared that no competing interests exist.

* E-mail: misako@ncgg.go.jp

❾ These authors contributed equally to this work.

Introduction

Tissue regeneration and maintenance is dependent on mesenchymal stem cells (MSCs) [1]. For the application of MSCs in tissue engineering and regenerative medicine, it is important to optimize their isolation and preserve their phenotypic properties. Moreover, it is necessary to determine the influence of donor age on MSCs [2]. Aging related changes consist of three distinct types: quantity (proliferation potential), quality (differentiation/regenerative potential) and mobilization potential [3]. More information about the age-related changes in MSCs is essential for the successful development of cell-therapies for the aged [4].

In a recent study on human bone marrow MSCs (BMSCs) and adipose tissue derived MSCs (ASCs), it has been shown that MSC numbers decline with donor age [5,6]. Aside from a decrease in overall expansion potential [7], several groups have also documented that aged MSCs have a decreased proliferation rate

compared to young MSCs from the initial cell passages and cellular senescence [6,8,9]. In addition, telomere length is decreased in aged MSCs compared to young MSCs [9], and this telomere shortening has been shown to inhibit the mobilization of stem cells out of their niche [10]. Furthermore, the migratory activity of periodontal ligament stem cells (PDLSCs) is decreased with age [11] and gene expression of pro-angiogenic factors including VEGF, PlGF, and HGF in MSCs is down-regulated with increasing age [9,12].

Results obtained from three different species -mouse, rat and human- clearly demonstrate a declining differentiation capability of MSCs with age [8,11,13,14]. On the other hand, no changes were observed in MSCs with age has been reported in their osteogenic and adipogenic differentiation potential *in vivo* [15,16] and *in vitro* [17,18]. Furthermore, isolated CD105+ MSCs from the aged does not influence the adipogenic, myogenic [19], and osteogenic potential [20]. Thus, there appears to be contradictory results in the literature regarding the phenotypic properties of aged stem cells. These apparent discrepancies may be attributed to variable methods of isolation of MSCs, resulting in the coexistence of various subsets of stem cells that vary in their differentiation potential and their vulnerability to senescence. In addition, there is not yet a clear understanding of the different cellular markers of MSCs [19,21].

Human dental pulp stem cells (DPSCs) represent a novel adult stem cell population that possesses the properties of high proliferative potential, self-renewal and multi-lineage differentiation [22]. The supply of autologous pulp tissue, however, is very limited with age, due to narrow root canals and the decrease in pulp tissue volumes due to physiological secondary dentin formation, pathological tertiary dentin formation and mineralization [23]. The older patients' teeth supply fewer colonies of human DPSCs than the younger patients' [24]. Human DPSCs from aged donors lose their proliferative activities and differentiation capabilities after repeated passages [25,26]. Hypoxic cultures, grown under 3% O2, however, have succeeded in overcoming this deficiency, indicating the possibility to obtain optimal numbers of human DPSCs from aged patients [24]. We have devised a method of isolation of mobilized dental pulp stem cells (MDPSCs) by G-CSF-induced mobilization that generates stem cell enriched subpopulations with increased expression of angiogenic/neurotrophic factors, with higher trophic effect on migration, immunomodulation and anti-apoptosis and attendant angiogenic, neurogenic and regenerative potential [27]. Thus, the evidence in the literature that isolated subfractions of MSCs from the aged showed no change in differentiation potential compared with that from the young [19,20] prompted us to determine whether the aged MDPSCs retain the quantity, quality and mobilization potential as the young MDPSCs useful for cell therapy.

Many factors are known to induce cellular senescence. These include dysfunctional telomeres, non-telomeric DNA damage, excessive mitogenic signals including those produced by oncogenes, perturbations to chromatin organization and stresses with an as-yet unknown etiology [28]. Generally, senescent cells display a characteristic enlarged, flattened morphology and are characterized by an irreversible G1 growth arrest involving the repression of genes that drive cell cycle progression and the up-regulation of cell cycle inhibitors like p53/p21 and p16/RB and by expression of senescence-associated β-galactosidase (SA-β-gal) activity [3,29]. However, the expression of CXCR2 and its ligands such as IL-8, GROα is also up-regulated in senescence cells [30].

In the present investigation, we have compared the biological properties of aged MDPSCs versus young MDPSCs, including their phenotypic stability and the expression of senescence markers in long-term cultures. In addition the regenerative potential was examined in ischemic hindlimb and ectopic tooth root models. The results demonstrated that MDPSCs are efficiently enriched and stable, secreting high levels of trophic factors with high proliferation, migration, and regenerative potential, and that these properties of the MDPSCs are independent of age.

Materials and Methods

This study was approved by the ethics committees and the animal care and use committees of National Center for Geriatrics and Gerontology, Research Institute and Aichi-gakuin University. All experiments were conducted using the strict guidelines of DNA Safety Programs.

Isolation of DPSCs by G-CSF induced chemotaxis

Normal human third molars were collected from young adult patients (19–30 years of age, n = 6) and older patients (44–70 years

of age, n = 6) at the Aichi-gakuin University Dental Hospital under approved guidelines set by School of Dentistry, Aichi-gakuin University and National Center for Geriatrics and Gerontology, Research Institute. Informed written consents were obtained from every donor for use of dental pulp tissue. Each dental pulp tissue were extracted from young and aged teeth and minced into pieces followed by enzymatic digestion using in 0.04 mg/ml Liberase (Roche, Mannheim, Germany) with slight modification of our previous method [31]. The number of isolated cells and their viability was determined by trypan blue staining of cells, and plated at 2–4×10^4 cells on 35 mm dishes (Asahi Technoglass, Funabashi, Japan) in Dulbecco's Modified Eagle's Medium (DMEM) (Sigma, St. Louis, MO) supplemented with 10% human serum collected from healthy consenting adult donors and basic fibroblast growth factor (bFGF) (Fibrast splay, Kaken Pharmaceutiical Co. Ltd.) (10 ng/ml). The dental pulp stem cells forming colonies (DPSCs) were detached by incubation with TrypLE Select (Invitrogen) prior to 70% confluency and subcultured at 1–2×10^5 cells on 10 cm dishes (Asahi Technoglass) in DMEM supplemented with 10% human serum.

The mobilized subpopulation of dental pulp stem cells, MDPSCs, was further isolated by our recently devised method utilizing G-CSF-induced stem cell mobilization [27]. Briefly, Costar Transwell (permeable support 8.0 μm polycarbonate membrane 6.5 mm Insert, Corning, Lowell, MA) as upper chamber was inserted into 24 well plate tissue culture plates (Falcon) as lower chamber. The membrane was modified chemically (Toray Industries, Inc., Tokyo) to prevent cell attachment. Young and aged DPSCs (2×10^4 cells/100 μl DMEM) at the third passage of culture were seeded into the upper chambers respectively, and 390 μl DMEM supplemented with 10% human serum and G-CSF (100 ng/ml) was added in the lower chambers. After 48 h incubation, the medium was changed into DMEM supplemented with 10% human serum without G-CSF, and the numbers of the cells attached to the dishes were counted. After 7 days culture, aggregates of ≥50 cells were scored as colonies. Once cells reached 60–70% confluence, they were detached and subcultured until senescence. To evaluate the colony forming efficiency of MDPSCs, 1×10^3 cells/ml of MDPSCs at the 4th passage were seeded into 35 mm dishes in DMEM supplemented with 10% human serum, and then incubated. After 4 days culture, aggregates of ≥10 cells were scored as colonies.

Flow cytometric analysis

Both young and aged MDPSCs were characterized by a flow cytometry FACSAria II (BD Biosciences, San Jose, CA) at the 5th passage of culture as described previously [27], and young and aged DPSCs from the same individuals at the same passage were also used as controls. They were immunolabeled for 60 min at 4°C with antibodies against CD29, CD31, CD44, CD73, CD90, CD105, CD146, CXCR4, and G-CSFR, respectively.

Induced differentiation

The differentiation of MDPSCs into angiogenic, neurogenic, odontogenic/osteogenic, and adipogenic lineages was induced and compared with that of DPSCs without the G-CSF induced migratory response [32].

Real-time RT-PCR

Total RNA was extracted using Trizol (Invitrogen) from young and aged MDPSCs, and from young and aged DPSCs at the 6th passage. First-strand cDNA synthesis was performed on total RNA of those cells by reverse transcription using the ReverTra Ace-α (Toyobo, Tokyo, Japan) after DNase I treatment (Roche

Diagnostics, Pleasanton, CA) at 37°C for 20 min. Real-time RT-PCR was performed as described previously [27] using the stem cell markers, *Oct3/4*, *Nanog*, *Sox2*, *Rex1*, *Stat3*, and *CXCR4*. To examine mRNA expression of angiogenic and neurotrophic factors, real-time RT-PCR amplifications of *granulocyte-monocyte colony-stimulating factor* (*GM-CSF*), *matrix metalloproteinase* (*MMP*)-*3*, *vascular endothelial growth factor* (*VEGF*), *brain-derived neurotrophic factor* (*BDNF*), *glial cell derived neurotrophic factor* (*GDNF*), *nerve growth factor* (*NGF*), and *neurotrophin-3* (*NT-3*) were also performed [27].

Proliferation and migration assay

To determine the proliferative activity in response to G-CSF, aged MDPSCs were compared with young MDPSCs at the 5th passage at 3×10^3 cells per 96 well in DMEM without serum. Young and aged DPSCs from the same individuals were used as controls. Ten μl of Tetra-color one (Seikagaku Kogyo, Co., Ltd) were added to the 96 well plate, and cell numbers were measured using a spectrophotometer at 450 nm absorbance at 2, 12, 24, 36, and 48 h of culture. Wells without cells served as negative controls.

To examine the migratory activity of young and aged MDPSCs, horizontal chemotaxis assay using TAXIScan-FL (Effector Cell Institute) was performed as described previously [33]. Young and aged DPSCs from the same individuals were also used as controls.

Effect of MDPSCs-conditioned medium

At 60% confluence, the culture medium was switched to DMEM without serum and the conditioned media from young and aged MDPSCs, and young and aged DPSCs at the 5th to 6th passage were collected 24 h later, and concentrated about 40 times by Amicon Ultra-15 Centrifugal Filter Unit with Ultracel-3 membrane (Millipore, Billerica, MA).

To assess the immunomodulatory effect of the conditioned medium (CM) of MDPSCs, a mixed lymphocyte reaction (MLR) assay was performed as described previously [34]. Autologous PBMCs and allogenic stimulator PBMCs were co-cultured at 10^4 cells per 96 well in RPMI-1640 without arginine, leucine, lysine, and phenol red (Sigma-Aldrich) supplemented 5 μg/ml of each CM. Cell numbers were measured at 0, 12, 24, and 36 h.

To assess the anti-apoptotic effect of the CM, NIH3T3 cells were incubated with 500 nM staurosporine (Sigma-Aldrich) in DMEM supplemented with 5 μg/ml of CM from young and aged MDPSCs and from young and aged DPSCs. After 3 h, NIH3T3 cells were harvested, and the cell suspensions were treated with Annexin V-FITC (Roche Diagnostics) and propidium iodide for 15 min, and analyzed by flow cytometry.

Stability of MDPSCs phenotype

To evaluate the stability of aged MDPSCs, the 6th passage of MDPSCs were compared with the 12th passage in the proliferation and migratory activities. Flow cytometric analysis of cell surface markers (CD29, CD31, CD44, CD73, CD90 and CD105) was also performed in young and aged MDPSCs to compare the 6th passage with the 12th passage.

Senescence associated (SA)-β-gal (Senescence Cells Histochemical Staining Kit, Sigma-Aldrich, St. Louis, MO, USA) staining assay and real-time RT-PCR analysis of senescence related genes (*p16*, *p21*, *Interleukin-1β* (*IL-1β*), *Interleukin-6* (*IL-6*), *Interleukin-8* (*IL-8*) and *Growth related oncogene-α* (*GROα*) were performed in the 6th and 20th passages of young MDPSCs and DPSCs in comparison with aged MDPSCs and DPSCs as described previously [27].

To analyze the karyotype of aged MDPSCs at the 7th passage, chromosomes prepared from cells were stained with quinacrine mustard (Sigma-Aldrich) and Hoechst 33258 (Sigma-Aldrich) dissolved in a McIlvane's buffered solution (pH 7.0) and examined under a fluorescence microscope. Suitable metaphases were photographed and karyotypes were analyzed.

The telomerase activity was determined with a Quantitative Telomerase detection kit (Allied Biotech, Inc., Vallejo, CA) as described previously [27]. Briefly, the 8th, 12th and 20th passages of MDPSCs and DPSCs from young and aged donors were lysed in Lysis buffer and the telomerase activity was determined with a Quantitative Telomerase detection kit (Allied Biotech, Inc., Vallejo, CA) by Applied Biosystems 7500 Real-time PCR system (Applied Biosystems, Foster City, CA) using whole-cell extract containing 0.5 μg of protein.

The telomere length was analyzed using the Telo TAGGG telomere Length Assay kit according to manufacturer's instructions (Roche Applied Science, Indianapolis, IN). Genomic DNA (gDNA) was extracted from the 8th, 12th and 20th passages of MDPSCs and DPSCs from young and aged donors using a DNA extraction kit (Life Technologies Corporation, Carlsbad, CA USA). One microgram of gDNA was digested with the mixture of HinfI and RsaI restriction endonucleases, electrophoresed through a 0.8% agarose gel, and transferred to a nylon membrane to be hybridized to a digoxigenin (DIG)-labeled telomeric oligonucleotide (TTAGGG)$_3$. The DNA/oligonucleotide hybridization products were visualized after reaction with a chemiluminescent substrate, using ImageQuant LAS4000 (GE Healthcare Life Sciences, Little Chalfont, UK).

Transplantation of MDPSCs into a mouse ischemic hindlimb model

The angiogenic potential of MDPSCs was examined in a murine model of hind limb ischemia in 5-week-old severe combined immunodeficient (SCID) mice (CB17, CLEA, Tokyo) as described previously [32]. In brief, 24 h after ligation of the left proximal portion of the femoral artery, 1×10^6 cells of young and aged MDPSCs, and young and aged DPSCs at the 6th passage after DiI (Sigma) labeling were injected intramuscularly. PBS injection was also used as negative control. Laser Doppler imaging (Perimed AB, Stockholm, Sweden) was performed 14 days after cell transplantation. The cryosections (12 μm thick) of isolated muscle tissue of ischemic hind limb were prepared and immunostained with Fluorescein *Griffonia (Bandeiraea) simplicifolia* Lectin 1/fluorescein-*Galanthus nivalis* (snowdrop) lectin (20 mg/ml; Vector Laboratories, Inc., Youngstown, OH). Microscopic digital images of six sections of every 120 μm were scanned in a frame composed of 500 μmx380 μm rectangle and statistical analyses was performed using software Dynamic cell count, BZ-HIC, on a fluorescein microscope BIOREVO, BZ-9000 (KEYENCE, Osaka, Japan). The co-localization of DiI-labeled transplanted cells and the newly formed BS-1 lectin-positive capillaries were observed using confocal laser microscopy (TCS SP5 conventional inverted microscope, Leica Microsystems, Wetzlar, Germany).

Subcutaneous implantation of human tooth root in SCID mice

An experimental model of human tooth root was used for the evaluation of ectopic pulp regeneration after subcutaneous implantation into SCID mice as described previously [27]. Human tooth roots were prepared, 6 mm in length, 1 mm in width, and one end was sealed with cement. Both young and aged MDPSCs, and young and aged DPSCs, respectively, at the 7th passage, 1×10^6 cells each, were injected into the root with collagen TE (Nitta Gelatin), and each 4 roots were transplanted subcutaneously into 5-week-old SCID mice (CB17, CLEA). The four roots in which only collagen TE was injected were also transplanted as a

4

Essentials of Clinical Geriatrics

control. Sixteen roots were harvested for histology after 21 days. The paraffin sections (5 μm in thickness) were stained with hematoxylin and eosin (HE), and the relative amounts of regenerated pulp tissue were morphometrically analyzed in each sample. For vascular staining, 5-μm-thick paraffin sections were immunostained with RECA1 (MONOSAN, UDEN, Netherlands) (1:500) and 2nd antibody (Vector) (1:200) and examined by confocal laser microscopy (TCS SP5 conventional inverted microscope, Leica). The ratio of RECA1 positive newly formed capillaries to the root canal area in the aged MDPSCs transplantation was compared with that in the young MDPSCs transplantation and the young DPSCs transplantation using a fluorescence microscope (BIOREVO, BZ-9000, KEYENCE).

For the analysis of regenerated dentin, *in situ* hybridization was performed using an odontoblastic marker, enamelysin. DIG signals were detected using a TSA system. Regenerated dentin width and enamelysin-positive cells along dentinal wall in the regenerated area on day 28 were calculated in three sections of each tooth ($n = 4$ teeth) by LAS AF software (Leica) using confocal laser microscopy.

Statistical Analyses

Data are reported as mean ± SD. *P* values were calculated using Student's *t* test and Tukey's multiple comparison test method in SPSS 21.0 (IBM, Armonk, NY http://www.ibm.com). The number of replicates in each experiment is indicated in the figure legends.

Results

Morphological analysis of young and aged MDPSCs

The efficiencies of attachment of young and aged mobilized DPSCs through membrane with G-CSF (MDPSCs) were 5% and 3%, respectively. Aged MDPSCs were morphologically similar to young MDPSCs, containing stellate cells with long process and spindle-shaped cells (**Figure S1**). Limiting dilution analysis at the third passage culture showed that the frequencies of colony forming unit (CFU) in young and aged MDPSCs were estimated to be 88% and 87%, respectively, and those in young and aged DPSCs were 70% and 68%, respectively.

Flow cytometric analysis of young and aged MDPSCs

Evaluation of the "stemness" of MDPSCs from aged donors was performed by flow cytometric analysis in comparison with that of young MDPSCs, and young and aged DPSCs. Young and aged MDPSCs and DPSCs were positive for CD29, CD44, CD73 and CD90, and negative for CD31, which are minimal criteria for MSCs. It is noteworthy, however, that the positive rates of CD105, CXCR4 and G-CSFR of young and aged MDPSCs were similar and were significantly higher than those of young and aged DPSCs. On the other hand, the positive rates of CD105 and G-CSFR of aged DPSCs were significantly lower compared to those of young DPSCs. These results suggested that aged MDPSCs contained similar numbers of pulp stem/progenitor cell populations to young MDPSCs, and that stemness may depend on the isolation method (**Table 1**).

Multi-lineage differential potential of aged MDPSCs

The multi-lineage differential potential of young and aged MDPSCs was compared to that of young and aged DPSCs. Aged MDPSCs formed extensive networks of cords and tube-like structures on a matrigel as early as 6 h like young MDPSCs (**Figure 1A, C**). However, no such formation was detected in aged DPSCs (**Figure 1D**). Fourteen days after neurogenic induction,

Table 1. Flow cytometric analysis of cell surface markers on MDPSCs compared with DPSCs isolated from young and aged donors.

| | Young (n=6) | | | | Aged (n=6) | | | |
| | MDPSCs | | DPSCs | | MDPSCs | | DPSCs | |
	Positive (%)	SD	Positive (%)	SD	Positive (%)	SD	Positive (%)	SD
CD29	97.8%	1.4	98.0%	1.5	97.3%	1.2	97.5%	2.1
CD31	0.1%	0.1	0.2%	0.2	0.2%	0.2	0.2%	0.2
CD44	98.8%	2.3	98.8%	2.2	99.5%	0.7	99.6%	0.5
CD73	98.0%	1.5	98.9%	1.0	97.5%	2.8	97.6%	2.5
CD90	98.0%	2.4	98.7%	1.4	97.0%	3.7	97.6%	3.0
CD105	##96.6%	2.2	**64.7%	7.6	##91.9%	2.9	48.6%	6.9
CD146	17.1%	8.1	16.4%	4.2	8.9%	3.7	21.4%	6.8
CXCR4	##16.5%	2.9	7.3%	1.8	##16.1%	2.0	7.6%	1.1
G-CSFR	56.7%	11.3	*26.0%	8.1	##44.2%	9.7	11.9%	3.7

##P<0.01, MDPSCs versus DPSCs;
**P<0.01,
*P<0.05, young DPSCs versus aged DPSCs.

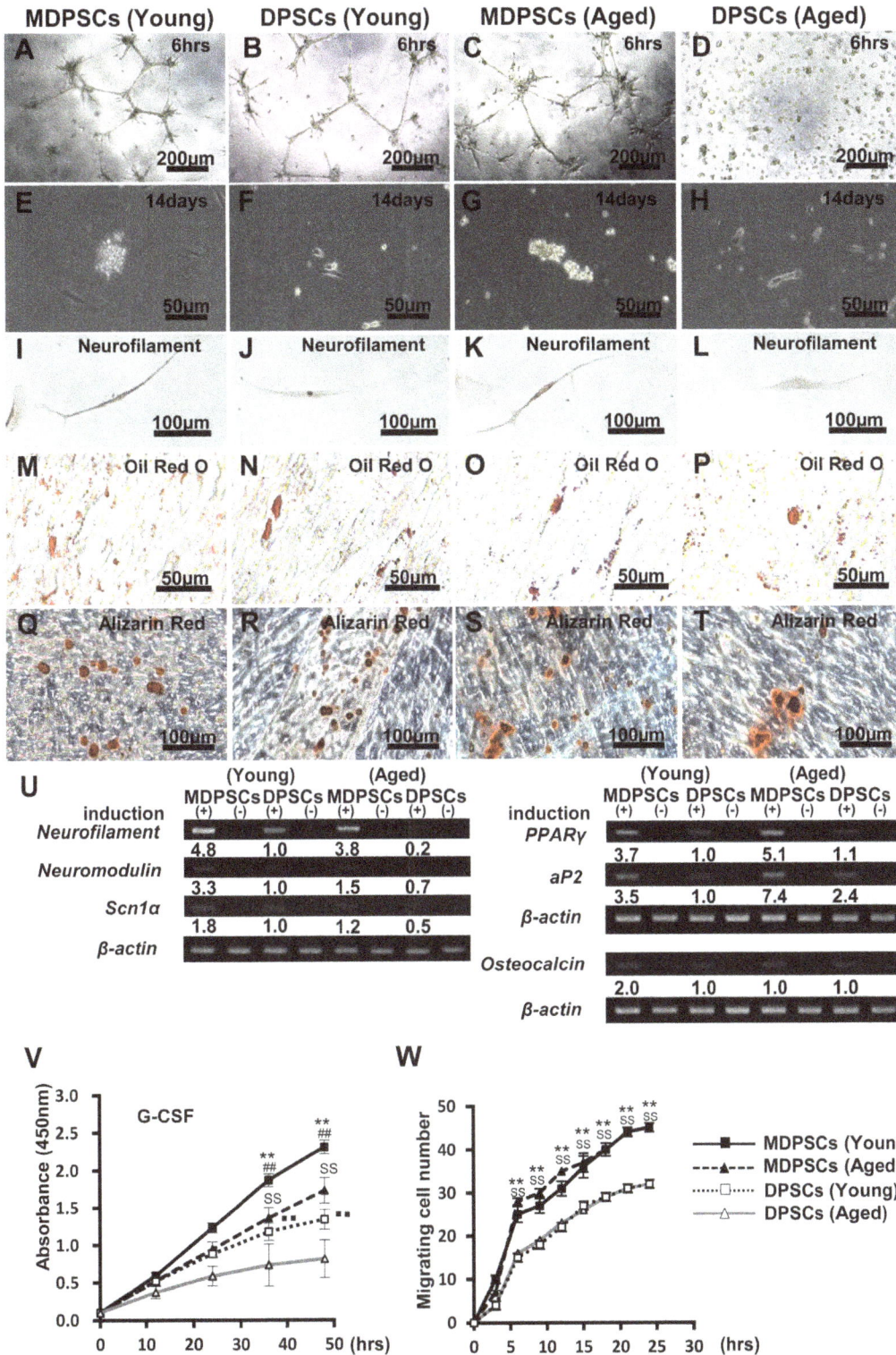

Figure 1. Multi-lineage differentiation potential and the characteristics. The aged dental pulp stem cells (DPSCs) mobilized by granulocyte-colony stimulating factor (G-CSF) (MDPSCs) were compared with aged colony-derived DPSCs (DPSCs), young MDPSCs and young DPSCs. (A–D) The endothelial differentiation potential using the matrigel assay. (E–H) Neurosphere formation, 14 days after induction. (I–L) Neuronal differentiation potential. Fourteen days after induction of dissociated neurosphere cells. (M–P) Adipogenic differentiation potential. (Q–T) Odontoblast differentiation potential. (U) Gene expression of *neurofilament*, *neuromodulin*, and *sodium channel, voltage-gated type I* α *(SCN1A)* for neuronal markers, *peroxisome proliferator-activated receptor* γ *(PPARγ)* and *adipocyte fatty acid binding protein 2* (*aP2*) for adipogenic markers, *osteocalcin* for a odonto/osteoblastic marker. (V) The proliferation analysis stimulated by 10% human serum (**$p<0.01$, young MDPSCs versus young DPSCs; $^{SS}p<0.01$, aged MDPSCs versus aged DPSCs; $^{##}p<0.01$, young MDPSCs versus aged MDPSCs; ■■$p<0.01$, young DPSCs versus aged DPSCs). (W) The migration analysis stimulated by G-CSF (10 ng/ml) (**$p<0.01$, young MDPSCs versus young DPSCs; $^{SS}p<0.01$, aged MDPSCs versus aged DPSCs). Data are expressed as the means ± SD of 6 determinations. The experiments were repeated six times (6 lots), and one representative experiment is presented.

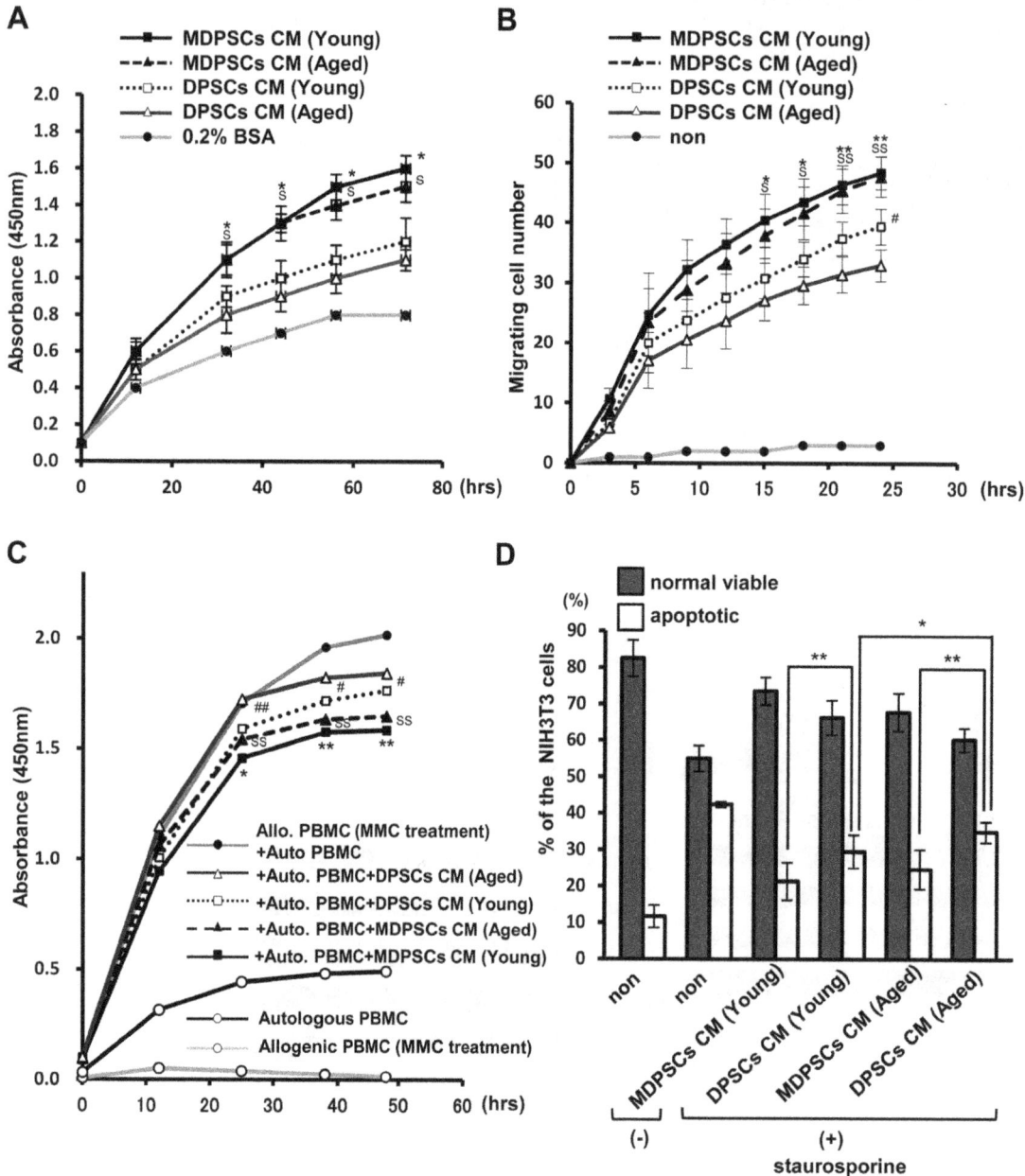

Figure 2. Effect of conditioned medium (CM) of aged MDPSCs. Effect of conditioned medium (CM) of the aged MDPSCs compared with those of aged DPSCs, young MDPSCs and young DPSCs. (A) The proliferative effect in NIH3T3 cells. (*$p<0.05$, young MDPSCs CM versus young DPSCs CM; $^Sp<0.05$, aged MDPSCs CM versus aged DPSCs CM). (B) The migratory effect in NIH3T3 cells (*$p<0.05$, **$p<0.01$, young MDPSCs CM versus young DPSCs CM; $^Sp<0.05$, $^{SS}p<0.01$, aged MDPSCs CM versus aged DPSCs CM; $^\#p<0.05$, young DPSCs CM versus aged DPSCs CM). (C) Mixed lymphocyte reaction (MLR) analysis. (*$p<0.05$, **$p<0.01$, young MDPSCs CM versus young DPSCs CM; $^{SS}p<0.01$, aged MDPSCs CM versus aged DPSCs CM; $^\#p<0.05$, $^{\#\#}p<0.01$, young DPSCs CM versus aged DPSCs CM). (D) The relative percentage of viable and apoptotic cells analyzed by flow cytometry by Annexin V staining. *$p<0.05$, **$p<0.01$. Data are expressed as the means ± SD of 6 determinations. The experiments were repeated three times (6 lots), and one representative experiment is presented.

clusters of proliferating neurospheres were more prevalent in aged MDPSCs and in young MDPSCs compared with DPSCs both from aged and young donors (**Figure 1E–H**). Following neuronal induction, neurite outgrowth and positive immunostaining for neurofilaments were found in aged MDPSCs as those in young MDPSCs (**Figure 1I, K**). The mRNA expression of the neuronal markers *neurofilament*, *neuromodulin*, and *sodium channel, voltage-gated type 1α* (*Scn1A*) in aged MDPSCs was similar to that of young MDPSCs and was higher compared with that of aged and young DPSCs (**Figure 1U**). As for the adipogenic induction, there was little difference among MDPSCs and DPSCs both from aged and young donors, as shown by the positive staining by Oil red O (**Figure 1M–P**) and the expression of the adipogenic markers *PPARγ* and *aP2* mRNA (**Figure 1U**). Aged MDPSCs, however, had the highest expression of these adipogenic markers (**Figure 1U**). Finally, 28 days after osteogenic/dentinogenic induction, the mineralized matrix was stained by alizarin red

Table 2. Relative mRNA expression of stem cell markers and angiogenic/neurotrophic factors in young MDPSCs, aged MDPSCs and aged DPSCs compared with young DPSCs.

Genes	Young		Aged	
	MDPSCs	DPSCs	MDPSCs	DPSCs
Oct3/4	2.6	1.0	1.2	0.6
Nanog	1.4	1.0	1.0	0.4
Sox2	6.7	1.0	7.9	0.5
Rex1	2.0	1.0	1.5	0.8
Stat3	2.8	1.0	1.6	0.6
CXCR4	14.4	1.0	5.6	0.1
GM-CSF	6.0	1.0	4.3	0.7
MMP3	25.5	1.0	24.9	0.8
VEGF	2.2	1.0	2.0	0.6
BDNF	2.3	1.0	1.1	0.7
GDNF	1.8	1.0	0.9	0.6
NGF	2.0	1.0	2.5	0.9
NT-3	1.3	1.0	1.4	0.4

The experiments were repeated three times (6 lots), and one representative experiment is presented.

(**Figure 1Q–T**), expressing the osteoblastic marker, *osteocalcin* mRNA, similarly in all cell populations (**Figure 1U**).

Biological characteristics of young and aged MDPSCs

The proliferation activity with human serum was higher in MDPSCs than in DPSCs from both young and aged donors. There were, however, significant differences between aged and young MDPSCs ($P<0.05$) (**Figure 1V**). The migratory activity with G-CSF was much higher in MDPSCs than in DPSCs and there was no significant difference between young and aged MDPSCs (**Figure 1W**).

Next, the ability of the conditioned medium (CM) from aged MDPSCs to accelerate cell proliferation and migration and suppress immunoreaction and apoptosis was investigated. The CM of aged MDPSCs was significantly more effective on proliferation compared to the CM of aged DPSCs. There was no significant difference in proliferation between the CM from aged and young MDPSCs (**Figure 2A**). The migratory effect of the CM from aged MDPSCs was higher than that from aged DPSCs when assayed on NIH3T3 cells. It is noteworthy that there was no significant difference between young and aged MDPSCs (**Figure 2B**). A significantly enhanced immunosuppression by the CM of MDPSCs was shown by MLR assay compared to the CM of DPSCs. No significant difference in immunosuppression between young and aged MDPSCs was found (**Figure 2C**). The survival rate of NIH3T3 cells was significantly enhanced by the CM of MDPSCs compared to the CM of DPSCs both from aged and young donors. The anti-apoptotic effect of the CM of aged MDPSCs was similar to that of the CM of young MDPSCs (**Figure 2D**). These results suggest that aged MDPSCs may induce similar trophic effects as young MDPSCs.

The mRNA expression of the stem cell markers, *Oct3/4, Nanog, Sox2, Rex1, Stat3* and *CXCR4* was similar in aged MDPSCs to those in young MDPSCs (Table 2), suggesting a similar stemness for aged MDPSCs and young MDPSCs. The expression of the angiogenic and/or neurotrophic factors *GM-CSF, MMP3, VEGF, BDNF, GDNF, NGF* and *NT-3* was similar or a little higher in young MDPSCs compared to aged MDPSCs (Table 2), suggesting

that MDPSCs may have similar angiogenic/vasculogenic and neurogenic potential. On the other hand, the expression of the stem cell markers, *Sox2* and *CXCR4*, and the angiogenic/neurotrophic factors, *GM-CSF, MMP3, VEGF, BDNF, GDNF* and *NT-3* was much higher in aged MDPSCs than in those in aged DPSCs. These results suggest a marked increase in the functionality and quality of MDPSCs compared with DPSCs from the aged donors.

Maintenance of the MDPSCs characteristics

The cumulative cell number of MDPSCs was much higher, and the proliferative life span of MDPSCs was longer than those of DPSCs both from aged and young donors. Aged MDPSCs showed a lower cumulative cell number compared to young MDPSCs (**Figure 3A**). To examine the stability of aged MDPSCs after prolonged *ex-vivo* culture, the proliferation activity, migratory activity, and cell surface markers in the 6th passage of aged MDPSCs were compared with those in the 12th passage. There was no significant difference between 6th and 12th passage of aged MDPSCs in proliferation activity (**Figure** 3B), migratory activity (**Figure 3C**) and percentages of cell surface markers (**Table S1**). The number of senescence associated (SA)-β-gal positive cells increased in DPSCs at the 20th passage, but both aged and young MDPSCs were negative for SA-β-gal expression at the 20th passage (**Figure 3D, E**). Furthermore, the expression of *p16, p21, IL-1β, IL-6, IL-8* and *Groα* was higher in aged DPSCs compared with that in aged MDPSCs at the 20th passage (**Figure 3F**). There were also no chromosomal abnormalities/aberrations in the karyotype of aged MDPSCs at the 7th passage (**Figure 3G**). Taken together, these results indicate stability of MDPSCs after cell expansion irrespective of age.

The telomerase enzyme activity of young and aged MDPSCs at the 8th, 12th and 20th passages was analyzed in comparison with that of young and aged DPSCs at each passage. Our results showed a reduction in both young and aged DPSCs compared to that in young and aged MDPSCs. In addition, the telomerase activity gradually decreased in MDPSCs with increasing passage number (**Figure 4A**). The telomere length was monitored using

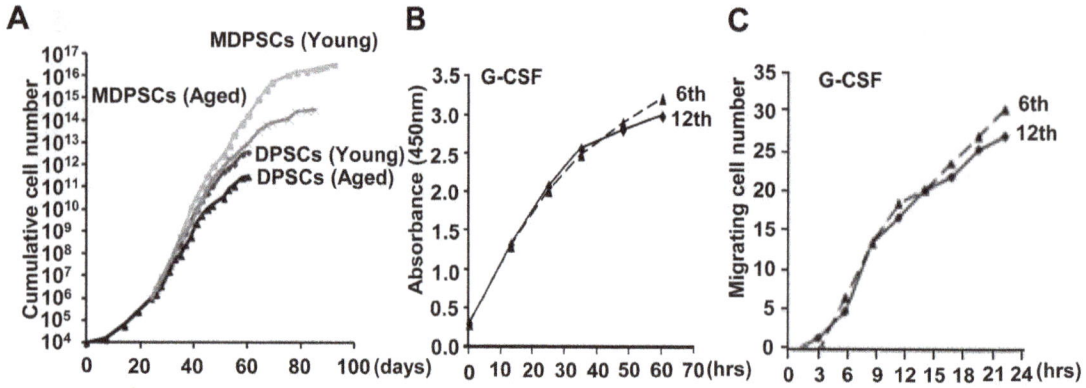

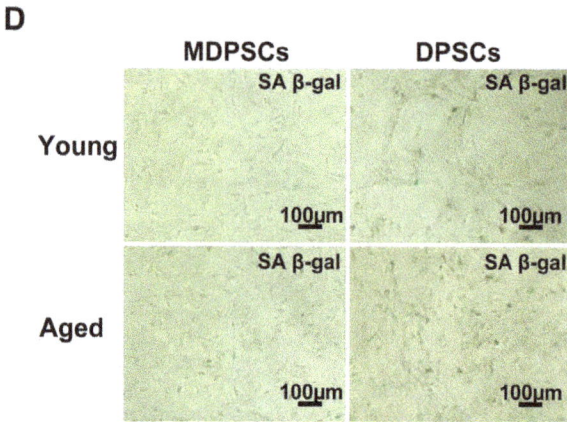

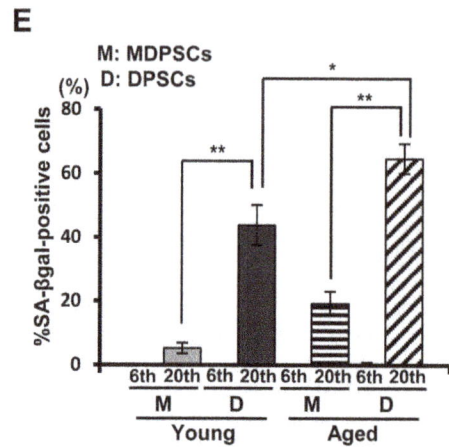

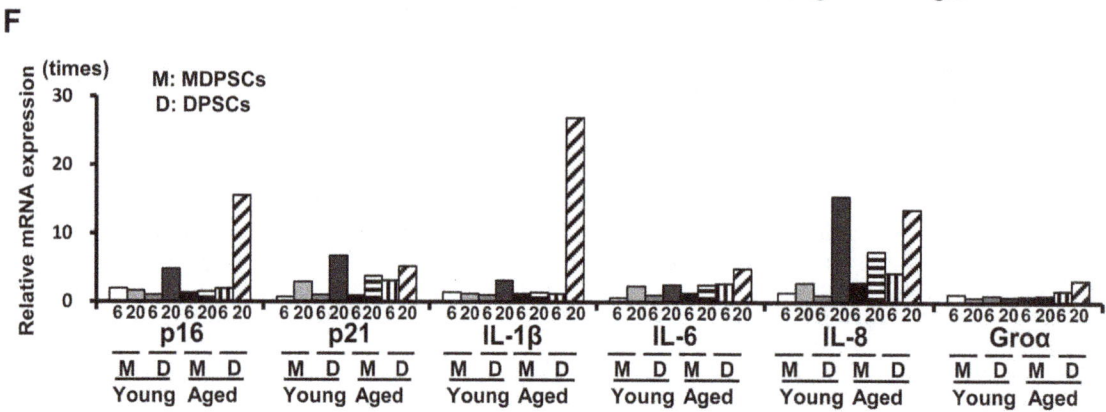

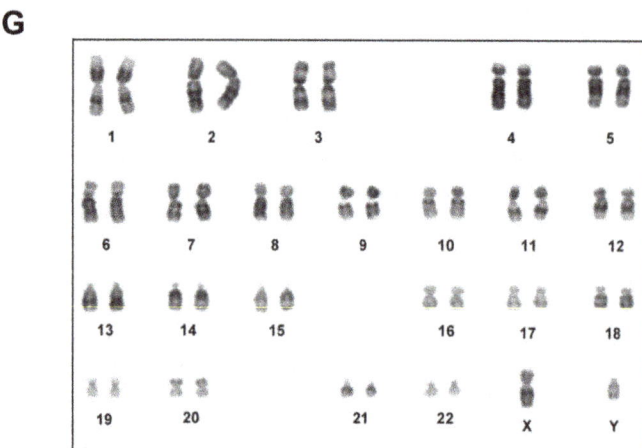

Figure 3. Maintenance of the stem cell properties of the aged MDPSCs with prolonged culture. (A) The cumulative cell number of aged MDPSCs, aged DPSCs, young MDPSCs and young DPSCs. (B) The proliferation of aged MDPSCs at the 6th and 12th passages by 10% human serum. (C) Migration of aged MDPSCs at the 6th and 12th passages. (D) Senescent associated (SA)-β-gal staining. (E) Percentage of SA-β-gal-positive cells of aged and young MDPSCs, and aged and young DPSCs at the 20th passage. *$p < 0.05$, **$p < 0.01$. Data are expressed as the means ± SD of 6 determinations. The experiments were repeated three times (6 lots), and one representative experiment is presented. (F) Relative mRNA expression of senescence-related genes, *p16, p21, IL-1β, IL-6, IL-8* and *Groα* in aged and young MDPSCs, and aged and young DPSCs at the 6th and 20th passages. The experiments were repeated six times (6 lots), and one representative experiment is presented. (G) Q-banding analysis for aged MDPSCs at the 7th passage showing normal karyotype.

the mean terminal restriction fragment (TRF) length of genomic DNA isolated from young and aged MDPSCs at the 8th, 12th and 20th passages in comparison with that of young and aged DPSCs at each passage. The telomere length was longer both in young and aged MDPSCs compared to that in young and aged DPSCs. With prolonged culture, the telomere length gradually decreased in MDPSCs (**Figure 4B**), consistent with the result of the telomerase activity.

Neovascularization in ischemic hindlimb with MDPSCs transplantation

Next, the regenerative potential of human MDPSCs was determined in a murine model of hindlimb ischemia. Fourteen days after transplantation of young and aged MDPSCs, the quantitative analysis of blood flow and capillary density was performed in comparison with young and aged DPSCs. Laser Doppler imaging revealed that blood flow was significantly increased approximately 1.4 and 2.0 times more in aged MDPSCs transplantation compared with aged DPSCs and PBS control without cells, respectively (**Figure 5C, D, E, F**). Capillary density in the ischemic region transplanted with aged MDPSCs increased 2.1 times higher than that with aged DPSCs (**Figure 5I, J, L**). There was no significant difference in blood flow and capillary density between young and aged MDPSCs (**Figure 5F, 5L**). Confocal microscopic analysis showed that DiI-labeled MDPSCs and DPSCs both from aged and young donors did not co-localize

with BS-1 lectin stained blood vessels (**Figure 5M–P**), implying their trophic effect on neovascularization.

Ectopic pulp regeneration by aged MDPSCs in the tooth root

We next evaluated pulp regenerative potential of human MDPSCs in an experimental model of ectopic tooth root transplantation in SCID mice. Pulp-like tissue with well-organized vasculature was regenerated in the tooth root 28 days after transplantation of MDPSCs and DPSCs from aged donors similar to young donors (**Figure 6A–H**). Statistical analysis showed that the regenerated pulp area was significantly larger (1.2-fold) in the transplantation of aged MDPSCs compared to the transplantations of aged DPSCs, and was similar to the comparison of young MDPSCs and DPSCs (**Figure 6U**). Neovascularization was observed in the regenerated pulp tissue after all the cell transplantations by immunofluorescent staining analysis with RECA1 antibody (**Figure 6I–L**). Statistical analysis showed that the vascularization areas were significantly larger (1.5-fold) in the transplantations of aged MDPSCs compared to aged DPSCs, and was similar to the comparison of young MDPSCs and young DPSCs (**Figure 6V**). Odontoblastic differentiation along the dentinal wall was also detected in the transplantations of aged MDPSCs with values similar to those of young MDPSCs and DPSCs, and was higher than that of aged DPSCs (**Figure 6M–T, W**), demonstrating higher dentin regeneration potential of aged MDPSCs compared with aged DPSCs.

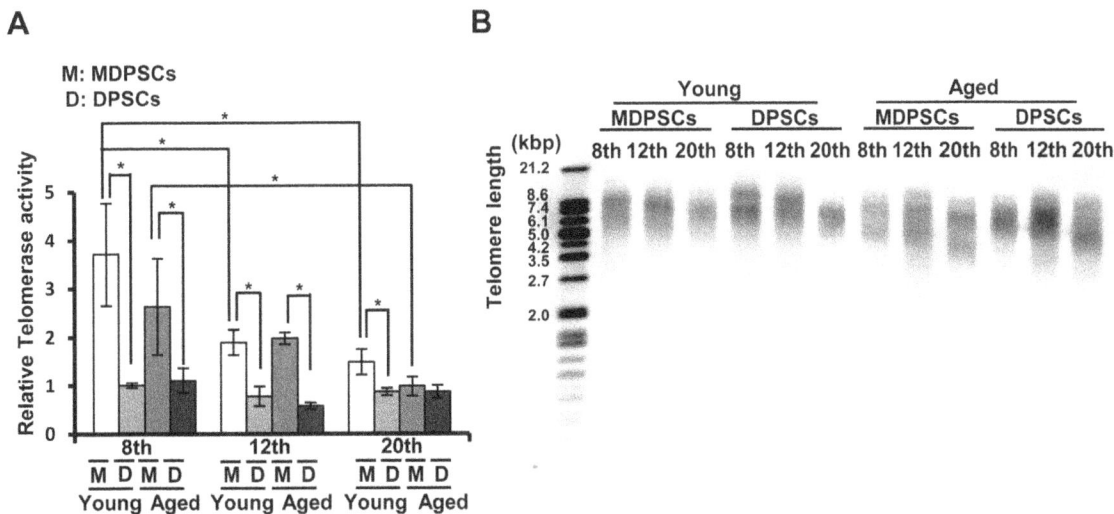

Figure 4. Changes of the telomerase activity and the telomere length with prolonged culture. (A) Relative telomerase activity in aged and young MDPSCs, and aged and young DPSCs at the 8th, 12th and 20th passages. *$p < 0.05$. Data are expressed as the means ± SD of 3 determinations. The experiments were repeated four times (4 lots), and one representative experiment is presented. (B) Southern blot analysis of telomeres in aged and young MDPSCs, and aged and young DPSCs at the 8th, 12th and 20th passages. Molecular sizes (kbp) are indicated on the left. The experiments were repeated four times (4 lots), and one representative experiment is presented.

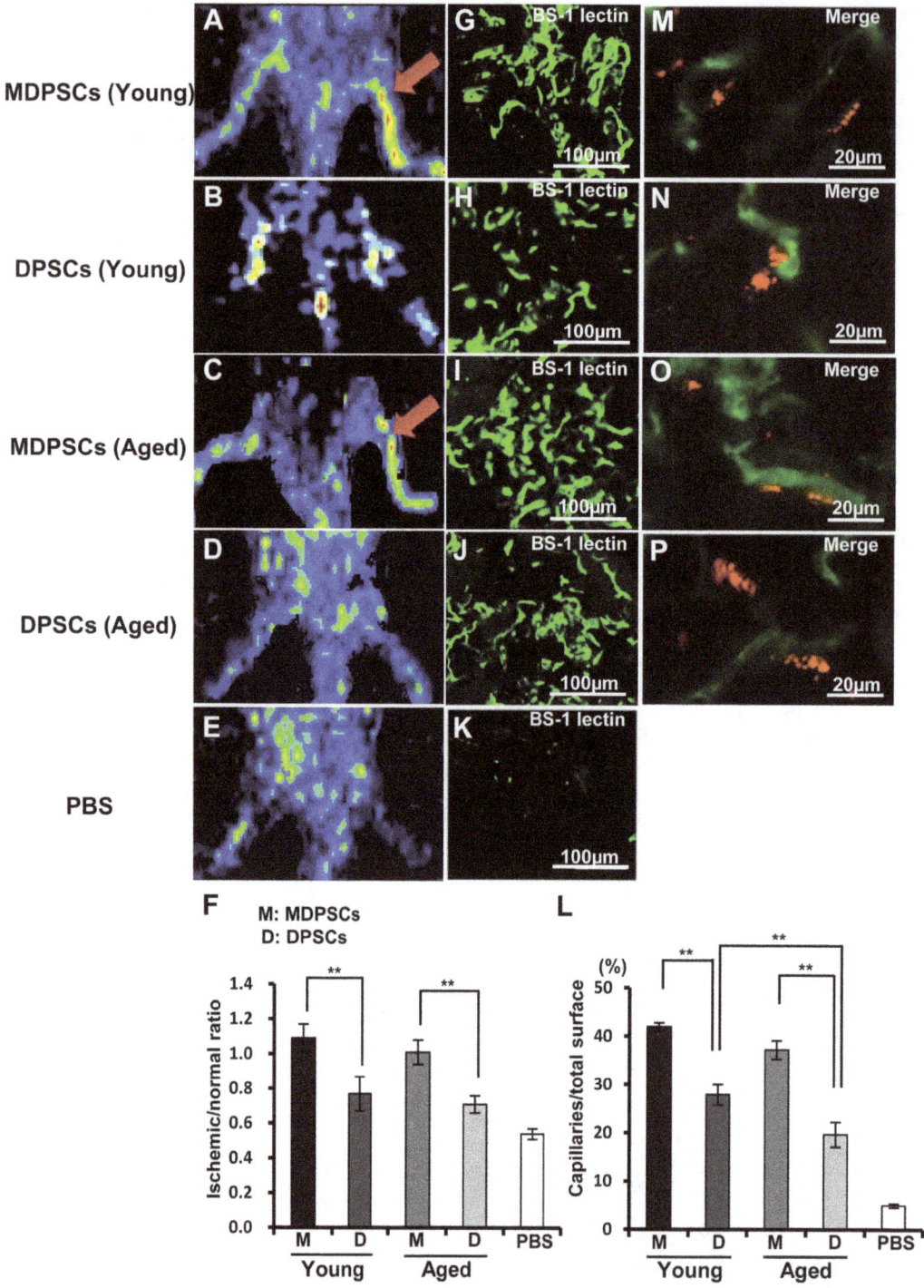

Figure 5. Neovascularization in the ischemic hindlimb 14 days after transplantation of aged MDPSCs. Neovascularization in the ischemic hindlimb 14 days after transplantation of aged MDPSCs compared with those of aged DPSCs, young MDPSCs and young DPSCs. (A–E) Laser Doppler imaging. Accelerated blood flow (arrows). (F) Quantification of blood flow in the ischemic versus normal limbs obtained from four mice in each group. **$p<0.01$. (G–K) Immunostaining of Fluorescein Griffonia (Bandeiraea) Simplicifolia Lectin 1/fluorescein-galanthus nivalis (snowdrop) lectin (BS-1 lectin) in the ischemic hindlimb. (L) Quantification and statistical analysis of the capillary density in the ischemic region using serial sections. Data are expressed as means ± SD of 4 determinations. **$p<0.01$. The experiments were repeated three times (3 lots), and one representative experiment is presented. (M–P) Localization of DiI-labeled transplanted cells and newly formed capillaries stained by BS-1 lectin.

Discussion

The aim of this investigation was to determine the influence of age on the mobilized dental pulp stem cells (MDPSCs). It is well known that there is a decline in MSCs properties [35]. In the present investigation, however, we have demonstrated that MDPSCs from aged donors are similar to young donors in their

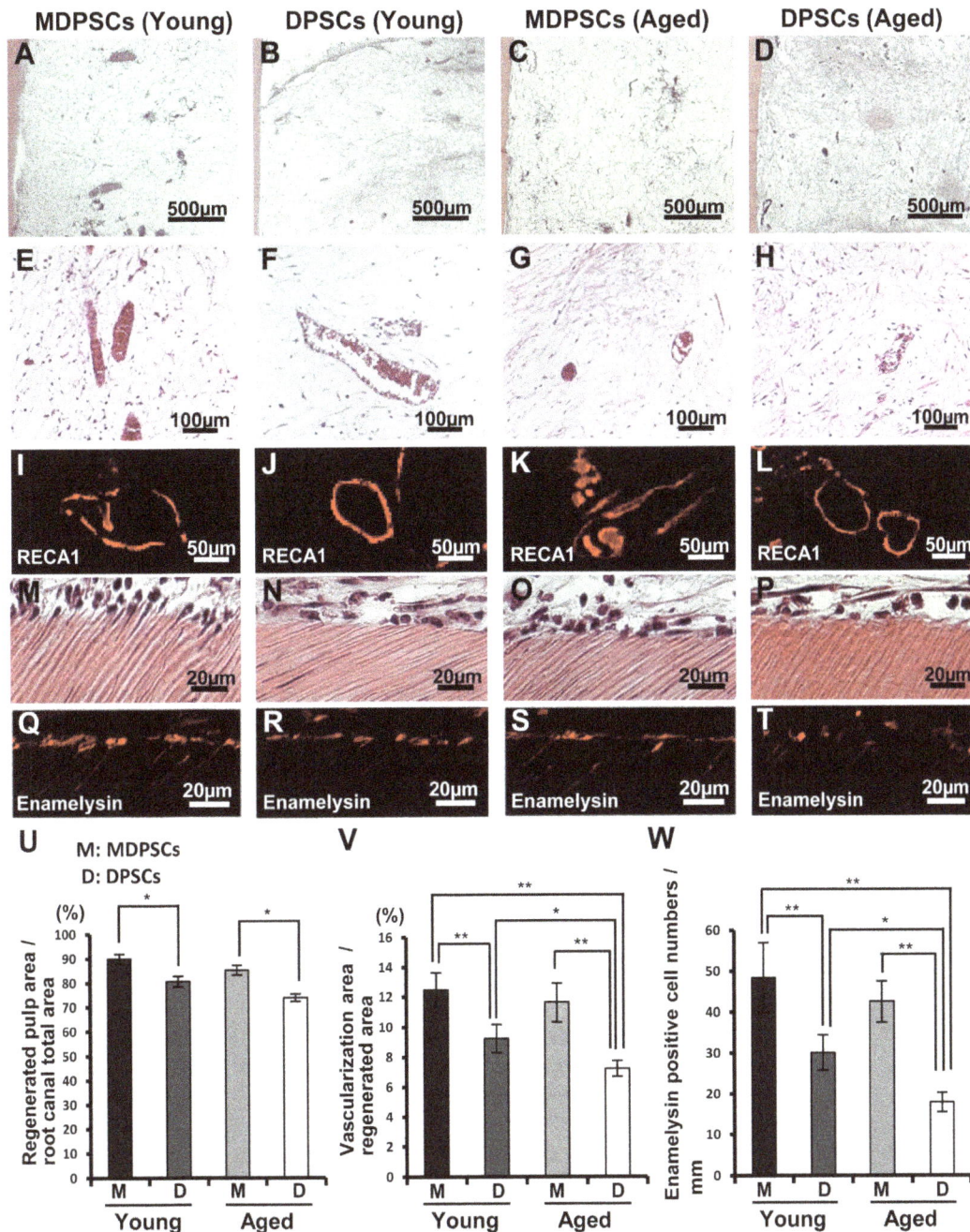

Figure 6. Regeneration of pulp tissue after ectopic tooth transplantation in severe combined immunodeficiency (SCID) mice. Aged MDPSCs, aged DPSCs, young MDPSCs and young DPSCs were injected into the emptied root canals. (A–L) Hematoxylin and Eosin (HE) staining. (I–L) Immunostaining with RECA1. (M–P) Odontoblast-like cells lining to the dentinal wall. (Q–T) In situ hybridization analysis with *enamelysin*. (U) Ratio of the regenerated area to the root canal area. Data are expressed as means ± SD of four determinations. *$p<0.05$. (V) Ratio of the vascularization area to the regenerated area. Data are expressed as means ± SD of four determinations. *$p<0.05$, **$p<0.01$. (W) *Enamelysin* positive cell number of the dentinal wall. Data are expressed as means ± SD of four determinations. *$p<0.05$, **$p<0.01$.

capacities for migration, differentiation, expression of angiogenic/ neurotrophic factors, trophic effects on proliferation and migration, and anti-apoptotic effects. MDPSCs from aged and young donors expressed stem cell markers, CD105, CXCR4 and G-CSFR. On the other hand, age-related changes of these capacities were demonstrated in colony-derived non- mobilized DPSCs. Similar age-independency in stemness has been reported in isolated MSCs [19,20]. Thus, isolation using G-CSF mobilization

renders the DPSCs to overcome the decline in stemness occurring with age. The present study demonstrated that the isolation utilizing G-CSF-induced stem cell mobilization [27] result in enrichment of G-CSFR positive DPSC subsets similarly both from young and aged donors. G-CSF promotes cell proliferation, migration, anti-apoptosis, endothelial cell differentiation and immunomodulation [27]. Thus, the present result that there was no significant difference in those stem cell properties between young MDPSCs and aged MDPSCs is plausible.

Tissue regeneration is dependent on stem cells and therefore, any loss in number or functionality due to aging will likely have a profound effect on regenerative capacity [36]. Aging of MSCs accompanied by a decline in the regenerative potential has been reported in many studies in vivo [11,24,37]. Therefore, in the present study, the regenerative potential for pulp/dentin and stem cell functionality of MDPSCs from the aged were examined in an ectopic tooth transplantation model compared with the young. It is noteworthy that no significant differences were found between them. On the other hand, a significant decline in pulp regenerative potential of DPSCs from the aged donors was demonstrated compared to that from the young donors. Thus, the induction of the migratory response by G-CSF in the DPSCs (MDPSCs) nullified the observed age dependent differences in the DPSCs. The angiogenic/vasculogenic potential of the aged MDPSCs transplanted in an ischemic hindlimb model was also similar to that of the young MDPSCs, while there was a significant difference between the aged and the young DPSCs. MSCs possess trophic activities including enhanced proliferation [38,39], enhanced migration [39], anti-inflammatory [40] and anti-apoptotic effects [41], and similar trophic activities have also been reported for MDPSCs [27]. In addition, the present study has shown that conditioned medium of aged MDPSCs had similar trophic effects *in vitro* as those from the young, whereas conditioned medium of aged DPSCs showed inferior trophic effects than those of the young. Furthermore, it has been shown that the regenerative potentials are dependent on trophic effects of MSCs [42]. Thus, the findings in this study suggest that donor age has no effect on the regeneration potential of MDPSCs and in their trophic effects.

Constitutive expression of telomerase RT (TERT) subunit gene prevents senescence and is responsible for the maintenance of MSCs properties. Telomere length, their shortening rate and activity of telomerase can be useful markers for aging evaluation [2,8]. Similarly, it has been well documented that the production of senescence-associated β-galactosidase, which is caused by related increased lysosomal activities and altered cytosolic pH, increases with aging [16,43]. In the present study, little accumulation of SA-β-gal was detected in aged MDPSCs even at the 20th passage, as in young MDPSCs, whereas an increased rate in aged DPSCs was observed. Gradual up-regulation of p16 and p21, which is associated with growth arrest [44], and pro-inflammatory cytokines IL-6 and IL-8, was also demonstrated in aged DPSCs but not in aged MDPSCs during cell expansion. These findings are consistent with a higher mRNA expression of telomerase RT (TERT) in aged MDPSCs compared with aged DPSCs, which prevents senescence and is responsible for the maintenance of stem cell properties. Telomeres are shortened by approximately 17 bps every year over a lifetime and make MSCs more sensitive to apoptotic stimuli [45]. There are, however, conflicting reports on the effect of aging on telomere length in MSCs [19,46]. The present study has demonstrated that telomere length was slightly shorter in aged MDPSCs at the 20th passage of culture compared with those at the 8th passage. These findings suggest that isolated MDPSCs might be superior to colony-derived DPSCs in inhibiting senescence and in maintaining functional characteristics of stemness during aging.

Finally, the proportion of people over age 60 is growing rapidly in industrial countries including Japan, and innovative strategies of stem cell therapy for the aged are a high priority. During aging, the status of MSCs changes with respect to their self-renewal capability, migration and differentiation potential, and the production of trophic factors that characterize their microenvironment [47]. Age-related modification of MSCs properties should be considered for suitable autologous cell transplantation. The method for isolation of DPSCs subsets on their migratory response to G-CSF is safe, efficacious and reproducible as described previously [27]. It is noteworthy, that in this investigation we have established unequivocally that the stem cell properties and their regenerative potential are significantly superior in aged MDPSCs compared to aged DPSCs, demonstrating their utility for potential clinical applications to autologous cell transplantation, especially in aged patients.

Conclusions

Comparison of human MDPSCs from aged donors to young donors demonstrated that there was a little age-related decline in stem cell properties including migration and differentiation potential, and in trophic effects on proliferation, migration, and anti-apoptosis. MDPSCs also showed a small age-dependent increase in senescence-associated β-galactosidase (SA-β-gal) production and senescence markers in long-term culture. Furthermore, the regenerative potential of aged MDPSCs was also similar to that of young MDPSCs in an ischemic hindlimb model and an ectopic tooth root model. Thus, these results demonstrated minimal alteration in human MDPSCs with aging, suggesting an immense utility for MDPSCs in clinical applications in dental pulp regeneration and ischemic diseases by autologous cell transplantation.

Supporting Information

Figure S1 Young and aged MDPSCs at the 3rd passage of culture forming a colony on day 3.

Table S1 Flow cytometric analysis of cell surface markers on young and aged MDPSCs at the 12 th passage compared with those at the 6 th passage. The experiments were repeated three times (3 lots), and one representative experiment is presented.

Acknowledgments

We thank Mr. Masaaki Shimagaki from Toray Industry Inc. for supplying the chemically treated transmembrane.

Author Contributions

Conceived and designed the experiments: MN. Performed the experiments: HH MM KI YH NT YT. Analyzed the data: HH MM YT. Contributed reagents/materials/analysis tools: HH YT KK MN. Wrote the paper: HH MN.

References

1. Kumar S, Chanda D, Ponnazhagan S (2008) Therapeutic potential of genetically modified mesenchymal stem cells. Gene Ther 15:711–5.

2. Bajek A, Czerwinski M, Olkowska J, Gurtowska N, Kloskowski T, et al. (2012) Does aging of mesenchymal stem cells limit their potential application in clinical practice? Aging Clin Exp Res 24:404–11.

3. Sethe S, Scutt A, Stolzing A (2006) Aging of mesenchymal stem cells. Ageing Res Rev 5:91–116.

4. Lepperdinger G, Brunauer R, Jamnig A, Laschober G, Kassem M (2008) Controversial issue: is it safe to employ mesenchymal stem cells in cell-based therapies? Exp Gerontol 43:1018–23.

5. Stolzing A, Jones E, McGonagle D, Scutt A (2008) Age-related changes in human bone marrow-derived mesenchymal stem cells: consequences for cell therapies. Mech Ageing Dev 129:163–73.

6. Alt EU, Senst C, Murthy SN, Slakey DP, Dupin CL, et al. (2012) Aging alters tissue resident mesenchymal stem cell properties. Stem Cell Res 8:215–25.

7. Mendes SC, Tibbe JM, Veenhof M, Bakker K, Both S, et al. (2002) Bone tissue-engineered implants using human bone marrow stromal cells: effect of culture conditions and donor age. Tissue Eng 8:911–20.

8. Baxter MA, Wynn RF, Jowitt SN, Wraith JE, Fairbairn LJ, et al. (2004) Study of telomere length reveals rapid aging of human marrow stromal cells following in vitro expansion. Stem Cells 22:675–82.

9. Efimenko A, Starostina E, Kalinina N, Stolzing A (2011) Angiogenic properties of aged adipose derived mesenchymal stem cells after hypoxic conditioning. J Transl Med 9: 10.

10. Flores I, Cayuela ML, Blasco MA (2005) Effects of telomerase and telomere length on epidermal stem cell behavior. Science 309:1253–6.

11. Zhang J, An Y, Gao LN, Zhang YJ, Jin Y, et al. (2012) The effect of aging on the pluripotential capacity and regenerative potential of human periodontal ligament stem cells. Biomaterials 33:6974–86.

12. Wu W, Niklason L, Steinbacher DM (2013) The effect of age on human adipose-derived stem cells. Plast Reconstr Surg 131:27–37.

13. Chen CS (2002) Phorbol ester induces elevated oxidative activity and alkalization in a subset of lysosomes. BMC Cell Biol 3:21.

14. Moerman EJ, Teng K, Lipschitz DA, Lecka-Czernik B (2004) Aging activates adipogenic and suppresses osteogenic programs in mesenchymal marrow stroma/stem cells: the role of PPAR-gamma2 transcription factor and TGF-beta/BMP signaling pathways. Aging Cell 3:379–89.

15. Justesen J, Stenderup K, Eriksen EF, Kassem M (2002) Maintenance of osteoblastic and adipocytic differentiation potential with age and osteoporosis in human marrow stromal cell cultures. Calcif Tissue Int 71:36–44.

16. Stenderup K, Justesen J, Clausen C, Kassem M (2003) Aging is associated with decreased maximal life span and accelerated senescence of bone marrow stromal cells. Bone 33:919–26.

17. Leskelä HV, Risteli J, Niskanen S, Koivunen J, Ivaska KK, et al. (2003) Osteoblast recruitment from stem cells does not decrease by age at late adulthood. Biochem Biophys Res Commun 311:1008–13.

18. Gala K, Burdzińska A, Idziak M, Makula J, Pączek L (2011) Characterization of bone-marrow-derived rat mesenchymal stem cells depending on donor age. Cell Biol Int 35:1055–62.

19. Roura S, Farré J, Soler-Botija C, Llach A, Hove-Madsen L, et al. (2006) Effect of aging on the pluripotential capacity of human CD105+ mesenchymal stem cells. Eur J Heart Fail 8:555–63.

20. Chang HX, Yang L, Li Z, Chen G, Dai G (2011) Age-related biological characterization of mesenchymal progenitor cells in human articular cartilage. Orthopedics 34:e382–88.

21. Lepperdinger G (2011) Inflammation and mesenchymal stem cell aging. Curr Opin Immunol 23:518–24.

22. Gronthos S, Brahim J, Li W, Fisher LW, Cherman N, et al. (2002) Stem cell properties of human dental pulp stem cells. J Dent Res 81:531–5.

23. Murray PE, Stanley HR, Matthews JB, Sloan AJ, Smith AJ (2002) Age-related odontometric changes of human teeth. Oral Surg Oral Med Oral Pathol Oral Radiol Endod 93:474–82.

24. Iida K, Takeda-Kawaguchi T, Tezuka Y, Kunisada T, Shibata T, et al. (2010) Hypoxia enhances colony formation and proliferation but inhibits differentiation of human dental pulp cells. Arch Oral Biol 55:648–54.

25. Takeda T, Tezuka Y, Horiuchi M, Hosono K, Iida K, et al. (2008) Characterization of dental pulp stem cells of human tooth germs. J Dent Res 87:676–81.

26. Bressan E, Ferroni L, Gardin C, Pinton P, Stellini E, et al. (2012) Donor age-related biological properties of human dental pulp stem cells change in nanostructured scaffolds. PLoS One 7:e49146.

27. Murakami M, Horibe H, Iohara K, Hayashi Y, Osako Y, et al. (2013) The use of granulocyte-colony stimulating factor induced mobilization for isolation of dental pulp stem cells with high regenerative potential. Biomaterials 34:9036–47.

28. Campisi J, d'Adda di Fagagna F (2007) Cellular senescence: when bad things happen to good cells. Nat Rev Mol Cell Biol 8:729–40.

29. Sebastian T, Johnson PF (2006) Stop and go: anti-proliferative and mitogenic functions of the transcription factor C/EBPbeta. Cell Cycle 5:953–7.

30. Acosta JC, O'Loghlen A, Banito A, Raguz S, Gil J (2008) Control of senescence by CXCR2 and its ligands. Cell Cycle 7:2956–9.

31. Nakashima M (1991) Establishment of primary cultures of pulp cells from bovine permanent incisors. Arch Oral Biol 36:655–63.

32. Iohara K, Zheng L, Wake H, Ito M, Nabekura J, et al. (2008) A novel stem cell source for vasculogenesis in ischemia: subfraction of side population cells from dental pulp. Stem Cells 26:2408–18.

33. Iohara K, Imabayashi K, Ishizaka R, Watanabe A, Nabekura J, et al. (2011) Complete pulp regeneration after pulpectomy by transplantation of CD105+ stem cells with stromal cell-derived factor-1. Tissue Eng Part A 17:1911–20.

34. Ishizaka R, Hayashi Y, Iohara K, Sugiyama M, Murakami M, et al. (2013) Stimulation of angiogenesis, neurogenesis and regeneration by side population cells from dental pulp. Biomaterials 34:1888–97.

35. Liu L, Rando TA (2011) Manifestations and mechanisms of stem cell aging. J Cell Biol 193:257–66.

36. Bellantuono I, Aldahmash A, Kassem M (2009) Aging of marrow stromal (skeletal) stem cells and their contribution to age-related bone loss. Biochim Biophys Acta 1792:364–70.

37. Khan M, Mohsin S, Khan SN, Riazuddin S (2011) Repair of senescent myocardium by mesenchymal stem cells is dependent on the age of donor mice. J Cell Mol Med 15:1515–27.

38. Kinnaird T, Stabile E, Burnett MS, Shou M, Lee CW, et al. (2004) Local delivery of marrow-derived stromal cells augments collateral perfusion through paracrine mechanisms. Circulation 109:1543–9.

39. Inukai T, Katagiri W, Yoshimi R, Osugi M, Kawai T, et al. (2013) Novel application of stem cell-derived factors for periodontal regeneration. Biochem Biophys Res Commun 430:763–8.

40. Ionescu L, Byrne RN, van Haaften T, Vadivel A, Alphonse RS, et al. (2012) Stem cell conditioned medium improves acute lung injury in mice: in vivo evidence for stem cell paracrine action. Am J Physiol Lung Cell Mol Physiol 303:967–77.

41. Mirotsou M, Zhang Z, Deb A, Zhang L, Gnecchi M, et al. (2007) Secreted frizzled related protein 2 (Sfrp2) is the key Akt-mesenchymal stem cell-released paracrine factor mediating myocardial survival and repair. Proc Natl Acad Sci U S A 104:1643–8.

42. Cantineaux D, Quertainmont R, Blacher S, Rossi L, Wanet T, et al. (2013) Conditioned medium from bone marrow-derived mesenchymal stem cells improves recovery after spinal cord injury in rats: an original strategy to avoid cell transplantation. PLoS One 8:e69515.

43. Zhou S, Greenberger JS, Epperly MW, Goff JP, Adler C, et al. (2008) Age-related intrinsic changes in human bone-marrow-derived mesenchymal stem cells and their differentiation to osteoblasts. Aging Cell 7:335–43.

44. Ksiazek K (2009) A comprehensive review on mesenchymal stem cell growth and senescence. Rejuvenation Res. 12: 105–16.

45. Fan M, Chen W, Liu W, Du GQ, Jiang SL, et al. (2010) The effect of age on the efficacy of human mesenchymal stem cell transplantation after a myocardial infarction. Rejuvenation Res 13:429–38.

46. Wagner W, Bork S, Horn P, Krunic D, Walenda T, et al. (2009) Aging and replicative senescence have related effects on human stem and progenitor cells. PLoS One 4:e5846.

47. Rosen CJ, Ackert-Bicknell C, Rodriguez JP, Pino AM (2009) Marrow fat and the bone microenvironment: developmental, functional, and pathological implications. Crit Rev Eukaryot Gene Expr 19:109–24.

2

A Novel ATM/TP53/p21-Mediated Checkpoint Only Activated by Chronic γ-Irradiation

Lili Cao[1,2,9], Hidehiko Kawai[2*,9], Megumi Sasatani[1], Daisuke Iizuka[1], Yuji Masuda[1,3], Toshiya Inaba[4], Keiji Suzuki[5], Akira Ootsuyama[6], Toshiyuki Umata[7], Kenji Kamiya[1], Fumio Suzuki[2]

1 Department of Experimental Oncology, Research Institute for Radiation Biology and Medicine, Hiroshima University, Hiroshima, Japan, 2 Department of Molecular Radiobiology, Research Institute for Radiation Biology and Medicine, Hiroshima University, Hiroshima, Japan, 3 Department of Genome Dynamics, Research Institute of Environmental Medicine, Nagoya University, Furo-cho, Chikusa-ku, Nagoya, Japan, 4 Department of Molecular Oncology & Leukemia Program Project, Research Institute for Radiation Biology and Medicine, Hiroshima University, Hiroshima, Japan, 5 Department of Radiation Medical Sciences, Atomic Bomb Disease Institute, Nagasaki University, Nagasaki, Japan, 6 Department of Radiation Biology and Health, School of Medicine, University of Occupational and Environmental Health, Kitakyushu, Japan, 7 Radioisotope Research Center, University of Occupational and Environmental Health, Kitakyushu, Japan

Abstract

Different levels or types of DNA damage activate distinct signaling pathways that elicit various cellular responses, including cell-cycle arrest, DNA repair, senescence, and apoptosis. Whereas a range of DNA-damage responses have been characterized, mechanisms underlying subsequent cell-fate decision remain elusive. Here we exposed cultured cells and mice to different doses and dose rates of γ-irradiation, which revealed cell-type-specific sensitivities to chronic, but not acute, γ-irradiation. Among tested cell types, human fibroblasts were associated with the highest levels of growth inhibition in response to chronic γ-irradiation. In this context, fibroblasts exhibited a reversible G1 cell-cycle arrest or an irreversible senescence-like growth arrest, depending on the irradiation dose rate or the rate of DNA damage. Remarkably, when the same dose of γ-irradiation was delivered chronically or acutely, chronic delivery induced considerably more cellular senescence. A similar effect was observed with primary cells isolated from irradiated mice. We demonstrate a critical role for the ataxia telangiectasia mutated (ATM)/tumor protein p53 (TP53)/p21 pathway in regulating DNA-damage-associated cell fate. Indeed, blocking the ATM/TP53/p21 pathway deregulated DNA damage responses, leading to micronucleus formation in chronically irradiated cells. Together these results provide insights into the mechanisms governing cell-fate determination in response to different rates of DNA damage.

Editor: Roberto Amendola, ENEA, Italy

Funding: Funding was provided by the Ministry of Education, Science, Sports and Culture of Japan (to HK). The funders had no role in study design, data collection and analysis, decision to publish, or preparation of the manuscript.

Competing Interests: The authors have declared that no competing interests exist.

* Email: kawaih@hiroshima-u.ac.jp

⑨ These authors contributed equally to this work.

Introduction

Lesions to genomic DNA, including modified bases, and single- and double-strand breaks, are constantly generated in living cells under physiological and environmental conditions [1]. DNA damage can result from internal or external sources and cause mutations to genomic DNA. These lesions and mutations to genomic DNA affect cell-fate outcomes (e.g., proliferation, cell-cycle arrest, senescence, differentiation, autophagy, transformation, and apoptosis), which are directly linked to human-health impairments, including cancer and aging [2]. The overall rate of spontaneous DNA damage in human cells is estimated to be tens of thousands of events per day, which is approximately equivalent to the rate induced by exposure to sparsely ionizing radiation (1.5–2.0 Gray (Gy)/day) [3,4]. Under these conditions, individual cells adopt particular cell fates to maintain homeostasis within the living organisms. As cell fates elicited by DNA damage responses may impact aging and age-associated diseases, it is important to understand the mechanisms governing DNA-damage associated cell-fate decisions.

It is possible that the loss of homeostasis between signaling networks affects cellular outcomes downstream of DNA damage responses, which would suggest that there are critical signaling thresholds determined by the level of DNA damage. For example, relatively high levels of DNA damage activate signaling pathways that regulate cell survival and apoptosis [5]. However, it is less clear how cell-fate decisions are made in cells exposed to chronic levels of DNA damage. Because individual cells must make cell-fate decisions under physiological and genotoxic conditions to maintain organismal homeostasis, it is important to determine how cells respond to the persistent induction and accumulation of DNA damage.

Here we exposed cultured cells or mice to various quantities and qualities of ^{137}Cs γ-irradiation. Automated fluorescence microscopy was used to monitor effects of this irradiation on numerous human cell types. This experimental system allowed us to

A

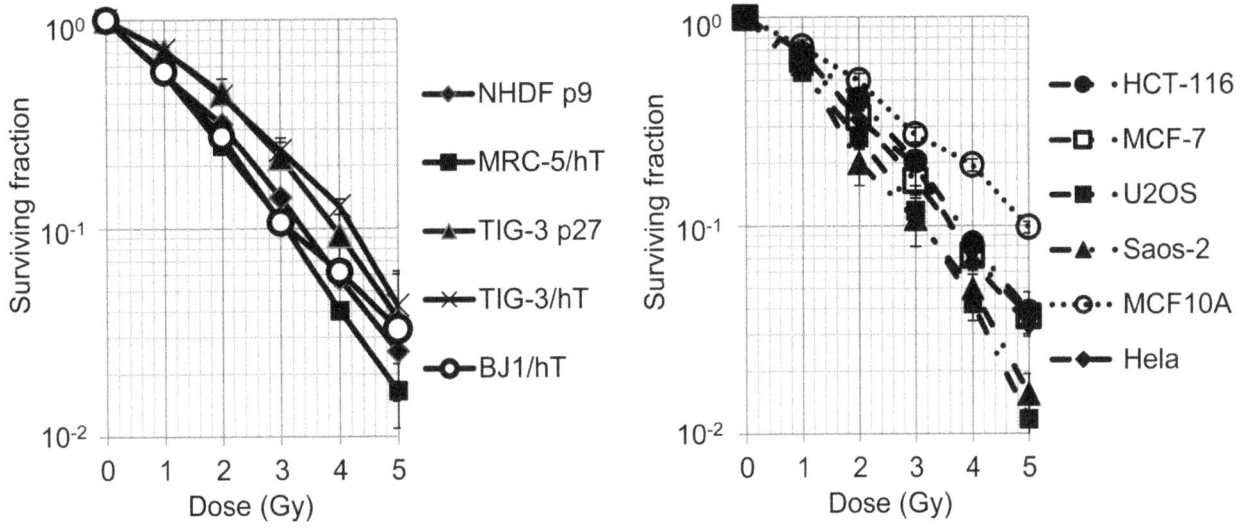

B

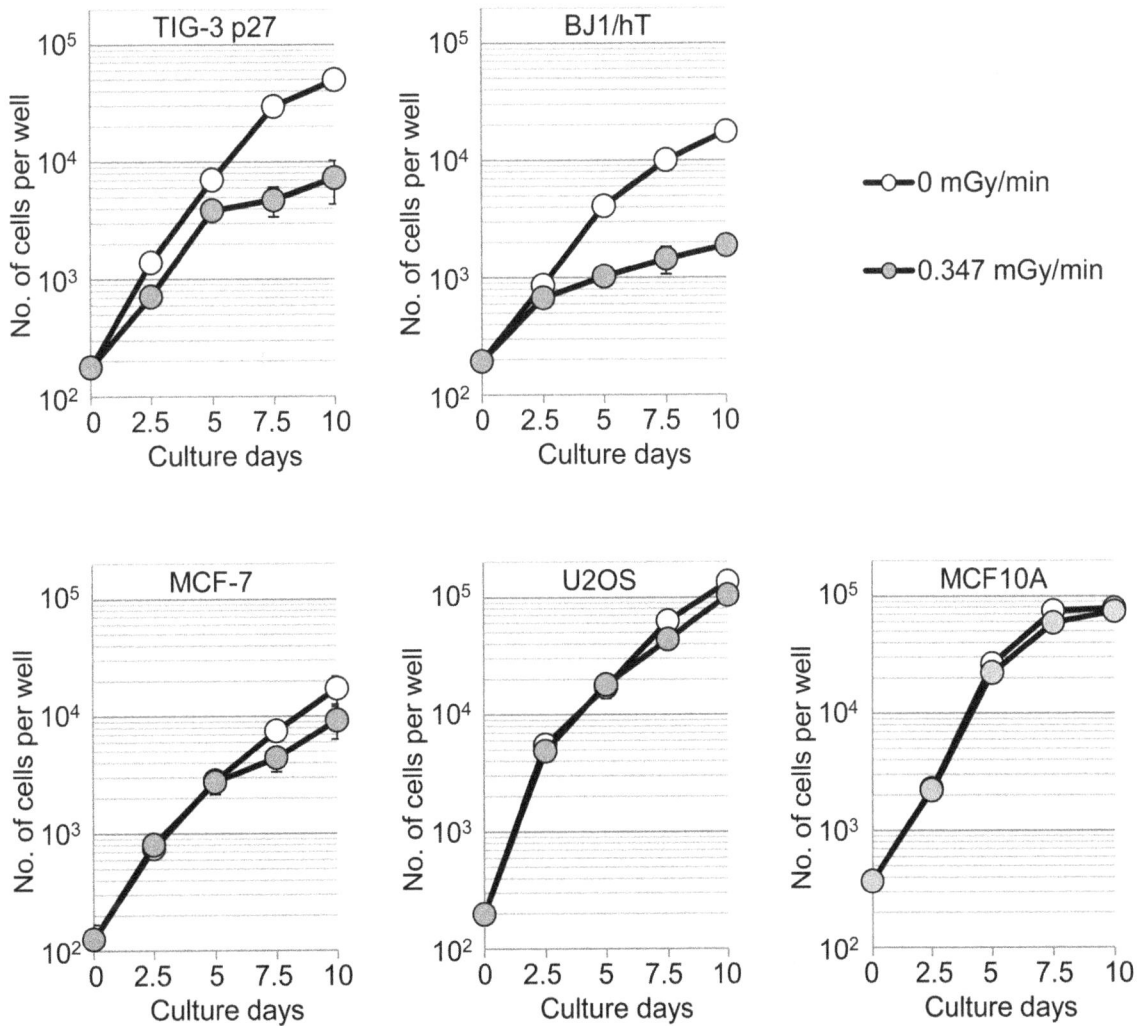

Figure 1. Different exposure conditions result in different sensitivities of proliferating cells to ionizing radiation. (A) Clonogenic survival of various human cell lines exposed to acute [137]Cs γ-irradiation (1 Gy/min). Surviving fractions are expressed relative to the plating efficiencies of non-irradiated cells. Values represent the mean ± SD of three independent experiments. (B) Cell proliferation of various human cell lines under chronic γ-irradiation conditions. Cells exposed to 0.347 mGy/min (grey circles) are compared to unirradiated controls (white circles).

quantitatively assess the dynamic behavior of cells exposed to a wide range of DNA damage, providing insights into cell-fate decisions that are determined by the dose rate of chronic γ-irradiation.

Materials and Methods

Cell lines and cell culture conditions

Primary human fibroblasts (passage 9, NHDF p9) [6], TIG-3 primary human fibroblast (passage 27, TIG-3 p27) [7], and the immortalized MRC-5/hT cells [7], TIG-3/hT cells [7] and BJ1/hT cells [8] transfected with hTERT were maintained in minimum essential medium eagle alpha modification (Sigma) supplemented with L-glutamine and 10% fetal bovine serum (FBS). Five human tumor cell lines obtained from ATCC, MCF-7 (a mammary carcinoma cell line), U2OS (an osteosarcoma cell line), Saos-2 (an osteosarcoma cell line), HCT-116 (a colorectal carcinoma cell line), and HeLa (a cervical carcinoma cell line) were cultured in minimum essential medium eagle alpha modification or McCoy's 5A medium (Sigma) supplemented with L-glutamine and 10% FBS. A spontaneously immortalized breast epithelial cell line (MCF10A) (ATCC) was cultured in mammary epithelium basal medium (Lonza) with supplements. All cells were maintained in a humidified 5% CO_2 atmosphere at 37°C. To optimize γ-irradiation conditions at different dose rates (0.007–0.694 mGy/min), cell culture incubators were placed at different distances from a ^{137}Cs radiation device (1.11 TBq) (Sangyo Kagaku). The dose rate associated with each incubator was measured using a GD-302M glass dosimeter (AGC Techno Glass). ATM kinase activity was inhibited by incubating cells with 10 μM KU55933 (Merck Millipore). DNA-PKcs kinase activity was inhibited by incubating cells with 10 μM NU7026 (Merck Millipore).

Colony formation and clonogenic survival assay

Colony formation assays with chronic γ-irradiation were performed by plating 100 or 200 cells in 60-mm culture dishes.

Cells were cultured at different dose rates (0.007–0.694 mGy/min) for indicated amounts of time and then allowed to form colonies for 6–10 days. Cells were stained with crystal violet. The sensitivity of cells to ionizing radiation was measured using a clonogenic survival assay as described [9]. Briefly, for acute irradiation 1–100×10^2 cells were seeded into 60-mm culture dishes and irradiated with a γ-ray dose that ranged from 1 to 5 Gy (^{137}Cs source, 148 TBq, Gammacell 40 Exactor, Best Theratronics). After 10–14 days of incubation, colonies were stained with crystal violet and counted. Only colonies containing ≥50 cells were scored as survivors. Survival fractions were calculated in each experiment as the average cloning efficiency after treatment from at least two parallel dishes. Survival fractions were corrected for plating efficiency.

Immunofluorescence staining and automated fluorescence microscope analysis

Cells plated on 96-well plates (μ-Plate, ibidi) were fixed with 4% paraformaldehyde in PBS for 30 min at room temperature, and then treated with 0.5% Triton X-100 in PBS for 20 min. Cells were immunolabeled using antibodies against TP53BP1 (1:20,000; BD Biosciences) or γ-H2AX (1:25,000; Millipore) and secondary antibodies conjugated with Alexa fluor 555 (1:2000; Life Technologies). Nuclei were labeled with Hoechst 33258. Fluorescence images were obtained using an automated fluorescence microscope (IN Cell Analyzer 2000; GE Healthcare BioScience). The number of TP53BP1 foci per cell was determined using the image-analysis software IN Cell Developer (GE Healthcare BioScience).

Cell cycle analysis

To analyze cell-cycle distributions, cells in S-phase were stained with EdU using a Click-It EdU Alexa Fluor 488 imaging kit (Life Technologies). Briefly, EdU was added to the growth medium (10 μM final concentration) for 30 min. Cells were then fixed with 4% paraformaldehyde, and labeled with a Click-It cocktail containing Alexa Fluor 488 azide and Hoechst dye. Fluorescence

Table 1. Comparison of colony forming abilities of different types of cells for acute versus chronic γ-irradiation (5 Gy).

Cell line	Surviving fraction[1] for acute γ-irradiation[2]	Surviving fraction for chronic γ-irradiation[3]
NHDF p9	0.026±0.003	0.069±0.015
BJ1/hT	0.033±0.005	0.041±0.013
TIG-3 p27	0.037±0.026	0.119±0.038
MCF10A	0.094±0.006	0.643±0.055
HCT-116	0.039±0.009	0.942±0.015
MCF-7	0.037±0.005	0.914±0.027
U2OS	0.012±0.003	0.933±0.010
Hela	0.033±0.003	0.924±0.068

Values represent the mean ± SD of three independent experiments.
[1]Survival fractions were determined based on crystal violet staining.
[2]Dose rate of 1.0 Gy/min for 5 min, total dose; 5 Gy. Cells were cultured for 10 days following acute γ-irradiation.
[3]Cells were cultured for 10 days at dose rate of 0.347 mGy/min, total dose; 5 Gy.

A

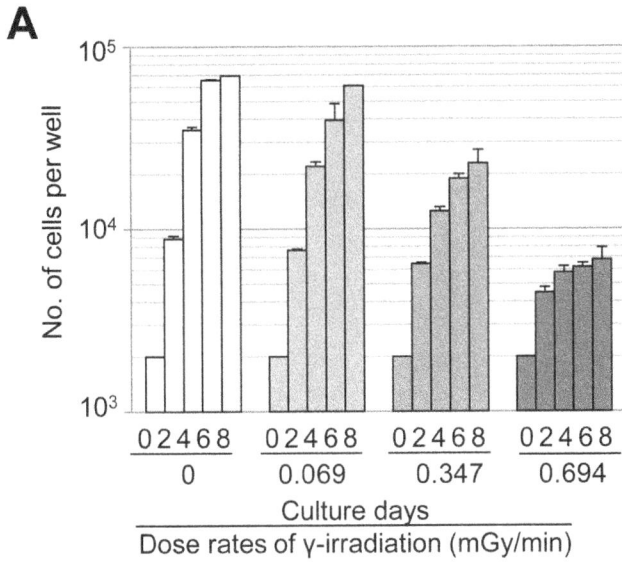

B

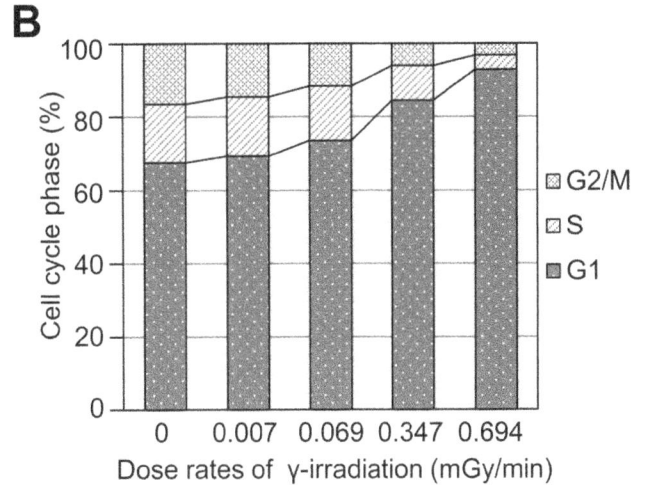

C

TIG-3 p27

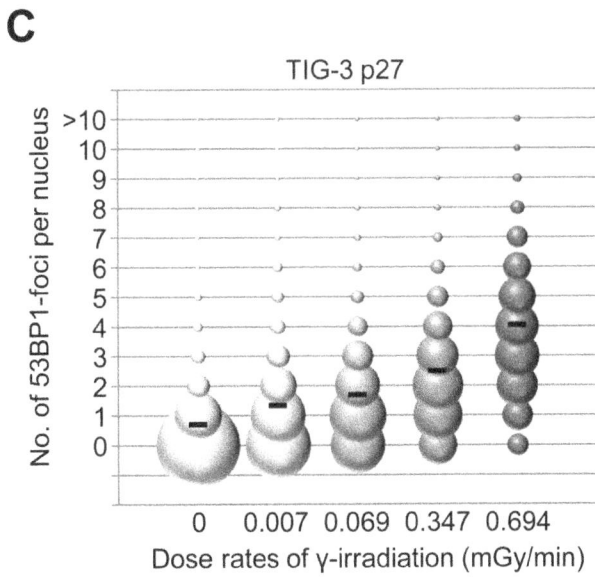

BJ1/hT

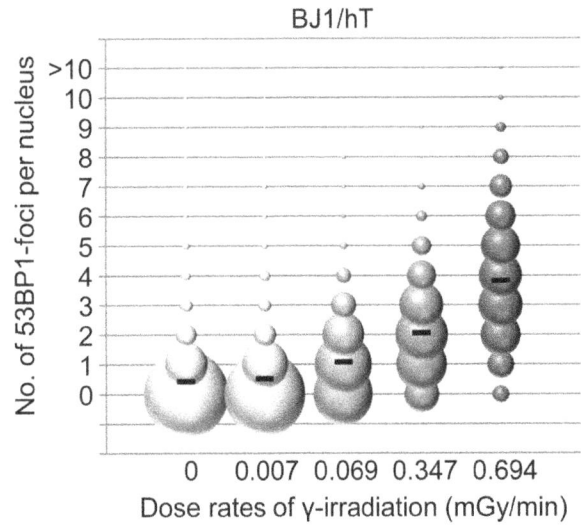

D

BJ1/hT (0.347 mGy/min)

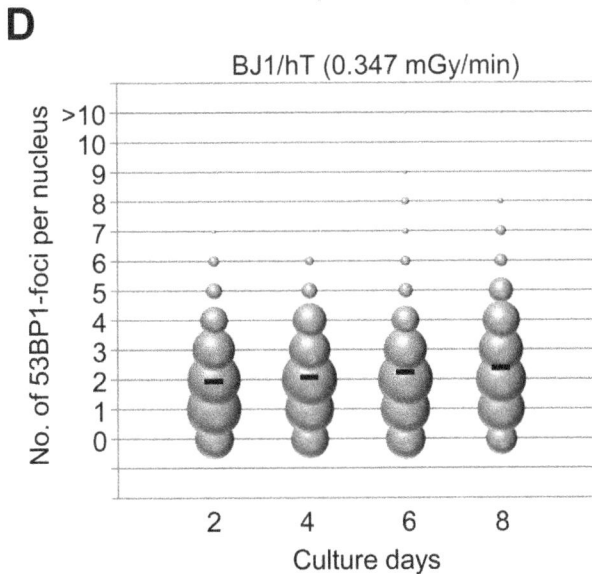

BJ1/hT (0.694 mGy/min)

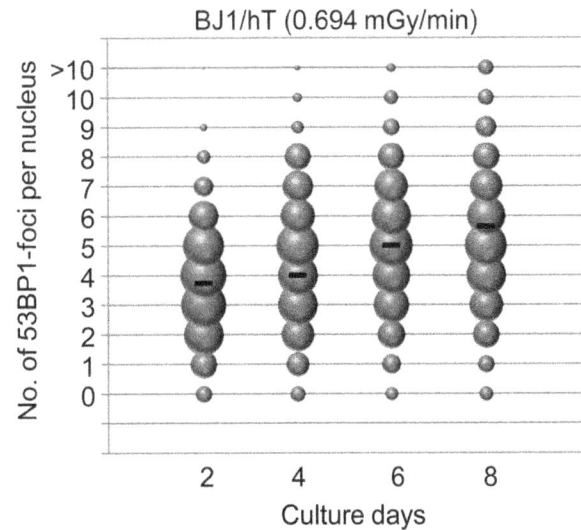

Figure 2. Chronic γ-irradiation suppresses the proliferation of human fibroblasts by inducing a G1 cell-cycle arrest. (A) Dose-dependent effect of chronic γ-irradiation on the proliferation of primary human fibroblasts (TIG-3 p27 cells). Values represent the mean ± SD of three independent wells. (B) Representative cell cycle distribution of TIG-3 p27 cells after 4 days of chronic γ-irradiation. (C) The frequency distribution of DNA damage-associated TP53BP1-foci in TIG-3 p27 (left) or BJ1/hT (right) cells exposed to 4 days of chronic γ-irradiation. At least 1×10^3 cells per well were examined to determine the frequency distribution. The size of the bubble is proportional to the number of cells with that number of TP53BP1-foci. Black bars indicate the mean number of TP53BP1-foci per cell. (D) Time-course analysis of TP53BP1 foci in BJ1/hT cell exposed to 0.347 (left) or 0.694 (right) mGy/min of chronic γ-irradiation.

images of nuclei were obtained using automated fluorescence microscopy. Cell-cycle distribution analyses were performed using IN Cell Developer software.

Mice and γ-irradiation

Female C57BL/6N mice that were 8–12 weeks old were purchased from Kyudo Co. (Saga, Japan). Mice were housed 5–10 animals per cage under specific pathogen-free conditions at 55–60% relative humidity and $22 \pm 2°C$. Mice were irradiated using a Gammacell 40 Exactor or in a chronic ^{137}Cs γ-irradiation area, as described for the cell culture experiments. The dose rate for the acute exposure was 1 Gy/min and dose rates for chronic exposures were 0.347, 0.694, or 1.388 mGy/min. Mice lacking *TP53* were obtained as described [10,11]. Female wild-type and *TP53*-null mice that were 8–12 weeks old were irradiated as described above. All mice were maintained according to Guiding Principles for the Care and Use of Animals. All experiments were approved in advance by the Ethics Committee of Animal Care and Experimentation at the University of Occupational and Environmental Health, Kitakyushu, Japan (Admission Number: AE04-047). All surgery was made to minimize suffering. Isolation of primary lung cells from irradiated mice were performed as described previously [12] with some modification. In briefly, the mice were sacrificed under diethyl ether anesthesia. After collection with lung tissue to tubes containing DMEM/F12 (Gibco)/10% FBS, lung tissue were minced with a sterile scalpel on a 100 mm-dish for about 3 min, then transferred into tubes filled with collagenase/hyaluronidase (Stem Cell Technologies)/Epicult medium (Stem Cell Technologies)/5% FBS and incubated under constant agitation in a shaker for 1 h at 37°C. After centrifugation, collected pellets were treated with pre-warmed trypsin/EDTA (Gibco) for 1 min at 37°C, mixed the content of the tubes up and down for at least 1 min. After centrifugation, added 5 ml of pre-warmed dispase (Stem Cell Technologies)/DNase and incubated for 1 min at 37°C. After centrifugation, added ammonium chloride (Stem Cell Technologies), centrifugated again, after adding DMEM/F12 medium, mononuclear cells were isolated by filtering suspension through a 40 μm mesh.

siRNA transfection

siRNA transfections were performed using Lipofectamine RNAiMAX (Life Technologies). TP53-specific siRNAs (VHS40366, s606, s607), P21-specific siRNAs (s416, s417), and non-targeting siRNA negative controls (AM4635, 4390846) were purchased from Life Technologies (Stealth RNAi or Silencer Select validated siRNAs).

Western blot analysis

Western blot analysis was performed using 10 μg of whole cell extracts as described [9], with modifications. Proteins were electrophoresed on a 5–20% sodium dodecyl sulfate polyacrylamide gradient gel (Atto). Blots were labeled using primary antibodies against TP53 (1:1000, Ab-6; Merck Millipore), phospho-TP53-Ser15 (1:1000; Cell Signaling), p21 (1:1000; BD Biosciences), MDM2 (1:200, SMP-14; Santa Cruz Biotech),

MDMX/HDMX (1:5000; Bethyl), CHEK2 (1:1000; Cell Signaling), phospho-CHEK2-Thr68 (1:1000; Cell Signaling), β-tubulin (1:1000; Sigma-aldrich), and β-actin (1:10,000; Sigma-aldrich).

Micronucleus assay

Irradiated cells in 96-well plates were fixed with 100% methanol at −20°C. Nuclei were stained with Hoechst 33258 and cytoplasms were visualized with the SYTO RNASelect green fluorescent cell stain (Life Technologies). Fluorescence images were obtained using an IN Cell Analyzer 2000. Micronuclei frequency was determined using In Cell Developer software.

Senescence detection assay

Irradiated cells were replated in triplicate in 6-well plates (1×10^4 cells per well) and cultured for 24 h in 5% CO_2 at 37°C. Senescence-associated β-gal activity was detected with a senescence detection kit (K320-250, Biovision). More than 300 cells per sample were counted to determine the percentage of senescent cells.

Results

Proliferating human fibroblasts are particularly sensitive to chronic γ-irradiation

It is generally accepted and well discussed that different types of cells exhibit different sensitivities to ionizing radiation, depending on the cell's origin, differentiation status, and genetic background [13,14]. For example, cells from patients with Ataxia-telangiectasia or Nijmegen breakage syndrome are particularly sensitive to ionizing radiation because a protein required for DNA damage responses is dysfunctional in these patients [15]. In this study, all types of cultured cells that we examined (human primary fibroblasts, telomerase reverse transcriptase (TERT)-immortalized fibroblasts, immortalized cell lines, and tumor cell lines) showed different, but relatively comparable, sensitivity to acute γ-irradiation exposure at a dose rate of 1.0 Gy/min (Figure 1A). The D_0 values (37% survival dose) were between 1.1 and 1.4 Gy. Individual cells treated with acute γ-irradiation determine an alternative cell fate at several decision points after massive and transient DNA damage [16]. Sustained DNA damage also causes individual cells to adopt a wider range of cell fates, including apoptosis, DNA-damage tolerance, or proliferation. In this context, the rates of induction and accumulation of DNA damage theoretically affect these cell-fate decisions. We therefore hypothesized that cells could tolerate low levels of DNA damage (chronic γ-irradiation) and would exhibit specific traits depending on their radiation sensitivity.

To test this hypothesis, we placed cell-culture incubators at different distances from a ^{137}Cs radiation source, allowing us to expose cells to chronic γ-irradiation at a wide range of dose rates (Figure S1A). We first exposed a number of cultured cell types to chronic γ-irradiation at a dose-rate of 0.347 mGy/min for 10 days (0.5 Gy/day, or 5 Gy in total). Cells were then analyzed for their colony forming ability. In contrast to results obtained with acute γ-irradiation, colony formation following chronic γ-irradiated was

A

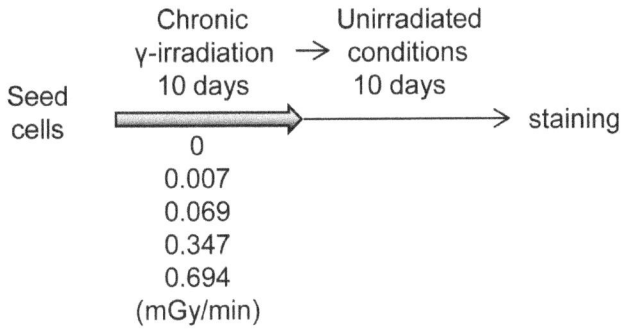

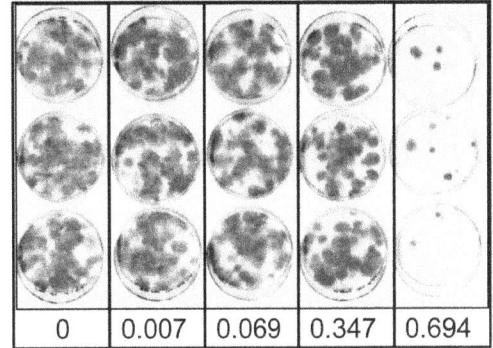

Dose rates of γ-irradiation (mGy/min)

B

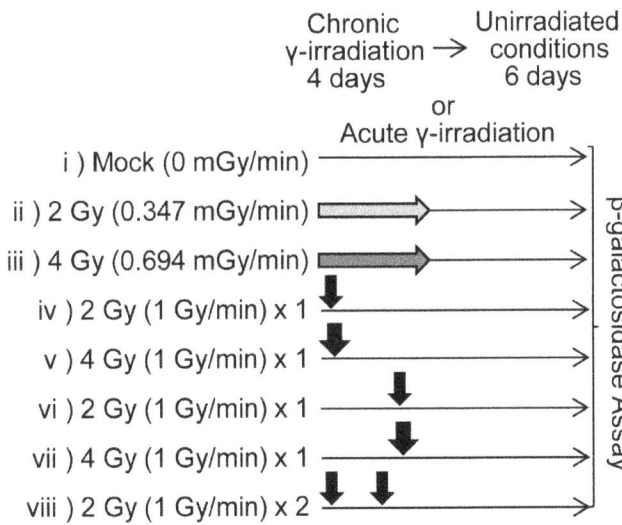

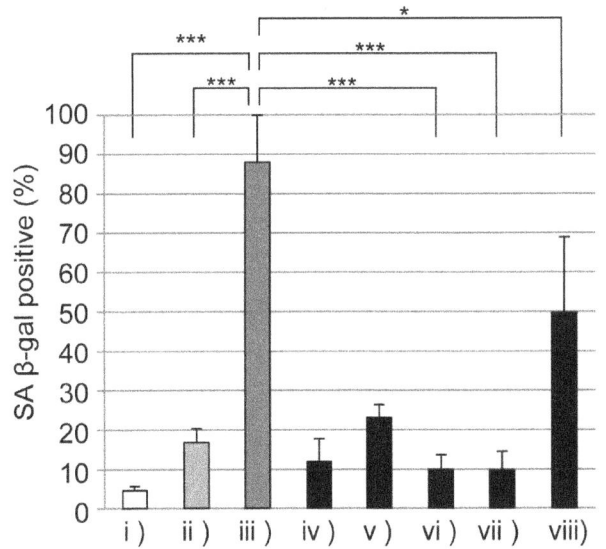

C

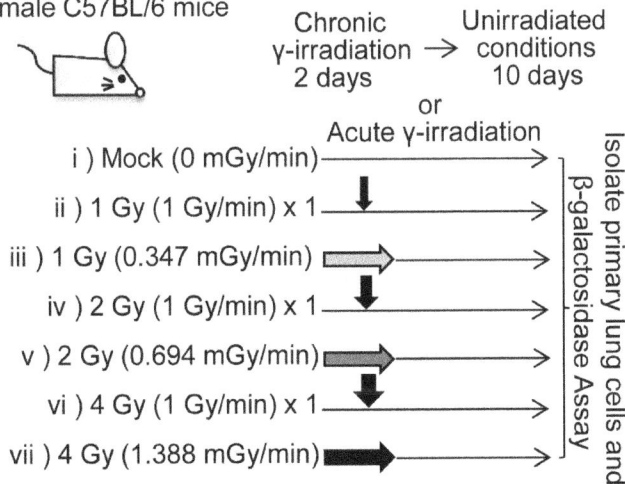

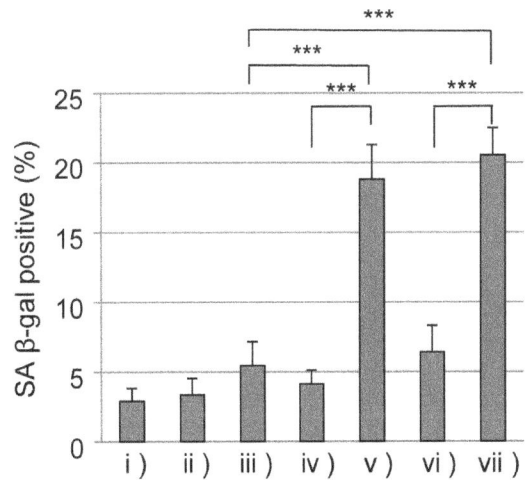

Figure 3. The dose rate of chronic γ-irradiation affects cell-fate decisions. (A) Colony-forming ability of fibroblasts following chronic γ-irradiation. The experimental scheme is illustrated to the left. TIG-3 p27 cells (2×10^2) were exposed to different dose-rates of γ-irradiation for 10 days and then allowed to grow under unirradiated conditions for an additional 10 days. Representative pictures of crystal violet-stained colonies are shown for each dose rate. **(B) Cellular senescence induced by acute or chronic γ-irradiation.** BJ1/hT cells (4×10^3) were exposed to the treatment condition indicated on the left. Grey arrows indicate chronic γ-irradiation at indicated dose rates. Black arrows indicate acute γ-irradiation of indicated doses. Following 1 day of recovery and 6 days of additional growth, cells were stained for β-gal activity to assess levels of senescence (right). Values represent the mean ± SD of three independent experiments. *$P < 0.05$, ***$P < 0.001$. **(C)** Cellular senescence induced by acute or chronic γ-irradiation *in vivo*. Female C57BL/6 mice were exposed to the treatment condition indicated to the left. Grey arrows indicate chronic γ-irradiation at indicated dose rates. Black arrows indicate acute γ-irradiation of indicated doses. Primary cells isolated from lungs of irradiated mice were stained for β-gal activity to assess levels of senescence (right). Values represent the mean ± SD of independent cultures from 2 mice. ***$P < 0.001$.

cell-type specific. Chronic γ-irradiation at a dose rate of 0.347 mGy/min had very little effect on tumor cell lines compared with unirradiated controls. Human fibroblasts, however, showed marked decreases in the number and size of macroscopic colonies (both primary and *hTERT*-immortalized fibroblasts; Figure S1B and Table 1).

To test whether insensitivity to low-dose irradiation was specific to transformed cells, we examined a spontaneously immortalized but non-transformed breast epithelial cell line (MCF10A). Similar to the cancer cell lines, MCF10A cells were not sensitive to chronic γ-irradiation at a dose rate of 0.347 mGy/min. When 8 cell lines were exposed to 5 Gy of γ-irradiation under acute or chronic conditions, all cells were sensitive to acute exposure, but only fibroblasts were affected by chronic exposure (Table 1). We next used automated fluorescence microscopy to assess the proliferation of different cell types exposed to chronic γ-irradiation (0.347 mGy/min). Consistent with colony-formation results, the proliferation of fibroblasts (TIG-3 p27, and BJ1/hT) was reduced compared to unirradiated controls, whereas other cell lines (MCF-7, U2OS, MCF10A) were not affected (Figure 1B). These results reveal a distinct sensitivity of human fibroblasts to chronic γ-irradiation.

Chronic γ-irradiation produces distinct effects on fibroblasts in a dose rate-dependent manner

To characterize the sensitivity of human fibroblasts to chronic γ-irradiation, we used automated fluorescence microscopy to quantitatively analyze dose rate-dependent effects. Cells were exposed to different dose rates of chronic γ-irradiation (0, 0.069, 0.347, or 0.694 mGy/min) for ≤10 days. The proliferation of human fibroblasts decreased in a dose rate-dependent manner (Figure 2A). Again, this effect was significant in human fibroblasts, as the proliferation of epithelial cells was less affected by chronic irradiation (Figure S2A). To determine the cell-cycle distribution of these fibroblasts, nuclei were labeled with Hoechst and the S-phase maker 5-ethynyl-2′-deoxyuridine (EdU). Under chronic γ-irradiation conditions, there were fewer mitotic cells but no increase in dead cells (Figure S2B), suggesting that cells were arrested in a slow- or non-cycling state. Furthermore, cells arrested in the G1 phase of the cell cycle in a dose rate-dependent manner (Figure 2B).

We next sought to determine whether different dose rates caused different levels of DNA-damage accumulation. Cells were exposed to chronic γ-irradiation for 4 days and then the number of tumor protein p53 binding protein 1 (TP53BP1) foci, which indicates DNA damage, was counted within each nucleus. In both TIG-3 p27 and BJ1/hT cell lines, chronic γ-irradiation caused a dose rate-dependent increase in TP53BP1 foci per nucleus (Figure 2C). Similar results were obtained when foci of phosphorylated histone H2AX (γ-H2AX), which is another marker of DNA damage, were analyzed (Figure S3A). Given that DNA damage can be repaired by a number of pathways, it was interesting that different dose rates caused different levels of DNA damage. We therefore sought to determine the irradiation dose rate that induced the accumulation of DNA damage. Cells were exposed to chronic γ-irradiation at dose rates of 0.347 or 0.694 mGy/min and the number of TP53BP1-foci was measured every 2 days. There was a clear difference in the level of DNA damage between these two dose rates. At 0.694 mGy/min, but not 0.347 mGy/min, we observed increased numbers of TP53BP1 and γ-H2AX foci in a time-dependent manner (Figure 2D and S3B). These data indicate that DNA damage begins to accumulate in cultured human fibroblasts when they are exposed to between 0.347 and 0.694 mGy/min of chronic γ-irradiation.

γ-irradiated cells undergo senescence when the dose rate exceeds the threshold for DNA-damage accumulation

We next wondered whether 0.347 and 0.694 mGy/min chronic γ-irradiation dose rates elicited different cellular responses. In particular, we sought to determine whether different dose rates resulted in reversible or irreversible cell-cycle arrest. Cells were exposed to different dose rates of γ-irradiation for 10 days, and then cultured for an additional 10 days (free from irradiation) to determine whether they could re-enter the cell cycle. Cells exposed to ≤0.347 mGy/min formed colonies during the irradiation-free culture period, but cells exposed to 0.694 mGy/min exhibited severe growth impairment (i.e., they were senescent; Figure 3A). In this experiment, differences between 0.347 and 0.694 mGy/min did not result from different total irradiation exposures because the same result was obtained when exposure times were adjusted to equalize the total irradiation dose (Figure S4A and B). When analyzed immediately following the irradiation exposure, cells exposed to 0.347 mGy/min arrested in G1 and did not form well-defined colonies (Figure S1B and S4C), but could re-enter the cell cycle when subsequently cultured in irradiation-free conditions. In contrast, cells exposed at 0.694 mGy/min could not form colonies following irradiation exposure suggesting that they had adopted an irreversible senescence-like growth arrest. We tested whether the 0.694 mGy/min dose rate induced senescence by measuring β-galactosidase (β-gal) activity [17]. Chronic γ-irradiation efficiently induced cellular senescence (i.e., β-gal activity) and 0.694 mGy/min was more potent than 0.347 mGy/min in this assay (Figure 3B). This result was consistent with results obtained using the colony survival assay (Figure 3A). Chronic irradiation at 0.694 mGy/min was considerably more effective than acute irradiation in inducing cellular senescence (Figure 3B).

To test the biological relevance of these results, we repeated these analyses in mice. Animals were irradiated with acute (1 Gy/min) or chronic (0.347–1.388 mGy/min) γ-rays and allowed to recover for 10 days (Figure 3C). Primary lung cells were then isolated from irradiated mice and stained for β-gal activity. At dose rates ≥0.694 mGy/min, chronic irradiation was more effective

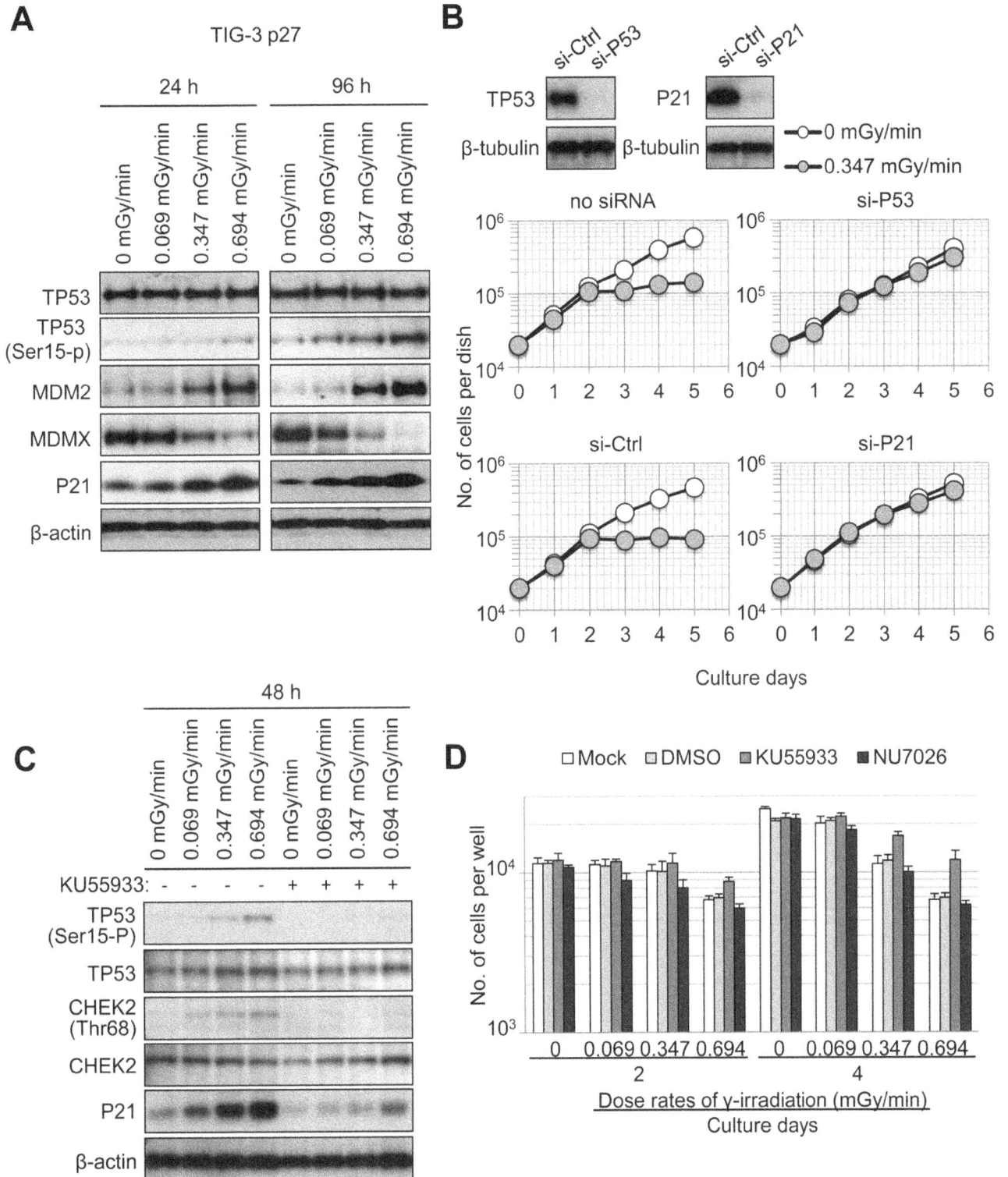

Figure 4. The ATM/TP53/p21 pathway mediates the effect of chronic γ-irradiation on cell proliferation. (A) Western blotting was used to determine levels of TP53, phosphorylated TP53 (Ser-15), MDM2, MDMX, and p21 in human fibroblasts (TIG-3 p27) cultured under chronic γ-irradiation conditions for 24 or 96 hours (dose rates are indicated). β-actin served as a loading control. (B) Knockdown of TP53 or p21 in BJ1/hT cells abolishes the growth inhibitory effect of chronic γ-irradiation. Western blot analysis of cells transfected with control siRNA (si-Ctrl), TP53-specific siRNA (si-P53), or P21-specific siRNA (si-P21) are shown (top). β-tubulin served as a loading control. Whole cell lysates were prepared 48 hours after the transfection. Forty-eight hours after transfection, BJ1/hT cells were placed into culture and grown under unirradiated control conditions (white circles) or a γ-irradiation dose rate of 0.347 mGy/min (grey circles). The number of cells per dish was counted after indicated periods of time. (C) ATM kinase is activated in response to chronic γ-irradiation. BJ1/hT cells were exposed to indicated dose rates of chronic γ-irradiation in the presence or absence of the ATM kinase inhibitor KU55933 (10 μM). ATM kinase activity was assessed by detecting phosphorylated TP53 (Ser15) or phosphorylated CHEK2

(Thr68) by Western blotting. TP53 activation and P21 induction by chronic γ-irradiation were examined by Western blotting. (D) Inhibition of ATM kinase, but not DNA-PKcs, attenuates the growth inhibitory effect of chronic γ-irradiation. BJ1/hT cells were cultured under chronic γ-irradiation conditions at indicated dose rates in the presence or absence of KU55933 (10 μM) or the DNA-PKcs inhibitor NU7026 (10 μM). Values indicate the mean ± SD of three independent wells.

than acute irradiation in inducing senescence (given equal total doses; Figure 3C), thus confirming the in vitro data.

The ATM/TP53/p21 pathway inhibits cellular growth in response to chronic γ-irradiation

The tumor suppressor protein p53 (TP53) regulates cell fate following DNA damage [18]. We therefore hypothesized that TP53 was involved in the G1 cell-cycle arrest induced by chronic γ-irradiation. To test this hypothesis, the expression of TP53 (and related proteins) in irradiated cells was analyzed by western blotting. Although TP53 levels were not affected by γ-irradiation (even at 0.694 mGy/min), γ-rays resulted in the phosphorylation of TP53 (at Ser 15), and increased levels of p21 and MDM2 oncogene, E3 ubiquitin protein ligase (MDM2), which are direct transcriptional targets of TP53 [19] (Figure 4A). In addition, MDMX, which negatively regulates TP53, was down-regulated in a dose rate-dependent manner. This result is consistent with a DNA damage response [9]. Notably, these inductions persisted for 96 hours, indicating sustained TP53 activity in response to chronic γ-irradiation. Interestingly, in other tumor cells also exhibit similar expression patterns in same proteins, but seem to be relatively insensitive especially when cells are irradiated at a dose-rate of 0.347 mGy/min (Figure S5).

To investigate the role of TP53 in cellular responses to chronic γ-irradiation, TP53 or p21 levels were knocked down in BJ1/hT fibroblasts. This treatment abolished the cell-proliferation inhibition induced by chronic γ-irradiation (0.347 mGy/min; Figure 4B). These results were confirmed in TIG-3 p27 cells (Figure S6A) and imply that the TP53/p21 pathway is required for chronic γ-irradiation-induced inhibition of cell proliferation in fibroblasts. Ataxia telangiectasia mutated (ATM) mediates cellular responses to ionizing radiation. In particular, ATM is involved in DNA-repair signaling, regulates multiple cell-cycle checkpoints, and acts upstream of TP53 following DNA damage [20]. We therefore asked whether inhibition of ATM affected the response of fibroblasts to chronic γ-irradiation. The ATM inhibitor KU55933 inhibited the phosphorylation of TP53 and checkpoint kinase 2 (CHEK2) (ATM kinase substrates) and reduced p21 induction in response to γ-irradiation (Figure 4C). In addition, KU55933 restored levels of cell proliferation in chronic γ-irradiated cells (Figure 4D for BJ1/hT cells and Figure S5B for TIG-3 p27 cells). In addition to ATM, DNA-PKcs also senses DNA damage and non-homologous end-joining repair of double-strand breaks [21]. However, the DNA-PKcs inhibitor NU7026 did not rescue proliferation of cells exposed to chronic γ-irradiation cells compared with mock- or DMSO-treated controls (Figure 4D for BJ1/hT cells and Figure S6B for TIG-3 p27 cells). These data indicate that ATM, but not DNA-PK, modulates cellular responses to DNA damage that are induced by chronic γ-irradiation.

The absence of TP53 abolishes chronic γ-irradiation-induced cellular senescence

Our data indicate that the dose rate of chronic γ-irradiation (in combination with the rate of DNA damage) affects cellular responses of fibroblasts (e.g., DNA-damage tolerance, reversible G1 cell-cycle arrest, or irreversible senescence). As the TP53/p21 pathway was required for growth arrest in response to chronic γ-

irradiation at 0.347 mGy/min (Figure 4B and Figure S6A), we asked whether TP53 or p21 were also essential for the induction of senescence at 0.694 mGy/min. Cells in which TP53 or p21 was knocked down were irradiated for 4 days and then analyzed for β-gal activity. Loss of TP53 or p21 reduced the number of β-gal-positive cells (Figure 5A). This data demonstrate that the TP53/p21 pathway is also essential for cellular senescence in response to chronic γ-irradiation. To confirm this result, colony formation and regrowth following 4 days of γ-irradiation were assessed for the two dose rates (Figure 5B and C). When BJ1/hT cells were exposed to chronic γ-irradiation at 0.694 mGy/min, knockdown of TP53 or p21 restored colony formation and regrowth compared to controls (Figure S7A). Similar results were observed for TIG-3 p27 cells (Figure S7B–D). To determine whether the TP53 pathway is essential for the induction of cellular senescence following chronic γ-irradiation in vivo, wild-type and TP53 null mice were irradiated at different doses and dose rates (Figure 3C) and levels of senescence were determined for primary cultured cells. Chronic γ-irradiation increased levels of senescence in wild-type cells but not in cells lacking TP53 (Figure 5D). Thus, the TP53 pathway regulated cell-fate responses to chronic γ-irradiation both in vitro and in vivo.

Finally, we examine the effect of the ATM/TP53/p21 pathway on genomic stability in fibroblasts exposed to chronic γ-irradiation. Genomic stability was assessed by measuring the frequency of micronucleus formation [22]. Fibroblasts transfected with TP53- or p21-specific siRNA were exposed to chronic γ-irradiation in the presence or absence of an ATM inhibitor for 4 days. Knockdown of TP53 or p21 increased the number of micronuclei compared to controls (Figure 5E), suggesting that the TP53/p21 pathway helps to maintain genomic stability in response to chronic γ-irradiation. In addition, ATM inhibition elevated the frequency of micronucleus formation in response to chronic γ-irradiation and abolished the difference between control and TP53/p21 deficient cells (Figure 5E). Thus, ATM is epistatic to the TP53/p21 pathway concerning cell-fate decisions in response to chronic γ-irradiation.

Discussion

DNA damage induced by ionizing radiation can significantly impact cell fate, i.e., affect whether a cell will proliferate, differentiate, become senescent, or apoptosis, for example [23,24]. In general, DNA-damage-associated cell-fate decisions are determined by a cell's properties (e.g., cell type and tissue of origin) [25]. In addition to cellular properties, the quantity and quality of DNA damage also affect these cell-fate decisions. The dose rate of sparsely ionizing radiation is particularly important, as lower dose rates produce smaller biological effects, even when the total dose is held constant [26]. The physiological properties of cells, including the abilities to sense, repair, and tolerate DNA damage, are likely important determinants of fate when cells are exposed to different rates of DNA damage. In this study, we tested whether the rate of DNA damage affects cell-fate decision in proliferating cells.

We discovered that different cell types exhibited different susceptibilities to chronic γ-irradiation, whereas these same cell types responded similarly to acute γ-irradiation. We defined susceptibility to γ-irradiation as the inability of exposed cells to

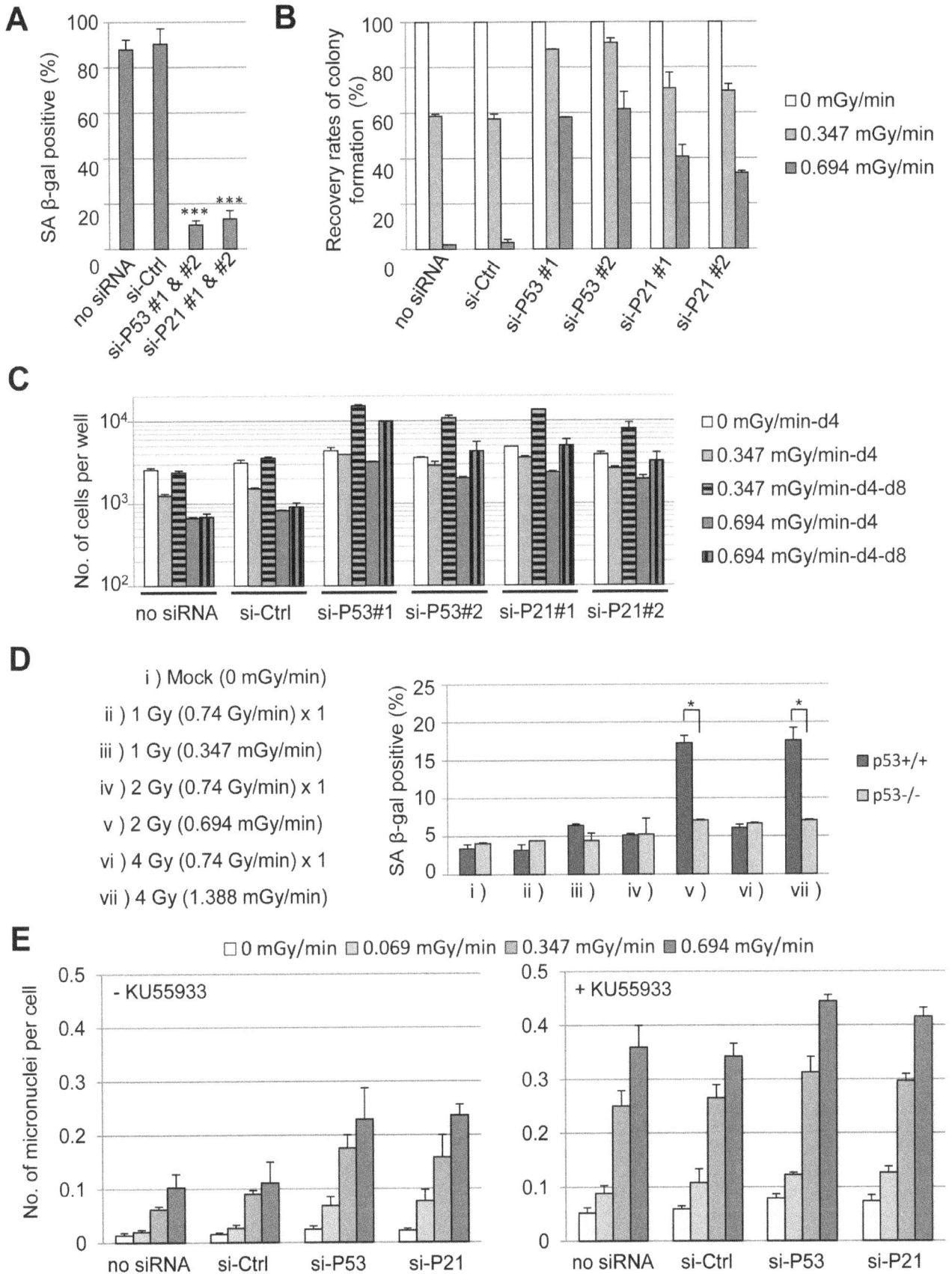

Figure 5. The ATM/TP53/p21 pathway maintains genomic integrity under chronic γ-irradiation conditions by regulating cell-fate decisions. (A) BJ1/hT cells were transfected with indicated siRNAs and cultured for 4 days under chronic γ-irradiation conditions (0.694 mGy/min). β-gal activity was used to assess cellular senescence. Values represent the mean ± SD of three independent experiments. ***P<0.001. (B) BJ1/hT cells were transfected with indicated siRNAs and then cultured under chronic γ-irradiation conditions at indicated dose rates for 4 days. After an additional 10 days of growth in unirradiated conditions, the number of macroscopic colonies was determined. Values were normalized to control and represent the mean ± SD of three independent experiments. (C) BJ1/hT cells were transfected with indicated siRNAs and then cultured under chronic γ-irradiation conditions at indicated dose rates for 4 days (-d4). Some cells were cultured an additional 4 days under unirradiated conditions (-d4-d8). Values represent the mean ± SD of three independent wells. (D) Wild-type or TP53 null mice were exposed to acute (ii, iv, vi) or chronic (iii, v, vii) γ-irradiation treatment conditions, as indicated on the left. β-gal activity was used to assess cellular senescence of primary lung cells isolated from these mice. Values represent the mean ± SD of independent cultures from 2 mice. *P<0.05. (E) BJ1/hT cells were transfected with indicated siRNA and then cultured without (left) or with (right) KU55933 (10 μM) under chronic γ-radiation conditions at indicated dose rates for 4 days. The number of micronuclei was then assessed. Values represent the mean ± SD of at least three independent experiments.

form a colony, i.e., cell death or senescence. However, when a population of cells is exposed to acute γ-irradiation cells within a single colony can exhibit quite heterogeneous behaviors [27], which may result from stochastic cellular responses to lethal and sub-lethal amounts of DNA damage. Interestingly, fibroblasts were most susceptible to chronic γ-irradiation. Susceptibility in this context was defined as a G0/G1 cell-cycle arrest, which is regulated by a number of cell-signaling pathways. Therefore, depending on the frequency of DNA damage and the period of exposure, cell-fate decisions are deterministic, rather than stochastic.

Here we discovered that two γ-irradiation dose rates induced different responses in fibroblasts, namely reversible or irreversible cell-cycle arrest. Precise regulation of proliferation and quiescence/senescence is essential for the development and homeostasis of multicellular organisms [28–30], and cellular stresses often promote cell-cycle exit [31]. A large number of proteins involved in cell-cycle progression and regulation have been identified, and complex interactions between these proteins during different cell-cycle stages and during checkpoint controls have been described [32,33]. However, the molecular mechanisms underlying cell-fate decisions under different cellular statuses remain unclear. Interestingly, our experimental system allowed us to deliver γ-irradiation at different dose rates, and cellular responses to this treatment likely reflected the DNA damage response systems work together to maintain genomic integrity, and help to determine cell fate in response to DNA damage. However, it is unclear how these systems are coordinate because the molecular events activated by DNA damage are complex and dynamic.

The TP53 regulates cellular responses (e.g., cell-cycle arrest, senescence, and apoptosis) to genotoxic stresses, thereby suppressing cellular malignancy and maintaining homeostasis within multicellular organisms [34,35]. We showed here that the TP53 pathway was a critical component of cellular responses to chronic γ-irradiation, and that these responses were triggered by the rate of DNA damage. Because TP53 regulates many physiological responses, the molecular mechanisms by which TP53 selectively induces sets of transcriptional targets to ensure appropriate cellular outcome have been extensively investigated [18]. We provide experimental evidences supporting the essential role of TP53 in cell-fate decisions to chronic γ-irradiation in vivo, using TP53 null mice. There are small molecule TP53 inhibitors that are able to modify the activity of TP53 in vivo [36], and that also will be useful tool for further studies of TP53 functions in cell-fate decisions. TP53 and its negative regulator MDM2 form a tight autoregulatory feedback loop, which regulates TP53 stability and activity [37,38]. ATM and wild type TP53-inducible phosphatase 1 (Wip1) phosphorylate and dephosphorylate TP53, respectively, thereby forming another autoregulatory feedback loop [39]. These feedback loops ensure that DNA damage-mediated TP53 activity is transient [40,41]. However, our data indicate that these

feedback loops also provide intrinsic tolerance to low levels of DNA damage. Overall cellular status and fate are dynamically regulated by nested signaling networks involving the TP53/MDM2 and ATM/Wip1 feedback loops [42]. A cell can respond to DNA damage by developing DNA-damage tolerance or by activating a DNA-damage response. Our data clearly demonstrated that the ATM/TP53/p21 pathway regulated the choice between DNA-damage tolerance and response when cells were exposed to chronic γ-irradiation and that this decision depended on the dose rate and the cell type. This decision is related to the balance between homeostasis and genomic stability, which is critical for the development and maintenance of viability of multicellular organisms [43]. It is therefore important to verify the hierarchy of the sensitive systems composed of the feedback loops in response to sustained low levels of DNA damage, as this information may shed light on the mechanisms of cancer and aging, for example. As we predicted, proliferating cells that are exposed to chronic γ-irradiation exhibit the most susceptible phenotype (cell-cycle arrest or senescence for fibroblasts) in response to the rate of DNA damage. Thus, we were able to distinguish between cell-fate decisions, allowing us to evaluate the mechanisms underlying this process. Future studies involving this system will provide insights into the molecular mechanisms governing cell-fate determination in response to DNA damage.

Supporting Information

Figure S1   Different cell types exhibit different radiation sensitivity when exposed to chronic γ-irradiation. (A) A diagram of the culture room containing a ^{137}Cs radiation source. Cubes indicate incubator positions. The dose rate for each incubator is indicated. (B) A variety of human cell lines were cultured for 10 days under control conditions (0) or chronic γ-irradiation conditions (0.347 mGy/min). Representative images of crystal violet-stained culture plates are shown.

Figure S2   Chronic γ-irradiation specifically suppresses the proliferation of fibroblasts via a G1 arrest. (A) A number of human cell lines were cultured under chronic γ-irradiation conditions at indicated dose rates. After 0, 2.5, 5, 7.5, or 10 days the number of cells in each well was determined. Values represent the mean ± SD of six independent wells. (B) Representative images of TIG-3 p27 cells after 4 days of chronic γ-irradiation (dose rates are indicated). Hoechst 33258 staining of DNA (blue) and EdU-Alexa Fluor488 (green) are shown. Scale bar is 250 μm.

Figure S3   Human fibroblasts undergo senescence when accumulated DNA damage exceeds a threshold. (A) BJ1/hT (left) or TIG-3 p27 (right) cells were cultured for 4 days under chronic γ-irradiation conditions at indicated dose rates. The number of γ-H2AX-foci per cell was then determined. The size of the bubble is proportional to the number of cells with that number of γ-H2AX-foci. Black bars indicate the mean number of foci per cell. (B) The number of γ-H2AX-foci increased over time in response to chronic γ-irradiation conditions. BJ1/hT (upper) or TIG-3 p27 (lower) cells were cultured under chronic γ-irradiation conditions at indicated dose rates for 2.5, 5, 7.5, or 10 days.

Figure S4 The chronic γ-irradiation dose rate affects cell-fate decisions in human fibroblasts. (A–C) Colony-forming ability of fibroblasts following chronic γ-irradiation. Experimental schemes are illustrated to the left. (A) TIG-3 cells (2×10^2) were cultured at indicated dose rates for 5 days and then grown under unirradiated conditions for an additional 10 days. Culture plates were then stained using crystal violet. Representative images are shown to the right. (B) TIG-3 p27 cells (2×10^2) were cultured for 10 days at 0.347 mGy/min or 5 days at 0.694 mGy/min (total dose of 5 Gy). Culture dishes were then incubated under unirradiated conditions for an additional 5 days and stained using crystal violet. Representative images of stained culture dishes are shown on the right. (C) TIG-3 p27 cells (2×10^2) were cultured at indicated dose rates for 10 days. Representative images of crystal violet-stained culture dishes are shown to the right.

Figure S5 TP53/p21 pathway is activated by chronic γ-irradiation in tumor cell lines. Changes in protein levels of TP53, phosphorylation of TP53 at Ser-15, MDM2, MDMX, and P21 in U2OS and MCF-7 cells cultured under chronic γ-irradiation for 24 and 96 hours at different dose-rates of background 0, 0.069, 0.347, 0.694 mGy/min were analyzed by Western blotting.

Figure S6 Inhibition of the ATM/TP53/p21 pathway attenuates chronic γ-irradiation induced growth inhibition. (A) TIG-3 p27 cells (2×103) were transfected with indicated siRNAs and cultured under chronic γ-irradiation conditions at indicated dose rates. The number of cells per well was determined at indicated time points. Values represent the mean ± SD of three

independent wells. (B) Inhibition of ATM kinase activity, but not DNA-PKcs activity, attenuates the growth inhibitory effect of chronic γ-irradiation. TIG-3 p27 cells were cultured for 2 or 4 days under chronic γ-irradiation conditions at indicated dose rates in the presence or absence of the ATM inhibitor KU55933 (10 μM) or the DNA-PKcs inhibitor NU7026 (10 μM). The number of Hoechst-stained nuclei was determined for each well. Values represent the mean ± SD of three independent wells.

Figure S7 Knock down of TP53 or p21 attenuates chronic γ-irradiation-induced senescence. (A) Western blot analysis of BJ1/hT cells transfected with control siRNA (si-Ctrl) or siRNA specific for *TP53* (si-P53 #1 or #2), or *P21* (si-P21 #1 or #2) (upper left). β-tubulin served as the loading control. Cells transfected with indicated siRNA were cultured under chronic γ-irradiation conditions at indicated dose rates for 4 days, and then incubated an additional 10 days under non-irradiated conditions (experimental scheme is illustrated lower left). Representative images of crystal violet-stained colonies are shown (right). (B) TIG-3 p27 cells were analyzed as in (A), except that cells were cultured for 6 days following γ-irradiation. (C–D) TIG-3 p27 cells transfected with indicated siRNAs were exposed to γ-irradiation at indicated dose rates. The ability of these cells to form colonies (C) or to proliferate (D) was subsequently assessed as shown in Figure 5 (B–C).

Acknowledgments

The authors thank Dr. Hidetoshi Tahara and Dr. Akira Shimamoto (Hiroshima University, Hiroshima, Japan) who kindly provided hTERT-immortalized fibroblasts. The authors also thank Mamiko Yano, Mariko Morozumi, Shinji Suga, and Shingo Sasatani for their assistance.

Author Contributions

Conceived and designed the experiments: HK YM. Performed the experiments: LC HK MS DI AO TU. Analyzed the data: LC HK. Contributed reagents/materials/analysis tools: TI KS KK. Contributed to the writing of the manuscript: HK FS.

References

1. Ciccia A, Elledge SJ (2010) The DNA damage response: making it safe to play withknives. Mol Cell 40: 179–204.
2. Campisi J (2013) Aging, cellular senescence, and cancer. Annu Rev Physiol 75: 685–705.
3. Lindahl T (1993) Instability and decay of the primary structure of DNA. Nature 362: 709–715.
4. Vilenchik MM, Knudson AG (2003) Endogenous DNA double-strand breaks: production, fidelity of repair, and induction of cancer. Proc Natl Acad Sci U S A 100: 12871–12876.
5. d'Adda di Fagagna F (2008) Living on a break: cellular senescence as a DNA-damage response. Nat Rev Cancer 8: 512–522.
6. Suzuki F, Nakao N, Nikaido O, Kondo S (1992) High resistance of cultured Mongolian gerbil cells to X-ray-induced killing and chromosome aberrations. Radiat Res 131: 290–296.
7. Tahara H, Kusunoki M, Yamanaka Y, Matsumura S, Ide T (2005) G-tail telomere HPA: simple measurement of human single-stranded telomeric overhangs. Nat Methods 2: 829–831.
8. Ojima M, Hamano H, Suzuki M, Suzuki K, Kodama S, et al. (2004) Delayed induction of telomere instability in normal human fibroblast cells by ionizing radiation. J Radiat Res 45: 105–110.
9. Kawai H, Wiederschain D, Kitao H, Stuart J, Tsai KKC, et al. (2003) DNA damage-induced MDMX degradation is mediated by MDM2. Journal of Biological Chemistry 278: 45946–45953.
10. Norimura T, Nomoto S, Katsuki M, Gondo Y, Kondo S (1996) p53-dependent apoptosis suppresses radiation-induced teratogenesis. Nat Med 2: 577–580.
11. Gondo Y, Nakamura K, Nakao K, Sasaoka T, Ito K, et al. (1994) Gene Replacement of the P53 Gene with the Lacz Gene in Mouse Embryonic Stem-Cells and Mice by Using 2 Steps of Homologous Recombination. Biochem Biophys Res Commun 202: 830–837.
12. Illa-Bochaca I, Fernandez-Gonzalez R, Shelton DN, Welm BE, Ortiz-de-Solorzano C, et al. (2010) Limiting-dilution transplantation assays in mammary stem cell studies. Methods Mol Biol 621: 29–47.
13. Hall EJ, Marchese MJ, Astor MB, Morse T (1986) Response of cells of human origin, normal and malignant, to acute and low dose rate irradiation. Int J Radiat Oncol Biol Phys 12: 655–659.
14. Michalowski A (1981) Effects of radiation on normal tissues: hypothetical mechanisms and limitations of in situ assays of clonogenicity. Radiat Environ Biophys 19: 157–172.
15. Shiloh Y (1997) Ataxia-telangiectasia and the Nijmegen breakage syndrome: related disorders but genes apart. Annu Rev Genet 31: 635–662.
16. Gudkov AV, Komarova EA (2003) The role of p53 in determining sensitivity to radiotherapy. Nat Rev Cancer 3: 117–129.
17. Debacq-Chainiaux F, Erusalimsky JD, Campisi J, Toussaint O (2009) Protocols to detect senescence-associated beta-galactosidase (SA-betagal) activity, a biomarker of senescent cells in culture and in vivo. Nat Protoc 4: 1798–1806.
18. Santoro R, Blandino G (2010) p53: The pivot between cell cycle arrest and senescence. Cell Cycle 9: 4262–4263.
19. Siliciano JD, Canman CE, Taya Y, Sakaguchi K, Appella E, et al. (1997) DNA damage induces phosphorylation of the amino terminus of p53. Genes Dev 11: 3471–3481.
20. Xu Y, Baltimore D (1996) Dual roles of ATM in the cellular response to radiation and in cell growth control. Genes Dev 10: 2401–2410.
21. Martin M, Terradas M, Tusell L, Genesca A (2012) ATM and DNA-PKcs make a complementary couple in DNA double strand break repair. Mutat Res.

22. Nussenzweig A (2007) Causes and consequences of the DNA damage response. Cell Cycle 6: 2339–2340.

23. Smith LE, Nagar S, Kim GJ, Morgan WF (2003) Radiation-induced genomic instability: radiation quality and dose response. Health Phys 85: 23–29.

24. McMillan TJ (1992) Residual DNA damage: what is left over and how does this determine cell fate? Eur J Cancer 28: 267–269.

25. Panganiban RAM, Snow AL, Day RM (2013) Mechanisms of Radiation Toxicity in Transformed and Non-Transformed Cells. International Journal of Molecular Sciences 14: 15931–15958.

26. Hall EJ, Bedford JS (1964) Dose Rate: Its Effect on the Survival of Hela Cells Irradiated with Gamma Rays. Radiat Res 22: 305–315.

27. Marin G, Bender MA (1966) Radiation-induced mammalian cell death: lapse-time cinemicrographic observations. Exp Cell Res 43: 413–423.

28. Munoz-Espin D, Canamero M, Maraver A, Gomez-Lopez G, Contreras J, et al. (2013) Programmed cell senescence during mammalian embryonic development. Cell 155: 1104–1118.

29. Rubin H (1997) Cell aging in vivo and in vitro. Mech Ageing Dev 98: 1–35.

30. Storer M, Mas A, Robert-Moreno A, Pecoraro M, Ortells MC, et al. (2013) Senescence Is a Developmental Mechanism that Contributes to Embryonic Growth and Patterning. Cell 155: 1119–1130.

31. Salama R, Sadaie M, Hoare M, Narita M (2014) Cellular senescence and its effector programs. Genes Dev 28: 99–114.

32. Kastan MB, Bartek J (2004) Cell-cycle checkpoints and cancer. Nature 432: 316–323.

33. Harper JW, Elledge SJ (2007) The DNA damage response: ten years after. Mol Cell 28: 739–745.

34. Wu XW, Bayle JH, Olson D, Levine AJ (1993) The P53 Mdm-2 Autoregulatory Feedback Loop. Genes Dev 7: 1126–1132.

35. Ashcroft M, Vousden KH (1999) Regulation of p53 stability. Oncogene 18: 7637–7643.

36. Gudkov AV, Komarova EA (2010) Pathologies associated with the p53 response. Cold Spring Harb Perspect Biol 2: a001180.

37. Levine AJ (1997) p53, the cellular gatekeeper for growth and division. Cell 88: 323–331.

38. Vousden KH, Prives C (2009) Blinded by the Light: The Growing Complexity of p53. Cell 137: 413–431.

39. Shreeram S, Demidov ON, Hee WK, Yamaguchi H, Onishi N, et al. (2006) Wip1 phosphatase modulates ATM-dependent signaling pathways. Mol Cell 23: 757–764.

40. Lu XB, Ma O, Nguyen TA, Joness SN, Oren M, et al. (2007) The Wip1 phosphatase acts as a gatekeeper in the p53-Mdm2 autoregulatory loop. Cancer Cell 12: 342–354.

41. Wagner J, Ma L, Rice JJ, Hu W, Levine AJ, et al. (2005) p53-Mdm2 loop controlled by a balance of its feedback strength and effective dampening using ATM and delayed feedback. Iee Proceedings Systems Biology 152: 109–118.

42. Purvis JE, Karhohs KW, Mock C, Batchelor E, Loewer A, et al. (2012) p53 dynamics control cell fate. Science 336: 1440–1444.

43. Harfouche G, Martin MT (2010) Response of normal stem cells to ionizing radiation: A balance between homeostasis and genomic stability. Mutation Research-Reviews in Mutation Research 704: 167–174.

3

Notch Signaling Regulates the Lifespan of Vascular Endothelial Cells via a p16-Dependent Pathway

Yohko Yoshida[1,9], Yuka Hayashi[1,9], Masayoshi Suda[1], Kaoru Tateno[2], Sho Okada[2], Junji Moriya[2], Masataka Yokoyama[2], Aika Nojima[2], Masakatsu Yamashita[3], Yoshio Kobayashi[2], Ippei Shimizu[1], Tohru Minamino[1,4]*

1 Department of Cardiovascular Biology and Medicine, Niigata University Graduate School of Medical and Dental Sciences, Niigata, Japan, 2 Department of Cardiovascular Medicine, Chiba University Graduate School of Medicine, Chiba, Japan, 3 Kazusa DNA Research Institute, Kisarazu, Chiba, Japan, 4 PRESTO, Japan Science and Technology Agency, Kawaguchi, Saitama, Japan

Abstract

Evolutionarily conserved Notch signaling controls cell fate determination and differentiation during development, and is also essential for neovascularization in adults. Although recent studies suggest that the Notch pathway is associated with age-related conditions, it remains unclear whether Notch signaling is involved in vascular aging. Here we show that Notch signaling has a crucial role in endothelial cell senescence. Inhibition of Notch signaling in human endothelial cells induced premature senescence via a p16-dependent pathway. Conversely, over-expression of Notch1 or Jagged1 prolonged the replicative lifespan of endothelial cells. Notch1 positively regulated the expression of inhibitor of DNA binding 1 (Id1) and MAP kinase phosphatase 1 (MKP1), while MKP1 further up-regulated Id1 expression by inhibiting p38MAPK-induced protein degradation. Over-expression of Id1 down-regulated p16 expression, thereby inhibiting premature senescence of Notch1-deleted endothelial cells. These findings indicate that Notch1 signaling has a role in the regulation of endothelial cell senescence via a p16-dependent pathway and suggest that activation of Notch1 could be a new therapeutic target for treating age-associated vascular diseases.

Editor: Ryuichi Morishita, Osaka University Graduate School of Medicine, Japan

Funding: This work was supported by a Grant-in-Aid for Scientific Research from the Ministry of Education, Culture, Sports, Science and Technology of Japan (grant numbers 2430195, 25126706, 25670382), and the grants from the Ono Medical Research Foundation, the Uehara Memorial Foundation, the NOVARTIS Foundation for the Promotion Science, the Japan Diabetes Foundation, the SENSHIN Medical Research Foundation, the Takeda Science Foundation, and the Mitsubishi Pharma Research Foundation, the Takeda Medical Research Foundation, the SUZUKEN Memorial Foundation (to TM), and the Japan Heart Foundation & Astellas/Pfizer Grant for Research on Atherosclerosis Update and the Japan Heart Foundation Dr. Hiroshi Irisawa & Dr. Aya Irisawa Memorial Research Grant (to YY). The funders had no role in study design, data collection and analysis, decision to publish, or preparation of the manuscript.

Competing Interests: The authors have declared that no competing interests exist.

* Email: t_minamino@yahoo.co.jp

9 These authors contributed equally to this work.

Introduction

The Notch pathway is a highly conserved signaling system that controls the fate and differentiation of cells during the development of various tissues. In mammals, the Notch signaling pathway is composed of four Notch receptors (Notch1 through 4) and five ligands (Jagged 1 and 2, and Delta-like 1, 3, and 4). All of the receptors and ligands are transmembrane proteins, so Notch signaling is often mediated by cell-cell interaction. Receptor-ligand interactions induce additional proteolytic cleavage, which frees the Notch intracellular domain (NICD) from the cell membrane. The NICD then translocates to the nucleus, where it associates with the DNA-binding protein CSL (Epstein-Barr virus latency C promoter binding factor 1 (CBF1; also known as RBPJ) in vertebrates, Suppressor of Hairless in Drosophila, and Lag1 in *C elegans*), displacing a histone deacetylase-co-repressor complex from CSL protein, so that transcription of Notch target genes is activated [1,2]. In the cardiovascular system, Notch signaling has been implicated in the regulation of cardiomyocyte differentiation, the epithelial-to-mesenchymal transition during heart valve development, and vascular development. Therefore, mutations of Notch receptors or ligands cause congenital cardiovascular disorders such as Alagille syndrome, cerebral autosomal dominant arteriopathy with subcortical infarcts and leukoencephalopathy (CADASIL), and bicuspid aortic valve [3–5]. In adults, Notch signaling is essential for neovascularization and has been reported to be involved in age-associated conditions such as cancer, neurodegenerative disorders, and impaired regeneration of aged skeletal muscle [6–10].

Vascular cells have a finite lifespan in vitro and eventually enter a state of irreversible growth arrest called cellular senescence that is associated with various morphological changes and increased expression of senescence-associated molecules such as p53 or p16 [11,12]. Accumulation of senescent vascular cells occurs in aged vessels, leading to an increase of inflammation combined with a decline of regenerative potential that promote vascular dysfunction and atherosclerosis [13]. Given that Notch signaling is involved in a wide range of pathophysiological processes, including age-associated conditions, we have examined the role of the Notch pathway in vascular aging.

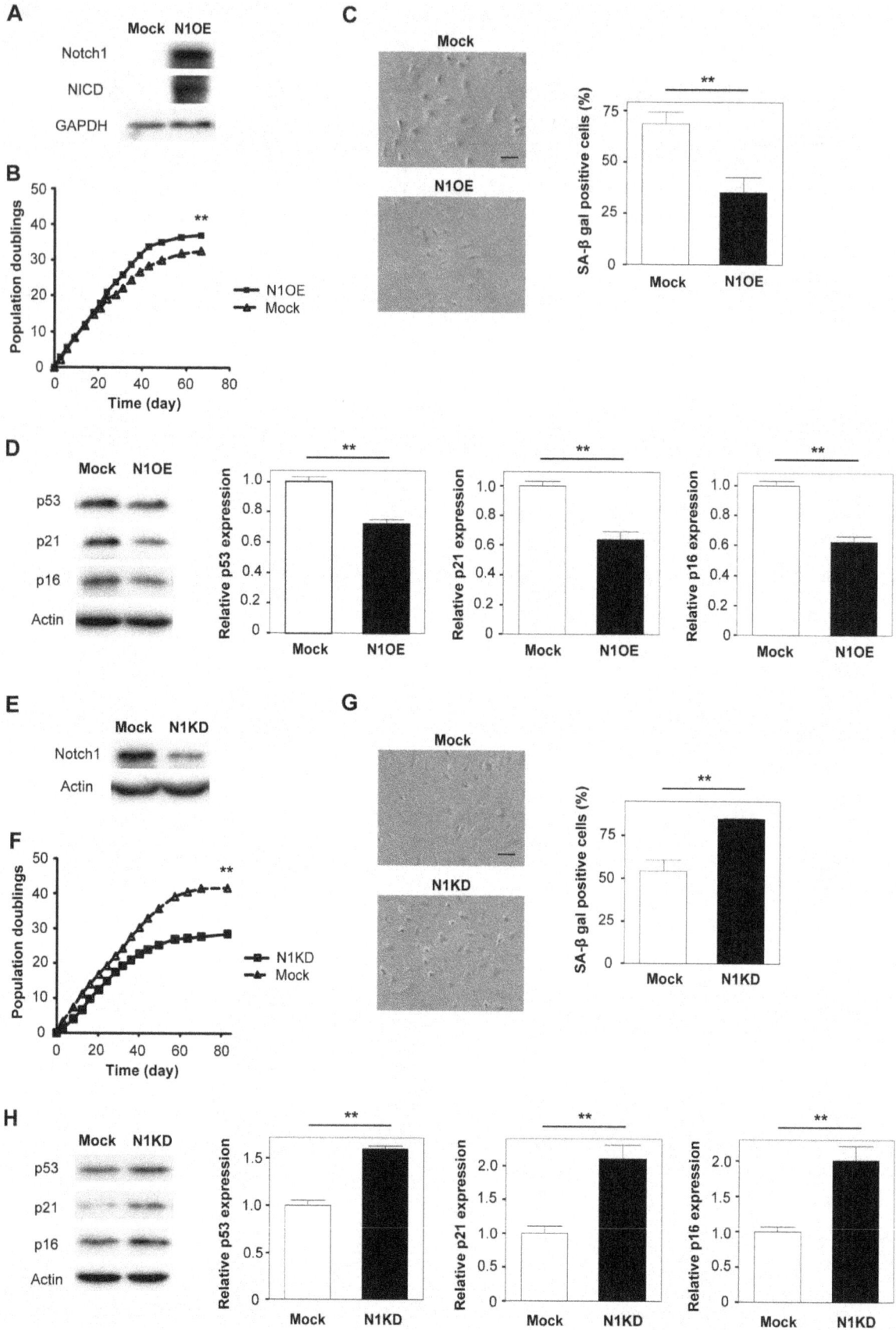

Figure 1. Over-expression of Notch1 prolongs the lifespan of vascular endothelial cells. (A) Western blot analysis of full length Notch1 (Notch1) and Notch intracellular domain (NICD) expression in human endothelial cells infected with a retroviral vector expressing Notch1 (N1OE) or the empty vector (Mock). GAPDH was used as the loading control. (B) Infected cells were passaged until senescence, and the total number of population doublings was determined (n = 3). (C) Senescence-associated β-galactosidase (SA-β gal) staining of endothelial cells prepared as in Figure 1A. Scale bar = 50 μm. The right graph shows quantitative data on SA-β gal-positive cells (n = 4). (D) Western blot analysis of p53, p21, and p16 expression in endothelial cells prepared as in Figure 1A. The right graph shows quantitative data on p53, p21, and p16 expression (n = 3). (E) Western blot analysis of full length Notch1 (Notch1) expression in human endothelial cells infected with a retroviral vector expressing Notch1 shRNA (N1KD) or sh-Control (Mock). (F) Infected cells were passaged until senescence, and the total number of population doublings was determined (n = 3). (G) Senescence-associated β-galactosidase (SA-β gal) staining of endothelial cells prepared as Figure 1E. Scale bar = 50 μm. The right graph shows quantitative data on SA-β gal positive cells (n = 4). (H) Western blot analysis of p53, p21, and p16 expression in endothelial cells prepared as in Figure 1E. The right graph shows quantitative data on p53, p21, and p16 expression (n = 3). All values represent the mean ± s.e.m. *P<0.05, **P< 0.01.

Here we show that Notch signaling has a crucial role in endothelial cell senescence. Mechanistically, activation of Notch signaling up-regulates inhibitor of DNA binding 1 (Id1) and MAPK phosphatase 1 (MKP1) expression and prolongs endothelial cell lifespan by inhibiting a p16-dependent pathway. We further demonstrated that Notch1-induced up-regulation of MKP1 stabilizes Id1 protein by inhibiting p38MAPK-induced degradation, leading to prolongation of the endothelial cell lifespan. Moreover, overexpression of Id1 significantly attenuated p16 expression and increased the proliferative activity of endothelial cells in *Notch1*-deficient mice. Taken together, our results suggest that activation of Notch1 could be a new therapeutic target for treating age-associated vascular diseases.

Materials and Methods

Cell culture and reagents

Human umbilical vein endothelial cells (HUVEC) were purchased from Lonza (Walkersville, MD, USA) and cultured according to the manufacturer's instructions. Endothelial cell proliferation was assessed by counting cell numbers after subculture. We defined senescent cells as those that did not increase in number and remained subconfluent after 2 weeks of culture. Senescence-associated β-galactosidase (SA-β-gal) staining was performed as described previously [14]. The number of population doublings (PD) was calculated as follows: PD = log (number of cells obtained/initial number of cells)/log 2. In some experiments, endothelial cells were treated with SB203580 (WAKO, Osaka, Japan, 10 μM), anisomycin (WAKO, 2 μM) or MG132 (WAKO, 0.5 μM).

Retroviral and lentiviral infection

The following plasmids were used for generating retroviral and lentiviral vectors: pLNCX or pLPCX (Clontech, Palo Alto, CA, USA) for a retroviral vector and pLVSIN (Takara, Tokyo, Japan) for a lentiviral vector. We created pLNCX-based vectors expressing full length Notch1, Notch1 intracellular domain (NICD), or Jagged1, and a pLPCX-based vector expressing inhibitor of DNA binding 1 (ID1), and a pLVSIN-based vector expressing inhibitor of DNA binding 1 (ID1). For knockdown experiments, we used the Knockout RNAi System (Clontech) or the MISSION lentiviral packaging system (Sigma, St. Louis, MO, USA), and generated retroviral or lentiviral vectors expressing short hairpin RNA (shRNA) targeting human Notch1, Jagged1, and INK4A according to the manufacturer's instruction. We used pLNCX, pLPCX, pSIREN-RetroQ, pLVSIN or pLKO.1 as negative control vectors. Human endothelial cells (passages 4–6) were plated at 5×10^5 cells in 100-mm diameter dishes at 24 hours before infection. Then the culture medium was replaced by retroviral or lentiviral stock supplemented with 8 μg/ml polybrene (Sigma). From 48 hours after infection, cells were selected by

culture in 500 μg/ml G418 (pLNCX-based vectors) or 0.5 μg/ml puromycin (pLPCX, pSIREN-RetroQ or pLKO.1-based vectors) for 7 days. After selection, 2×10^5 cells were seeded in 100-mm diameter dishes on the 8th day post-infection, which was designated as day 0. For double infection, endothelial cells were infected with pLNCX-based vectors, purified with 500 μg/ml G418 for 7 days, and then subjected to infection with the second vector as described above.

Animal models

All animal study protocols were approved by the Chiba University and Niigata University review boards. C57BL/6NCr mice were purchased from SLC Japan (Shizuoka, Japan) and Tie2-cre mice were obtained from Jackson Laboratories (Bar Harbor, ME, USA). Floxed Notch-1 mice have been described elsewhere [15]. Deletion of Notch1 in endothelial cells (EC) was accomplished by crossing male Tie2-cre$^+$ mice with female *Notch1*$^{lox/lox}$ mice (Tie2-cre$^+$; *Notch1*$^{lox/+}$, N1KO), and the corresponding littermates without the Cre transgene (Tie2-cre$^-$; *Notch1*$^{lox/+}$) served as controls.

Aortic ring assay

An *ex vivo* angiogenesis assay was performed as described previously[16] with slight modifications. Briefly, descending thoracic aortas from 8- to 10-week-old N1KO mice and littermate control mice were harvested and placed in Opti-MEM (GIBCO, Tokyo, Japan). The adventitia was dissected away and each aorta was cut into 1-mm rings under a dissecting microscope, which were cultured in Opti-MEM with lentivirus stock for 24 hours to introduce Id1 or Mock. Then the aortic rings were embedded in type I collagen gel in a 96-well plate supplemented with EGM-2 (Lonza) and 20 ng/ml VEGF, and cultured at 37°C. On day 7, cultured aortic rings were fixed with 4% formalin and stained with BS1 lectin-FITC (Sigma). Quantitative analysis of endothelial sprouting was performed by using images obtained with a Biorevo (Keyence Co., Osaka, Japan).

Western blot analysis

Lysates were resolved by SDS-polyacrylamide gel electrophoresis. Proteins were transferred to a polyvinylidene difluoride membrane (Millipore, Bedford, MA, USA), which was incubated with the primary antibody followed by incubation with anti-rabbit, anti-mouse, or anti-goat immunoglobulin-G conjugated with horseradish peroxidase (Jackson ImmunoResearch, West Grove, PA, USA). Specific proteins were detected by using enhanced chemiluminescence (GE Healthcare, Backinghamshire, UK). The primary antibodies for Western blotting were as follows: anti-Notch1 antibody (Santa Cruz, Dallas, TX, USA), anti-Jagged1 antibody (Santa Cruz), anti-p53 antibody (DO-1) (Santa Cruz), anti-p21 antibody (Millipore, Billerica, MA, USA), anti-p16 antibody (BD Pharmingen, San Jose, CA, USA), anti-ID1

A

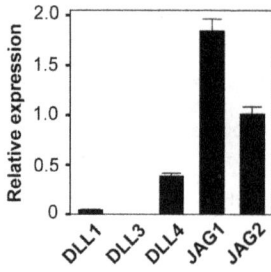

B

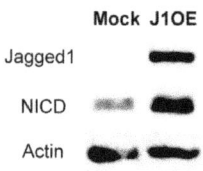

C

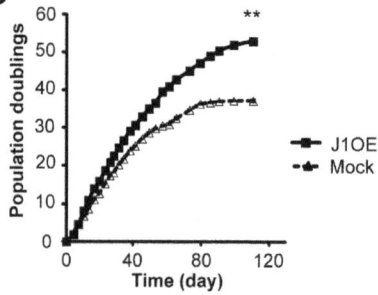

D

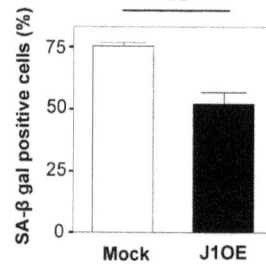

E

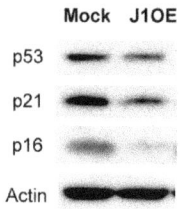

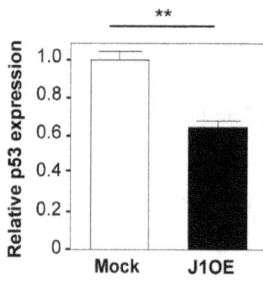

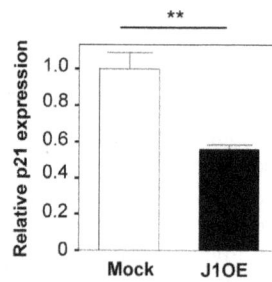

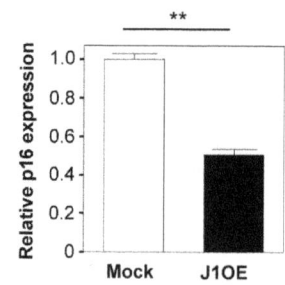

F

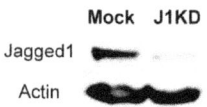

G

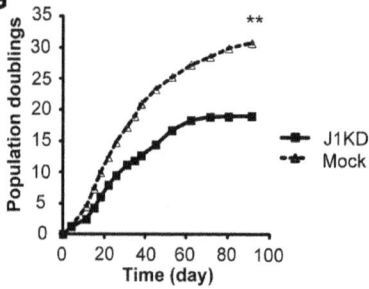

H

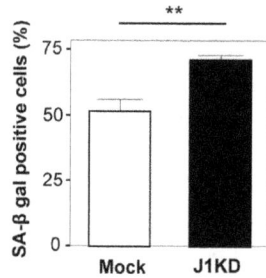

I

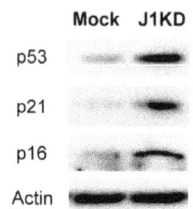

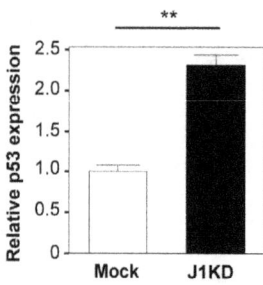

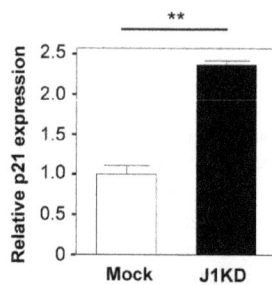

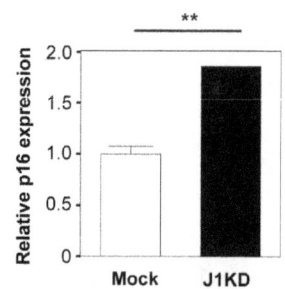

Figure 2. Over-expression of Jagged1 prolongs the lifespan of vascular endothelial cells. (A) Real-time PCR analysis showing the relative expression of Notch ligands (*DLL1, DLL3, DLL4, JAG1,* and *JAG2*) in human endothelial cells (n = 5). (B) Western blot analysis of Jagged1 and Notch intracellular domain (NICD) expression in human endothelial cells infected with a retroviral vector encoding Jagged1 (J1OE) or an empty vector (Mock). Actin was used as the loading control. (C) Infected cells were passaged until senescence, and the total number of population doublings was determined (n = 3). (D) Senescence-associated β-galactosidase (SA-β gal) staining of endothelial cells prepared as in Figure 2B. The graph shows quantitative data on SA-β gal-positive cells (n = 4). (E) Western blot analysis of p53, p21, and p16 expression in endothelial cells prepared as in Figure 2B. The right graphs show quantitative data on p53, p21, and p16 expression (n = 3). (F) Western blot analysis of Jagged1 in human endothelial cells infected with a retroviral vector expressing human Jagged1 shRNA (J1KD) or shControl (Mock). (G) Infected cells were passaged until senescence, and the total number of population doublings was determined (n = 3). (H) Senescence-associated β-galactosidase (SA-β gal) staining of endothelial cells prepared as in Figure 2F. The graph shows quantitative data on SA-β gal-positive cells (n = 4). (I) Western blot analysis of p53, p21, and p16 in endothelial cells prepared as in Figure 2F. The right graphs show quantitative data on p53, p21, and p16 expression (n = 3). All values represent the mean ± s.e.m. *P<0.05, **P<0.01.

antibody (Santa Cruz), anti-phospho p38MAPK (Thr180/Tyr182) antibody (Cell signaling, Boston, MA, USA), anti-p38MAPK antibody (Cell signaling), anti-phospho SAPK/JNK (Thr183/Tyr185) antibody (Cell Signaling), anti-JNK1/3 antibody (Santa Cruz), anti-actin antibody (Cell signaling), anti-GAPDH antibody (Santa Cruz), anti-phosphoserine antibody (Abcam, Cambridge, UK) and anti-phosphothreonine antibody (Cell signaling). To assess the phosphorylation level of Id1, cell lysates were immunoprecipitated with FLAG M2 agarose (Sigma).

RNA analysis

Total RNA (1 μg) was isolated from endothelial cells with RNA-Bee (TEL-TEST INC, Freindswood, TX, USA). Real-time PCR was performed by using a Light Cycler 480 (Roche, Basel, Swiss) with the Universal Probe Library and the Light Cycler 480 Probes Master (Roche) according to the manufacturer's instruction.

DNA microarray analysis

HUVEC were infected with retroviral vectors encoding Jagged1, Jagged1-shRNA or Notch1-shRNA, or empty vector as control. Total RNA of them were isolated from HUVEC with RNA-Bee (TEL-TEST INC). Cyanine-3 (Cy3) labeled cRNA was prepared from 0.5 ug RNA using the One-Color Low RNA Input Linear Amplification PLUS kit (Agilent, Santa Clara, CA, USA) according to the manufacturer's instructions, and the resulting probes were hybridized to Agilent Whole Human Genome Oligo Microarrays (G4112F). The scanned images were normalized by Agilent GeneSpring GX software and differentially expressed genes were identified via the fold-change (FC) and p values of the t-test. Gene expression data is available through the Gene Expression Omnibus database (GSE40403).

Measurement of telomere length

Telomere length was measured as described previously [17]. Briefly, genomic DNA was extracted from endothelial cells and telomeres were measured by real-time PCR using a Light Cycler 480 (Roche) with the LightCycler FastStart DNA Master SYBR Green kit (Roche) according to the manufacturer's instruction.

The single-copy gene 36B4 (which encodes acidic ribosomal phosphor-protein) was used as the internal control.

Chromatin immunoprecipitation assay

Chromatin immunoprecipitation (ChIP) was performed using chromatin prepared from Flag-tagged Notch1 over-expressing human endothelial cells or control cells (Mock). Sonicated chromatin was immunoprecipitated with antibodies targeting FLAG M2 (Sigma Aldrich), or normal mouse immunoglobulin G (IgG; Sigma Aldrich), and the precipitates were collected on protein A/G Sepharose beads (GE Healthcare). Real-time PCR was performed with the following primer pairs for CBF1 (forward: 5′-ttaattgatgatgtctctctcttttga-3′; reverse: 5′-tcaggaaaccaggaaaacca-3′) and beta-globin (forward: 5′-tgcaggctgcctatcagaa-3′; reverse: 5′-gcgagcttagtgatacttgtgg-3′).

Statistical analysis

Data are shown as the mean ± SEM. Differences between groups were examined by Student's *t*-test or ANOVA followed by Bonferroni's correction for comparison of means. For all analyses, *P*<0.05 was considered statistically significant.

Results

Over-expression of Notch1 prolongs the lifespan of vascular endothelial cells

To examine the role of the Notch pathway in endothelial senescence, we infected human endothelial cells with a retroviral vector encoding *NOTCH1* cDNA or an empty vector. Western blot analysis revealed that introduction of this construct led to stable up-regulation of Notch1 and its activation, as shown by up-regulation of Notch intracellular domain (NICD) (Figure 1A and Figure S1A). We examined the replicative lifespan of infected cells and found that up-regulation of Notch1 prolonged the lifespan of endothelial cells along with a decrease of senescence-associated β-galactosidase (SA-β-gal) activity and decreased expression of senescence-associated molecules such as p53, p21, and p16 (Figure 1B–D). We next examined the effect of Notch1 deletion on the lifespan of endothelial cells by using a retroviral vector

Gene symbol	Ref Seq Accesion	Jagged1 OE		Jagged1 KD		Notch1 KD	
		FC	p-value	FC	p-value	FC	p-value
ID1	NM_002165	2.2989	0.0002	0.7473	0.0015	0.9275	0.0448
DUSP1	NM_004417	1.5863	0.0051	0.8523	0.0464	0.7690	0.0055

(FC; Fold change vs. Control)

Figure 3. Microarray analysis in human endothelial cells. Microarray analysis of human endothelial cells showing that the Notch signaling positively regulates the expression of *ID1* and *DUSP1*. OE; over-expression, KD; knock-down.

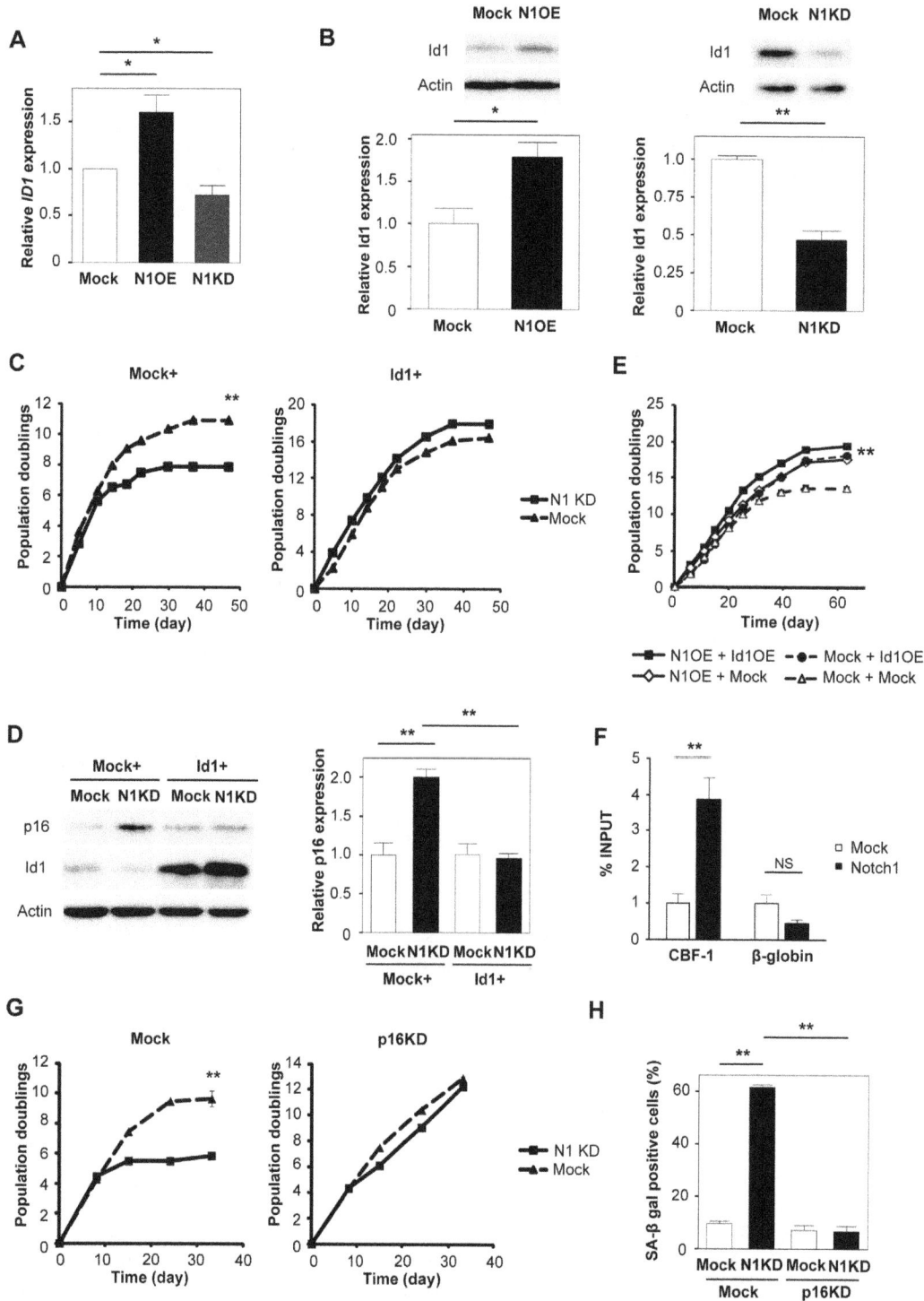

Figure 4. Up-regulation of Id1 inhibits premature senescence induced by Notch1 disruption. (A) Real-time PCR for the expression of *ID1* in Notch1 over-expressing endothelial cells (N1OE), Notch1 knockdown cells (N1KD), and Mock-infected cells (Mock) (n = 12). (B) Western blot analysis of Id1 in endothelial cells prepared as in Figure 4A. The graphs display quantitative data on Id1 expression (n = 3). (C) Human endothelial cells were infected with a retroviral vector encoding Notch1 shRNA (N1KD) or an empty vector (Mock). Infected cells were then transduced with pLNCX-Id1 (Id1+) or an empty vector (Mock+) and subjected to the proliferation assay as described in the legend for Figure 1B (n = 3). (D) Western blot analysis of p16 and Id1 expression in endothelial cells prepared as in Figure 4C. The right graph displays quantitative data on p16 expression (n = 3). (E) Human endothelial cells were co-infected with retroviral vectors encoding Notch1 and Id1. Infected cells were passaged until senescence, and the total number of population doublings was determined (n = 3). (F) ChIP assay of the direct association between Notch1 and Id1 in Notch1 overexpressing cells (Notch1) or mock-infected cells (Mock) (n = 5). The amount of activated Notch1 localized to the CBF1-binding element was estimated by real-time PCR. The β-globin locus was used as a negative control. (G) Human endothelial cells were infected with a lentiviral vector encoding p16 shRNA (p16KD) or an empty vector (Mock). Infected cells were then transduced with a retroviral vector encoding Notch1 shRNA (N1KD) or an empty vector (Mock) and subjected to the proliferation assay as described in the legend for Figure 1B. (H) Senescence-associated β-galactosidase (SA-β gal) staining

of endothelial cells prepared as in Figure 4G. The graph displays quantitative data on SA-β gal-positive cells (n = 4). All values represent the mean ± s.e.m. *P<0.05, **P<0.01.

encoding short hairpin RNA for Notch1. Disruption of Notch1 markedly reduced the maximum number of population doublings together with an increase of SA-β-gal activity and up-regulation of the expression of p53, p21, and p16 (Figure 1E–H). One widely discussed hypothesis of cellular senescence is the telomere hypothesis. Telomerase activity declines with aging because of a decrease in telomerase catalytic component (TERT) expression, leading to telomere shortening and cellular senescence. We examined telomere length and TERT expression and found that over-expression of Notch1 did not affect either of these factors (Figure S2A, B), suggesting that Notch signaling regulates vascular aging via a telomere-independent mechanism. We also found that introduction of NICD led to premature senescence of human endothelial cells along with up-regulation of negative regulators of cell cycle (Figure S1A-C), suggesting that constitutive activation of the Notch pathway negatively regulates cell lifespan.

Over-expression of Jagged1 prolongs the lifespan of vascular endothelial cells

Because Notch signaling is induced by a receptor-ligand interaction, we speculated that Notch ligands could also be related to vascular aging. To test this concept, we infected endothelial cells with a retroviral vector encoding the Notch ligand Jagged1, which is most highly expressed by endothelial cells among the various Notch ligands (Figure 2A). Western blot analysis revealed that over-expression of Jagged1 activated Notch signaling (Figure 2B). Similar to Notch1 over-expressing cells, up-regulation of Jagged1 extended the replicative lifespan of endothelial cells along with a decrease of SA-β-gal activity, and decreased the expression of senescence-associated molecules such as p53, p21, and p16 (Figure 2C-E). Conversely, knockdown of Jagged1 by shRNA induced premature senescence with an increase of SA-β-gal activity, increased expression of p53, p21, and p16 (Figure 2F-I). These results suggest that Notch signaling induced by receptor-ligand interactions, especially that of Notch1 with Jagged1, has a crucial role in endothelial cell senescence.

Up-regulation of Id1 inhibits premature senescence induced by Notch1 disruption

To further investigate the mechanism by which disruption of Notch signaling induces premature senescence of endothelial cells, we performed DNA microarray analysis and identified inhibitor of DNA binding 1 (Id1) as a potential target of the Notch signaling (Figure 3). Consistent with the results of microarray analysis, real-time PCR and western blotting showed that Id1 expression was increased in Notch1 over-expressing endothelial cells, whereas it was decreased in Notch1 knockdown cells (Figure 4A, B). Id1 is a basic helix-loop-helix (bHLH) protein that lacks a basic DNA-binding domain but is able to form heterodimers with other bHLH proteins, thereby inhibiting DNA binding and the transcriptional activity of these proteins. Since Id1 was reported to negatively regulate the expression of p16 [18,19], we speculated that down-regulation of Id1 induced by the disruption of Notch1 led to up-regulation of p16 and premature senescence of endothelial cells. To test this hypothesis, we co-infected human endothelial cells with retroviral vectors encoding Id1 and Notch1 shRNA. Over-expression of Id1 inhibited premature senescence induced by knockdown of Notch1 and normalized p16 expression (Figure 4C, D). We also examined the effects of co-expression of Notch1 and

Id1 on cell lifespan and found no additive or synergic effects (Figure 4E), suggesting that Id1 is a crucial regulator for Notch1-induced extension of endothelial cell lifespan. When Notch signaling was activated, cleaved NICD underwent translocation to the nucleus and bound to CBF1 protein. This binding of NICD facilitated displacement of transcriptional repressors from CBF1 and recruited transcriptional co-activators, thereby leading to transcription of target genes. Our *in silico* assay identified a putative CBF1-binding site in the promoter region of *ID1*. The chromatin immunoprecipitation (ChIP) assay showed that activated Notch1 has a high affinity for the CBF1-binding element in the *ID1* promoter (Figure 4F). To investigate whether Notch1 deletion induced endothelial cell senescence via a p16-dependent pathway, we co-infected human endothelial cells with the p16 shRNA and Notch1 shRNA vectors. Notch1 deletion led to premature senescence of mock-infected cells but not p16 shRNA-infected cells (Figure 4G, H), suggesting that disruption of Notch1 promotes endothelial cell senescence via an Id1/p16-dependent pathway.

Inhibition of p38MAPK prevents induction of premature senescence by Notch1 disruption

We also found that expression of MAPK phosphatase 1 (MKP1, also known as DUSP1), which inactivates p38MAPK, was associated with the Notch1 signaling, as demonstrated by DNA microarray analysis (Figure 3). Consistent with this finding, the expression of *DUSP1* was significantly up-regulated in Notch1 over-expressing cells and was down-regulated in Notch1 knockdown cells (Figure 5A). Expression of phosphorylated p38MAPK was decreased by over-expression of Notch1 and increased by knockdown of Notch1 (Figure 5B). Since MKP-1 is also reported to inactivate c-Jun N-terminal kinase (JNK) in some settings [20,21], we examined whether MKP-1 inhibits phosphorylation of JNK and found that expression of phosphorylated JNK was unchanged by the knockdown of Notch1 or Jagged1 (Figure S3). Treatment of Notch1 knockdown cells with SB203580, an inhibitor of p38MAPK, significantly improved premature senescence induced by disruption of Notch1 along with a decrease of p16 expression (Figure 5C, D). Interestingly, although transcription of *ID1* was not altered by treatment with SB203580 (Figure 5E), expression of Id1 protein in Notch1 knockdown cells was significantly increased (Figure 5D). Expression of Id1 protein in Notch1 knockdown cells was also increased by treatment with MG132, a proteasome inhibitor (Figure 5F). Conversely, treatment with anisomycin, which activates p38MAPK, down-regulated Id1 protein expression (Figure 5G). Moreover, treatment with the proteasome inhibitor inhibited anisomycin-induced down-regulation of Id1 protein expression (Figure 5H). Activation of p38MAPK increased serine/threonine phosphorylation of Id1 protein (Figure 5I), suggesting that p38MAPK phosphorylates this protein and down-regulates Id1 expression by promoting its proteasomal degradation.

Up-regulation of Id1 improved the phenotypic changes induced by Notch1 disruption

Expression of *Cdkn2a* (the gene encoding p16 protein) in the aortas of mice was up-regulated with aging (Figure 6A). To investigate whether Notch signaling was involved in vascular aging, we performed the aortic ring assay in endothelial cell-

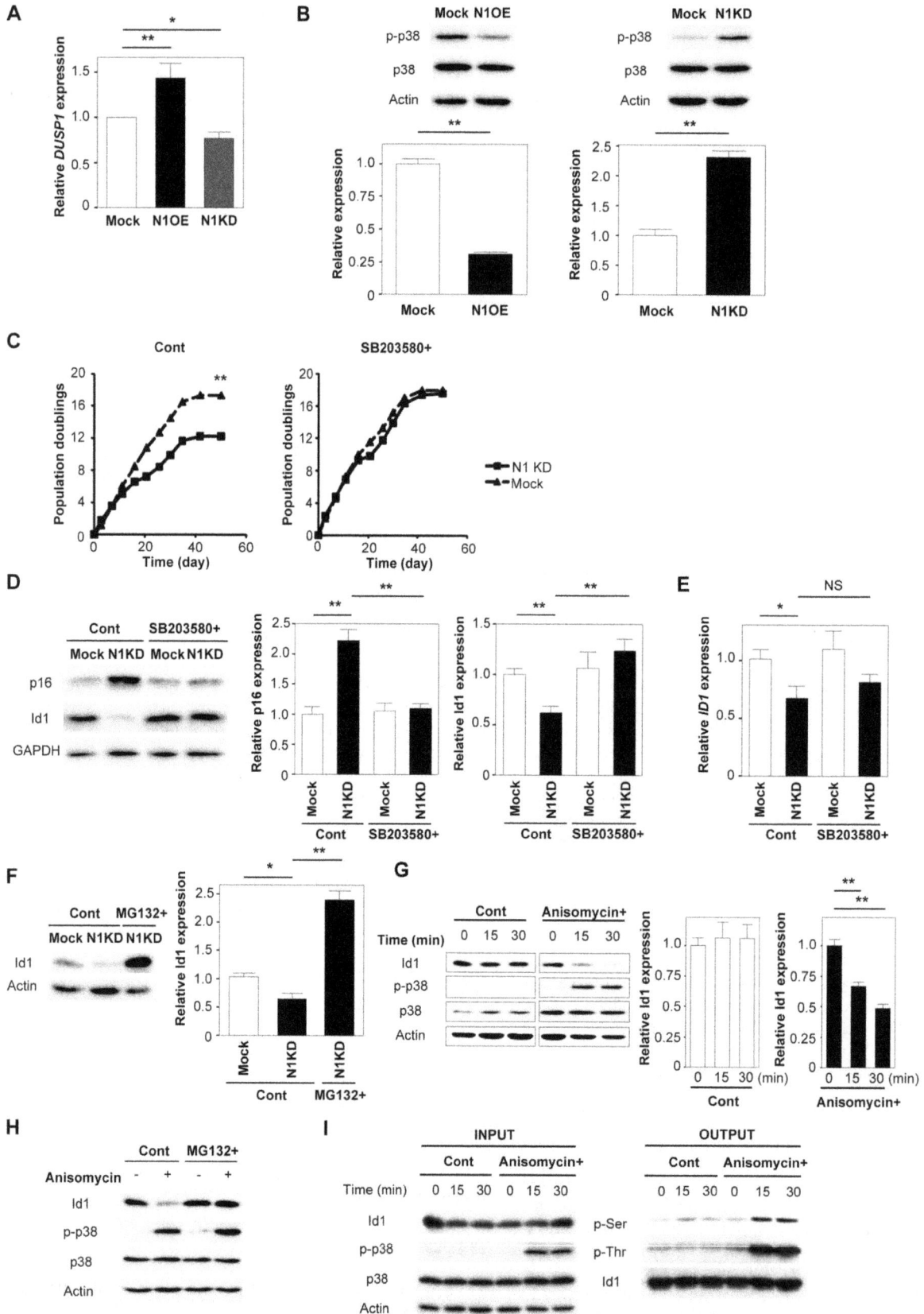

Figure 5. Inhibition of p38MAPK prevents induction of premature senescence by Notch1 disruption. (A) Real-time PCR for the expression of *DUSP1* (MKP1) in Notch1 over-expressing endothelial cells, Notch1 knockdown cells, and Mock-infected cells (n = 8). (B) Western blot analysis of phospho-p38MAPK (p-p38) and whole p38MAPK expression. The graphs show quantitative data on phospho-p38 expression (n = 3). (C)

Human endothelial cells were infected with a retroviral vector encoding Notch1 shRNA (N1KD) or an empty vector (Mock). Infected cells were then treated with vehicle (Cont) or SB203580 (SB203580+) and subjected to the proliferation assay as described in the legend for Figure 1B (n = 3). (D) Western blot analysis of p16 and Id1 expression. The right graphs show the quantitative data on p16 and Id1 expression (n = 3). (E) Real-time PCR for the expression of *ID1* (n = 6). (F) Human endothelial cells were infected with a retroviral vector encoding Notch1 shRNA (N1KD) or an empty vector (Mock) and were treated with vehicle (Cont) or proteasome inhibitor MG132 (MG132+), after which the expression of Id1 was assessed by western blot analysis. The right graph shows quantitative data on Id1 expression (n = 3). (G) Human endothelial cells were treated with vehicle (Cont) or anisomycin (Anisomycin+) for 0, 15 or 30 minutes, after which the expression of Id1, phosphorylated p38MAPK (p-p38), and whole p38MAPK was determined by western blot analysis. The right graph shows quantitative data on Id1 expression (n = 3). (H) Western blot analysis of the expression of Id1, phosphorylated p38MAPK (p-p38), and whole p38MAPK in human endothelial cells pre-incubated with vehicle (Cont) or MG132 for 1 hour followed by treatment with or without anisomycin for 15 minutes. (I) Flag-tagged Id1 over-expressing cells were pre-incubated with MG132 for 1 hour, followed by treatment with vehicle (Cont) or anisomycin (Anisomycin+) for 0, 15, or 30 minutes. Cell lysates were immunoprecipitated with FLAG M2 agarose. Then the levels of serine phosphorylated Id1 (p-Ser), threonine phosphorylated Id1 (p-Thr), and whole Id1 were assessed by western blot analysis (right; OUTPUT). Expression of Id1, phosphorylated p38MAPK (p-p38), and whole p38 MAPK was also estimated before immunoprecipitation (left; INPUT). All values represent the mean ± s.e.m. *P<0.05, **P<0.01.

specific *Notch1* heterozygous knockout (Tie2-cre⁺ *Notch1*ˡᵒˣ/⁺, (N1KO)) mice. We utilized Tie2-cre⁺ *Notch1*ˡᵒˣ/⁺ mice in our study because Tie2-cre⁺ *Notch1*ˡᵒˣ/ˡᵒˣ mice show embryonic lethality[22]. The expression of *Notch1* was significantly down-regulated in the aortas of N1KO mice (Figure 6B). Consistent with the *in vitro* data on Notch1 knockdown cells, aortic expression of *Cdkn2a* was significantly higher in N1KO mice than in littermate controls (Figure 6B). Consequently, endothelial cell proliferation was markedly impaired in *ex vivo* aortic cultures derived from N1KO mice compared with their littermate controls (Figure 6C). Introduction of Id1 with a lentiviral vector significantly increased cell proliferation in N1KO mice together with decreased expression of *Cdkn2a* (Figure 6B, C), indicating that Notch signaling positively regulates the lifespan of endothelial cells via the down-regulation of p16.

Discussion

In the present study, we demonstrated that the Notch signaling pathway is crucially involved in the process of vascular aging. Down-regulation of Notch signaling reduced Id1 and MKP1 expression and also accelerated endothelial cell senescence via a p16-dependent pathway. It has been reported that down-regulation of Notch signaling is related to various age-associated conditions. A recent study revealed that Notch signaling is down-regulated in aged skeletal muscle, and a decline of Notch activity was shown to impair the proliferation of muscle precursor cells and their production of myoblasts for muscle regeneration [9,10].

The role of Notch signaling in endothelial cell proliferation has been controversial. A study by Venkatesh et al. showed that up-regulation of Notch signaling by NICD inhibits the proliferation of endothelial cells [23]. In line with our results, Notch activation was reported to down-regulate expression of p21 [24]. It is well accepted that Notch signaling plays a crucial role in the development of various malignancies [25–27]. Activating Notch mutations have been reported in human leukemia and breast cancer. It also has been reported that oncogenic stimuli provoke premature senescence in a variety of human somatic cells [28]. For example, constitutive activation of Ras or Akt has been shown to cause premature senescence [29,30], and both of these signaling molecules are known to promote cell proliferation and contribute to tumorigenesis. In this regard, cellular senescence is thought to be a defensive mechanism against malignant transformation. We found that introduction of NICD led to premature senescence of human endothelial cells along with up-regulation of negative regulators of the cell cycle including p16, whereas introduction of Notch1 prolonged the lifespan of endothelial cells. Thus, constitutive activation of the Notch signaling pathway with NICD could act as an oncogenic stimulus that leads to premature senescence, whereas activation of this pathway at a physiological

level by full length Notch1 may result in extension of the cellular lifespan. Although activation of Notch signaling was reported to reduce telomerase activity [31], we did not find any differences of telomere length or telomerase expression between Notch1-infected and mock-infected cells. Because it is well-known that mice have high telomerase activity and long telomeres [32,33], it is unlikely that Notch signaling regulates endothelial cell proliferation by modulating telomerase activity in mice.

Tip cells are non-proliferative highly motile cells that are restricted to the tips of sprouts [34]. In contrast, stalk cells are highly proliferative and form the trunks of new blood vessels [34]. In vascular sprouts, the tip cells express a high level of delta-like (Dll) 4 and a low level of Notch1, while the stalk cells show high expression of both Notch1 and Jagged1 [35]. There have been previous reports demonstrating that inhibition of Dll4-mediated Notch signaling leads to an increase in the number of filopodia and sprouting tips, and that Jagged1 antagonizes the effects of Dll4 on sprouting angiogenesis [36–38]. The genetic models used in these studies included endothelial-specific Notch1 homozygous knockout mice (an inducible model) and Dll4 heterozygous knockout mice. We utilized endothelial cell-specific Notch1 heterozygous knockout (Tie2-cre⁺ *Notch1*ˡᵒˣ/⁺) mice and obtained the opposite results. Consistent with our findings, however, it has been reported that endothelial cell-specific or systemic Notch1 heterozygous knockout results in impairment of postnatal angiogenesis [39,40]. Our *in vitro* experiments clearly demonstrated that activation of the Jagged1/Notch1 pathway promotes endothelial cell proliferation. Collectively, these results suggest that strong inhibition of the Notch1 signaling promotes vascular sprouting by attenuating Dll4-dependent signaling in the tip cells, while moderate inhibition of this pathway leads to significant reduction of Jagged1-dependent signaling in the stalk cells that results in impaired angiogenesis, but does not affect Dll4-dependent signaling in the tip cells.

We also found that the Notch pathway positively regulates Id1 and MKP1 expression. Some evidence has been published suggesting a potential association between Notch and Id1 [41,42], and our results indicate that *ID1* is a target gene of Notch1. In agreement with the results of our microarray analysis, Kondoh et al. showed that Notch signaling suppresses p38MAPK activity via induction of MKP1 during myogenesis [43]. We further demonstrated that Notch1-induced up-regulation of MKP1 stabilized Id1 protein by inhibiting p38MAPK-induced degradation, leading to prolongation of the endothelial cell lifespan. Taken together, our results suggest that activation of Notch1 could be a new therapeutic target for treating age-associated vascular diseases.

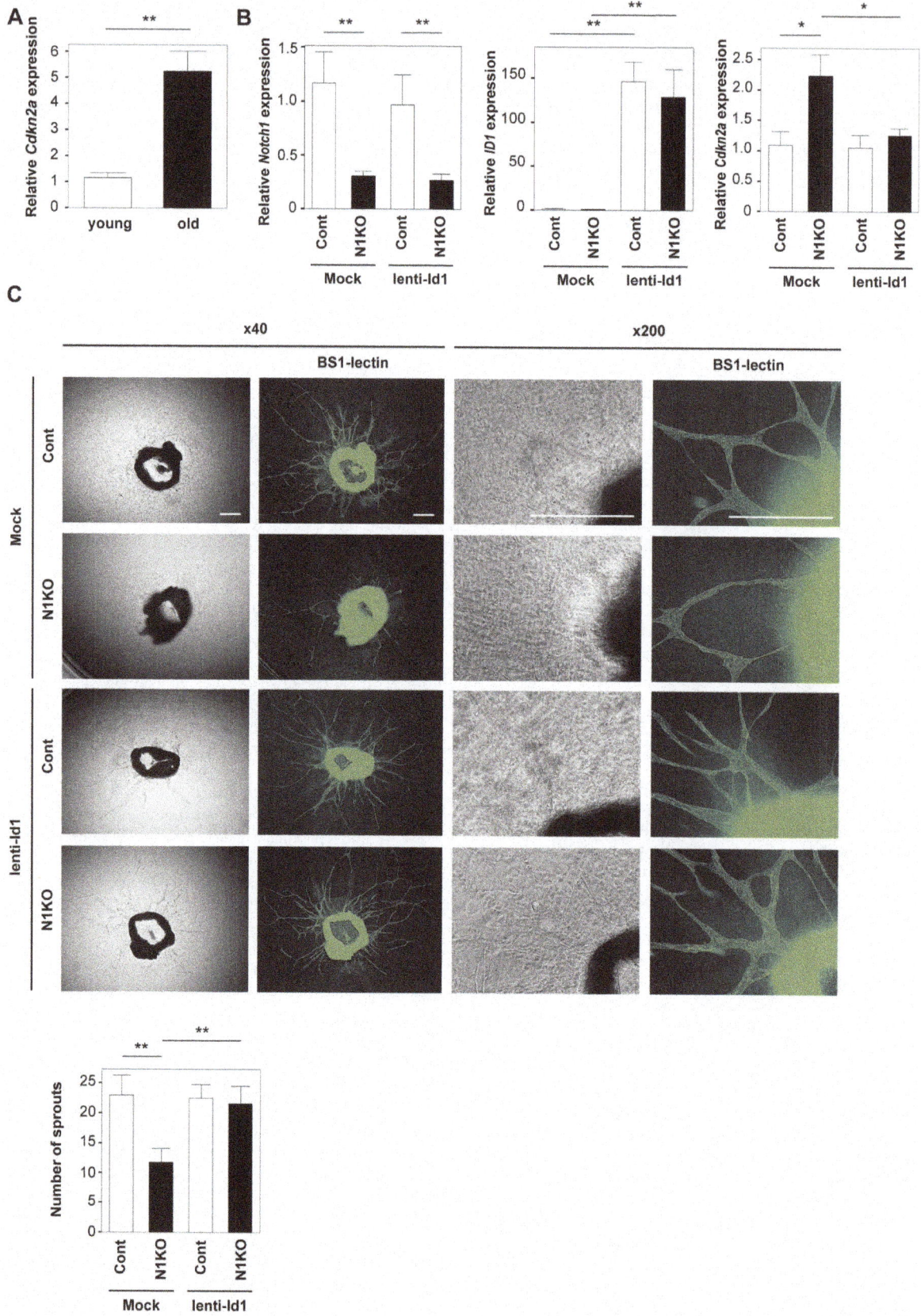

Figure 6. Up-regulation of Id1 improved the phenotypic changes induced by Notch1 disruption. (A) Real-time PCR analysis showing the expression of *Cdkn2a* (p16) in the aortas of young mice (12–15 weeks) or old mice (50–55 weeks) (n = 6). (B) Real-time PCR analysis showing the expression of *Notch1*, *ID1*, and *Cdkn2a* (p16) in aortas prepared as in Figure 6C (n = 6). (C) Aortic ring assay performed in endothelial cell-specific

Notch1 heterozygous knockout mice (N1KO) and their littermate controls (Cont) infected with lentivirus expressing human Id1 (lenti-Id1) or an empty vector (Mock). Cultured aortic rings were immunostained with BS1 lectin-FITC (Green). Scale bar = 100 µm. The graph displays the quantitative data for the number of sprouting cells (n = 14). All values represent the mean ± s.e.m. *P<0.05, **P<0.01.

Supporting Information

Figure S1 The effects of NICD overexpression. (A) Western blot analysis for the expression of Notch intracellular domain (NICD) and p16 in endothelial cells infected with Notch1 (N1OE), NICD, or an empty vector (Mock). (B) Population doublings of endothelial cells infected with Notch1 (N1OE), NICD, or an empty vector (Mock) (n = 3). **P<0.01 vs. Mock. (C) Real-time PCR analysis showing the expression of p53 (*TP53*), p21 (*CDKN1A*), and p16 (*CDKN2A*) in cells as prepared in Figure S1B (n = 5–9). The results of N1OE and Mock are also shown in Figure 1A. Data are shown as the mean ± s.e.m. *P<0.05, **P<0.01.

Figure S2 The effect of Notch1 overexpression on endothelial cell senescence is independent of telomere shortening. (A) Real-time PCR for the relative expression of telomerase reverse transcriptase (TERT) in endothelial cells infected with Notch1 (N1OE) or an empty vector (Mock) (n = 6).

PC3 (PC3) is a human prostate cancer cell line that was used for a positive control. (B) Relative telomere length in endothelial cells infected with Notch1 (N1OE) or an empty vector (Mock) (n = 4). All data are shown as the mean ± s.e.m. *P<0.05, **P<0.01.

Figure S3 The expression of phosphorylated JNK of Notch1 or Jagged1 knock-down cells. Western blot analysis of phospho-JNK (p-JNK) and whole JNK expression in Notch1 (N1KD) or Jagged1 (J1KD) knock-down cells. The graphs indicate the quantification relative to whole JNK (n = 7). Values are the mean ± s.e.m.

Author Contributions

Conceived and designed the experiments: YY YH TM. Performed the experiments: YY YH MS M. Yamashita. Analyzed the data: YY YH KT SO JM M. Yokoyama AN YK IS. Wrote the paper: YY TM.

References

1. Kopan R, Ilagan MX (2009) The canonical Notch signaling pathway: unfolding the activation mechanism. Cell 137: 216–233.
2. Andersson ER, Sandberg R, Lendahl U (2011) Notch signaling: simplicity in design, versatility in function. Development 138: 3593–3612.
3. High FA, Epstein JA (2008) The multifaceted role of Notch in cardiac development and disease. Nat Rev Genet 9: 49–61.
4. Gridley T (2007) Notch signaling in vascular development and physiology. Development 134: 2709–2718.
5. Niessen K, Karsan A (2007) Notch signaling in the developing cardiovascular system. Am J Physiol Cell Physiol 293: C1–11.
6. Lobry C, Oh P, Aifantis I (2011) Oncogenic and tumor suppressor functions of Notch in cancer: it's NOTCH what you think. J Exp Med 208: 1931–1935.
7. Ables JL, Breunig JJ, Eisch AJ, Rakic P (2011) Not(ch) just development: Notch signalling in the adult brain. Nat Rev Neurosci 12: 269–283.
8. Ethell DW (2010) An amyloid-notch hypothesis for Alzheimer's disease. Neuroscientist 16: 614–617.
9. Conboy IM, Conboy MJ, Smythe GM, Rando TA (2003) Notch-mediated restoration of regenerative potential to aged muscle. Science 302: 1575–1577.
10. Carey KA, Farnfield MM, Tarquinio SD, Cameron-Smith D (2007) Impaired expression of Notch signaling genes in aged human skeletal muscle. J Gerontol A Biol Sci Med Sci 62: 9–17.
11. Faragher RG, Kipling D (1998) How might replicative senescence contribute to human ageing? Bioessays 20: 985–991.
12. Campisi J (2005) Senescent cells, tumor suppression, and organismal aging: good citizens, bad neighbors. Cell 120: 513–522.
13. Minamino T, Komuro I (2007) Vascular cell senescence: contribution to atherosclerosis. Circ Res 100: 15–26.
14. Minamino T, Miyauchi H, Yoshida T, Ishida Y, Yoshida H, et al. (2002) Endothelial cell senescence in human atherosclerosis: role of telomere in endothelial dysfunction. Circulation 105: 1541–1544.
15. Mancini SJ, Mantei N, Dumortier A, Suter U, MacDonald HR, et al. (2005) Jagged1-dependent Notch signaling is dispensable for hematopoietic stem cell self-renewal and differentiation. Blood 105: 2340–2342.
16. Baker M, Robinson SD, Lechertier T, Barber PR, Tavora B, et al. (2012) Use of the mouse aortic ring assay to study angiogenesis. Nat Protoc 7: 89–104.
17. Gil ME, Coetzer TL (2004) Real-time quantitative PCR of telomere length. Mol Biotechnol 27: 169–172.
18. Ohtani N, Zebedee Z, Huot TJ, Stinson JA, Sugimoto M, et al. (2001) Opposing effects of Ets and Id proteins on p16INK4a expression during cellular senescence. Nature 409: 1067–1070.
19. Alani RM, Young AZ, Shifflett CB (2001) Id1 regulation of cellular senescence through transcriptional repression of p16/Ink4a. Proc Natl Acad Sci U S A 98: 7812–7816.
20. Vandevyver S, Dejager L, Van Bogaert T, Kleyman A, Liu Y, et al. (2012) Glucocorticoid receptor dimerization induces MKP1 to protect against TNF-induced inflammation. J Clin Invest 122: 2130–2140.
21. Hirsch DD, Stork PJ (1997) Mitogen-activated protein kinase phosphatases inactivate stress-activated protein kinase pathways in vivo. J Biol Chem 272: 4568–4575.
22. Limbourg FP, Takeshita K, Radtke F, Bronson RT, Chin MT, et al. (2005) Essential role of endothelial Notch1 in angiogenesis. Circulation 111: 1826–1832.
23. Venkatesh D, Fredette N, Rostama B, Tang Y, Vary CP, et al. (2011) RhoA-mediated signaling in Notch-induced senescence-like growth arrest and endothelial barrier dysfunction. Arterioscler Thromb Vasc Biol 31: 876–882.
24. Noseda M, Chang L, McLean G, Grim JE, Clurman BE, et al. (2004) Notch activation induces endothelial cell cycle arrest and participates in contact inhibition: role of p21Cip1 repression. Mol Cell Biol 24: 8813–8822.
25. Ranganathan P, Weaver KL, Capobianco AJ (2011) Notch signalling in solid tumours: a little bit of everything but not all the time. Nat Rev Cancer 11: 338–351.
26. South AP, Cho RJ, Aster JC (2012) The double-edged sword of Notch signaling in cancer. Semin Cell Dev Biol 23: 458–464.
27. Guo S, Liu M, Gonzalez-Perez RR (2011) Role of Notch and its oncogenic signaling crosstalk in breast cancer. Biochim Biophys Acta 1815: 197–213.
28. Serrano M, Blasco MA (2001) Putting the stress on senescence. Curr Opin Cell Biol 13: 748–753.
29. Serrano M, Lin AW, McCurrach ME, Beach D, Lowe SW (1997) Oncogenic ras provokes premature cell senescence associated with accumulation of p53 and p16INK4a. Cell 88: 593–602.
30. Miyauchi H, Minamino T, Tateno K, Kunieda T, Toko H, et al. (2004) Akt negatively regulates the in vitro lifespan of human endothelial cells via a p53/p21-dependent pathway. EMBO J 23: 212–220.
31. Liu ZJ, Tan Y, Beecham GW, Seo DM, Tian R, et al. (2012) Notch activation induces endothelial cell senescence and pro-inflammatory response: implication of Notch signaling in atherosclerosis. Atherosclerosis 225: 296–303.
32. Blasco MA, Lee HW, Hande MP, Samper E, Lansdorp PM, et al. (1997) Telomere shortening and tumor formation by mouse cells lacking telomerase RNA. Cell 91: 25–34.
33. Lee HW, Blasco MA, Gottlieb GJ, Horner JW, 2nd, Greider CW, et al. (1998) Essential role of mouse telomerase in highly proliferative organs. Nature 392: 569–574.
34. Garcia A, Kandel JJ (2012) Notch: a key regulator of tumor angiogenesis and metastasis. Histol Histopathol 27: 151–156.
35. Thomas JL, Baker K, Han J, Calvo C, Nurmi H, et al. (2013) Interactions between VEGFR and Notch signaling pathways in endothelial and neural cells. Cell Mol Life Sci 70: 1779–1792.
36. Hellstrom M, Phng LK, Hofmann JJ, Wallgard E, Coultas L, et al. (2007) Dll4 signalling through Notch1 regulates formation of tip cells during angiogenesis. Nature 445: 776–780.
37. Benedito R, Roca C, Sorensen I, Adams S, Gossler A, et al. (2009) The notch ligands Dll4 and Jagged1 have opposing effects on angiogenesis. Cell 137: 1124–1135.
38. Eilken HM, Adams RH (2010) Turning on the angiogenic microswitch. Nat Med 16: 853–854.
39. Takeshita K, Satoh M, Ii M, Silver M, Limbourg FP, et al. (2007) Critical role of endothelial Notch1 signaling in postnatal angiogenesis. Circ Res 100: 70–78.

40. Kikuchi R, Takeshita K, Uchida Y, Kondo M, Cheng XW, et al. (2011) Pitavastatin-induced angiogenesis and arteriogenesis is mediated by Notch1 in a murine hindlimb ischemia model without induction of VEGF. Lab Invest 91: 691–703.

41. Nobta M, Tsukazaki T, Shibata Y, Xin C, Moriishi T, et al. (2005) Critical regulation of bone morphogenetic protein-induced osteoblastic differentiation by Delta1/Jagged1-activated Notch1 signaling. J Biol Chem 280: 15842–15848.

42. Chadwick N, Zeef L, Portillo V, Fennessy C, Warrander F, et al. (2009) Identification of novel Notch target genes in T cell leukaemia. Mol Cancer 8: 35.

43. Kondoh K, Sunadome K, Nishida E (2007) Notch signaling suppresses p38 MAPK activity via induction of MKP-1 in myogenesis. J Biol Chem 282: 3058–3065.

4

Adipose Tissue-Derived Mesenchymal Stem Cells in Long-Term Dialysis Patients Display Downregulation of PCAF Expression and Poor Angiogenesis Activation

Shuichiro Yamanaka[1,2], Shinya Yokote[2], Akifumi Yamada[3], Yuichi Katsuoka[1], Luna Izuhara[1], Yohta Shimada[4], Nobuo Omura[5], Hirotaka James Okano[1], Takao Ohki[5], Takashi Yokoo[2]*

1 Division of Regenerative Medicine, Department of Internal Medicine, The Jikei University School of Medicine, Tokyo, Japan, 2 Division of Nephrology and Hypertension, Department of Internal Medicine, The Jikei University School of Medicine, Tokyo, Japan, 3 Department of Pediatrics, The Jikei University School of Medicine, Tokyo, Japan, 4 Department of Gene Therapy, Institute of DNA Medicine, The Jikei University School of Medicine, Tokyo, Japan, 5 Department of Surgery, The Jikei University School of Medicine, Tokyo, Japan

Abstract

We previously demonstrated that mesenchymal stem cells (MSCs) differentiate into functional kidney cells capable of urine and erythropoietin production, indicating that they may be used for kidney regeneration. However, the viability of MSCs from dialysis patients may be affected under uremic conditions. In this study, we isolated MSCs from the adipose tissues of end-stage kidney disease (ESKD) patients undergoing long-term dialysis (KD-MSCs; mean: 72.3 months) and from healthy controls (HC-MSCs) to compare their viability. KD-MSCs and HC-MSCs were assessed for their proliferation potential, senescence, and differentiation capacities into adipocytes, osteoblasts, and chondrocytes. Gene expression of stem cell-specific transcription factors was analyzed by PCR array and confirmed by western blot analysis at the protein level. No significant differences of proliferation potential, senescence, or differentiation capacity were observed between KD-MSCs and HC-MSCs. However, gene and protein expression of p300/CBP-associated factor (PCAF) was significantly suppressed in KD-MSCs. Because PCAF is a histone acetyltransferase that mediates regulation of hypoxia-inducible factor-1α (HIF-1α), we examined the hypoxic response in MSCs. HC-MSCs but not KD-MSCs showed upregulation of PCAF protein expression under hypoxia. Similarly, HIF-1α and vascular endothelial growth factor (VEGF) expression did not increase under hypoxia in KD-MSCs but did so in HC-MSCs. Additionally, a directed *in vivo* angiogenesis assay revealed a decrease in angiogenesis activation of KD-MSCs. In conclusion, long-term uremia leads to persistent and systematic downregulation of PCAF gene and protein expression and poor angiogenesis activation of MSCs from patients with ESKD. Furthermore, PCAF, HIF-1α, and VEGF expression were not upregulated by hypoxic stimulation of KD-MSCs. These results suggest that the hypoxic response may be blunted in MSCs from ESKD patients.

Editor: Ariela Benigni, IRCSS - Istituto di Ricerche Farmacologiche Mario Negri, Italy

Funding: This work was supported by grants from the Ministry of Education, Culture, Sports, Science and Technology and Ministry of Health, Labour and Welfare of Japan. The funders had no role in study design, data collection and analysis, decision to publish, or preparation of the manuscript.

Competing Interests: The authors have declared that no competing interests exist.

* Email: tyokoo@jikei.ac.jp

Introduction

The number of end-stage kidney disease (ESKD) patients is increasing worldwide [1]. Dialysis therapy for ESKD results in heavy physical and mental burdens, and associated annual medical expenses are very high [2]. Development of a treatment method that does not involve dialysis is therefore desirable to reduce expenses and increase the quality of life of patients. Kidney transplantation significantly prolongs the life expectancy of chronic kidney disease (CKD) patients [3], [4] and is less expensive than dialysis, but there is a shortage of organs available for transplantation, and lifetime immunosuppressant therapy is required for patients [5].

This critical shortage of organs has driven new technologies such as tissue engineering and regenerative medicine to achieve functional kidney replacement [5], [6]. Our previous studies showed that a xenobiotic developmental process for growing xenoembryos allows exogenous human mesenchymal stem cells (MSCs) to undergo epithelial conversion and form a nephron that produces urine and erythropoietin [7]–[9]. These findings suggested that MSCs might be a cell source for future renal regeneration. Furthermore, MSCs are easy to obtain in large numbers and are not costly to establish [10], [11].

Previously, we used bone marrow-derived MSCs from healthy volunteers, although it is unclear whether these differ from MSCs from dialysis patients. This is because patients with terminal renal failure have been exposed to uremic toxins over long periods, which may affect the viability and regenerative capacity of MSCs, suggesting that they may be unsuitable for kidney regeneration. Similarly, some reports have suggested that the regenerative capacity of adult stem cells in patients with chronic renal failure is inferior to those in patients with normal renal function [12], [13]. However, a recent report found that adipose tissue-derived MSCs (ASCs) of patients with renal disease have similar characteristics and functionality to those from healthy individuals in terms of their

Table 1. Characteristics of patients at time of adipose tissue sampling.

	Healthy controls (n = 6)	End-stage kidney disease patients (n = 9)
Sex (F/M)	2/4	2/7
Age, years (mean, range)	56.2 (50–63)	52.6 (37–64)
BMI (mean, range)	23.5 (18.4–27.3)	22.6 (17.0–30.1)
Creatinine, mg/dl (mean, range)	0.79 (0.53–1.01)	11.9 (6.8–16.5)
eGFR, ml/min per 1.73m2 (mean, range)	73.5 (62–89)	4.0 (3–6)
Duration of RRT (months, range)		72.3(±26.3)
Diabetes mellitus	1/6	4/9
Hypertension	5/6	7/9
Medication		
Anti-hypertensive drugs	5/6	7/9
Erythropoiesis-stimulating agents	NA	7/9
Anti-platelet drugs	0/6	2/9
Cholesterol-lowering drugs	1/6	2/9
Prednisone	0/6	0/9
Insulin	0/6	3/9
KTx indication		
RPGN		1
IgA nephropathy		1
Adult-onset polycystic kidney disease		1
Diabetic nephropathy		4
von Gierke's disease		1
unknown		1

immunosuppressive capacities, and expression of pro-inflammatory and anti-inflammatory factors [14]. Despite these findings, the previous report did not analyze the expression of stemness genes in ASCs.

Previously, we evaluated the differentiation capabilities and gene expression profiles of bone marrow-derived MSCs and ASCs from normal rats and those with adenine-induced renal failure [15]. Although the uremic toxin has only a small effect on the gene expression and differentiation of MSCs, we used a rat model of CKD and the exposure time to the toxin was shorter than in human ESKD because of the short lifespan of the rat. Actual ESKD patients have a much longer duration of renal insufficiency.

In this study, to clarify the effect of long-term CKD on ASCs, we explored differences in the expression profiles of stemness and other important genes in ESKD patients (KD-MSCs) and healthy controls (HC-MSCs) using RT-PCR array analysis. We hypothesized that downregulation of p300/CBP-associated factor (PCAF) in the long-term uremic state might render KD-MSCs as an inappropriate cell source for kidney regenerative therapy.

Materials and Methods

Ethics Statement

This study was conducted according to the principles of the Declaration of Helsinki and approved by the Ethics Committee of The Jikei University School of Medicine. All donors provided written informed consent for collection of samples and subsequent analyses.

Isolation and Culture of Human MSCs

Patient characteristics are shown in Table 1 (glomerular filtration rate was calculated using the modification of diet in the renal disease study equation). Subcutaneous or mesenteric adipose tissue was surgically removed from ESKD patients ($n = 9$, mean age: 52.6 years; mean glomerular filtration rate: 4 ml/min/ 1.73 m^2) and healthy controls ($n = 6$, mean age: 56.2 years; mean glomerular filtration rate: 73.5 ml/min/1.73 m^2). All ESKD patients were undergoing dialysis (CKD stage 5D). Experiments were independently performed for each donor.

Tissues were placed in Hanks' balanced salt solution (Gibco Life Technologies, Grand Island, NY) with 100 IU/ml penicillin and 100 mg/ml streptomycin (Gibco Life Technologies). MSCs were isolated from the adipose tissues of all 15 participants by a previously described culture method [16], [17] and used for KD-MSCs (ESKD patients; $n = 9$) and HC-MSCs (healthy controls; $n = 6$). After mincing and washing with phosphate-buffered saline (PBS) (Gibco Life Technologies), the adipose tissues were enzymatically dissociated with 1 ml of 0.1% collagenase (type I) (Wako, Osaka, Japan) in PBS for 1 h at 37°C. The dissociated tissue was combined with 8 ml α-minimum essential medium (Gibco Life Technologies) supplemented with 20% fetal bovine serum (FBS) (Invitrogen, Carlsbad, CA) and then centrifuged at 300 g for 5 min at room temperature. After washing with PBS, the isolated adipose cells including MSCs were cultured in α-minimum essential medium supplemented with 20% FBS to prevent the inclusion of serum from renal disease patients. MSCs of passage numbers 3–5 were analyzed after 14–28 days following isolation from adipose tissue.

Flow Cytometric Analysis of MSCs

The International Society for Cell Therapy previously suggested the following minimal criteria to define human MSCs [18]:

Table 2. Differences in mRNA expression between KD-MSCs and HC-MSCs by RT-PCR analysis.

GeneBank No.	Gene Name	Gene Symbol	Fold Change	T-Test	
			KDMSC/HCMSC	p Value	* p<0.05
Stemness Markers					
NM_002006	Fibroblast growth factor 2 (basic)	FGF2 (bFGF)	0.7953	0.6199	
NM_000207	Insulin	INS	1.5621	0.1746	
NM_002309	Leukemia inhibitory factor	LIF	0.8646	0.8617	
NM_002701	Octamer-binding transcription factor 4	OCT4	1.4192	0.4964	
NM_003106	SRY (sex determining region Y)-box 2	SOX2	0.8048	0.6364	
NM_198253	Telomerase reverse transcriptase	TERT	0.8910	0.7668	
NM_033131	Wingless-type MMTV integration site family, member 3A	WNT3A	0.6201	0.1349	
NM_174900	Zinc finger protein 42 homolog (mouse)	ZFP42	0.8237	0.4309	
MSC-Specific Markers					
NM_001627	Activated leukocyte cell adhesion molecule	ALCAM	1.3080	0.8221	
NM_001150	Alanyl (membrane) aminopeptidase	ANPEP	0.7301	0.0570	
NM_004346	Caspase 3	CASP3	0.9429	0.6789	
NM_000610	CD44 molecule (Indian blood group)	CD44	0.7366	0.1873	
NM_000118	Endoglin	ENG	0.8326	0.1912	
NM_004448	V-erb-b2 erythroblastic leukemia viral oncogene homolog 2, neuro/glioblastoma derived oncogene homolog (avian)	ERBB2 (HER2)	1.4973	0.2182	
NM_002033	Fucosyltransferase 4	FUT4	2.7344	0.1352	
NM_003508	Frizzled family receptor 9	FZD9	1.0164	0.9788	
NM_000210	Integrin, alpha 6	ITGA6	0.7706	0.0587	
NM_002210	Integrin, alpha V	ITGAV	0.6457	0.1285	
NM_006500	Melanoma cell adhesion molecule	MCAM	2.3341	0.2525	
NM_002507	Nerve growth factor receptor	NGFR	2.1012	0.6663	
NM_002526	5'-nucleotidase, ecto (CD73)	NT5E	0.7620	0.4739	
NM_002609	Platelet-derived growth factor receptor, beta polypeptide	PDGFRB	2.1955	0.1926	
NM_006017	Prominin 1	PROM1	0.8566	0.9428	
NM_006288	Thy-1 cell surface antigen	THY1	1.4852	0.8937	
NM_001078	Vascular cell adhesion molecule 1	VCAM1	1.4291	0.3592	
Other Genes Associated with MSC					
NM_001154	Annexin A5	ANXA5	0.7301	0.0570	
NM_001709	Brain-derived neurotrophic factor	BDNF	0.6672	0.1248	
NM_199173	Bone gamma-carboxyglutamate (gla) protein	BGLAP (Osteocalcin)	0.8570	0.3911	
NM_001719	Bone morphogenetic protein 7	BMP7	1.0223	0.8279	
NM_000088	Collagen, type I, alpha 1	COLA1	0.9038	0.6852	
NM_000758	Colony stimulating factor 2 (granulocyte-macrophage)	CSF2	0.8835	0.7697	
NM_000759	Colony stimulating factor 3 (granulocyte)	CSF3	0.5650	0.4167	
NM_001904	Catenin (cadherin-associated protein), beta 1, 88kDa	CTNNB1	0.8108	0.1780	
NM_001963	Epidermal growth factor	EGF	1.1041	0.3717	
NM_000148	Fucosyltransferase 1 (galactoside 2-alpha-L-fucosyltransferase, H blood group)	FUT1	1.0851	0.9881	
NM_002097	General transcription factor IIIA	GTF3A	0.7706	0.0587	
NM_000601	Hepatocyte growth factor (hepapoietin A; scatter factor)	HGF	1.0719	0.7792	
NM_000201	Intercellular adhesion molecule 1	ICAM1	0.9367	0.2667	
NM_000619	Interferon, gamma	IFNG	0.8852	0.6453	

Table 2. Cont.

GeneBank No.	Gene Name	Gene Symbol	Fold Change	T-Test	
			KDMSC/HCMSC	p Value	* p<0.05
NM_000618	Insulin-like growth factor 1 (somatomedin C)	IGF1	0.6575	0.4696	
NM_000572	Interleukin 10	IL10	0.8646	0.7706	
NM_000576	Interleukin 1, beta	IL1B	1.1277	0.6064	
NM_000600	Interleukin 6 (interferon, beta 2)	IL6	0.5735	0.3332	
NM_002211	Integrin, beta 1	ITGB1	0.8252	0.1995	
NM_003994	KIT ligand	KITLG	1.3767	0.4027	
NM_004530	Matrix metallopeptidase 2	MMP2	0.8092	0.9990	
NM_006617	Nestin	NES	2.8428	0.1399	
NM_007083	Nudix (nucleoside diphosphate linked moiety X)-type motif 6	NUDT6	0.6588	0.0966	
NM_033198	Phosphatidylinositol glycan anchor biosynthesis, class S	PIGS	0.7380	0.0112	*
NM_002838	Protein tyrosine phosphatase, receptor type, C	PTPRC	0.9385	0.4442	
NM_012434	Solute carrier family 17 (anion/sugar transporter), member 5	SLC17A5	0.7650	0.2122	
NM_003239	Transforming growth factor, beta 3	TGFB3	2.8015	0.0747	
NM_000594	Tumor necrosis factor alpha	TNFA	1.3130	0.9124	
NM_003380	Vimentin	VIM	1.0246	0.6979	
NM_000552	Von Willebrand factor	VWF	0.7469	0.9309	
MSC Differentiation Markers					
NM_000927	ATP-binding cassette, sub-family B, member 1	ABCB1	0.6870	0.2662	
NM_001613	Actin, alpha 2, smooth muscle, aorta	ACTA2	1.1200	0.3465	
NM_001200	Bone morphogenetic protein 2	BMP2	0.7372	0.3316	
NM_130851	Bone morphogenetic protein 4	BMP4	0.4244	0.0318	*
NM_001718	Bone morphogenetic protein 6	BMP6	0.5956	0.2765	
NM_004465	Fibroblast growth factor 10	FGF10	0.8527	0.8111	
NM_000557	Growth differentiation factor 5	GDF5	1.1011	0.7284	
NM_001001557	Growth differentiation factor 6	GDF6	0.8882	0.3208	
NM_182828	Growth differentiation factor 7	GDF7	1.5621	0.1746	
NM_004864	Growth differentiation factor 15	GDF15	1.5164	0.4034	
NM_003642	Histone acetyltransferase 1	HAT1	0.6457	0.1285	
NM_004964	Histone deacetylase 1	HDAC1	1.0645	0.6023	
NM_000545	HNF1 homeobox A	HNF1A	1.3150	0.2274	
NM_000887	Integrin, alpha X (complement component 3 receptor 4 subunit)	ITGAX	1.3150	0.2274	
NM_000214	Jagged 1	JAG1	0.9097	0.9708	
NM_002253	Kinase insert domain receptor (a type III receptor tyrosine kinase)	KDR	0.7721	0.4877	
NM_017617	Notch 1	NOTCH1	1.2610	0.6630	
NM_003884	KAT2B K acetyltransferase 2B (p300/CBP-associated factor)	KAT2B (PCAF)	0.7324	0.0187	*
NM_015869	Peroxisome proliferator-activated receptor gamma	PPARG	2.8549	0.2081	
NM_005607	PTK2 protein tyrosine kinase 2	PTK2	0.9267	0.9863	
NM_001664	Ras homolog gene family, member A	RHOA	0.7527	0.0553	
NM_004348	Runt-related transcription factor 2	RUNX2	0.8218	0.8104	
NM_005359	SMAD family member 4	SMAD4	0.9616	0.8781	
NM_020429	SMAD specific E3 ubiquitin protein ligase 1	SMURF1	1.2223	0.2759	
NM_022739	SMAD specific E3 ubiquitin protein ligase 2	SMURF2	0.6907	0.0917	

Table 2. Cont.

GeneBank No.	Gene Name	Gene Symbol	Fold Change	T-Test	
			KDMSC/HCMSC	p Value	* p<0.05
NM_000346	SRY (sex determining region Y)-box 9	SOX9	0.6700	0.8982	
NM_181486	T-box 5	TBX5	2.3522	0.4270	
NM_000660	Transforming growth factor, beta 1	TGFB1	1.1680	0.4280	
House Keeping Gene					
NM_001101	Actin, beta	ACTB	1.0199	0.7951	
NM_004048	Beta-2-microglobulin	B2M	1.0868	0.5985	
NM_002046	Glyceraldehyde-3-phosphate dehydrogenase	GAPDH	1.2408	0.1401	
NM_000194	Hypoxanthine phosphoribosyltransferase 1	HPRT1	0.7455	0.0567	
NM_001002	Ribosomal protein, large, P0	RPLP0	0.9754	0.7501	

*p<0.05 between HC-MSCs (n = 6) and KD-MSCs (n = 9).

expression of CD105, CD73, and CD90, and no expression of CD45, CD34, CD14, CD11b, CD79α, CD19, or HLA-DR surface molecules. Cells were harvested by treatment with 0.05% trypsin-EDTA (Sigma-Aldrich, St Louis, MO) for 3 min at 37°C, recovered by centrifugation at $400\times g$ for 5 min, washed twice in ice-cold PBS containing 2% FBS, and re-suspended at 1×10^5 cells/antibody test. The expression of specific MSC markers was assessed using the following antibodies: CD14-FITC, CD31-PE, CD105-FITC, CD34-PE, CD45-PE, CD73-PE, and CD90-APC (all purchased from Abcam, Cambridge, UK). Negative control staining was performed using FITC/PE/APC-conjugated mouse IgG_1 isotype antibodies (Abcam). After incubation for 30 min at room temperature in the dark, the cells were washed with PBS, resuspended in 100 μL PBS, and analyzed by a MACSQuant flow cytometer (Miltenyi Biotec, Gladbach, Germany).

Senescence-associated β-galactosidase (SA-β-gal) Staining and Cell Proliferation Assay

The senescence assay was performed using a senescence β-galactosidase staining kit (Cell Signaling Technologies, Danvers, MA) according to the manufacturer's instructions. Cells from passages 5, 8, and 10 were observed under a light microscope (Nikon, Tokyo, Japan) for blue coloration, and a minimum of 100 cells were counted in 10 random fields to determine the percentage of β-galactosidase-positive cells [19], [20].

Senescence-associated beta-heterochromatic foci (SAHF) analysis was performed by culturing cells and fixing them with 4% paraformaldehyde (Wako). After washing with PBS, cells were permeabilized with 0.2% Triton X-100 (Nacalai Tesque, Kyoto, Japan)/PBS for 10 min. DNA was visualized after DAPI (1 μg/ml) staining (Life Technologies) for 1 min, and washing twice with PBS as previously described [20]. DAPI-stained MSCs were observed under a light microscope (Nikon).

Proliferation rates of MSCs were determined by counting cell numbers and calculating population doubling (PD). Cells were cultured in 60-mm tissue culture dishes at 2×10^4 cells/dish. At confluency, they were trypsinized and counted by a cell counter (Luna automated cell counter; Logos Biosystems, Gyunggi, Korea). At passages 5–10, PD was determined by the formula: $PD = [\log10(NH)-\log10(NI)]/\log10(2)$ where NI is the initial cell number and NH is the cell number at harvest [21]. The cumulative PD level was the sum of PDs in culture. The mean and SD were calculated from three independent experiments.

Statistical analysis was carried out using a t-test. P-values of less than 0.05 were considered significant. All senescence assay measurements were performed in duplicate.

Induction of Adipogenesis, Osteogenesis, and Chondrogenesis

Passage 3–5 MSCs were trypsinized and re-seeded in induction medium with various hMSC differentiation Kits (Poietics human mesenchymal stem cells; Lonza, Walkersville, MD) for adipogenic, osteogenic, or chondrogenic induction. MSCs were maintained in culture according to the manufacturer's protocols.

Detection of Adipogenesis and Osteogenesis

Adipogenic and osteogenic differentiation of MSCs were evaluated by measuring glycerol-3-phosphate dehydrogenase (GPDH) and alkaline phosphatase (ALP) activity, respectively. The GPDH assay kit (MK426) was obtained from Takara Bio (Shiga, Japan), and the ALP assay kit was from Wako. Assay plates were analyzed using a microplate reader (SH-1000; Hitachi High-Technologies, Tokyo, Japan). GDPH and ALP activities were normalized to the protein concentration determined by a DC protein assay kit (Bio-Rad, Hercules, CA).

Histopathological Examination

Adipocytes differentiated from MSCs were stained with Sudan III. Osteoblasts differentiated from MSCs were stained by the von Kossa method. Chondrocytes differentiated from MSCs were stained with Safranin O, Fast green, and Toluidine blue using a Cartilage Staining Kit (Takara Bio). The cells were photographed under a microscope.

RT-PCR Array Analysis

Gene expression profiles of stem cell-specific transcription factors of MSCs at passages 3–5 were analyzed by RT-PCR Array (PAHS-082ZA; Qiagen, Hilden, Germany) in accordance with the manufacturer's recommendations of 84 key genes and five housekeeping genes (Table 2). Briefly, total RNA was extracted using an RNeasy Mini Kit (Qiagen), and 1 μg total RNA was used to generate cDNA (First Strand Kit, Qiagen). Real-time PCR was performed using an ABI 7300 Real-time PCR System (Applied Biosystems, Foster City, CA) with RT2 SYBR Green qPCR Master mix (Qiagen) and a Human Mesenchymal Stem Cell PCR Array (Qiagen) according to the manufacturer's instructions.

A

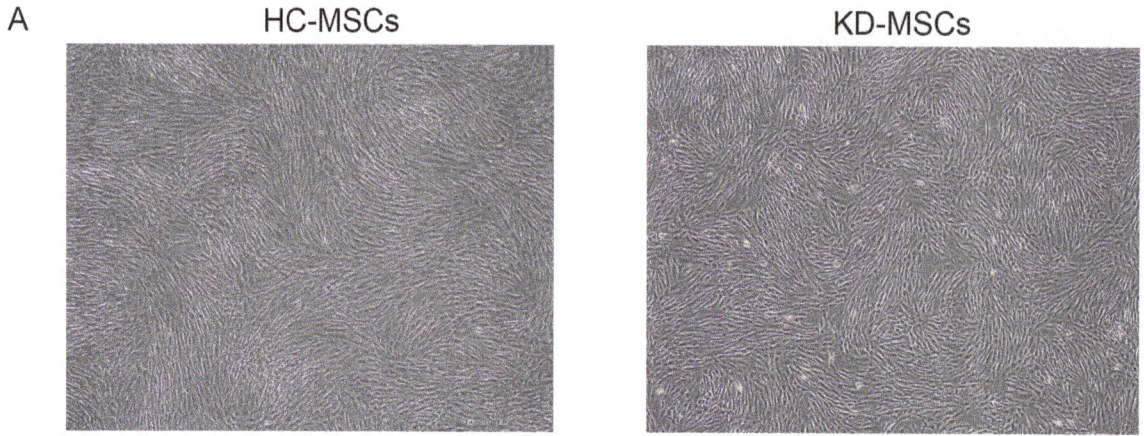

HC-MSCs   KD-MSCs

B

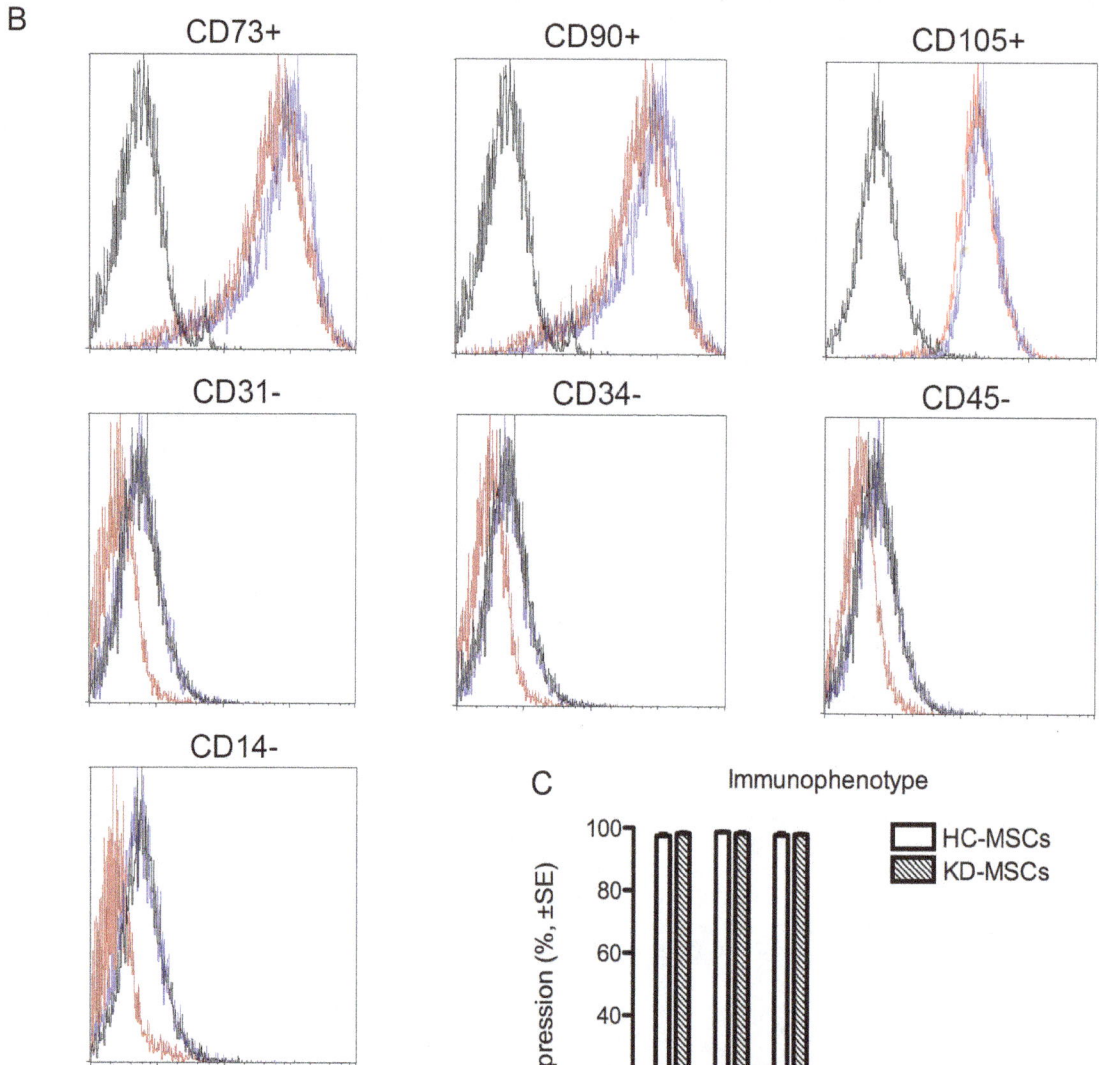

C

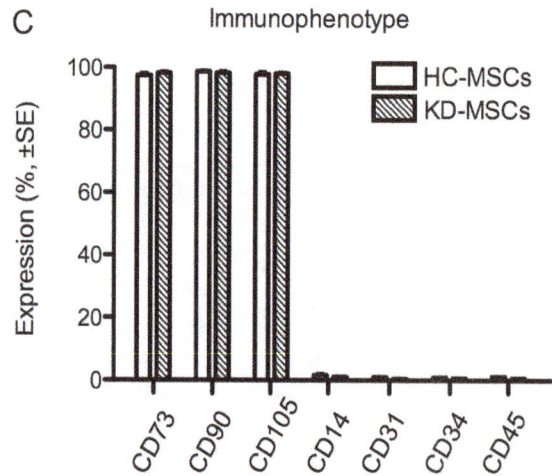

Figure 1. Characteristics of mesenchymal stem cells from healthy controls (HC-MSCs) and patients with ESKD (KD-MSCs). (A) Representative images of HC-MSCs (left) and KD-MSCs (right; original magnification, ×100). (B) Flow cytometric analysis of cell surface marker expression of HC-MSCs (solid lines; $n = 6$) and KD-MSCs (dashed lines; $n = 9$). Isotype-matched IgG controls are represented by solid histograms. (C) Comparison of cell surface marker expression in HC-MSCs ($n = 6$) and KD-MSCs ($n = 9$). The percentages of positive cells are shown. Data are the mean ± SE. There were no significant differences.

Briefly, the cDNA was diluted and mixed with an equal amount of SYBR Green Master mix, which was previously aliquoted (25 μl) into each well of a 96-well PCR array plate containing predispensed gene-specific primer sets. PCR was then performed according to the manufacturer's instructions. The thermal cycling conditions were: 95°C for 10 min, followed by 45 cycles of 95°C for 15 s then 56°C for 1 min. Data (fold changes in C_t values of all genes) were analyzed using Qiagen software. P-values were calculated based on the Student's t-test of replicate $2^{\wedge}(-\Delta Ct)$ values for each gene in control and treatment groups.

Quantitative RT-PCR Analysis of PCAF Expression

Total RNA was extracted using an RNeasy Mini Kit, and cDNA was synthesized using a RT2 First Strand Kit (Qiagen). An RT2 qPCR Primer Assay (Cat. No: PPH02176F; Qiagen) was used to analyze PCAF expression. PCR was performed using the ABI 7300 Real-time PCR System and RT2 SYBER Green Master Mix. All samples were tested in duplicate. Dissociation curves were analyzed after each reaction to assess quantification specificity. All samples were normalized to β-actin expression using the relative standard curve method.

Western Blot Analysis

Protein samples for western blot analysis were prepared as described previously [22]. Briefly, MSCs (passages 3–5) were washed three times with ice-cold PBS and then treated with lysis buffer (50 mM Tris-HCl, pH 7.5, containing 2% SDS (Sigma-Aldrich) and a protease inhibitor cocktail (Roche, Mannheim, Germany). Samples were centrifuged for 1 h at $18,000 \times g$ at 4°C. The supernatants were collected as whole cell lysates. Protein concentrations were estimated using a DC protein assay (Bio-Rad) with a bovine serum albumin standard. Equal amounts of proteins (10 μg) were resolved by SDS-polyacrylamide gel electrophoresis on 4–20% acrylamide gradient gels (Bio-Rad) and then transferred onto a polyvinylidene fluoride microporous membrane (Millipore, Billerica, MA). The membranes were blocked with a blocking reagent (Toyobo, Tokyo, Japan) and then incubated with each primary antibody. The primary antibodies used were: rabbit anti-PCAF, rabbit anti-HIF-1α (Cell Signaling Technology), rabbit anti-VEGF (Santa Cruz Biotechnology, Santa Cruz, CA) and rabbit anti-β-actin (Cell Signaling Technology). After washing, the membranes were incubated with a peroxidase-labeled secondary antibody (Nichirei, Tokyo, Japan) and visualized using Immunostar LD (Wako). Images were captured digitally using a ChemiDoc XRS+ (Bio-Rad) and analyzed by Image Lab 2.0.1 software (Bio-Rad).

PCAF, HIF-1α, and VEGF Expression under Hypoxia

Because PCAF acetylates HIF-1α under hypoxic conditions and modulates the activity and protein stability of HIF-1α [22], we investigated the effect of hypoxia on HIF-1α expression in HC-MSCs and KD-MSCs. Quantitative RT-PCR and western blotting were used to analyze PCAF, HIF-1α, and VEGF expression in HC-MSCs and KD-MSCs at 24 h under normoxia and hypoxia (1% O_2).

Statistical Analysis

Experiments were performed using independently isolated MSCs from all 15 participants. All data are presented as means ± SE. Data were analyzed using the (two-tailed) paired t-test or unpaired t-test. Statistical significance was defined as $P<0.05$. Experimental data were analyzed using GraphPad Prism version 5.0 software (Graphpad Software, San Diego, CA) and Microsoft Excel (Microsoft, Redmond, WA).

Directed *In Vivo* Angiogenesis Assay

A directed *in vivo* angiogenesis assay (DIVAA; Trevigen, Gaithersburg, MD) was performed according to the manufacturer's protocol. Briefly, implant-grade silicone cylinders closed at one end (angioreactors) were filled with 18 μl Trevigen's basement membrane extract (Trevigen) with 37.5 ng VEGF and 12.5 ng basic fibroblast growth factor (bFGF; positive control, $n = 8$), PBS (negative control, $n = 8$), or 1×10^6 HC/KD-MSCs in serum-free αMEM ($n = 8$). MSCs were selected from one cell line each of HC-MSCs and KD-MSCs at passage 3. The angioreactors were implanted subcutaneously into 8-week-old nude mice (Sankyo Laboratory Service, Tokyo, Japan). At 9 days after implantation, the mice were sacrificed and the angioreactors were removed, photographed, and stained with FITC-labeled lectin as an endothelial cell-selective reagent [23] to quantify the invasion of endothelial cells into the angioreactors [24]. Fluorescence was measured in 96-well black plates (Thermo Fisher Scientific, Roskilde, Denmark) using an ARVO MX model spectrofluorometer (485 nm excitation and 510 nm emission; Perkin Elmer, Boston, MA). The mean relative fluorescence ± S.E. were determined for triplicate assays. Statistical analysis (Unpaired t-test) was performed using GraphPad Prism version 5.0 software (Graphpad Software, San Diego, CA).

Results

MSC Isolation

MSCs were successfully isolated from all six healthy controls (HC-MSCs) and nine ESKD patients (KD-MSCs). MSC donor characteristics are depicted in Table 1. All ESKD patients had received standard dialysis therapy for renal insufficiency. Additionally used medications are listed in Table 1.

Characterization of MSCs

HC-MSCs and KD-MSCs cultured in standard culture medium showed a similar spindle-shaped morphology (Figure 1A). Surface markers of all the established MSC lines were characterized by flow cytometric analysis. Both HC-MSCs and KD-MSCs were positive for CD73, CD90, and CD105, and negative for CD14, CD31, CD34, and CD45. MSC surface markers CD73, CD105, and CD90 were expressed in >95% of cell populations (Figure 1B), and CD14, CD31, CD34, and CD45 were expressed in <2% of cell populations (Figure 1B). No differences were found in the immunophenotypes of cultured HC-MSCs and KD-MSCs (Figure 1C).

A

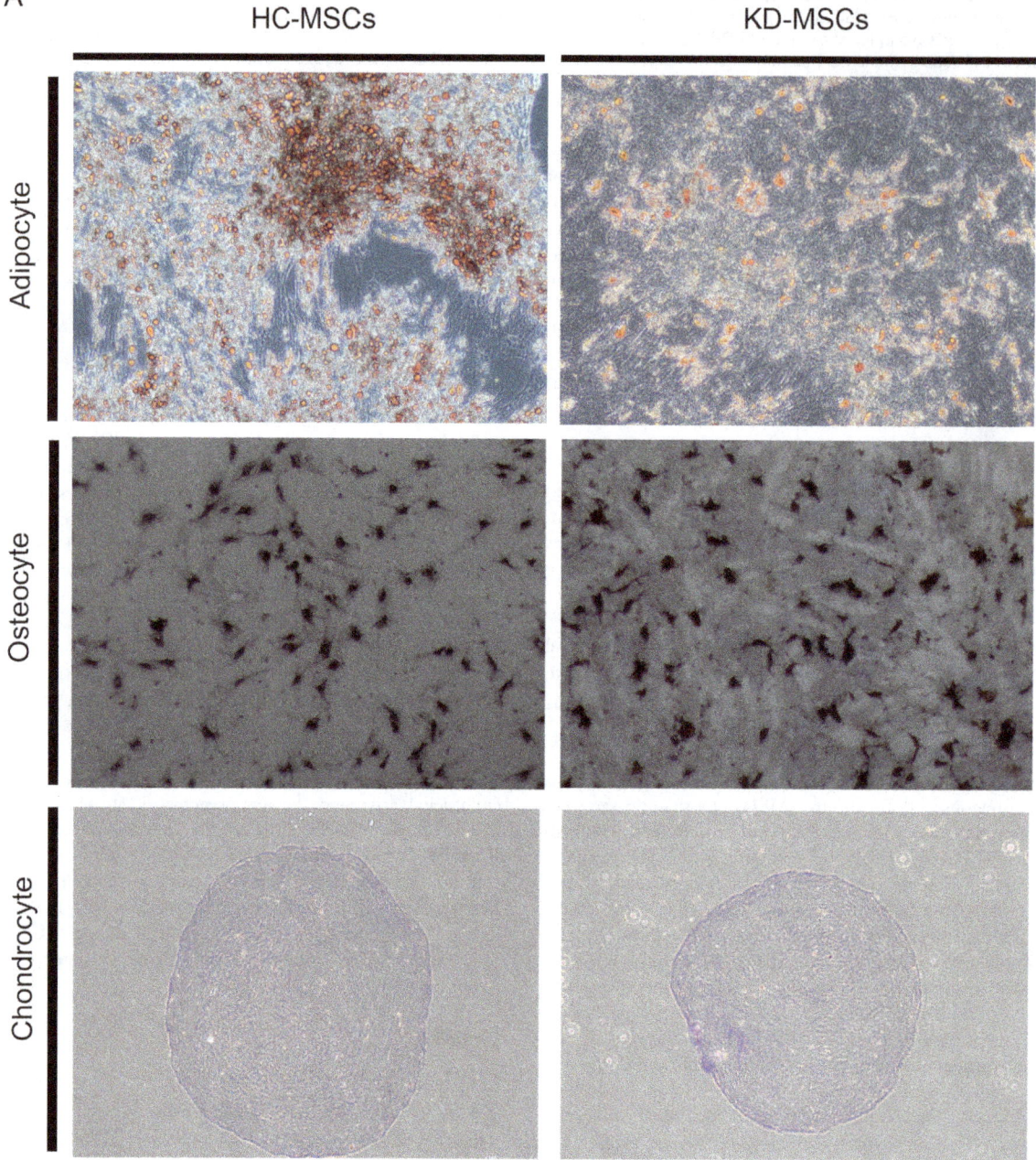

B

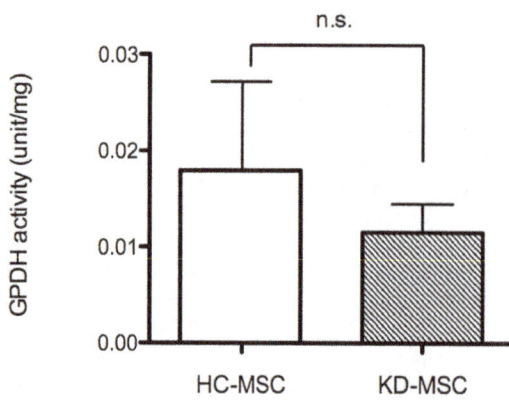

C

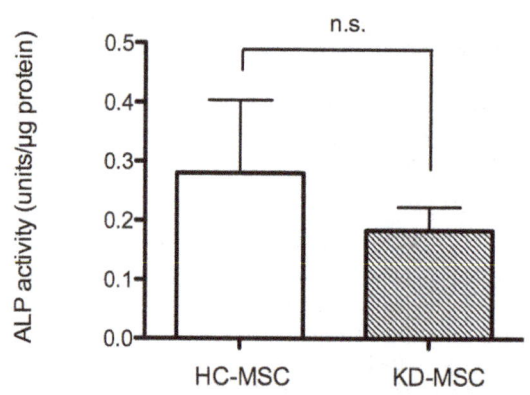

Figure 2. Differentiation capacities of HC-MSCs and KD-MSCs. (A) Adipogenic differentiation of HC-MSCs (top and left) and KD-MSCs (top and right) was examined after 2 weeks of culture under adipogenic conditions by Sudan III staining (original magnification, ×100). Osteogenic differentiation of HC-MSCs (second from top and left) and KD-MSCs (second from top and right) was examined after 4 weeks of culture under osteogenic conditions by von Kossa staining (original magnification, ×100). Chondrogenic differentiation of HC-MSCs (bottom and left) and KD-MSCs (bottom and right) was examined after 3 weeks of culture under chondrogenic conditions by Safranin O/Fast green staining (original magnification, ×100). (B) GPDH activity of cells was measured to compare the adipogenic differentiation capacities of HC-MSCs ($n = 5$) and KD-MSCs ($n = 5$). Data are expressed as the mean ± standard error (SE). $^*P < 0.05$. (C) ALP activity of the cells was measured to indicate their osteogenic differentiation capacity ($n = 4$). Data are expressed as the mean ± SE. $^*P < 0.05$.

Adipogenic, Osteogenic, and Chondrogenic Differentiation

Histopathological examination by Sudan III, von Kossa, Safranin O, and Fast green staining was performed to identify adipogenic, osteogenic, and chondrogenic lineages, respectively (Figure 2A). We also found no significant differences in GPDH ($n = 5$ for KD-MSCs and HC-MSCs) or ALP ($n = 5$ for KD-MSCs and HC-MSCs) activities, representing adipogenic and osteogenic differentiation, respectively, in HC-MSCs and KD-MSCs (Figure 2B and 2C).

MSC Senescence and Proliferation

MSCs possess a limited lifespan during *in vitro* culture because they undergo senescence [19], characterized by cell cycle arrest, telomere shortening, and altered morphology. To assess the percentage of cells undergoing senescence, we used SA-β-gal as a senescence marker. The percentages of β-galactosidase-positive cells increased from passage 5 to 10, but there was no significant difference in β-galactosidase positivity in HC-MSCs ($n = 4$) and KD-MSCs ($n = 4$) at passages 5, 8, and 10 (Figure 3A and 3B). These results suggest that there was no significant difference in the proliferation or senescence of HC-MSCs and KD-MSCs.

A second senescence assay determined the formation of SAHF, which are visible as microscopically discernible, punctate DNA foci in DAPI-stained senescent cells [25]. As shown in Figure 3A (right columns), late passage (P10) MSCs showed punctuated DNA foci, while early passage (P5) MSCs displayed several small nucleoli and a more uniform DAPI staining pattern. We observed a similar formation of SAHF between HC-MSCs and KD-MSCs in early and late passages.

The proliferation potentials of HC-MSCs and KD-MSCs were evaluated over six passages and PD levels were measured from passage 5–10. HC-MSCs and KD-MSCs displayed similar cumulative PDs with a peak of 10.89±1.52 and 10.71±1.26, respectively, at passage 10 ($P < 0.05$ versus controls) (Figure 3C). Cell proliferation rates of HC-MSCs ($n = 5$) and KD-MSCs ($n = 5$) showed no significant difference.

RT-PCR Array Analysis of MSCs

Quantitative RT-PCR array analysis profiled the expression of 84 key genes, including those involved in stemness and self-renewal of MSCs (Table 2), and revealed distinct expression patterns in HC-MSCs ($n = 6$) and KD-MSCs ($n = 9$). Compared with HC-MSCs, we found significantly lower expression of *PCAF*, *BMP4*, and *PIGS* (fold differences: 0.73, 0.42, and 0.72, respectively) in KD-MSCs (Figure 4A, Table 2), suggesting a functional difference in HC-MSCs and KD-MSCs. There were no significant differences in expression of the other 81 genes (Table 2).

Quantitative RT-PCR and Western Blot Analyses of MSCs

Quantitative RT-PCR was performed to verify the downregulation of *PCAF* expression in KD-MSCs, and confirmed that *PCAF* expression levels were significantly downregulated in KD-MSCs ($n = 6$, $^*P < 0.05$, Figure 4B). Similarly, PCAF protein expression

was significantly decreased in KD-MSCs ($n = 9$) compared with HC-MSCs ($n = 6$) as shown by western blotting ($^*P < 0.05$, Figure 4C).

Downregulation of PCAF, HIF-1α, and VEGF Gene and Protein Expression in KD-MSCs Cultured under Hypoxic Conditions

We hypothesized that PCAF in human MSCs would be upregulated under hypoxia, so investigated the gene and protein expression of PCAF, HIF-1α, and the downstream factor VEGF in HC-MSCs and KD-MSCs under normoxia (21% O_2) and hypoxia (1% O_2) at 24 h. PCAF protein expression was significantly upregulated under hypoxia (1% O_2, 24 h) in HC-MSCs ($n = 6$, $P < 0.05$, Figure 5A, 5B), but this was not observed in KD-MSCs ($n = 9$, $P < 0.05$, Figure 5A, 5B). Similarly, HIF-1α expression was significantly upregulated under hypoxia in HC-MSCs ($n = 6$, $P < 0.05$, Figure 5C), but not in KD-MSCs ($n = 9$, $P < 0.05$, Figure 5C). Furthermore, the enhancement of VEGF expression under hypoxic conditions, which is regulated by HIF-1α [26], was significantly decreased in KD-MSCs under hypoxia ($n = 9$, $P < 0.05$ Figure 5D). We demonstrated that KD-MSCs did not upregulate the protein expression of PCAF, HIF-1α, or VEGF under hypoxia, suggesting that the hypoxic response might be blunted in KD-MSCs.

DIVAA of MSCs

Because a previous study has proposed that PCAF is a key regulator of angiogenesis [27], we tested angiogenesis activation of HC-MSCs and KD-MSCs *in vivo*. A DIVAA assesses angiogenesis activation, which provides quantitative and reproducible results [28]. The results showed significant blood vessel growth into angioreactors containing HC-MSCs, which was similar to that seen in positive controls (VEGF/bFGF). However, we observed only slight growth into angioreactors containing KD-MSCs (Fig. 6, lower panel). Thus, HC-MSCs showed better angiogenesis activation than that of KD-MSCs.

Furthermore, measurement of FITC-lectin bound to the endothelial contents of angioreactors supported these findings and demonstrated reduced fluorescence in angioreactors containing KD-MSCs compared with the strong fluorescence seen in angioreactors containing HC-MSCs (Fig. 6, bar graph). These results support the notion that KD-MSCs with low expression of PCAF exhibit lower angiogenesis activation than that of HC-MSCs.

Discussion

Stem cells from patients with ESKD are needed for kidney regeneration, but it is not yet known if stem cells exposed to long-term uremic conditions will function normally. To explore whether the acquired disease environment causes long-term changes and influences the cell environment, we compared MSCs from ESKD patients and those with normal kidney function by RT-PCR array. After culturing KD-MSCs under normal condi-

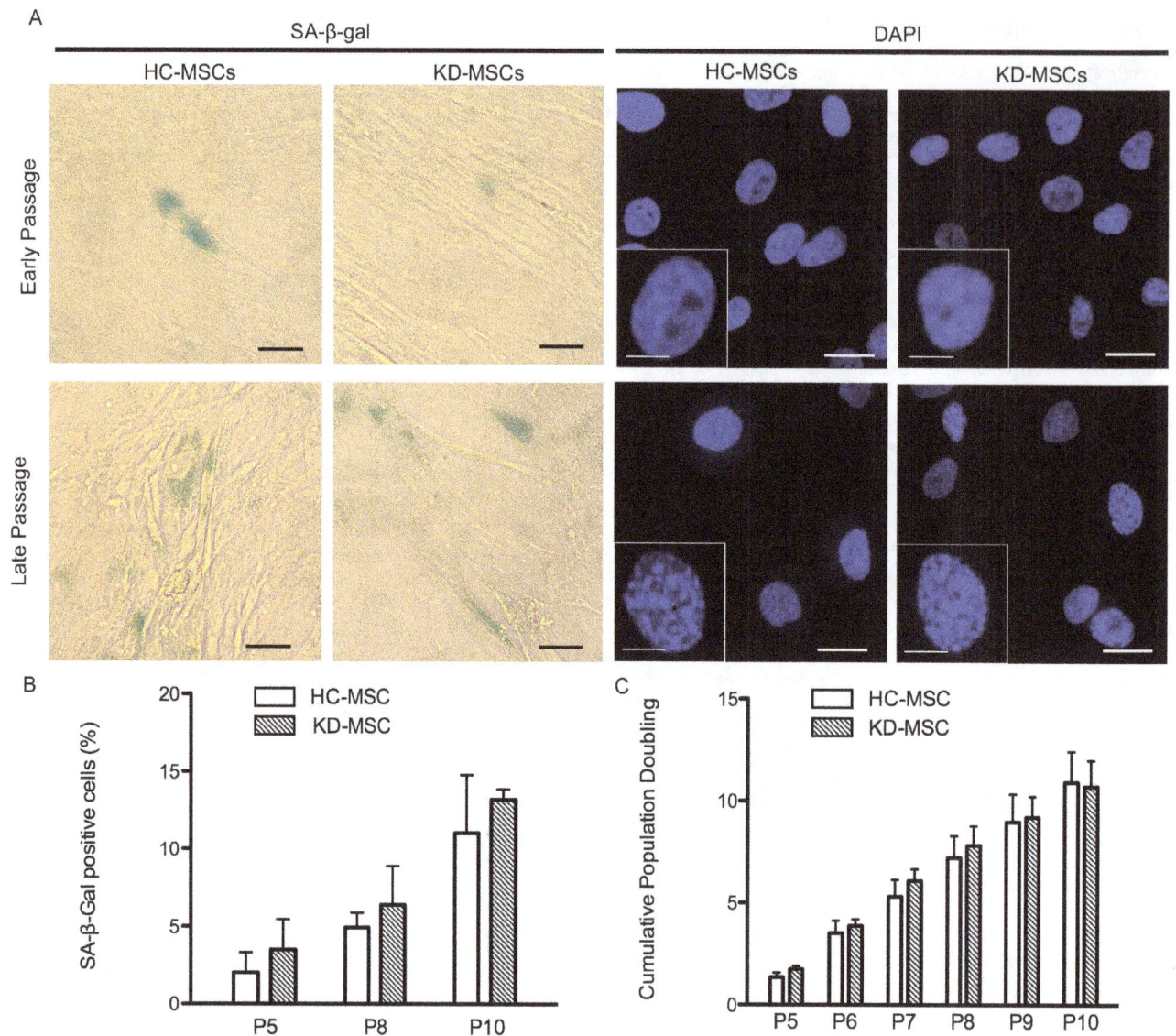

Figure 3. Proliferation and senescence of HC-MSCs and KD-MSCs. (A) Representative images of HC-MSCs and KD-MSCs (magnification, ×40). Left columns show assessment of senescence using the senescence biomarker SA-β-gal (green) in HC-MSCs and KD-MSCs. Black scale bars represent 50 μm. Right columns show DAPI staining of senescence-associated heterochromatic foci (SAHF) in MSC DNA foci. White scale bars represent 10 μm. Insets show an enlargement of DAPI staining (white scale bars represent 5 μm). Early passage: P5; late passage: P10. (B) Quantitative assessment of SA-β-gal positive cells. Data are the mean ± SE ($n = 4$). $^*P<0.05$. (C) Cumulative population doublings (PDs) of HC-MSCs ($n = 5$) and KD-MSCs ($n = 5$) from passage 5–10. Data are expressed as the mean ± SE. $^*P<0.05$. Experiments were performed in triplicate.

tions for 2–3 weeks, *PCAF*, *PIGS*, and *BMP4* expression was shown to differ significantly between HC-MSCs and KD-MSCs.

PCAF plays a role in the regulation of differentiation, angiogenesis, cell cycle progression, and gluconeogenesis [27], [29], [30], and is one of the many factors involved in epigenetics [31]. However, the mechanisms behind its actions have not yet been elucidated, particularly its role in angiogenesis. A previous study of PCAF$^{-/-}$ mice indicated that PCAF acts as a master switch for effective arteriogenesis [27], while another report demonstrated a role for PCAF in angiogenic tubule formation because human umbilical vein endothelial cells transfected with PCAF siRNA showed a significant reduction of angiogenic tubule formation [32].

A previous study used proteomics to show that PCAF was upregulated under hypoxia in the rat kidney fibroblast NRK-49F cell line [33]. Additionally, PCAF acetylates HIF-1α under hypoxic conditions, which fine tunes its transcriptional activity, increases its protein stability, and causes modulation of cellular responses [20], [33]–[35]. HIF-1α is known to be a key regulator of angiogenesis and controls the expression of multiple angiogenic factors including VEGF [26], [36].

Interestingly, we found that PCAF expression under hypoxia was increased in HC-MSCs (Figure 5A and 5B), but not KD-MSCs in the present study. Previously, studies in other animal cell types have suggested that PCAF is upregulated under hypoxia [37], but no investigations have been carried out into the hypoxic response and the influence of long-term uremic conditions on PCAF in human MSCs. Because PCAF is a facilitator for HIF-1α and VEGF [29], [38], we investigated the hypoxic responses of HIF-1α and VEGF by western blotting and detected low levels of

A

RT-PCR array analysis of MSCs

B

qPCR of PCAF

C

Western blot of PCAF

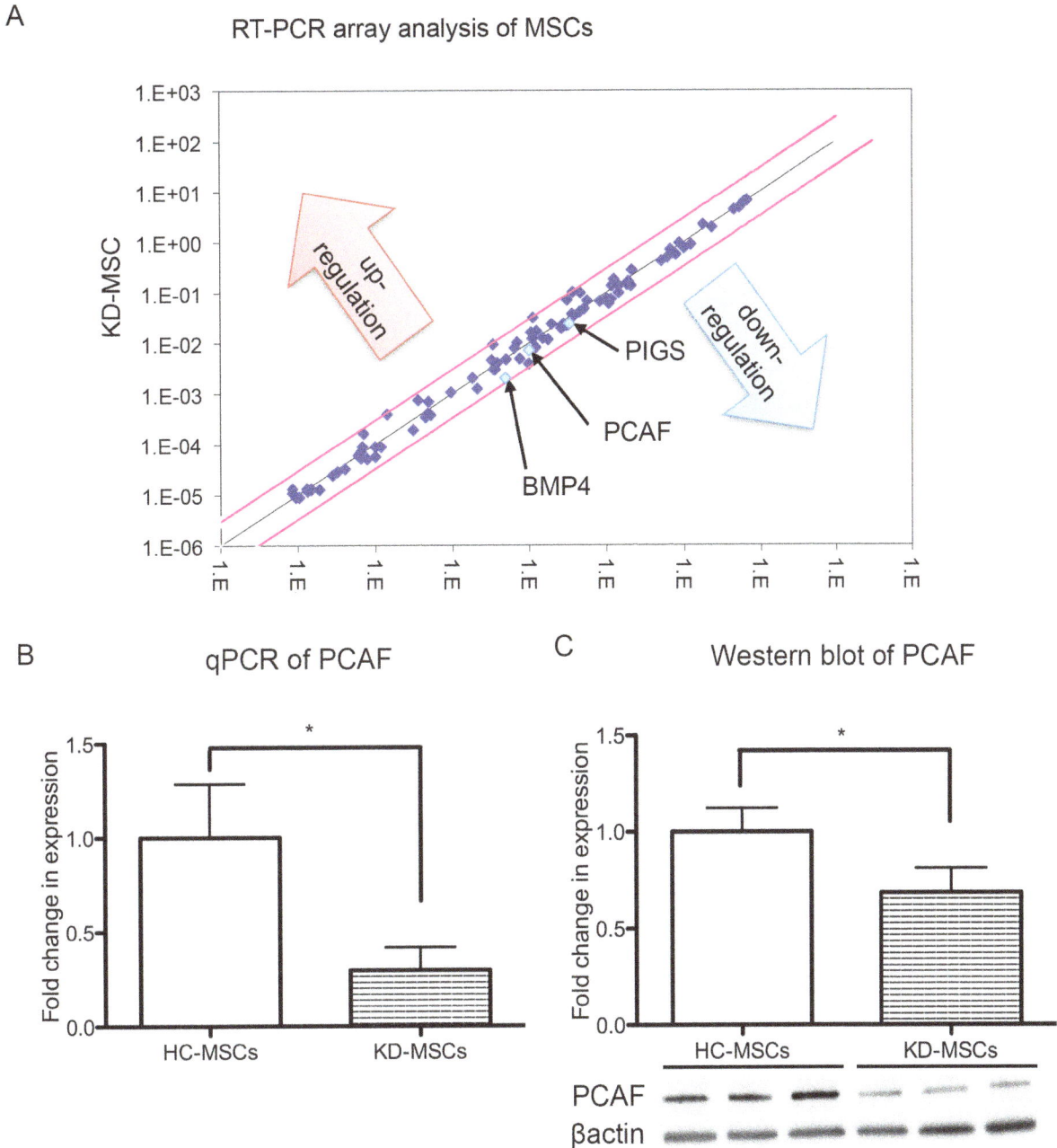

Figure 4. Real-time PCR array, quantitative PCR, and western blot analyses of MSCs. (A) Downregulation of multiple stem cell-relevant transcription factors in KD-MSCs ($n = 9$) compared with HC-MSCs ($n = 6$). The fold change $[2^{\wedge}(-\Delta\Delta Ct)]$ is the normalized gene expression $[2^{\wedge}(-\Delta Ct)]$ in KD-MSCs relative to that in HC-MSCs. P-values were calculated based on the Student's t-test of replicate $2^{\wedge}(-\Delta Ct)$ values for each gene in HC-MSCs and KD-MSCs. $P < 0.05$ is indicated with black arrows. (B) Quantitative PCR was performed to measure the levels of gene expression in HC-MSCs ($n = 6$) and KD-MSCs ($n = 6$). Data are expressed as the mean $\pm$ SE. $^{*}P < 0.05$. (C) Western blot analysis of PCAF in KD-MSCs and HC-MSCs. PCAF expression was decreased in KD-MSCs ($n = 9$) compared with HC-MSCs ($n = 6$). PCAF protein levels are expressed relative to β-actin. Data are expressed as the mean $\pm$ SE. $^{*}P < 0.05$.

HIF-1α and VEGF protein expression in KD-MSCs under hypoxic conditions (Figure 5C and 5D). Consequently, it appears that the hypoxic response is significantly blunted in KD-MSCs with low PCAF expression, but not in HC-MSCs.

A previous report found that uremic conditions decreased HIF-1α and VEGF expression under hypoxia in mice [13]. However, this study did not refer to PCAF, and it was thought that Akt phosphorylation might underlie abnormal cell survival and the

angiogenic functions of MSCs in uremia. Uremia is an illness accompanying kidney failure that cannot be explained by alteration of the extracellular volume, inorganic ion concentrations, or lack of known renal synthetic products [39]. The precise mechanisms have yet to be identified for uremia and hypoxia, but the finding that KD-MSCs show downregulation of PCAF expression, poor angiogenesis activation *in vivo*, and blunting of

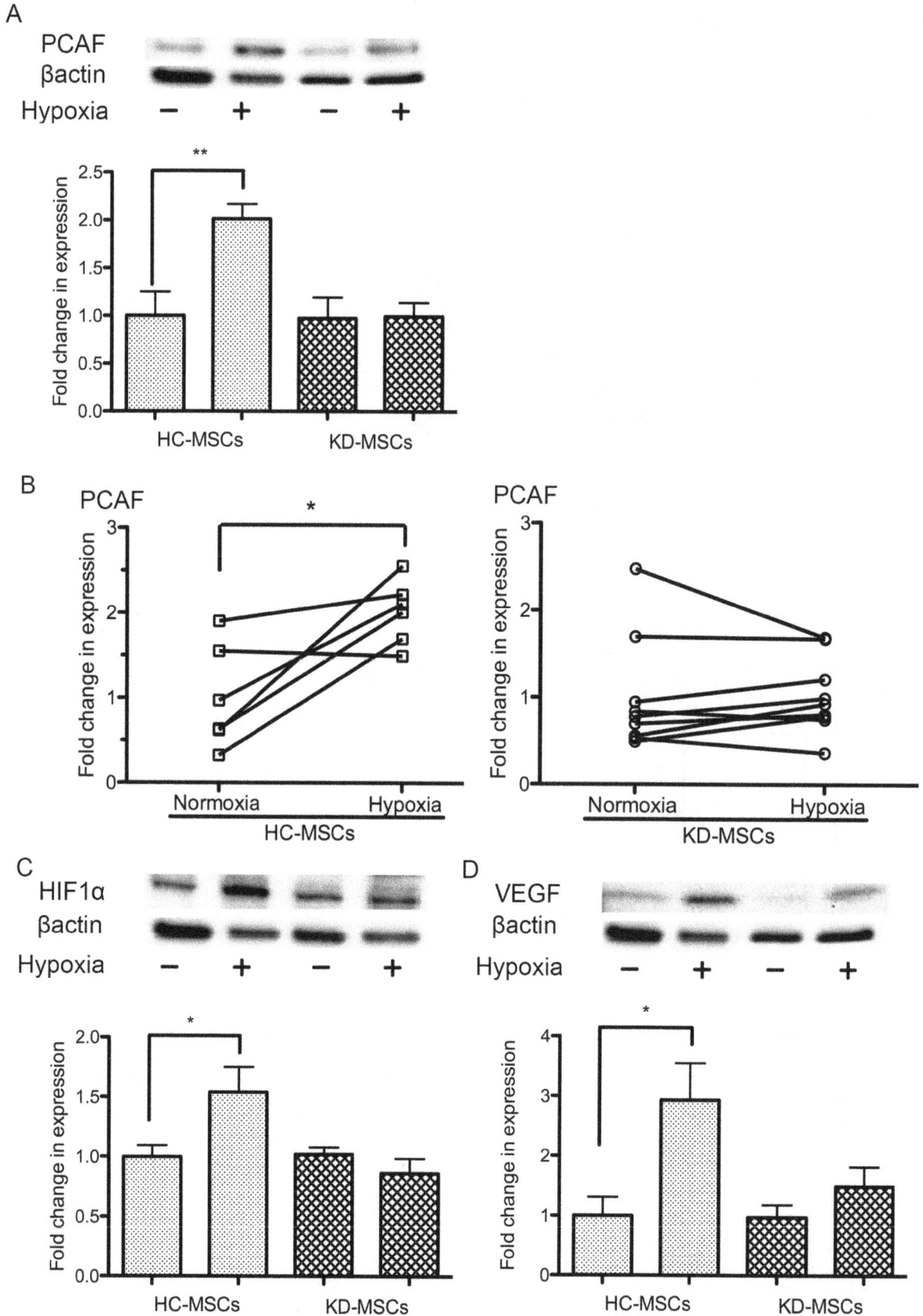

Figure 5. Western blot analysis of PCAF, HIF-1α, and VEGF expression under hypoxia and normoxia. (A) Western blot analysis of PCAF expression in KD-MSCs ($n = 9$) and HC-MSCs ($n = 6$) under normoxia and hypoxia (1% O_2). Data are the mean ± SE. **$P < 0.01$ normoxia versus hypoxia in HC-MSCs (two-tailed, unpaired t-test). (B) Western blot analysis of PCAF expression at 24 h under hypoxia showed it to be clearly upregulated in

HC-MSCs. There was no change in PCAF in KD-MSCs under hypoxia. Data are the mean ± SE (HC-MSCs $n=6$, KD-MSCs $n=9$; $^*P<0.05$ versus normoxia, two-tailed, paired t-test). (C) Western blot analysis of HIF-1α expression in KD-MSCs ($n=9$) and HC-MSCs ($n=6$) under normoxia and hypoxia. Data are the mean ± SE. $^*P<0.05$ versus normoxia (two-tailed, unpaired t-test). (D) Western blot analysis of VEGF expression in KD-MSCs ($n=9$) and HC-MSCs ($n=6$) under normoxia and hypoxia. Data are the mean ± SE. $^*P<0.05$ versus normoxia (two-tailed, unpaired t-test). (A–D) MSC lines were isolated independently.

the hypoxic response might be helpful in their elucidation in ESKD patients.

Kidney development is associated with coordinated branching of the renal tubular and vascular systems, and hypoxia has been proposed as a major regulatory factor in this process [40]. We have developed a regeneration method involving transplantation of a metanephros into the omentum to attract the host veins into the graft and generate urine in hypoxic tissues [7]–[9]. Because angiogenesis and hypoxia might play a role in kidney regeneration, it is important to investigate the hypoxic responses of PCAF, HIF-1α, and VEGF in KD-MSCs and HC-MSCs. Furthermore, PCAF is a member of the histone acetyltransferases (HATs). HATs promote an open chromatin configuration and transcriptional activation. Epigenetic modifications by HATs and histone deacetylases (HDACs) have a direct effect on gene regulation, cell differentiation, and cellular stability during renal development [41]. In fact, even though the role of HDACs is well studied [42], little is known about the role of HATs during metanephric kidney development [41].

There are currently no available assays to directly test for PCAF activity, so we cannot exclude histone acetyltransferase activity as an underlying mechanism for the effect of PCAF. Our data suggest that, within the context of the hypoxic response, it is more likely that PCAF functions as a transcriptional coactivator to regulate HIF-1α expression. The involvement of global gene expression and epigenetic effects is also unclear and should be investigated further. While it would be useful to demonstrate the regeneration of kidney tissue from KD-MSCs using our previous methods [7]–[9], and directly compare the differences between KD-MSCs and HC-MSCs, this technique is very difficult. The cell transplantation efficiency has a 3% success rate and only about 30% of transplantations generate a neo-kidney. Thus, we did not apply this method in the current study because of its very low success rate.

In conclusion, we demonstrated differences in the gene and protein expression of MSCs from ESKD patients and healthy individuals using a PCR array and western blot analysis. We found that long-term uremic conditions led to persistent and systematic

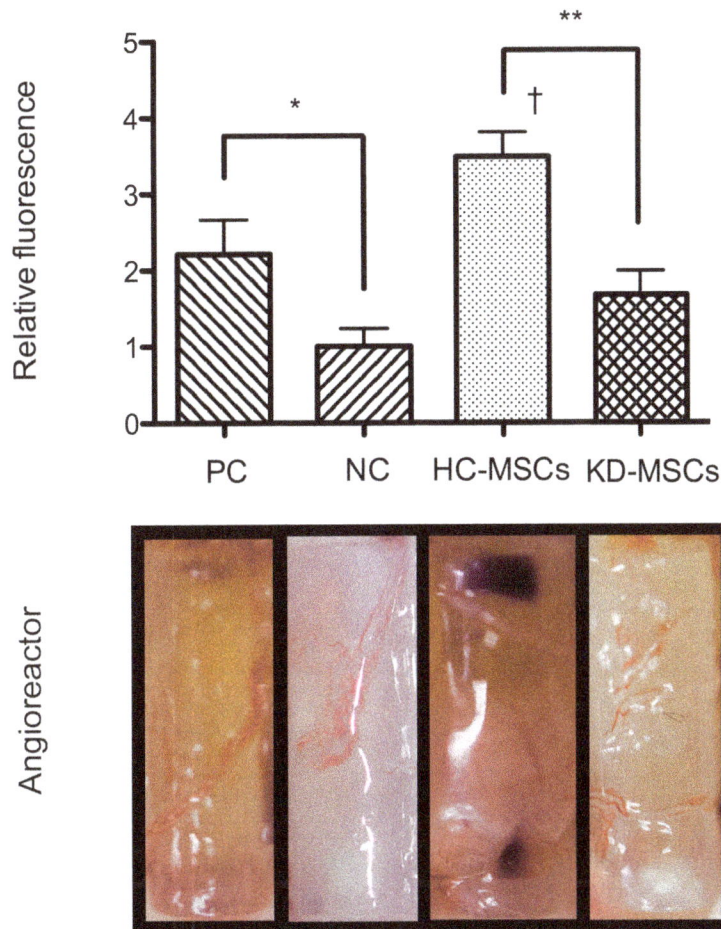

Figure 6. Directed *in vivo* angiogenesis assay. Angioreactors containing HC-MSCs ($n=8$), KD-MSCs ($n=8$), 37.5 ng VEGF and 12.5 ng bFGF (positive control, $n=8$), or PBS (negative control, $n=8$) were used in a DIVAA. The photographs show blood vessel growth into the angioreactors. The bar graph shows the average ± S.E. of triplicates. $^{**}P<0.01$, HC-MSCs versus KD-MSCs; $^*P<0.05$, PC versus NC; $^†P<0.05$, HC-MSCs versus PC. PC: Positive control; NC: Negative control.

downregulation of *in vitro* gene and protein expression of PCAF and poor *in vivo* angiogenesis activation of MSCs from patients with ESKD. Furthermore, we demonstrated that the hypoxic responses of PCAF, HIF-1α, and VEGF were significantly blunted in MSCs from ESKD patients. We propose that the transcriptional regulation by low levels of PCAF might be inappropriately controlled by environmental factors representing long-term ESKD. Low expression of PCAF induced by long-term ESKD may lead to downregulation of HIF-1α and VEGF in KD-MSCs under hypoxia. These findings should help to elucidate the mechanisms of the effects of uremic toxins. Further studies are needed to clarify the relationship of CKD and the downregulation of PCAF. Moreover, based on our study, the role of PCAF may be investigated further in epigenetic mechanisms during kidney development.

Acknowledgments

We are grateful to Yudo Tanno and Nanae Matsuo for their role in collecting adipose tissue samples.

Author Contributions

Conceived and designed the experiments: S. Yamanaka TY. Performed the experiments: S. Yamanaka S. Yokote AY YK LI YS. Analyzed the data: S. Yamanaka. Contributed reagents/materials/analysis tools: NO HJO TO. Wrote the paper: S. Yamanaka TY.

References

1. The Japanese Society of Nephrology (2012) Clinical practice guidebook for diagnosis and treatment of chronic kidney disease. Jpn J Nephrol 54: 1031–1189.
2. Berger A, Edelsberg J, Inglese GW, Bhattacharyya SK, Oster G (2009) Cost comparison of peritoneal dialysis versus hemodialysis in end-stage renal disease. Am J Manag Care 15: 509–518.
3. Wolfe RA, Ashby VB, Milford EL, Ojo AO, Ettenger RE, et al. (1999) Comparison of mortality in all patients on dialysis, patients on dialysis awaiting transplantation, and recipients of a fiomp cadaveric transplant. N Engl J Med 341: 1725–1730.
4. Sonoda T, Takahara S, Takahashi K, Uchida K, Ohshima S, et al. (2003) Outcome of 3 years of immunosuppression with tacrolimus in more than 1,000 renal transplant recipients in Japan. Transplantation 75: 1999–024.
5. Badylak SF, Taylor D, Uygun K (2011) Whole-organ tissue engineering: decellularization and recellularization of three-dimensional matrix scaffolds. Annu Rev Biomed Eng 15: 27–53.
6. Xinaris C, Benedetti V, Rizzo P, Abbate M, Corna D, et al. (2012) In vivo maturation of functional renal organoids formed from embryonic cell suspensions. J Am Soc Nephrol 23: 1857–1868.
7. Yokoo T, Ohashi T, Shen JS, Sakurai K, Miyazaki Y, et al. (2005) Human mesenchymal stem cells in rodent whole embryo culture are reprogrammed to contribute kidney tissues. Proc Natl Acad Sci U S A 102: 3296–3300.
8. Yokoo T, Fukui A, Ohashi T, Miyazaki Y, Utsunomiya Y, et al. (2006) Xenobiotic kidney organogenesis from human mesenchymal stem cells using a growing rodent embryo. J Am Soc Nephrol 17: 1026–1034.
9. Yokoo T, Fukui A, Matsumoto K, Ohashi T, Sado Y, et al. (2008) Generation of transplantable erythropoietin producer derived from human mesenchymal stem cells. Transplantation 85: 1654–1658.
10. Aust L, Devlin B, Foster SJ, Halvorsen YD, Hicok K, et al. (2004) Yield of human adipose-derived adult stem cells from liposuction aspirates. Cytotherapy 6: 7–14.
11. Gonzalez-Cruz RD, Fonseca VC, Darling EM (2012) Cellular mechanical properties reflect the differentiation potential of adipose-derived mesenchymal stem cells. Proc Natl Acad Sci U S A 12: E1523–1529.
12. Drewa T, Joachimiak R, Kaznica A, Flisinski M, Brymora A, et al. (2008) Bone marrow progenitors from animals with chronic renal failure lack capacity of in vitro proliferation. Transplant Proc 40: 1668–1673.
13. Noh H, Yu MR, Kim HJ, Jeon JS, Kwon SH, et al. (2012) Uremia induces functional incompetence of bone marrow-derived stromal cells. Nephrol Dial Transplant 27: 218–225.
14. Roemeling-van Rhijn M, Reinders ME, de Klein A, Douben H, Korevaar SS, et al. (2012) Mesenchymal stem cells derived from adipose tissue are not affected by renal disease. Kidney Int 82: 748–758.
15. Yamada A, Yokoo T, Yokote S, Yamanaka S, Izuhara L, et al. (2014) Comparison of multipotency and molecular profile of MSCs between CKD and healthy rats. Hum Cell 27: 59–67.
16. Zuk PA, Zhu M, Mizuno H, Huang J, Futrell JW, et al. (2001) Multilineage cells from human adipose tissue: implications for cell-based therapies. Tissue Eng 7: 211–228.
17. Banas A, Teratani T, Yamamoto Y, Tokuhara M, Takeshita F, et al. (2007) Adipose tissue-derived mesenchymal stem cells as a source of human hepatocytes. Hepatology 46: 219–228.
18. Dominici M, Le Blanc K, Mueller I, Slaper-Cortenbach I, Marini F, et al. (2006) Minimal criteria for defining multipotent mesenchymal stromal cells. The International Society for Cellular Therapy position statement. Cytotherapy 8: 315–317.
19. Wagner W, Horn P, Castoldi M, Diehlmann A, Bork S, et al. (2008) Replicative senescence of mesenchymal stem cells: a continuous and organized process. PLoS One 3: e2213.
20. Huang J, Gan Q, Han L, Li J, Zhang H, et al. (2008) SIRT1 overexpression antagonizes cellular senescence with activated ERK/S6k1 signaling in human diploid fibroblasts. PLoS One 5: e1710.
21. Nekanti U, Dastidar S, Venugopal P, Totey S, Ta M (2010) Increased proliferation and analysis of differential gene expression in human Wharton's jelly-derived mesenchymal stromal cells under hypoxia. Int J Biol Sci 9: 499–512.
22. Shimada Y, Nishida H, Nishiyama Y, Kobayashi H, Higuchi T, et al. (2011) Proteasome inhibitors improve the function of mutant lysosomal α-glucosidase in fibroblasts from Pompe disease patient carrying c.546G>T mutation. Biochem Biophys Res Commun 415: 274–278.
23. Sahagun G, Moore SA, Fabry Z, Schelper RL, Hart MN (1989) Purification of murine endothelial cell cultures by flow cytometry using fluorescein-labeled griffonia simplicifolia agglutinin. Am J Pathol 134: 1227–32.
24. Basile JR, Holmbeck K, Bugge TH, Gutkind JS (2007) MT1-MMP controls tumor-induced angiogenesis through the release of semaphorin 4D. J Biol Chem 2: 6899–905.
25. Narita M, Nûnez S, Heard E, Narita M, Lin AW, et al. (2003) Rb-mediated heterochromatin formation and silencing of E2F target genes during cellular senescence. Cell 13: 703–16.
26. Okuyama H, Krishnamachary B, Zhou YF, Nagasawa H, Bosch-Marce M, et al. (2006) Expression of vascular endothelial growth factor receptor 1 in bone marrow-derived mesenchymal cells is dependent on hypoxia-inducible factor 1. J Biol Chem 281: 15554–15563.
27. Bastiaansen AJ, Ewing MM, de Boer HC, van der Pouw Kraan TC, de Vries MR, et al. (2013) Lysine acetyltransferase PCAF is a key regulator of arteriogenesis. Arterioscler Thromb Vasc Biol 33: 1902–1910.
28. Guedez L, Rivera AM, Salloum R, Miller ML, Diegmueller JJ, et al. (2003) Quantitative assessment of angiogenic response by the Directed In Vivo Angiogenesis Assay. American J Pathol 162: 1431–1439.
29. Xenaki G, Ontikatze T, Rajendran R, Stratford IJ, Dive C, et al. (2008) PCAF is an HIF-1alpha cofactor that regulates p53 transcriptional activity in hypoxia. Oncogene 27: 5785–5796.
30. Ravnskjaer K, Hogan MF, Lackey D, Tora L, Dent SY, et al. (2013) Glucagon regulates gluconeogenesis through KAT2B- and WDR5-mediated epigenetic effects. J Clin Invest 123: 4318–4328.
31. Ferrari R, Pellegrini M, Horwitz GA, Xie W, Berk AJ, et al. (2008) Epigenetic reprogramming by adenovirus e1a. Science 321: 1086–1088.
32. Pillai S, Kovacs M, Chellappan S (2010) Regulation of vascular endothelial growth factor receptors by Rb and E2F1: role of acetylation. Cancer Res 70: 4931–4940.
33. Lim JH, Lee YM, Chun YS, Chen J, Kim JE, et al. (2010) Sirtuin 1 modulates cellular responses to hypoxia by deacetylating hypoxia-inducible factor 1alpha. Mol Cell 38: 864–878.
34. Jin Y, Zeng SX, Dai MS, Yang X-J, Lu H (2002) MDM2 inhibits PCAF-mediated p53 acetylation. J Biol Chem 277: 30838–30843.
35. Linares LK, Kiernan R, Triboulet R, Chable-Bessia C, Latreille D, et al. (2007) Intrinsic ubiquitination activity of PCAF controls the stability of the oncoprotein Hdm2. Nat Cell Biol 9: 331–338.
36. Kelly BD, Hackett SF, Hirota K, Oshima Y, Cai Z, et al. (2003) Cell type-specific regulation of angiogenic growth factor gene expression and induction of angiogenesis in nonischemic tissue by a constitutively active form of hypoxia-inducible factor 1. Circ Res 93: 1074–1081.
37. Shakib K, Norman JT, Fine LG, Brown LR, Godovac-Zimmermann J (2005) Proteomics profiling of nuclear proteins for kidney fibroblasts suggests hypoxia, meiosis, and cancer may meet in the nucleus. Proteomics 5: 2819–2838.
38. Martínez-Balbás MA, Bauer UM, Nielsen SJ, Brehm A, Kouzarides T (2000) Regulation of E2F1 activity by acetylation. EMBO J 19: 662–671.
39. Meyer TW, Hostetter TH (2007) Uremia. N Engl J Med 27: 1316–1325.
40. Bernhardt WM, Schmitt R, Rosenberger C, Munchenhagen PM, Grone HJ, et al. (2006) Expression of hypoxia-inducible transcription factors in developing human and rat kidneys. Kidney Int 69: 114–122.
41. Bechtel-Walz W, Huber TB (2014) Chromatin dynamics in kidney development and function. Cell Tissue Res 356: 601–608.
42. Chen S, Bellew C, Yao X, Stefkova J, Dipp S, et al. (2011) Histone deacetylase (HDAC) activity is critical for embryonic kidney gene expression, growth, and differentiation. J Biol Chem 286: 32775–32789.

5

Modulation of PPARγ Provides New Insights in a Stress Induced Premature Senescence Model

Stefania Briganti[⬥], Enrica Flori[⬥], Barbara Bellei, Mauro Picardo*

Laboratory of Cutaneous Physiopathology, San Gallicano Dermatologic Institute, Istituto di Ricovero e Cura a Carattere Scientifico, Rome, Italy

Abstract

Peroxisome proliferator-activated receptor gamma (PPARγ) may be involved in a key mechanism of the skin aging process, influencing several aspects related to the age-related degeneration of skin cells, including antioxidant unbalance. Therefore, we investigated whether the up-modulation of this nuclear receptor exerts a protective effect in a stress-induced premature senescence (SIPS) model based on a single exposure of human dermal fibroblasts to 8-methoxypsoralen plus + ultraviolet-A-irradiation (PUVA). Among possible PPARγ modulators, we selected 2,4,6-octatrienoic acid (Octa), a member of the parrodiene family, previously reported to promote melanogenesis and antioxidant defense in normal human melanocytes through a mechanism involving PPARγ activation. Exposure to PUVA induced an early and significant decrease in PPARγ expression and activity. PPARγ up-modulation counteracted the antioxidant imbalance induced by PUVA and reduced the expression of stress response genes with a synergistic increase of different components of the cell antioxidant network, such as catalase and reduced glutathione. PUVA-treated fibroblasts grown in the presence of Octa are partially but significantly rescued from the features of the cellular senescence-like phenotype, such as cytoplasmic enlargement, the expression of senescence-associated-β-galactosidase, matrix-metalloproteinase-1, and cell cycle proteins. Moreover, the alterations in the cell membrane lipids, such as the decrease in the polyunsaturated fatty acid content of phospholipids and the increase in cholesterol levels, which are typical features of cell aging, were prevented. Our data suggest that PPARγ is one of the targets of PUVA-SIPS and that its pharmacological up-modulation may represent a novel therapeutic approach for the photooxidative skin damage.

Editor: Andrzej T. Slominski, University of Tennessee, United States of America

Funding: This work has been partly supported by a research grant provided by Giuliani Pharma, Milan, Italy. The funders had no role in study design, data collection and analysis, decision to publish, or preparation of the manuscript. No additional funding received for this study.

Competing Interests: The authors received an unrestricted research grant from Giuliani Pharma Milan, thus they declare a financial competing interest.

* Email: picardo@ifo.it

⬥ These authors contributed equally to this work.

Introduction

Ultraviolet (UV) radiation elicits premature aging of the skin and cutaneous malignancies [1]. UVA rays generate reactive oxygen species (ROS) via photodynamic actions [2], resulting in skin degeneration and aging [3,4] and, in particular, oxidative damage to lipids, proteins, and DNA [5–7]. Moreover, UVA-induced ROS regulate the gene expression of matrix metallo-proteinases (MMPs), which are the main enzymes responsible for dermal extracellular matrix degradation [8–10]. As a result, the incidence of skin photoaging and skin cancer dramatically increases with increased exposure to UVA rays [11]. To protect its structure against UV, skin has developed several defence systems which include pigmentation, antioxidant network and neuro-immune-endocrine functions, which are tightly networked to central regulatory system and are involved in the protection and in the maintenance of global homeostasis, through the production of cytokines, neurotransmitters, neuroendocrine hormones [12]. Thus, UV would stimulate production and secretion of α-melanocyte-stimulating hormone, proopiomelanocortin-derived β-endorphin, adrenocorticotropin, corticotrophin releasing factor, and glucocorticoids [13]. An unbalance between pro-inflammato-ry or anti-inflammatory responses activated by these mediators may be related to cellular degeneration in aged skin.

A way to investigate *in vitro* aging process is the study of cellular senescence, a loss of proliferative capacity attributed to telomere shortening during cell replication or after exposure to pro-oxidant stimuli and closely interconnected with aging, longevity and age-related disease [14,15]. Due to the key role of oxidative stress in the photoaging process, the change of proliferating skin cells to photo-aged cells resembles premature senescence under conditions of artificially increased ROS levels. Consistently, stress-induced premature senescence (SIPS) models can represent useful tools with which to investigate the biological and biochemical mecha-nisms involved in photo-induced skin damage and photocarcino-genesis and to evaluate the potential protective effects of new molecules. SIPS can be induced in human skin dermal fibroblasts (HDFs) by a single subcytotoxic exposure to UVA-activated 8-methoxypsoralen (PUVA) [16], widely used in the treatment of different skin disorders like psoriasis, T-cell lymphoma and other inflammatory skin disorders. We previously reported that oxida-tive stress and cell antioxidant capacity are involved in both the induction and maintenance of PUVA-SIPS and supplementation with low-weight antioxidants abrogated the increased ROS generation and rescued fibroblasts from the PUVA-dependent changes in the cellular senescence phenotype [17]. Moreover, PUVA treatment induced a prolonged expression of interstitial collagenase/MMP-1, leading to connective tissue damage, a hallmark of premature aging [17], confirming this experimental model as a useful tool to investigate in vitro the mechanisms of skin ageing. The function of nuclear receptors has been reported to be involved in the molecular mechanisms controlling the aging process. The peroxisome proliferator-activated receptor (PPAR) family regulates the function and expression of complex gene networks, especially involved in energy homeostasis and inflammation [18–20], and modulate the balance between MMP activity and collagen expression to maintain skin homeostasis [21]. In particular, PPARγ has been implicated in the oxidative stress response, an imbalance between antithetic pro-oxidation and antioxidation, and in this delicate and intricate game of equilibrium, PPARγ stands out as a central player specializing in the quenching and containment of damage and fostering cell survival. Moreover, PPARγ activation has been reported to restore the "youthful" structure and function of mitochondria that are structurally and functionally impaired by excessive oxidant stress [22]. However, PPARγ does not act alone, but is interconnected with various pathways, such as the nuclear factor erythroid 2-related factor 2 (NRF2), Wnt/β-catenin, and forkhead box protein O (FoxO) pathways [23]. PPARγ activation has been reported to be a link to melanocyte differentiation pathways, as suggested by the ability of PPARγ ligands to regulate Microphthalmia-associated transcription factor gene and Wnt/β-catenin levels, promoting differentiation and growth arrest of melanoma cells [24]. Given these features, PPARγ is emerging as an important regulator of skin photodamage.

Among anti-aging agents, topical all-trans-retinoic acid (AtRA) inhibits MMP expression [25] and has a significant diminishing effect on UV-induced photoaging, such as wrinkles, water loss, and reduced wound healing [26]. However, irritant reactions, such as burning, scaling, or dermatitis, limit the acceptance of AtRA by patients [27]. To minimize these side effects, various novel drug delivery systems have been developed; in addition, screening to discover new natural or synthetic retinoid-like molecules has been conducted. Psittacofulvins are a mixture of polyenals identified exclusively in the red plumage of the Ara macao [28], indicating that these compounds are produced at the feather bulb for defense against environmental insults. Parrodienes, congeners of psittaco-fulvins that are considered retinoid-like molecules, as they possess a polyene structure and an alcohol functional group, have been synthesized to investigate the biological effects of psittacofulvins. Studies have shown that parrodienes possess antioxidant [29] and anti-inflammatory activities and are able to inhibit the lipoperox-idation of cell membranes induced by CCl_4 [30]. Among the parrodiene family members, 2,4,6-octatrienoic acid (Octa) pro-motes melanogenesis and antioxidant defense in normal human melanocytes, and its mechanism of action involves the modulation of PPARγ [31]. We added Octa to PUVA-treated HDFs to evaluate Octa's ability to counteract PUVA-SIPS and to investigate whether PPARγ is involved in photo-induced cell senescence.

Materials and Methods

Standards and reagents

Dulbecco's modified Eagle's medium (DMEM), penicillin and streptomycin were purchased from Gibco, Life Technologies Italia, Milan, Italy. Octa was furnished by Giuliani Pharma, Milan, Italy. Crystalline 8-methoxypsoralen (8-MOP), dimethyl-sulfoxide (DMSO), 3-(4,5 dimethylthiazol)-2,5-diphenyl tetrazoli-um bromide (MTT), butylated hydroxytoluene (BHT), 6-hydroxy-2,5,7,8-tetramethylchromane-2-carboxylic acid (Trolox), N-ethyl-maleimide (NEM), thiosalicylic acid (TSA), sodium methoxide, potassium hydroxide (KOH), retinol (ReOH) and all-trans retinoic acid AtRA were from Sigma-Aldrich, Milan, Italy. 2′,7′-dichlor-odihydrofluorescein diacetate ($DCFH_2$-DA) was from Molecular Probes (Eugene, OR, USA). All organic solvents used were of HPLC-grade.

Cell culture and treatments

Human Dermal Fibroblasts (HDFs) were derived from neonatal foreskin of healthy male caucasian individuals (n = 3), phototype III, ranged from 4 to 7 years old and were isolated as previously described [16]. Cells were grown in DMEM supplemented with 10% FBS, penicillin (100 U/ml) and streptomycin (100μg/ml) and used between passage 2 and 8. Institutional Research Ethic committee (Istituti Fisioterapici Ospitalieri) approval was obtained to collect sample of human material for research. The Declaration of Helsinki Principle was followed and due to the fact that the study included children participants their parents gave written informed consent. Stock solutions (10 mM) of Octa was prepared in DMSO. The maximum concentration of Octa, without affecting cell viability or proliferation, was determined by MTT assay and Trypan blue exclusion test (data not shown). Moreover we did not observe any relevant modification of protein content in Octa treated cells (data not shown).

PUVA treatment

8-MOP (25 ng/ml) was added to the cell culture medium overnight. Cell were washed twice with phosphate-buffered saline (PBS) containing 8-MOP 25 ng/ml. HDFs were irradiated at a dose of 6 J/cm^2 using a Bio-Sun irradiation apparatus (Vilbert Lourmat, Marnè-la-Vallée, France) with maximum emission at 365nm in the UVA spectral region (340 to 450 nm). Following irradiation, PBS was replaced by fresh medium which was changed every three days. Octa was diluted in cell culture medium at a final concentration of 2 μM and added to HDFs immediately following PUVA and twice a week thereafter.

Cell morphology

To monitor fibroblast morphology after PUVA treatment, fibroblasts were fixed and stained with Comassie brilliant Blue as previously described [32].

Senescence associated beta-galactosidase (SA-β-gal) staining

SA-β-gal staining was performed as previously described [33]. The proportion of cells positive for SA-β-gal activity are given as percentage of the total number of fibroblasts counted in each dish. Triplicates were performed. The stained dishes were photo-graphed, positive fibroblasts counted and the results expressed as mean ± S.D. of SA-β-gal positive fibroblasts in% of total fibroblast number.

MMP-1 ELISA

MMP-1 total release (proMMP-1, active MMP-1 and MMP-1/TIMP-1 complex) was measured using an Human, Biotrack ELISA immunoassay (Amersham Pharmacia Biotech, Milan, Italy), according to the manufacturer's instructions, and was normalized against protein concentration, determined by Quick Start Bradford Dye Reagent (Bio-Rad, Hercules, CA, USA). The results are the mean ± S.D. of experiments performed in each donor (n = 3) in triplicate.

Determination of ROS generation

The generation of intracellular ROS was determined by employing the cell-permeable fluorogenic probe DCFH-DA. In brief, DCFH-DA is diffused into cells and deacetylated by cellular esterases to non fluorescent $2'$, $7'$-dichlorofluorescin (DCFH), which is rapidly oxidazed to highly fluorescent $2'$, $7'$-dichloro-fluorescein (DCF). The fluorescence intensity of the supernatant was measured with a multiplate reader (DTX 880 Multimode Detector; Beckman Coulter Srl, Milan, Italy) at 485nm excitation and 535 nm emission. Cellular oxidant levels were expressed as relative DCF fluorescence per microgram of protein. The results are the mean ± S.D. of experiments performed in each donor (n = 3) in triplicate.

JC-1 assay for mitochondrial membrane potential

Mitochondrial trans-membrane potential ($\Delta\Psi_m$) was assessed in live HDFs using the lipophilic cationic probe 5,5′,6,6′-tetrachloro-1,1′,3,3′-tetraethylbenzimidazolcarbocyanine iodide (JC-1, Molecular Probes). For quantitative fluorescence measurements, cells were rinsed once after JC-1 staining and scanned with a Flow cytometer (FACS-Calibur, Becton Dickinson, San José, CA, USA) at 485 nm excitation, and 530 and 570 nm emission, to measure green and orange-red JC-1 fluorescence, respectively. Results of experiments performed in each donor (n = 3) in triplicate are expressed as percentage of variation (± SD) respect to control values of the orange-red/green fluorescence intensity ratio.

Catalase (Cat) activity

Fibroblasts were lysed in PBS by repeated freezing and thawing, in the presence of protease inhibitors. Cat activity was determined by spectrophotometric monitoring the rate of disappearance of H_2O_2 at 240 nm [34]. A standard curve was obtained with bovine catalase (Sigma-Aldrich, Srl Milan, Italy). Units were normalized for protein content. Results of experiments performed in each donor (n = 3) in triplicate are given as% of relative units of Cat per mg protein ± S.D.

Biological Antioxidant Potential (BAP) Assay

BAP was measured with a commercially available assay kit (Diacron srl, Grosseto Italy). The principle of the test is to measure the color change upon reduction of Fe^{3+} to Fe^{2+} by the reducing components in the sample. The optical density was measured at 505 nm by a microplate reader. The data were obtained by interpolating the absorbance on a calibration curve obtained with Trolox (30–1000 μM). Results of experiments performed in each donor (n = 3) in triplicate are expressed as medium percentage of variation (± S.D.) respect to control values of untreated cells.

Glutathione (GSH) measurement

GSH levels were determined in cell lysates by high-performance liquid chromatography-mass spectrometry (HPLC-MS) as previously described [35]. The mean value of experiments performed in each donor (n = 3) in triplicate is given as GSH in nmol/mg of total protein ± S.D.

Alpha-tocopherol (α-Toc) analysis

Cells were extracted in hexane:ethanol 3:1 in the presence of γ and δ tocopherol (Sigma-Aldrich, Milan, Italy), as internal standards, and the tocopherols were analysed by gas chromatography-mass spectrometry (GC-MS) as previously described [36]. The mean value of experiments performed in each donor (n = 3) in duplicate is expressed as nanogram per milligram of proteins ± S.D.

Assessment of cell membrane phospholipids polyunsaturated fatty acids

Cell pellets were extracted twice in chloroform/methanol (2:1, v:v) in the presence of tricosanoic acid methyl ester (Sigma Aldrich, Milan Italy), as internal standard. Fatty acids of cell total lipid extract were analysed by GC-MS on a capillary column (FFAP, 60 m×0.32 μm×0.25 mm, Hewlett Packard, Palo Alto, CA, USA), as previously reported [36]. Results of experiments performed in each donor (n = 3) in triplicate are given as mean percentage ± S.D.

Conjugated Dienes

Conjugated diene level was evaluated as described by Kurien and Scofield [37] with modification. Cells were extracted with 3 ml chloroform/methanol (2:1, v/v). After centrifugation at 3,000 rpm for 15 min, 2 ml of organic phase was transferred into another tube and dried at 45°C. The dried lipids were dissolved in 2 ml of methanol and absorbance at 234 nm was determined. It corresponds to the maximum absorbance of the extracted compounds. Results of experiments performed in each donor (n = 3) in triplicate are given as mean percentage ± S.D.

Lipid peroxidation (LP) evaluation

After treatment with PUVA, cells were trypsinized and collected. Suspensions with approximately $1,5\times10^6$ cells ml^{-1} were centrifuged (8000 rpm for 5 min) and the pellet was suspended in 0,5 ml of PBS and extracted twice in chloroform/methanol (2:1, v:v). Measurement of LP was assessed according to the thiobarbituric acid (TBA) method [38] with slight modifications. The spectrum was recorded in the 400–600 nm range showing a maximum at 532 typical for the MDA-TBA complex. Optical density at 532 nm was corrected for background absorption by interpolation. The standard curve was constructed using 1,1,1,3-tetraethoxypropane, after hydrolysis with 1% H_2SO_4, as external standard. The levels of lipid peroxides were expressed as nmol of TBA reactive species (TBARS)/mg protein. The results are the means of three different assays performed in each donor (n = 3).

Analyses of cell membrane cholesterol and oxysterols

HDFs were suspended extracted with methanol containing BHT 100 μM and 5-α-cholestane 100 ng (Sigma-Aldrich, Milan, Italy) as internal standard. Cholesterol (CH) was measured by GC-MS as previously described [39]. Selected ion monitoring (SIM) was carried out by monitoring m/z 329 and 458 for CH, 454 for 7β-OH-cholesterol (7β-OH-CH), 456 for 7-keto-cholesterol (7-keto-CH), 217 and 357 for 5α-cholestane (IS). The mean value of experiments performed in each donor (n = 3) in duplicate is expressed as microgram (for CH) or as nanogram (for 7β-OH-CH and 7-keto-CH) for per milligram of proteins ± S.D.

Western Blot analysis of cell cycle proteins

Samples were lysed in RIPA buffer with protease inhibitors. Aliquotes of cell proteins (30 μg) were resolved on SDS-polyacrilamide gel and transferred to nitrocellulose membrane and then treated with anti-p53 (clone DO-1, Dako, Milan, Italy; diluted 1:3000 in TBS-T), anti p21 (Santa Cruz Biotechnology Inc., Santa Cruz, CA, USA; diluted 1:3000 in TBS-T), anti phospho-p38 (Cell Signaling Technology Inc., Danvers, MA, USA; diluted 1:3000 in TBS-T), or anti IκB-alpha (Santa Cruz Biotechnology Inc., Santa Cruz, CA, USA; diluted 1:1000 in TBS-T) overnight at 4°C. Horseradish-peroxidase-conjugated goat anti-mouse or anti-rabbit immuglobulins (Santa Cruz, Biotechnology

Inc., Santa Cruz, CA, USA) were used as secondary antibodies. Antibodies complexes were visualized using the ECL Chemiluminescence Luminol Reagent (Santa Cruz Biotechnology Inc., Santa Cruz, CA, USA). As a loading control, the blots were reprobed with an anti-β-tubulin or anti- glyceraldehyde-3-phosphate dehydrogenase (GAPDH) antibody (Sigma-Aldrich, Milan, Italy).

RARE Transfection and luciferase assays

Cells were plated in a 24-well plate at a density of 2×10^4 cells/well and left to grow overnight. Afterwards cells were transfected with retinoid responsive element (RARE) reporter, negative control and positive control (CignalTM RARE Reporter Assay Kit; Superarray Bioscience Corp., Frederick, USA). After 24 h, cells were treated with 5μM ReOH for 6 h, 5μM AtRA for 6–48 h, and 4μM Octa for 6–48 h. Measurement of luciferase activity was carried out at the end of the treatments. Cells were harvested in 100 μl of lysis buffer and soluble extracts assayed for luciferase and Renilla activities by using Dual-Luciferase Reporter Assay System (Promega Corp., Madison, USA) according to the manufacturer's procedure.

RNA extraction and real time RT-PCR

Total RNA was isolated using an RNeasy Mini kit (Qiagen, Hilden, Germany). Following DNAse I treatment, cDNA was synthesized from 1 μg of total RNA using ImProm-II Reverse Transcriptase (Promega Corporation, Madison, WI) according to the manufacturer's instructions. Real time RT-PCR was performed with SYBR Green PCR Master Mix (Bio-Rad, Hercules, CA) and 200 nM concentration of each primer. Sequences of all primers used are indicated in Table S1. Reactions were carried out in triplicates using the Real-Time Detection System (iQ5 Bio-Rad, Milan, Italy) supplied with iCycler IQ5 optical system software version 2.0 (BioRad). The thermal cycling conditions comprised an initial denaturation step at 95°C for 3 minutes, followed by 40 cycles at 95°C for 10 seconds and 60°C for 30 seconds. Levels of gene expression in each sample were quantified applying the $2^{-\Delta\Delta C_T}$ method, using GADPH as an endogenous control.

PPARγ transactivation assay

HDFs were transfected with pGL3-(Jwt)3TKLuc reporter construct [40] using Amaxa human fibroblasts Nucleofector kit (Lonza, Basel, Switzerland) according to the manufacturer's instructions. Twenty-four and forty-eight hours after treatment with PUVA ± Octa, cells were harvested and assayed for luciferase activity using Promega's Dual Luciferase (Promega) according to the manufacturer's protocol. The renilla luciferase plasmid was also transfected as an internal control for monitoring transfection efficiency and for normalizing the firefly luciferase activity. The mean value of luciferase activity performed in each donor (n = 3) in duplicate is expressed as fold of the activity ± S.D. obtained in cells treated divided by luciferase activity from non-stimulated cells.

RNA interference experiments

For the RNA interference experiments, HDFs were transfected with 100 pmol (h) siRNA specific for PPARγ (sc-29455; Santa Cruz Biotechnology). An equivalent amount of non-specific siRNA (sc-44234; Santa Cruz Biotechnology) was used as a negative control. Cells were transfected using the Amaxa human fibroblasts Nucleofector kit (Lonza) according to manufacturer's instructions. To ensure identical siRNA efficiency among the plates, cells were transfected together in a single cuvette and plated immediately after nucleofection. Twenty-four hours following

transfection, HDFs were treated with PUVA and post-incubated with 2μM Octa in agreement with the experimental design.

Statistical analysis

Statistically significant differences were calculated using Student's t-test. The minimal level of significance was $p \leq 0.05$.

Results

Identification of a specific PPARγ modulator as a useful tool to study possible interference with PUVA-induced damage

To investigate the role of PPARγ modulation in PUVA-SIPS, we used Octa, a compound we previously reported to activate PPARγ in human melanocytes [31]. Because the chemical structure of Octa resembles the polyene chain of carotenoids, we evaluated the ability of this molecule to modulate the retinoid-mediated signaling in HDFs to study the activation of retinoic acid receptor (RAR) and the subsequent transcriptional activation of RARE. We compared the effects with those caused by the specific retinoid receptor ligands AtRA and ReOH. Both ReOH and AtRA induced an early (6 h) and relevant enhancement of the expression of the RARE-driven reporter, whereas Octa showed a mild capacity to transactivate RARE only after 48 h (Fig. 1A). Moreover, Octa treatment did not exhibit any ability to induce the mRNA expression of cellular retinoic acid binding protein 2 (CRABPII) or cytochrome P450 hydroxylase (CYP26), two genes that contain RARE reporter promoters, which are directly involved in the proliferative response elicited by retinoid-like molecules, whereas atRA induced a relevant up-regulation of both genes (Fig. 1B). In contrast, Octa was more effective than atRA in inducing the expression of PPARγ and fatty acid binding protein-5 (FABP5), a carrier protein for PPAR ligands, at the evaluated time points (6 and 24 h) (Fig. 1C). Consistently, a luciferase assay using the pGL3-(Jwt)TKLuc reporter construct [40] showed that Octa enhanced luciferase expression at 24 and 48 h (Fig. 1D).

PUVA induced a significant reduction of PPARγ expression and activity

A reduction of PPARγ expression in H_2O_2-SIPS HDFs has been reported to reflect age-related inflammation and aging progression [41]. We previously demonstrated that azelaic acid, a natural compound that is able to act as a ligand of PPARγ, was able to revert, at least in part, PUVA-induced decrease in PPARγ activation [42]. To confirm that PPARγ represents a main biological target of PUVA-SIPS, we performed photo-irradiated HDFs RT-PCR analysis and luciferase assay to evaluate the changes in PPARγ expression and/or activity induced by PUVA treatment. Our results showed that PUVA exposure induced an early reduction of PPARγ expression (at 6 and 24 h) as well as a significant decrease in transcriptional activity (at 24 and 48 h) (Fig. 2A and 2B). Octa treatment significantly counteracted the decreased expression and inhibition of PPARγ (Fig. 2C and 2D).

PUVA-induced ROS production and mitochondria damage are counteracted by PPARγ modulation

Exposure of HDFs to PUVA induces mitochondrial membrane damage with a persistent intracellular ROS accumulation [17]. To determine whether PPARγ modulation has a protective effect, ROS generation was determined at 24 h, 48 h, and 1 week after PUVA exposure using the $DCFH_2$-DA assay. PUVA led to a significant time-dependent ROS increase in HDFs, and post-incubation with Octa significantly decreased ($p < 0.01$) ROS

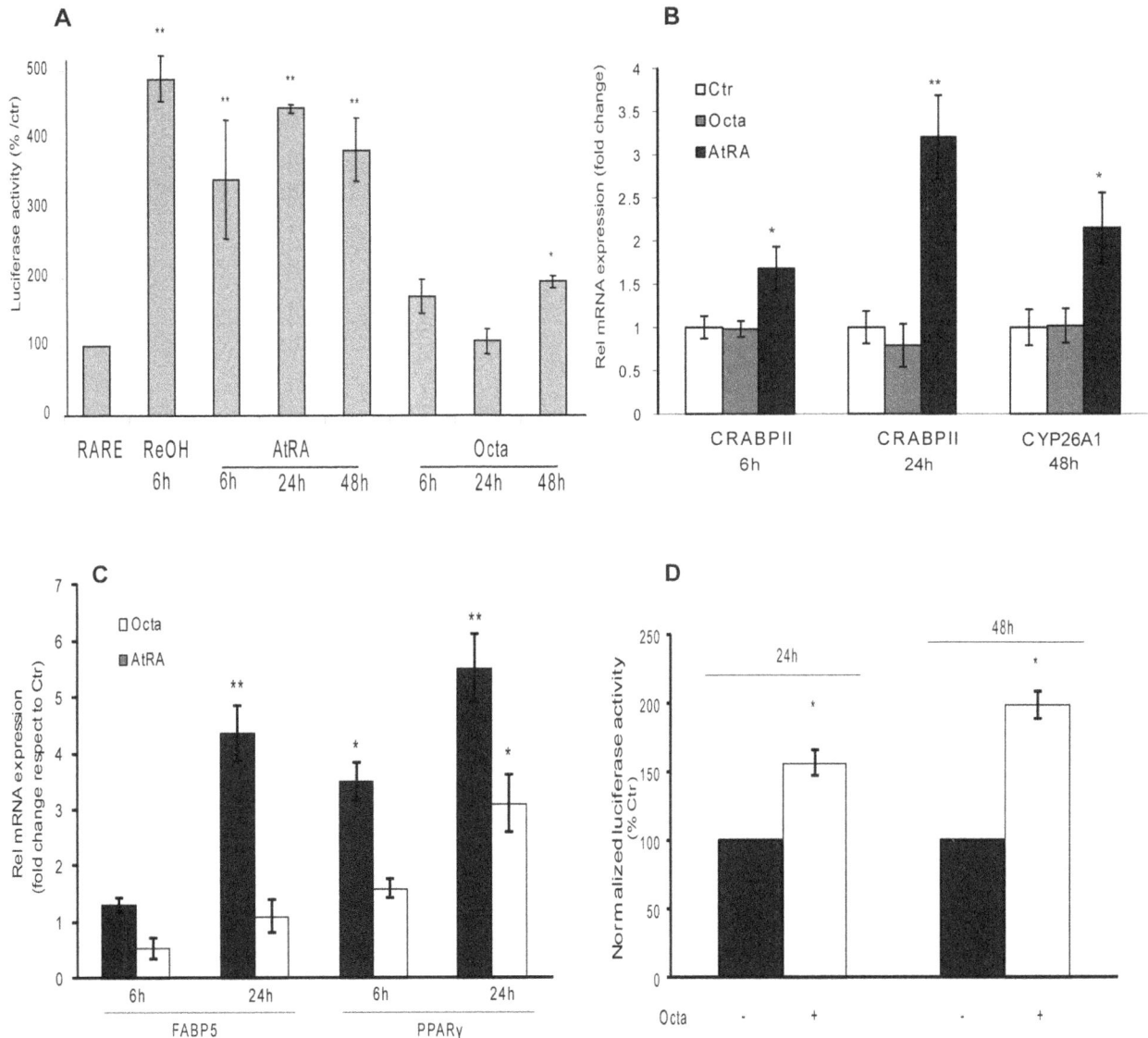

Figure 1. Evidence for Octa-mediated activation of PPARγ-linked signal transduction. (A) Activation of RARE. Cells (2×10^4 cells/well) were plated in a 24-well plate and after 24 h they were transfected with RARE. After 24 h, cells were treated with 5μM ReOH for 6 h, 5μM AtRA for 6–48 h, and 2μM Octa for 6–48 h. Measurement of luciferase activity was assessed as reported in **Materials and Methods**. (B) Quantitative real-time RT-PCR was performed to measure the expression of CRABPII and CYP26A1 mRNA at various time points after treatment with 2μM Octa or 5 μM AtRA. The values were normalized to GAPDH mRNA levels. (C) Quantitative real-time RT-PCR was performed to measure the expression of FABP5 and PPARγ mRNA at various time points after treatment with 2μM Octa or 5μM AtRA. The values were normalized to GAPDH mRNA levels. (D) Luciferase activity analysis of cells transfected with pGL3-(Jwt)3TKLuc reporter construct. After 24 h of transfection, cells were treated with 2μM Octa. The measurement of luciferase activity was carried out 24 h and 48 h after treatment. *p<0.05; **p<0.001 respect to untreated control cells.

production at all evaluated time points (Fig. 3A). ROS generation was correlated with a decrease in mitochondrial $\Delta\Psi_m$ based on JC-1 staining. Consistent with the literature [43], PUVA determined a progressive decline in the ratio of orange-red/green fluorescent JC-1 density compared with sham-irradiated fibroblasts after 24 h, 48 h, and 1 week. PPARγ modulation induced a significant improvement of mitochondrial $\Delta\Psi_m$ (Fig. 3B).

PPARγ modulation counteracted the imbalance of the redox system in PUVA-treated HDF

The PUVA-induced imbalance in the intracellular redox environment was investigated by analyzing the following: a) BAP, an index of overall antioxidant status; b) Cat activity, which

is directly involved in the persistent accumulation of hydrogen peroxide in senescent cells; c) GSH, a major endogenous antioxidant; and d) α-Toc, which protects the cell membrane lipid layer by acting as a chain anti-breaking antioxidant. Because our aim was to investigate the ability of PPARγ modulation to interfere with already activated cell senescence, we did not incubate fibroblasts with Octa before PUVA exposure and we considered untreated fibroblasts as the controls. Up to 1 week, PUVA caused a decline in BAP (p<0.01), GSH levels, and α-Toc content, which were recovered by post-treatment with Octa (Fig. 4A, 4C, 4D). Moreover, PUVA led to a relevant and long-lasting decrease in Cat activity to 50% of the baseline value after 24 h, which was still reduced to 47% after 1 week. Octa protected

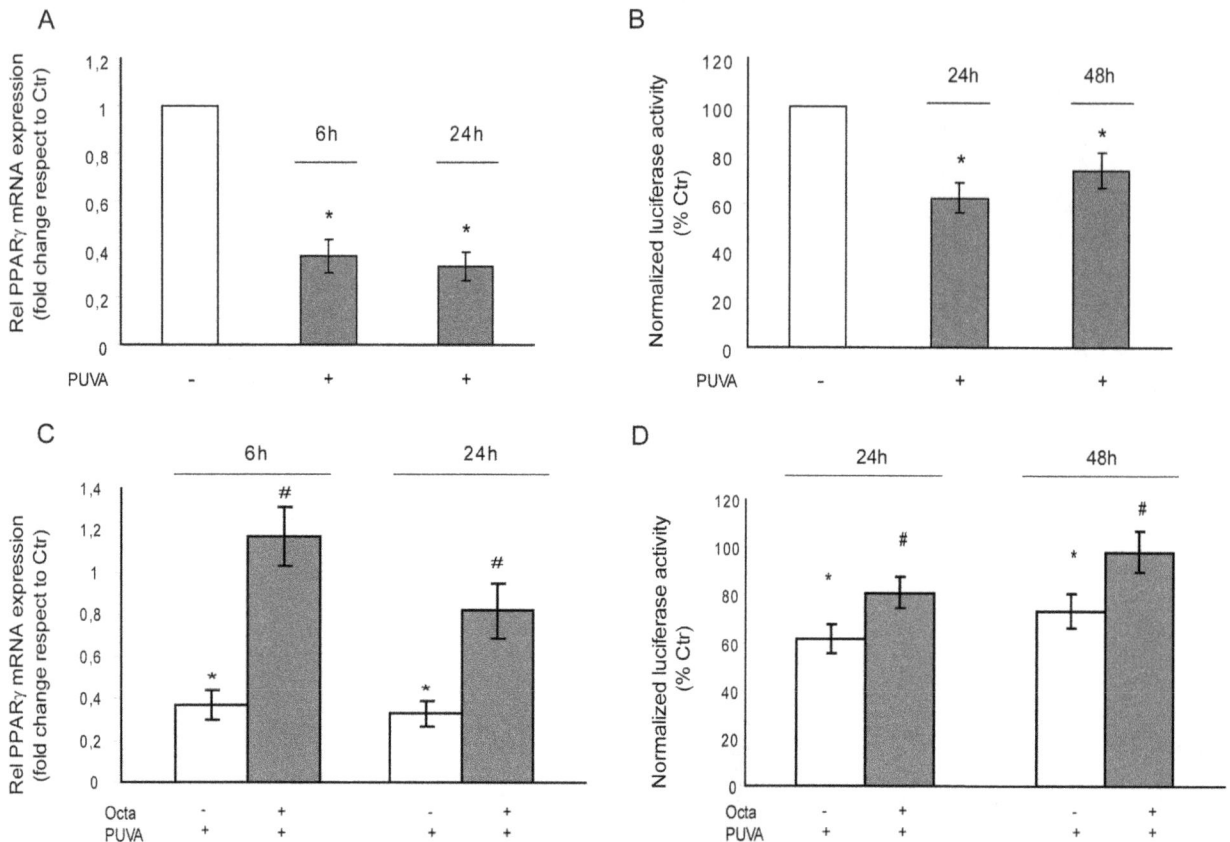

Figure 2. Evaluation of PUVA induced effects on PPARγ expression and activity. (A) Real-time RT-PCR was performed to measure the expression of PPAR-γ mRNA 6 h and 24 h after PUVA exposure. The level of PPAR-γ mRNA was normalized to the expression of GAPDH and is expressed relative to untreated control cells (*$p < 0.05$ respect to Ctr). (B) Luciferase activity analysis of cells transfected with pGL3-(Jwt)3TKLuc reporter construct. After 24 h of transfection, cells were treated with PUVA. The measurement of luciferase activity was carried out 24 h and 48 h after treatment (*$p < 0.05$ respect to Ctr). (C) Real-time RT-PCR was performed to measure the effect of Octa post-treatment on the expression of PPAR-γ mRNA 6 h and 24 h after PUVA exposure. The level of PPAR-γ mRNA was normalized to the expression of GAPDH and is expressed relative to untreated control cells (*$p < 0.05$ respect to Ctr; #$p < 0.05$ respect to PUVA). (D) Luciferase activity analysis of cells transfected with pGL3-(Jwt) 3TKLuc reporter construct. After 24 h of transfection, cells were treated with PUVA and post-incubated with Octa. The measurement of luciferase activity was carried out 24 h and 48 h after treatment (*$p < 0.05$ respect to Ctr; #$p < 0.05$ respect to PUVA).

against enzyme damage, leading to a recovery of Cat activity within 1 week (Fig. 4B).

PPARγ activation is needed to promote cell antioxidant defense

In parallel, we treated non-irradiated fibroblasts with Octa to evaluate its capacity to enhance basal antioxidant defense. Endogenous antioxidants and, in particular, total antioxidant capacity and Cat activity in sham-irradiated cells were significantly increased by supplementation with Octa (Fig. 5A). Considering that PPARγ regulates the expression of catalase via functional PPREs identified in its promoter [44], we investigated the implication of PPARγ in the activation of this endogenous antioxidant by Octa in both sham-irradiated and PUVA exposed HDFs, that were transiently transfected with PPARγ siRNA (siPPARγ) (Fig. 5B). As expected, Octa significantly increased Cat activity in siCtr cells but failed to up-regulate Cat in PPARγ-silenced HDFs (Fig. 5C). Furthermore, in PPARγ-deficient HDFs, Octa failed to counteract the decrease in Cat activity caused by PUVA (Fig. 5C), indicating that the increase in the antioxidant enzyme was PPARγ dependent.

Possible interference of PPARγ against the PUVA-induced modulation of the cellular stress response system

The activation of nuclear factor erythroid-related factor 2 (NRF2) and subsequent induction of NRF2-dependent genes are part of an efficient adaptive response mechanism to electrophilic and oxidant stress, as occurs upon UVA irradiation [45]. Quantitative PCR results indicated that the copy of the cellular NRF2 mRNA increased 2.3 and 5.1-fold, 6 h and 24 h, respectively, after PUVA treatment (Fig. 6A). Cells supplemented with Octa after PUVA exposure showed a significant reduction ($p < 0.01$) of NRF2 mRNA, and no significant modifications of basal level of NRF2 mRNA were observed in HDFs treated with Octa (Fig. 6A). Moreover, NRF2 plays a key role in the UVA-induced up-modulation of heme oxygenase 1 (HO-1), which is considered an immediate cellular response to oxidative insults [46,47]. However, whereas modest HO-1 expression is cytoprotective, the exacerbation of oxidative injury correlates with high HO-1 expression [48]. In HDFs, the basal level of HO-1 expression was low and PPARγ modulation did not induce relevant changes (Fig. 6B). In response to PUVA, HO-1 expression increased significantly in a time-dependent manner up to 40-fold after 24 h (Fig. 6B), indicating a promotion by the persistent oxidative stress, and Octa treatment significantly reduced ($p < 0.001$) this effect.

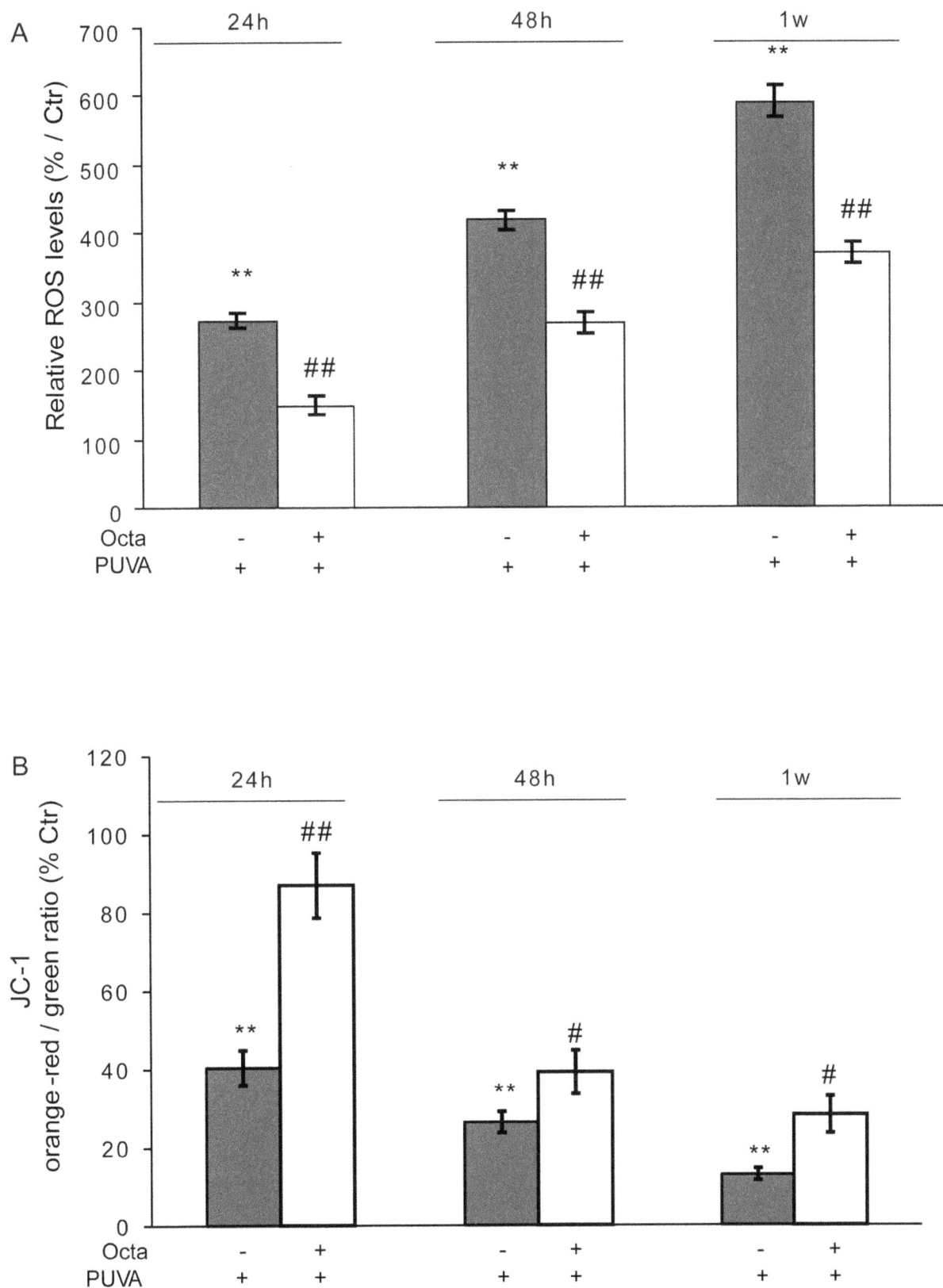

Figure 3. Effects of PPARγ modulation against PUVA-induced intracellular ROS accumulation and mitochondria damage. HDFs were treated with PUVA or left untreated (Ctr). Immediately after irradiation PBS was replaced by fresh medium with or without Octa 2μM for 24 h, 48 h or 1 week. (A) Intracellular oxidative stress was assessed by Flow cytometry using the fluorescent probe DCFH$_2$-DA. The median value of fluorescence was used to evaluate the intracellular content of DCF as a measure of the ROS formation. (B) $\Delta\Psi_m$ was assessed in live HDFs using the lipophilic cationic probe JC-1. For quantitative fluorescence measurements, cells were rinsed once after JC-1 staining and scanned with a Flow cytometer **p< 0.001 statistically different from unirradiated cells; ##p<0.001 compared with PUVA-treated fibroblasts.

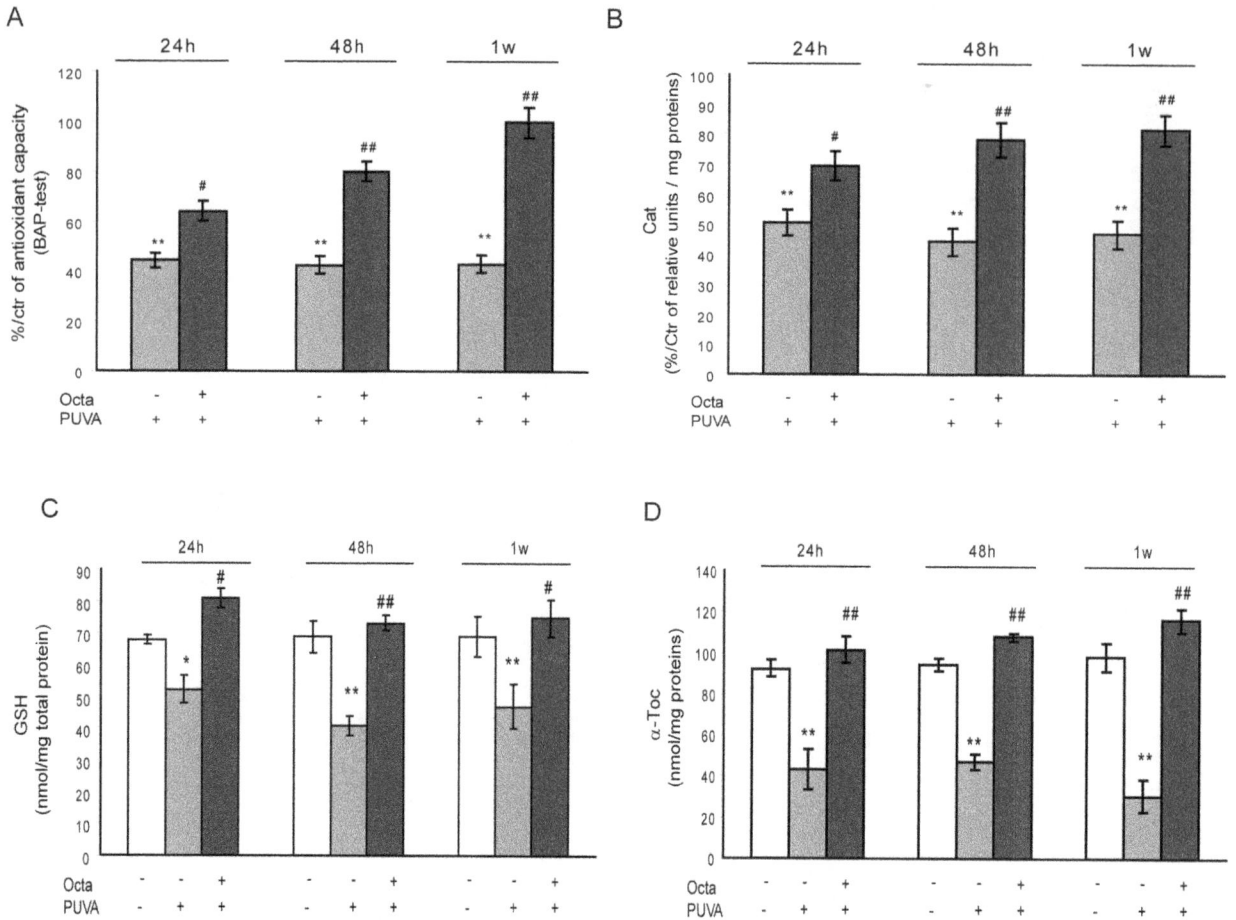

Figure 4. Protective action of PPARγ modulation on PUVA-induced imbalance of cell antioxidant system. HDFs (1×10^6) were lysed in PBS and protease inhibitor cocktail. Cell lysates were used for analytical determinations. (A) Total antioxidant capacity (TAC) was assessed by BAP-test as described under **Materials and Methods** section. (B) Cat enzyme activity was determined by spectrophotometry as described under **Materials and Methods**. (C) GSH concentrations were determined by HPLC-MS as described in **Materials and Methods**. (D) α-Toc is measured by GC-MS as described in **Materials and Methods**. *$p < 0.05$; **$p < 0.001$ respect to control fibroblasts; #$p < 0.05$; ##$p < 0.001$ compared with PUVA-treated fibroblasts.

Consistent with the incapacity of Octa to increase the basal level of NRF2 mRNA, we observed only a slight increase in basal intracellular GSH, which is synthesized by glutamate cysteine ligase, an NRF2-dependent gene (Fig. 6C). As discussed above, PUVA exposure caused a strong and long-lasting GSH depletion and Octa significantly counteracted this effect (Fig. 4C).

The FoxO1 is a transcription factor that is directly involved in cell responses to ROS [49], and it plays a substantial role in skin photoaging [50]. Moreover, a regulatory feedback loop involving PPARγ and FoxO and characterized by a transrepression mechanism has been described [51]. In this set of experiments, PUVA-treated HDFs showed a significant increase in FoxO1a mRNA expression, and PPARγ stimulation was able to reverse this effect (Fig. 6D), suggesting that this molecule promotes an antioxidant defense response by also interfering with the FoxO-induced repression of PPARγ.

PPARγ modulation reduced the senescence-like phenotype in PUVA-treated HDFs

We showed that an altered expression and activity of PPARγ is an early effect determined by PUVA and may be implicated in the appearance of the PUVA-induced cell-senescent phenotype. The

interference of PPARγ in PUVA-induced cell senescence was also investigated by examining its effect on typical senescence features, such as cell morphology, SA-β-gal expression, MMP-1 release, and regulatory cell cycle protein expression. PPARγ modulation was able to rescue, at least in part, the enlarged and flattened senescent fibroblast morphology observed 4 weeks after PUVA exposure (Fig. 7A). SA-β-gal is a β-galactosidase whose activity is detectable at pH 6.0 in cultured cells undergoing replicative or induced senescence but whose activity is absent from proliferating cells [33]. In HDFs exposed to PUVA, SA-β-gal activity was detected after 1 week followed by a steady increase up to 4 weeks, when virtually all of the fibroblasts exhibited *de novo* activity of SA-β-gal (insert in Fig. 7B). The total number of cells was not significantly different, but the percentage of SA-β-gal-positive fibroblasts was significantly suppressed (approximately 40%) by post-treatment with Octa (Fig. 7B). In HDFs, PUVA induced a strong and persistent release of MMP-1, the main metalloproteinase induced by UV exposure [52,53], with a maximum at 48 h after photo-irradiation and an approximately 10-fold (SE ± 0.42) higher amount compared to that of non-irradiated control cells (Fig. 7C). Octa caused a mild but significant decrease of MMP-1 release with a maximum reduction of 21% at 48 h (Fig. 7C);

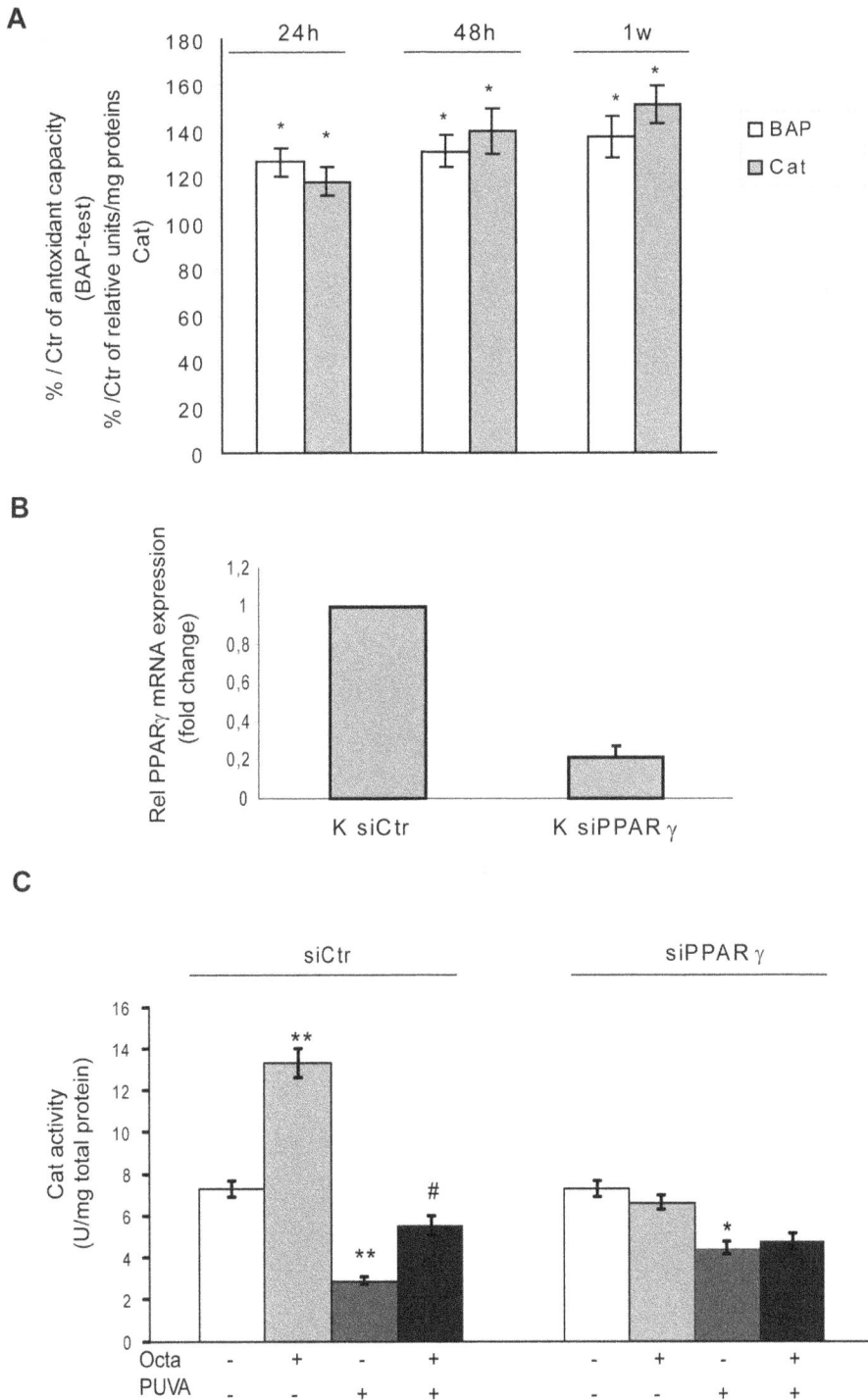

Figure 5. Evidence for PPARγ-induced promotion of cell antioxidant defence. (A) Octa treatment for 24 h, 48 h and 1 week determined a significant increase of antioxidant cell response. TAC was assessed by BAP-test and Cat enzyme activity was determined by spectrophotometry as described under **Materials and Methods** section. (B) HDFs were transfected with siRNA specific for PPARγ (siPPARγ) or non-specific siRNA (siCtr). PPARγ level was evaluated by real-time RT-PCR (C) The activity of Cat was assessed in HDFs transfected with siPPARγ or siCtr and exposed to 2μM Octa for 6 h. In parallel Cat activity was measured in HDFs transfected with siPPARγ or siCtr and exposed to PUVA w/o post-incubation with 2μM Octa. *p<0.05; **p<0.001 respect to control fibroblasts; #p<0.05 compared with PUVA-treated fibroblasts.

however, it had no effect on the basal secretion of MMP-1 (data not shown). Growth arrest is an important feature of cellular senescence and stress-induced premature senescence. We observed a strong expression of p53 and p21 proteins starting from 24 h

after PUVA that was still elevated after 1 week (Fig. 7D). p53 and p21 were not detectable in untreated and Octa-treated control cells. Octa significantly reversed the up-regulation of p53 protein expression after 24 h and p21 after 1 week (0.65-fold and 0.7-fold

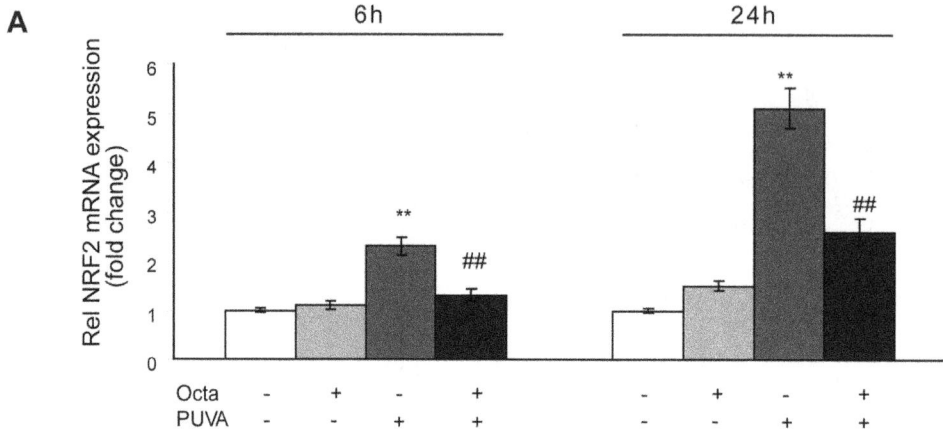

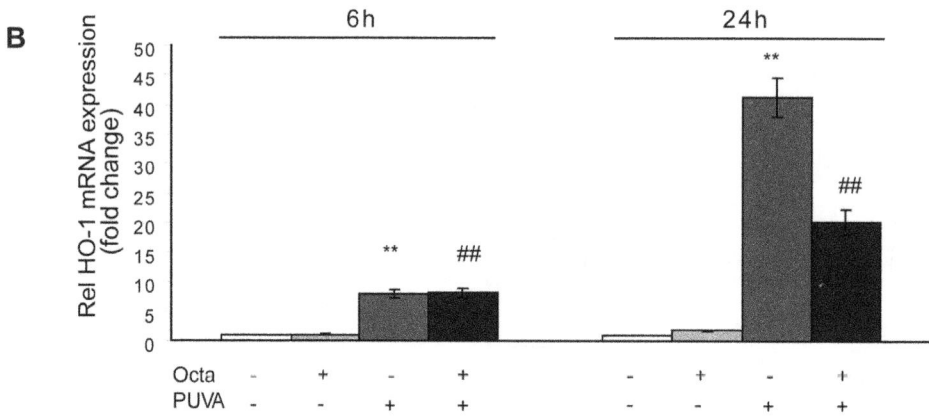

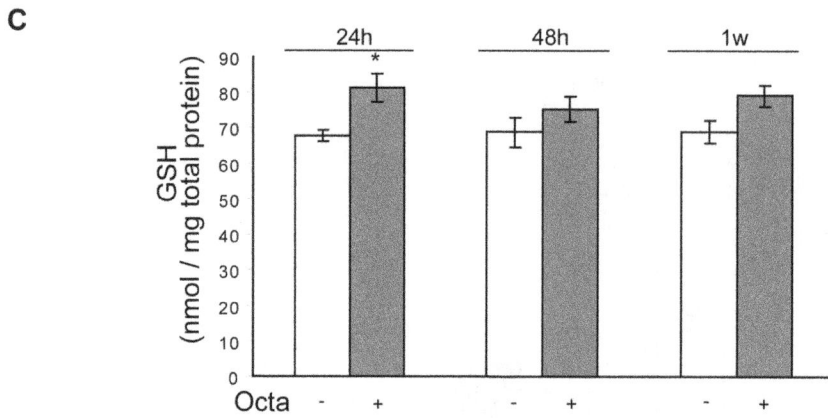

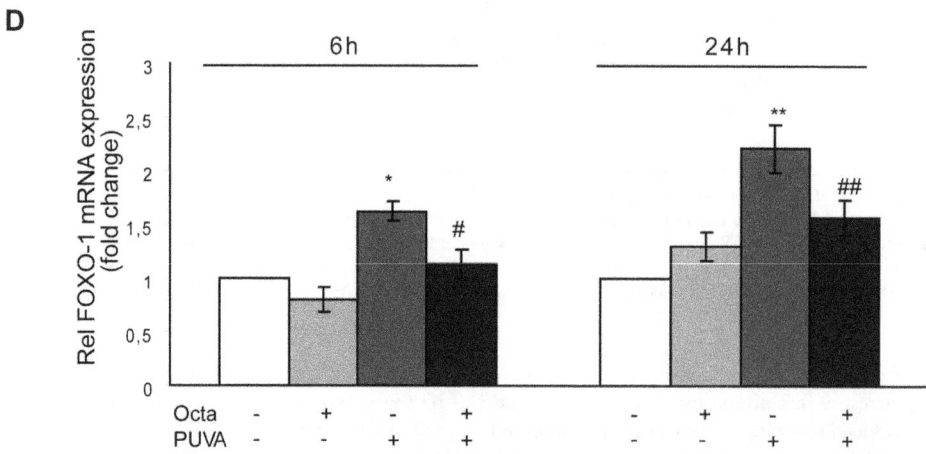

Figure 6. Possible interference of PPARγ against PUVA induced modulation of the cellular stress response system. (A) RT-PCR was performed to measure the expression of NRF2 mRNA 6 and 24 h after PUVA exposure, w/o Octa post-incubation. The level of NRF2 mRNA was normalized to the expression of GAPDH and is expressed relative to untreated control cells (**p<0.001 respect to Ctr; ##p<0.001 compared with PUVA-treated fibroblasts). (B) RT-PCR was performed to measure the expression of HO-1 mRNA 6 and 24 h after PUVA exposure, w/o Octa post-incubation. The level of HO-1 mRNA was normalized to the expression of GAPDH and is expressed relative to untreated control cells (**p<0.001 respect to Ctr; ##p<0.001 compared with PUVA-treated fibroblasts). (C) GSH concentrations were determined by HPLC-MS as described in **Materials and Methods** (*p<0.05 respect to control fibroblasts). (D) RT-PCR was performed to measure the expression of FoxO1 mRNA 6 and 24 h after PUVA exposure, w/o Octa post-incubation. The level of FoxO1 mRNA was normalized to the expression of GAPDH and is expressed relative to untreated control cells. *p<0.05 respect to control fibroblasts; #p<0.05 compared with PUVA-treated fibroblasts.

compared to PUVA-treated samples, respectively) (Fig. 7D). In addition, we detected a moderate expression of p16 in PUVA-treated cells, but Octa post-treatment did not induce a significant reduction (data not shown).

PPARγ modulation interferes with changes in cellular membrane lipids in PUVA-treated HDFs

Unsaturated lipids in cell membranes, including phospholipids and cholesterol, are well-known targets of oxidative modification, which can be induced by a variety of stresses, including UVA-induced photodynamic stress. To evaluate the modifications of the plasma membrane induced by PUVA oxidative damage, we assessed the content of polyunsaturated fatty acids of membrane phospholipids (Pl-PUFA) and the level of CH as the main lipid component of raft domains of cell membranes. PUVA induced a significant modification of the fatty acid composition of cell membrane lipids, with a strong reduction in the Pl-PUFA percentage, which was detectable immediately after irradiation (data not shown) and was still reduced at 1 week (Fig. 8A); this was accompanied a bi-modal alteration in the CH level, with an early (up to 48 h) reduction followed by a relevant accumulation 1 week after photo-irradiation (Fig. 8B). PUVA-induced lipid alterations were almost completely reversed by Octa (Fig. 8A and 8B). Moreover, we evaluated the formation of oxidative products, such as conjugated dienes, fatty acid hydroperoxides, TBARS, and oxysterols (7β-hydroxycholesterol (7-β-OH-CH) and 7-ketocholesterol (7-Keto-CH)), in photo-irradiated cells. PUVA-treated HDFs showed a time-dependent accumulation of lipid peroxidation products. In particular, conjugated dienes were the early products of PUVA-induced lipoperoxidation, and their levels peaked after 3 h (Fig. 8C), whereas both TBARS and oxysterols constantly increased up to 1 week after photo-irradiation (Fig. 8D, 8E, and 8F). Octa significantly reduced the PUVA-induced generation and accumulation of these cell membrane oxidation products (Fig. 8C, 8D, 8E, and 8F). Interestingly, oxysterols were reported to induce the expression of p21 and modulation of the phosphorylation signaling involved in the activation of nuclear factor κB (NF-κB), a transcription factor involved in the induction of pro-inflammatory cytokines. [54]. Considering that these processes are implicated in the aging process and age-related inflammatory responses, we hypothesize that the Octa-mediated reduction of oxysterols plays a key role in the disruption of PUVA-SIPS by Octa.

PPARγ interfered with the PUVA-induced phosphorylation pathway and NF-kB activation

The UV-induced inflammatory process in the skin is characterized by ROS-mediated phosphorylation of mitogen-activated proteins kinases (MAPKs), including p38 kinase, and the subsequent activation of NF-κB, To determine the alterations of the phosphorylation pathway and NF-κB activation in the PUVA-SIPS model and the possible protective effect of PPARγ modulation, phosphorylation of p38 and expression of IκBα were

evaluated by Western Blot. PUVA-treated HDFs showed an increased phosphorylation of p38 (Fig. 9A) and a decreased expression of IκBα (Fig. 9B), indicating that the activation of the pro-inflammatory response is involved in the senescence-like phenotype. Octa post-treatment inhibited p38 phosphorylation and decreased IκBα expression at 24 h and 48 h after PUVA treatment, respectively (Fig. 9A and 9B). The ability of Octa to interfere with the PUVA-induced activation of the phosphorylation pathway and the activation of NF-κB at later time points compared to its effects on PPARγ activation and generation of cell membrane lipid peroxidation products suggests that p38 and NF-κB are not direct targets of Octa, but they can be modified by the Octa-induced activation of PPARγ and a reduction of the ROS-induced lipoperoxidation process.

Discussion

PUVA-SIPS is characterized by the persistent induction of ROS and stable alteration of the cell redox system inducing robust aging markers, including morphological changes, increased staining of SA-β galactosidase, and MMP-1 release, thereby representing a suitable tool for the analysis of photoaging-related mechanisms *in vitro* [17]. The imbalance of the antioxidant network is crucial for propagating PUVA-induced oxidative stress, as demonstrated by the ability of antioxidant molecules to counteract the phenomenon [17], most likely not exclusively due to scavenging ROS but also to the modulation of cell signaling pathways.

To further investigate the mechanism mediating the imbalance of the cell-redox system, we focused on possible cell targets and transcription factors involved in the induction of PUVA-SIPS. We previously reported that azelaic acid, a modulator of PPARγ, interfered with PUVA-induced cell responses, and here we sought to determine whether this nuclear receptor represents a "conductor" of PUVA-SIPS. PPARs regulate the expression of genes involved in multiple biological pathways, including cellular lipid metabolism, inflammation, differentiation, and proliferation [18–20]. Therefore, these nuclear receptors are possible regulators of mitochondrial functions, inflammatory responses, and antioxidant imbalances observed in premature cell senescence. Reduced activity of the proteins PPARγ coactivator-1α (PGC-1α) and PPARγ coactivator-1β (PGC-1β), which are master regulators of PPARγ, is associated with mitochondrial dysfunction and reduced expression of numerous ROS-detoxifying enzymes [22]. We investigated the possible interplay among PPARγ modulation and the PUVA-induced senescence-like phenotype by employing Octa, a polyunsaturated acid with retinoid-like molecular features. Despite its reported features in common with retinoids [29], the molecule caused only a weak activation of RARE and was not associated with the modulation of RA target genes, such as CYP26, which is a cytochrome P450 isoenzyme that specifically metabolizes RA [55], or CRABPII, which transports retinoids to the nucleus [56]. In contrast, Octa significantly activated PPARγ and FABP5, which is an intracellular protein that binds lipid molecules and transports them to PPARs [57]. Consistent with the

A

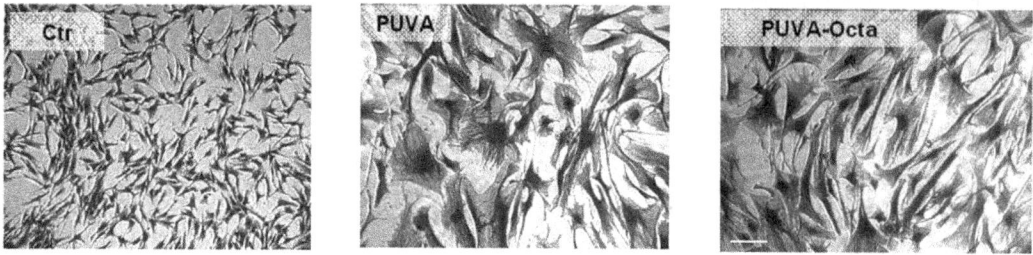

B

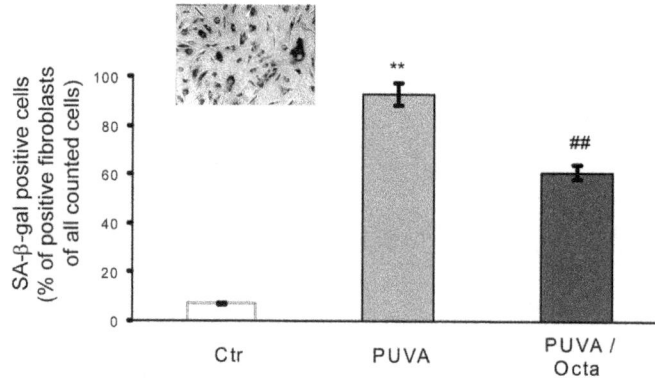

C

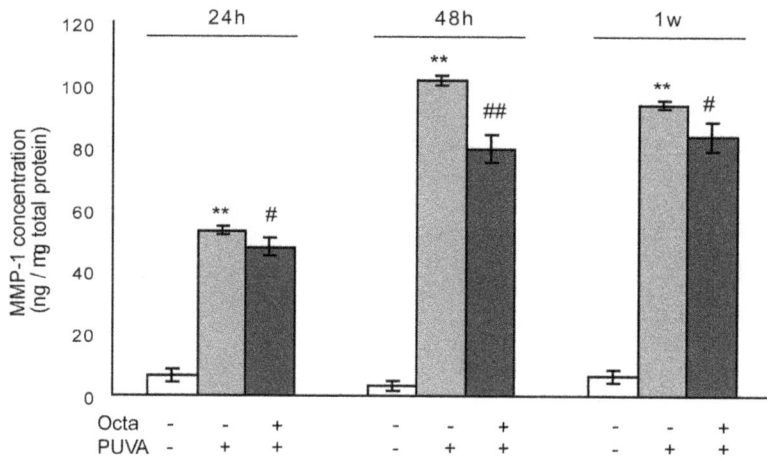

D

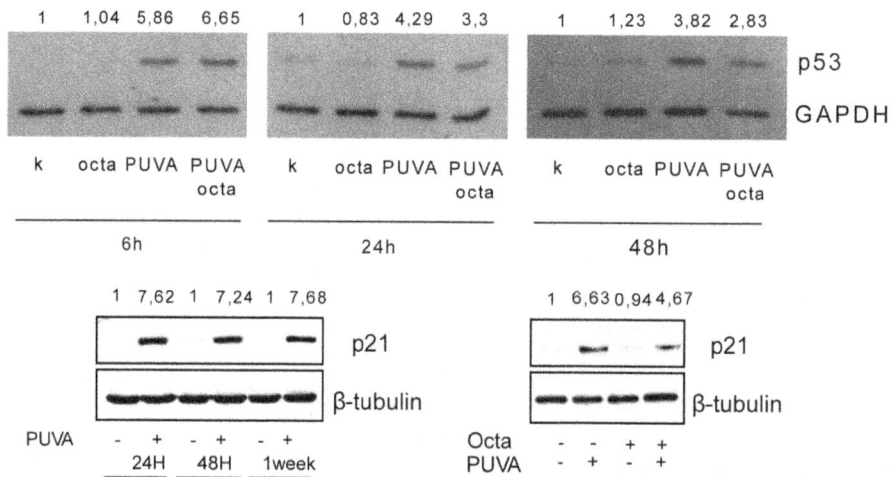

Figure 7. Effect of PPARγ modulation on PUVA-induced expression of senescence-like phenotype in HDFs. After PUVA treatment, HDFs were cultured in the absence or in the presence of 2μM Octa. The medium was changed every 3 days to ensure efficient antioxidant capacity. (A) To evaluate fibroblast morphology, 2 weeks after PUVA in the absence or presence of Octa treatment, cells were fixed and stained with Comassie Brilliant Blue. Scale bar 50 μm. (B) SA-β-gal expression was detected as described in **Materials and Methods**. The *inset* represents fibroblasts after PUVA-treatment revealing a senescent phenotype with enlarged cytoplasmic morphology and SA-β-gal expression. The number of SA-β-gal positive fibroblasts is shown as mean ± SD of three independent experiments. **p<0.001 as compared with mock treated controls; ##p<0.001 as compared with PUVA-treated fibroblasts. (C) Supernatants were collected from mock-treated fibroblasts, at 24 h, 48 h and 1 week post PUVA-treatment. MMP-1 release was assessed by ELISA-kit. Three independent experiments in each donor (n=3) were performed to determine specific MMP-1 protein concentrations in the supernatants. **p<0.001 as compared with mock-treated fibroblasts; #p<0.05; ##p<0.001 as compared with PUVA-treated fibroblasts. (D) Total cellular proteins (30μg/lane) were subject to 10% SDS-PAGE. Variation of protein loading was determined by reblotting membrane with an anti-β-tubulin antibody. Western Blot assays are representative of at least three experiments. Increase of p53 and p21 proteins expression is remarkable 24 h after irradiation as well as until 7 days. Octa treatment decreased PUVA-induced expression of p53 protein (at 24 and 48 h) and of its target gene p21 (at 1 week).

results reported for H_2O_2-SIPS [41], PUVA-treated HDFs showed an immediate decrease in the expression and activity of PPARγ, indicating a relevant role of this receptor in the biological modifications induced by senescence-like phenotype. Octa mitigated the PUVA effects, indicating that PPARγ modulation may be responsible for the protective mechanism. Because PPARγ promotes mitochondrial function and endogenous antioxidants, we evaluated the effects of the nuclear receptor modulation against PUVA-induced damage to these cellular targets. Mitochondrial oxidative stress, characterized by the reduction of the oxidative phosphorylation efficiency and $\Delta\Psi_m$, promotes the senescence of skin cells both *in vitro* [58] and *in vivo* [59]. In PUVA-treated HDFs, we observed a progressive accumulation of intracellular ROS and a decline in $\Delta\Psi_m$, indicating that mitochondria are involved in the senescence-like phenotype. However, the excessive ROS generation induced by PUVA overwhelmed the cell redox system. Because antioxidant enzymes are themselves targets of oxidative modifications [60], PUVA-SIPS mimics the alterations observed in photoaged cells [61]. In particular, PUVA-treated HDFs showed a dramatic decline in Cat activity and a significant reduction in intracellular GSH, which are both critical for preserving cellular redox balances, with a very low recovery to basal values. Despite the reported antioxidant action of Octa [29], the compound reduced but did not abrogate PUVA-induced intracellular ROS accumulation and the alteration of mitochondrial integrity, suggesting that scavenging ability is only partly involved in the protective effect of Octa. Octa treatment promoted the increase of both Cat activity and GSH levels in both untreated and PUVA-exposed HDFs, interfering with their biosynthetic pathways.

PPARγ is directly involved in the regulation of the expression of Cat via functional PPREs identified in its promoter [44], and the activation of PPARγ by Octa was functionally relevant for the induction of catalase activity, as the use of a specific PPARγ siRNA abolishes this effect. Moreover, silencing the PPARγ receptor significantly reduced the PUVA-induced decrease in Cat activity and completely abrogated the protection of Octa against this damage.

PPARγ regulates antioxidant defense and counteracts mitochondrial damage in close connection with other transcription factors involved in the oxidative stress response [23]. In the activation of cellular defense against the oxidative stress antioxidant response, PPARγ cooperates with NRF2, a transcription factor that regulates the expression of antioxidant genes, including HO-1 and the glutamate cysteine ligase, which is the rate-limiting enzyme for the cellular biosynthesis of GSH [23]. PUVA induced an increased expression of NRF2, indicating the attempt of the cells to activate an adaptive response against oxidative stress. Among the target genes of NRF2, HO-1 acts as a general marker of oxidative stress [47]. The activation by UVA is an emergency

stress response that results in the clearance of excess heme levels. However, HO-1 overexpression has deleterious consequences if the excess free heme is not quickly catabolized [48]. The balance of expression is particularly delicate for UVA, which itself damages heme-containing proteins and releases labile iron. Moreover, the induction of HO-1 by the ROS-generating system occurs in association with the depletion of intracellular GSH and may be enhanced by the chemical depletion of GSH [62,63]. Octa significantly reduced NRF2 and HO-1 mRNA expression in PUVA-treated HDFs, suggesting an attempt to interrupt the persistent activation of detoxifying genes, which may indicate a compromised redox homeostasis in photo-irradiated cells. Although the mRNA expression of NRF2 was increased in photo-irradiated cells, a stable decline in intracellular GSH was observed, whereas Octa effectively counteracted this damage, indicating its ability to promote the maintenance of the NRF2 signaling pathway, leading to the up-modulation of the GSH level. These findings strongly suggest a relationship between NRF2 and PPARγ in the PUVA-induced senescence-like phenotype. However, the mechanisms that regulate the reciprocal feedback circuit between these transcription factors require further investigation. Moreover, PPARγ acts at an intersection of the intracellular signaling pathways activated by FoxO1, a transcription factor that plays a pivotal role in cell fate decisions because it regulates and is regulated by oxidative stress [49]. FoxO1 may modulate PPARγ at the mRNA and protein levels [51], acting as a transcriptional repressor binding to the PPARγ promoter [64] and reducing PPARγ activity through a transrepression mechanism that involves a direct protein-protein interaction [65]. Octa decreases the PUVA-induced nuclear concentration of FoxO1, ROS accumulation, and mitochondrial damage, suggesting an interference with the regulatory feedback loop between PPARγ and FoxO proteins. Moreover, due to their ability to cross talk with the p53 tumor suppressor gene, FoxOs can participate in ROS-induced cell cycle arrest, a typical feature of cell senescence [50]. PUVA activates p53 stabilization, phosphorylation, and nuclear localization as well as the induction of p21 (Waf/Cip1), which is needed for the entry into the growth arrest state [66,67]. Octa interfered with the increase of p53 and p21, interrupting the positive axis between FoxO1 and cell cycle proteins. The evidence that the molecule did not interfere with immediate (up to 6 h) PUVA-induced ROS generation (data not shown) and p53 expression indicates that scavenger ability is not relevant for Octa interference with the senescence-like phenotype. In contrast, the compound effectively counteracted typical features of PUVA-induced cell senescence, such as enlarged cell shape, the up-modulation of MMPs and the subsequent malfunction of the connective tissue remodeling process, and a steady increase in SA-β-gal expression, suggesting that the up-modulation of PPARγ can effectively contribute to its "anti-senescence" action.

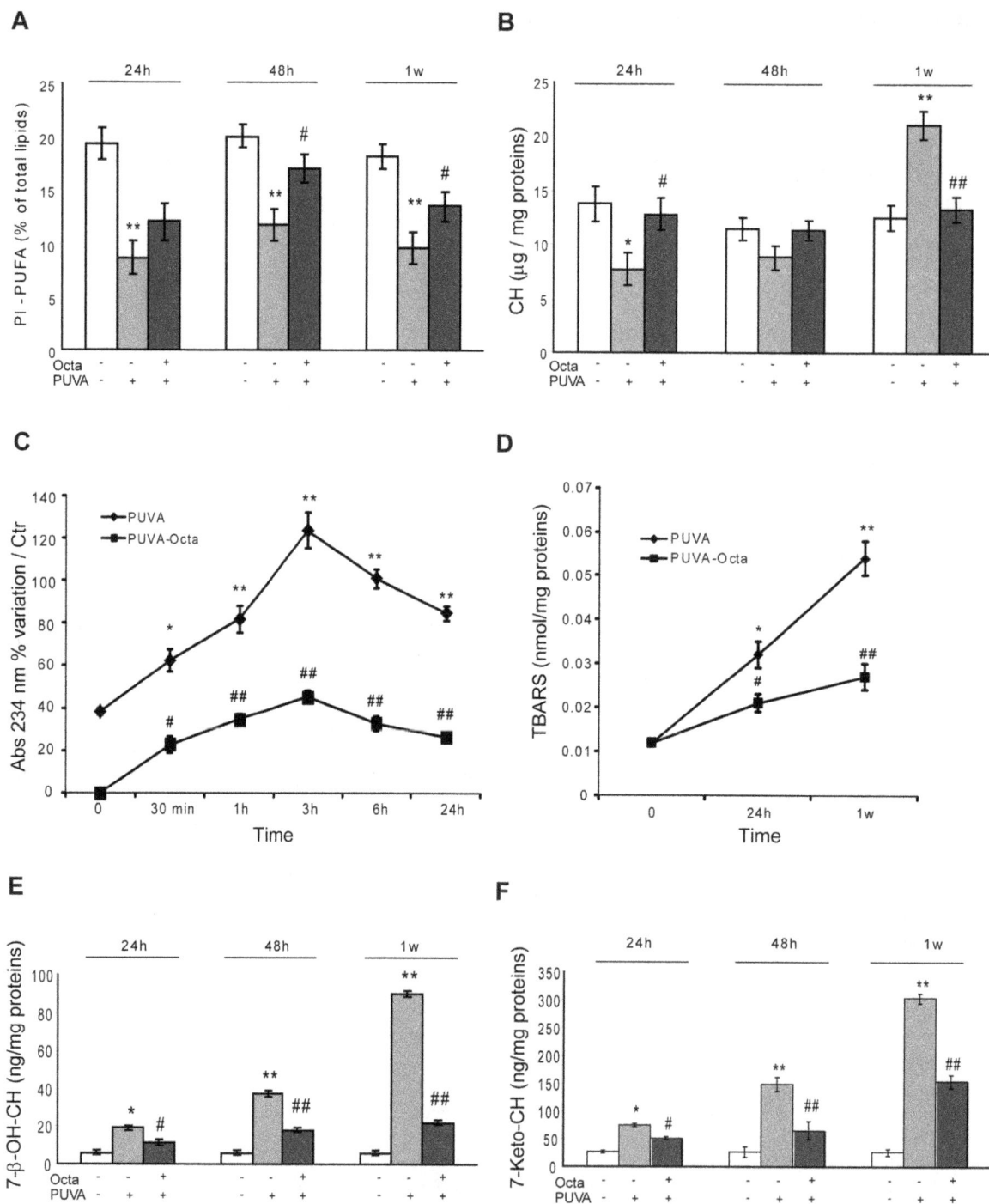

Figure 8. Octa counteracts alteration of lipid cell membrane homeostasis in PUVA treated HDFs. (A) Polyunsaturated fatty acids of membrane phospholipids (Pl-PUFA) in PUVA-treated HDFs were assessed GC-MS as described in **Materials and Methods**. (B) Chol content was analyzed by GC-MS as described in **Materials and Methods**. (C) Early lipid peroxidation products were assessed by the spectrophotometric evaluation of conjugated diene levels as described in **Materials and Methods**. (D) End products of lipid peroxidation were measured according to TBA assay as described in **Materials and Methods**. (E) and (F) Chol oxidation was evaluated by assessing 7β-OH-CH and 7-keto-CH as described in **Materials and Methods**. *p<0.05; **p<0.001 respect to control fibroblasts; #p<0.05; ##p<0.001 compared with PUVA-treated fibroblasts.

Since PPARγ is a key player in lipid metabolism and because damage to cellular lipids is involved in the imbalance of the antioxidant network, we investigated the consequences of PUVA treatment for lipid composition and the possible interference of Octa against this damage. Among the cell compartments, membrane phospholipids play a causal role in the aging process by modulating oxidative stress and molecular integrity [68,69]. 8-MOP can permeate cell membranes and establish photochemical cross-links between its furan or pyrone ring and unsaturated lipid molecules [70], and the subsequent UVA exposure disturbs the

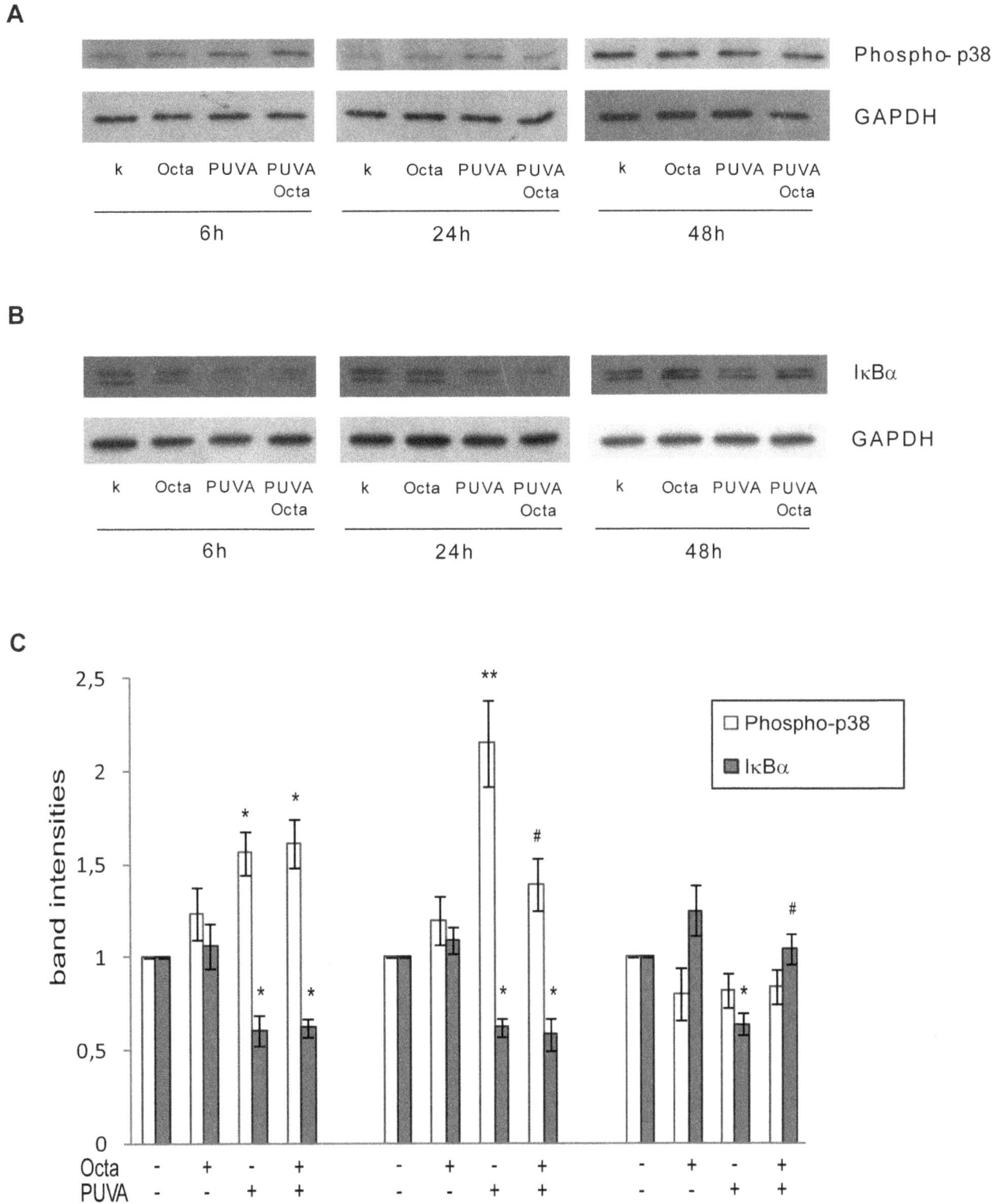

Figure 9. PPARγ interference with PUVA-induced phosphorylation pathway and NF-κB activation. Total cellular proteins (30μg/lane) were subject to 10% SDS-PAGE. Variation of protein loading was determined by reblotting membrane with an anti-GADPH antibody. PUVA-treated HDFs showed an increased phosphorylation of p38 (A) and a decreased expression of IkBα (B). Octa post-treament inhibited p38 phosphorylation (A) as well as decrease of IkBα expression (B) 24 h and 48 h after PUVA treatment, respectively. (C) Densitometric scanning of band intensities obtained from two separate experiments performed in each donor were used to quantify change of protein expression (control value taken as 1-fold in each case). *p<0.05; **p<0.001 respect to control fibroblasts; #p<0.05 compared with PUVA-treated fibroblasts.

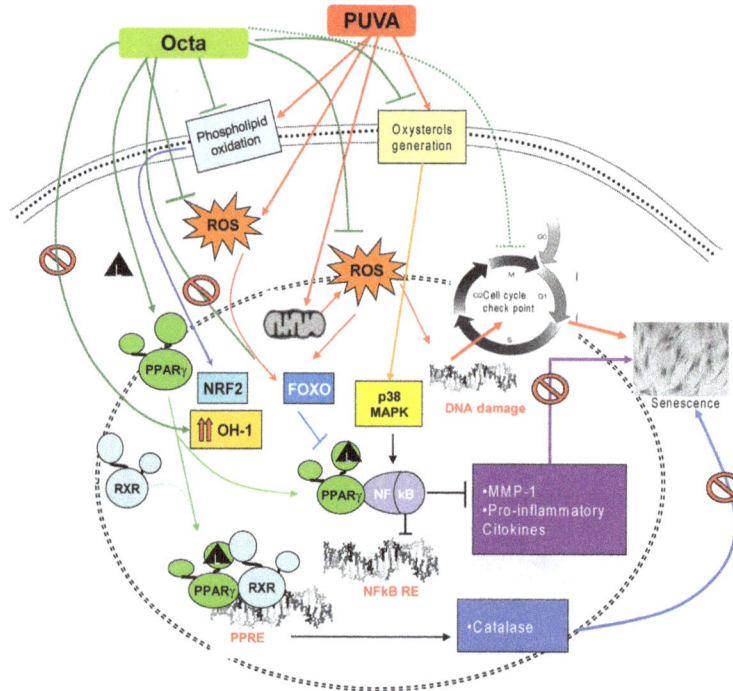

Figure 10. Summary scheme of possible role of PPARγ modulation in counteracting PUVA-SIPS of HDFs. PUVA exposure induced intracellular generation of ROS, alteration of mitochondria function, activation of antioxidant stress response and MAPK phosphorylation pathway, dysregulation of membrane lipid metabolism, DNA-oxidative damage and altered expression of cell cycle regulators. PPARγ modulation by Octa may counteract PUVA-induced senescence-like phenotype. Moreover, Octa ability to reduce phospholipid oxidation and oxysterol generation contributes to the reduction of PUVA-induced inflammatory response and redox imbalance.

integrity of HDF membrane lipids, as demonstrated by the early and permanent decrease in the Pl-PUFA content and the relevant generation of both early and end-products of lipid peroxidation. The oxidative products of cellular lipids diffuse in the cytosol, interacting with intracellular organelles and determining a propagation of the oxidative stress reaction. Phospholipid oxidation products have been reported to activate NRF2 and HO-1 as a compensatory reaction of cells against oxidative stress [71]. However, the accumulation of lipoperoxidation products induced by PUVA can lead to an excessive over-expression of HO-1, shifting the emergency stress response to a deleterious effect against the cell structure. Therefore, the Octa-induced reduction of PUVA-induced phospholipids oxidation products may contribute to the regulation of NRF2 and HO-1 and the subsequent preservation of cell integrity. In addition to phospholipids, CH plays an indispensable role in regulating the properties of cell membranes and the fluidity and the integrity of lipid rafts [72,73]. CH accumulation has been observed in fibroblasts obtained from aged skin [74] as well as *in vitro* senescent cells [75]. The pro-oxidant effect of PUVA caused an early decrease in CH and the immediate generation of oxysterols, peroxidation products of CH metabolism representing reliable markers of oxidative stress *in vivo* [76]. Moreover, the stable appearance of the senescence-like phenotype was associated with a time-dependent accumulation of CH and oxysterols. The observed effect of PUVA on CH metabolism prompted us to investigate the role of PPARγ in controlling the activation of the inflammatory response by chronic oxidative stress which is associated with the induction of cell senescence. The age-related inflammatory chronic state has been associated with a reduction of PPARγ function and an increased generation of oxysterols, which act as secondary messengers in

MAPK signaling pathways [77], an important component of the pathway that regulates cellular senescence as well as the inflammatory response [78]. PUVA-SIPS was characterized by a progressive generation of oxysterols and the up-modulation of phosphorylation signaling involved in NF-κB activation and, in particular, the increase in phosphorylated p38 and the decrease in IκBα, leading to NF-κB activation. In PUVA-exposed cells, the ability of Octa to counteract the accumulation of oxysterols and the changes in the level of CH may contribute to the observed interference with the phosphorylation pathway. It has been suggested that oxysterols act as signaling molecules [79] by influencing lipid membrane integrity as well as the structure and function of PPAR and RXR receptors and their subsequent modulation of the antioxidant response and inflammation [80]. Therefore, PUVA-SIPS contributes to the identification of how biochemical modulators are integrated in the induction of the chronic inflammation state that is typical of aged skin and provides new insights in the activation of nuclear receptors as novel therapeutic approaches for photo-aging (Fig. 10).

Conclusions

Taken together, our data suggest that PUVA-SIPS involves a complex interplay of various cellular transcription factors activated by sustained and long-lasting oxidative stress. Mitochondria are the most probable cell targets, and the modulation of PPARγ provides relevant insights into the mechanism of PUVA-SIPS. The reciprocal influences of PUVA-induced signaling pathways have been investigated by employing Octa due to its ability to increase the trans-activation of PPARγ by acting as a partial agonist and interfering with ROS-dependent cellular signaling mechanisms. Interestingly, Octa counteracts certain molecular markers of

PUVA-SIPS by improving physiological defense mechanisms without significant changes to the cell redox environment.

Supporting Information

Table S1   List of primers used for quantitative real time PCR. Sequences of primers indicated with an F correspond to sense strands and with an R correspond to anti-sense.

Acknowledgments

The pGL3-(Jwt)3TKLuc reporter construct was kindly provided by Dr R. Ballotti and Dr S. Rocchi (INSERM U895, Centre Méditerranéen de Médecine Moléculaire, Nice, France).

Author Contributions

Conceived and designed the experiments: SB MP. Performed the experiments: SB EF BB. Analyzed the data: SB EF MP. Wrote the paper: SB.

References

1. Halliday GM (2005) Inflammation, gene mutation and photoimmunosuppression in response to UVR-induced oxidative damage contributes to photocarcinogenesis. Mutat Res 571: 107–120.
2. Bruls WA, Van Weedlden H, Van der Leun JC (1984) Transmission of UV-irradiation through human epidermal layers as a factor influencing the minimal erythema dose. Photochem Photobiol 39: 63–67.
3. El-Domyati M, Attia S, Saleh F, Brown D, Birk DE, et al. (2002) Intrinsic aging vs. photoaging: a comparative histopathological, immunohistochemical, and ultrastructural study of skin. Exp Dermatol 11: 398–405.
4. Yasui H, Sakurai H (2002) Age-dependent generation of reactive oxygen species in the skin of live hairless rats exposed to UVA light. Exp Dermatol 12: 655–661.
5. Cunningham ML, Krinsky NI, Giovanazzi SM, Peak MJ (1985) Superoxide anion is generated from cellular metabolites by solar radiation and its components. Free Radic Biol Med 1: 381–385.
6. Hanson KM, Clegg RM (2002) Observation and quantification of ultraviolet-induced reactive oxygen species in ex vivo human skin. Photochem Photobiol 76: 57–63.
7. Vile GF, Tyrrell RM (1995) UVA radiation-induced oxidative damage to lipids and proteins in vitro and in human skin fibroblasts is dependent on iron and singlet oxygen. Free Radic Biol Med 18: 721–730.
8. Berneburg M, Grether-Beck S, Kurten V, Ruzicka T, Briviba K, et al. (1999) Singlet oxygen mediates the UVA-induced generation of the photoaging-associated mitochondrial common deletion. J Biol Chem 274: 15345–15349.
9. Scharffetter-Kochanek K, Brenneisen P, Wenk J (2000) Photoaging of the skin from phenotype to mechanisms. Exp Gerontol 35: 307–316.
10. Wenk J, Brenneisen P, Meewes C (2001) UV-induced oxidative stress and photoaging. Curr Probl. Dermatol 29: 74–82.
11. Pinnel SR (2003) Cutaneous photo-damage, oxidative stress and topical antioxidant protection. J Am Acad Dermatol. 48: 1–22.
12. Slominski AT, Zmijewski MA, Skobowiat C, Zbytek B, Slominski RM, et al. (2012) Sensing the Environment: Regulation of Local and Global Homeostasis by the Skin's Neuroendocrine System. Advances in Anatomy, Embriology and Cell Biology. New York: Springer-Verlag Berlin Heidelberg. 115p.
13. Nejati R, Kovacic D, Slominski A (2013) Neuro-immune-endocrine functions of the skin: an overview. Expert Rev Dermatol 8: 581–583.
14. Chen JH, Hales NC, Ozanne SE (2007) DNA damage, cellular senescence and organismal ageing: causal or correlative? Nucleic Acids Res 35: 7417–7428.
15. Herbig U, Ferreira M, Condel L, Carey D, Sedivy JM (2006) Cellular senescence in aging primates. Science 311: 1257.
16. Hermann G, Brenneisen P, Wlaschek M, Wenk J, Faisst K, et al. (1998) Psoralen photoactivation promotes morphological and functional changes in fibroblasts in vitro reminiscent of cellular senescence. J Cell Sci 111: 759–767.
17. Briganti S, Wlaschek M, Hinrichs C, Bellei B, Flori E, et al. (2008) Small molecular antioxidants effectively protect from PUVA-induced oxidative stress responses underlying fibroblast senescence and photoaging. Free Radic Biol Med 45: 636–644.
18. Desvergne B, Wahli W (1999) Peroxisome proliferator-activated receptors: nuclear control of metabolism. Endocrine Reviews 20: 649–688.
19. Varga T, Czimmerer Z, Nagy L (2011) PPARs are a unique set of fatty acid regulated transcription factors controlling both lipid metabolism and inflammation. Biochimica Biophysica Acta 1812: 1007–1022.
20. Qq Kwak BR, Mulhaupt F, Mach F (2002) The role of PPARγ ligands as regulators of the immune response. Drug News Perspectives 15: 325–332.
21. Ham SA, Kang ES, Lee H, Hwang JS, Yoo T, et al. (2013) PPARδ inhibits UVB-induced secretion of MMP-1 through MKP-7 mediated suppression of JNK signaling. J Invest Dermatol 133: 2593–2600.
22. McCarty MF, Barroso-Aranda J, Contreras F (2009) The "rejuvenatory" impact of lipoic acid on mitochondrial function in aging rats may reflect induction and activation of PPAR-γ coactivator-1α. Medical Hypotheses 72: 29–33.
23. Polvani S, Tarocchi M, Galli A (2012) PPARγ and Oxidative Stress: Con(β) Catenating NRF2 and FOXO. PPAR Res 2012: 641087.
24. Grabacka M, Placha W, Urbanska K, Laidler P, Płonka PM, et al. (2008) PPAR gamma regulates MITF and beta-catenin expression and promotes a differentiated phenotype in mouse melanoma S91. Pigment Cell Melanoma Res 21: 388–396.
25. Jurzak M, Latocha M, Gojniczek K, Kapral M, Garncarczyk A, et al. (2008) Influence of retinoids on skin fibroblasts metabolism in vitro. Acta Pol Pharm 65: 85–91.
26. Weiss JS, Ellis CN, Headington JT, Voorhees JJ (1988) Topical tretinoin in the treatment of aging skin. J Am Acad Dermatol 19: 169–175.
27. Kim BH, Lee YS, Kang KS (2003) The mechanism of retinol-induced irritation and its application to anti-irritant development. Toxicol Lett 146: 65–73.
28. Stradi R, Pini E, Celentano G (2001) The chemical structure of pigments in Ara macao plumage. Comp Biochem Physiol Part B 130: 57–63.
29. Morelli R, Loscalzo R, Stradi R, Bertelli A, Falchi M (2003) Evaluation of the antioxidant activity of new carotenoid-like compounds by electron paramagnetic resonance. Drugs Exp Clin Res 29: 95–100.
30. Pini E, Bertelli A, Stradi R, Falchi M (2004) Biological activity of parrodienes, a new class of polyunsaturated linear aldehydes similar to carotenoids. Drugs Exp Clin Res 30: 203–206.
31. Flori E, Mastrofrancesco A, Kovacs D, Ramot Y, Briganti S, et al. (2011) 2,4,6-Octatrienoic acid is a novel promoter of melanogenesis and antioxidant defence in normal human melanocytes via PPAR-γ activation. Pigment Cell. Melanoma Res. 24: 618–630.
32. Bayreuther K, Francz PI, Rodemann HP (1992) Fibroblasts in normal and pathological terminal differentiation, aging, apoptosis and transformation. Arch. Geront. Geriatr. Suppl 3: 47–74.
33. Dimri GP, Lee X, Basile G, Acosta M, Scott G, et al. (1995) A biomarker that identifies senescent human cells in culture and in aging skin in vivo. Proc Nat Acad Sci USA 92: 9363–9367.
34. Claiborne A (1985) Catalase activity. In: Greewald RA, editors. Handbook of Methods for Oxygen Radical Research. Boca Raton, FL: CRC. pp. 283–284.
35. Camera E, Rinaldi MR, Briganti S, Picardo M, Fanali S (2001) Simultaneous determination of reduced and oxidized glutathione in peripheral blood mononuclear cells by liquid chromatography-electrospray mass spectrometry. J Chromatogr B Biomed App 757: 69–78.
36. Picardo M, Grammatico P, Roccella F, Roccella M, Grandinetti M, et al. (1996) Imbalance in the antioxidant pool in melanoma cells and normal melanocytes from patients with melanoma. J Invest Dermatol 107: 322–326.
37. Kurien BT, Scofield RH (2003) Free radical mediated peroxidative damage in systemic lupus erythematosus. Life Sciences 73: 1655–1666.
38. Stocks J, Dormandy TL (1971) The autooxidation of human red cell lipids induced by hydrogen peroxide. British J Haematol 20: 95–111.
39. Saito Y, Yoshida Y, Niki E (2007) Cholesterol is more susceptible to oxidation than linoleates in cultured cells under oxidative stress induced by selenium deficiency and free radicals. FEBS Lett. 581: 4349–4354.
40. Rocchi S, Picard F, Vamecq J, Gelman L, Potier N, et al. (2001) A unique PPAR-gamma ligand with potent insulin-sensitizing yet weak adipogenic activity. Mol Cell 8: 737–747.
41. Lee YH, Lee NH, Bhattarai G, Yun JS, Kim TI, et al. (2010) PPARgamma inhibits inflammatory reaction in oxidative stress induced human diploid fibroblast. Cell Biochem Funct 28: 490–496.
42. Briganti S, Flori E, Mastrofrancesco A, Kovacs D, Camera E, et al. (2013) Azelaic acid reduced senescence-like phenotype in photo-irradiated human dermal fibroblasts: possible implication of PPARγ. Exp Dermatol 22: 41–47.
43. Canton M, Caffieri S, Dall'Acqua F, Di Lisa F (2002) PUVA-induced apoptosis involves mitochondrial dysfunction caused by the opening of the permeability transition pore. FEBS Lett 522: 168–172.
44. Okuno Y, Matsuda M, Miyata Y, Fukuhara A, Komuro R, et al. (2010) Human catalase gene is regulated by peroxisome proliferator activated receptor gamm through a response element distinct from that of mouse. Endocr J 57: 303–309.
45. Tian FF, Zhang FF, Lai XD, Wang LJ, Yang L, et al. (2011) Nrf2-mediated protection against UVA radiation in human skin keratinocytes. Biosci Trends 5: 23–29.
46. Raval CM, Zhong JL, Mitchell SA, Tyrrell RM (2012) The role of Bach1 in ultraviolet A-mediated human heme oxygenase 1 regulation in human skin fibroblasts. Free Radic Biol Med 52: 227–236.
47. Zhong JL, Edwards GP, Raval C, Li H, Tyrrell RM (2010) The role of Nrf2 in ultraviolet A mediated heme oxygenase 1 induction in human skin fibroblasts. Photochem Photobiol Sci 9: 18–24.
48. Suttner DM, Dennery PA (1999) Reversal of HO-1 related cytoprotection with increased expression is due to reactive iron. Faseb J 13: 1800–1809.
49. Essers MA, Weijzen S, de Vries-Smits AM, Saarloos I, de Ruiter ND, et al. (2004) FOXO transcription factor activation by oxidative stress mediated by the small GTPase Ral and JNK. The EMBO Journal 23: 4802–4812.

50. Tanaka H, Murakami Y, Ishi I, Nakata S (2009) Involvement of a forkhead transcription factor, FOXO1a, in UV-induced changes of collagen metabolism. J Invest Dermatol Symposium Proceedings 14: 60–62.

51. Dowell P, Otto CT, Adi S, Lane MD (2003) Convergence of peroxisome proliferator-activated receptor γ and Foxo1 signaling pathways. J Biol Chem 278: 45485–45491.

52. Naru E, Suzuki T, Moriyama M, Inomata K, Hayashi A, et al. (2005) Functional changes induced by chronic UVA irradiation to cultured dermal fibroblasts. Br J Dermatol 153: 6–12.

53. Brenneisen P, Sies H, Scharffetter-Kochanek K (2002) Ultraviolet-B irradiation and matrix metalloproteinases: from induction via signalling to initial events. Ann N Y Acad Sci 973: 31–43.

54. McCubrey JA, Lahair MM, Franklin RA (2006) Reactive oxygen species-induced activation of the MAP-kinase signalling pathways. Antiox Redox Signal 8: 1775–1789.

55. Thatcher JE, Isoherranen N (2009) The role of CYP26 enzymes in retinoic acid clearance. Expert Opin Drug Metab Toxicol 5: 875–886.

56. Mongan NP, Gudas LJ (2007) Diverse actions of retinoid receptors in cancer prevention and treatment. Differentiation 75: 853–870.

57. Furuhashi M, Hotamisligil GS (2008) Fatty acid-binding proteins: role in metabolic diseases and potential as drug targets. Nat Rev Drug Discov 7: 489–503.

58. Chiba Y, Yamashita Y, Ueno M, Fujisawa H, Hirayoshi K, et al. (2005) Cultured murine dermal fibroblast-like cells from senescence-accelerated mice as in vitro model for higher oxidative stress due to mitochondrial alterations. J Gerentol A Biol Sci Med Sci 60: 1087–1098.

59. Koziel R, Greussing R, Maier AB, Declercq L, Jansen-Dürr P (2011) Functional interplay between mitochondrial and proteasome activity in skin aging. J Invest Dermatol 131: 594–603.

60. Afaq F, Mukhtar H (2001) Effects of solar radiation on cutaneous detoxification pathways. J Photochem Photobiol B 63: 61–69.

61. Shin MH, Rhie GE, Kim YK, Park CH, Cho KH, et al. (2005) H$_2$O$_2$ accumulation by catalase reduction changes MAP kinase signaling in aged human skin in vivo. J Invest Dermatol 125: 221–229.

62. André M, Felley-Bosco E (2003) Heme oxygenase-1 induction by endogenous nitric oxide: influence of intracellular glutathione. FEBS Lett 546: 223–227.

63. Lehmann JC, Listopad JJ, Rentzsch CU, Igney FH, von Bonin A, et al. (2007) Dimethylfumarate induces immunosuppression via glutathione depletion and subsequent induction of heme oxygenase 1. J Invest Dermatol 127: 835–845.

64. Armoni M, Harel C, Karni S, Chen H, Bar-Yoseph F, et al. (2006) FOXO1 represses peroxisome proliferator-activated receptor-gamma1 and -gamma2 gene promoters in primary adipocytes. A novel paradigm to increase insulin sensitivity. J Biol Chem 281: 19881–19891.

65. Fan W, Yanase T, Morinaga H, Okabe T, Nomura M, et al. (2007) Insulin-like growth factor 1/insulin signaling activates androgen signaling through direct interactions of Foxo1 with androgen receptor. J Biol Chem 282: 7329–7338.

66. Santamaria AB, Davis DW, Nghiem DX, McConkey DJ, Ullrich SE, et al. (2002) p53 and Fas ligand are required for psoralen and UVA-induced apoptosis in mouse epidermal cells. Cell Death Differ 9: 549–560

67. Waldman T, Kinzler KW, Vogelstein B (1995) p21 is necessary for the p53-mediated G1 arrest in human cancer cells. Cancer Res 55: 5187–5190.

68. Pamplona R (2008) Membrane phospholipids, lipoxidative damage and molecular integrità: A causal role in aging and longevity. Biochim Biophys Acta 1777: 1249–1262.

69. Park HY, Youm JK, Kwon MJ, Park BD, Lee SH, et al. (2008) K6PC-5, a novel sphingosine kinase activator, improves long-term ultraviolet light-exposed aged murine skin. Exp Dermatol 17: 829–836.

70. dos Santos DJ, Eriksson LA (2006) Permeability of psoralen derivatives in lipid membranes. Biophys J 91: 2464–2474.

71. Gruber F, Mayer H, Lengauer B, Mlitz V, Sanders JM, et al. (2010) NF-E2-related factor 2 regulates the stress response to UVA-1-oxidized phospholipids in skin cells. FASEB J 24: 39–48.

72. Brown DA, London E (2000) Structure and function of of sphingolipid- and cholesterol-rich membrane rafts. J Biol Chem 275: 17221–17224.

73. Simons K, Toomre D (2000) Lipid raftes and signal transduction. Mol Cell Biol 1: 31–39.

74. Park WY, Park JS, Cho KA Kim DI, Ko YG, et al. (2000) Up-regulation of caveolin attenuates epidermal growth factor signaling in senescent cells. J Biol Chem 275: 20847–20852.

75. Maeda M, Scaglia N, Igal RA (2009) Regulation of fatty acid synthesis and Delta9-desaturation in senescence of human fibroblasts. Life Sci 84: 119–124.

76. Schroepfer GJ (2000) Oxysterols: Modulators of cholesterol metabolism and other processes. Physiol Rev 80: 361–554.

77. Anticoli S, Arciello M, Mancinetti A, De Martinis M, Ginaldi L, et al. (2010) 7-ketocholesterol and 5,6-secosterol modulate differently the stress-activated mitogen-activated protein kinases (MAPKs) in liver cells. J CellPhysiol 222: 586–595.

78. Wada T, Stepniak E, Hui L, Leibbrandt A, Katada T, et al. (2008) Antagonistic control of cell fates by JNK and p38-MAPK signaling. Cell Death Differ 15: 89–93.

79. Feingold KR, Jiang YJ (2011) The mechanisms by which lipids coordinately regulate the formation of the protein and lipid domains of the stratum corneum: Role of fatty acids, oxysterols, cholesterol sulfate and ceramides as signaling molecules. Dermatoendocrinol 3: 113–118.

80. Palozza P, Simone R, Catalano A, Monego G, Barini A, et al. (2011) Lycopene prevention of oxysterol-induced proinflammatory cytokine cascade in human macrophages: inhibition of NF-kB nuclear binding and increase in PPARγ expression. J Nutr Biochem 22: 259–268.

6

Prostaglandin E$_2$ Promotes Features of Replicative Senescence in Chronically Activated Human CD8+ T Cells

Jennifer P. Chou[1], Christina M. Ramirez[3], Danielle M. Ryba[1], Megha P. Koduri[1], Rita B. Effros[1,2]*

1 Department of Pathology & Laboratory Medicine, David Geffen School of Medicine, University of California Los Angeles, Los Angeles, California, United States of America, **2** UCLA AIDS Institute, David Geffen School of Medicine, University of California Los Angeles, Los Angeles, California, United States of America, **3** Department of Biostatistics, Fielding School of Public Health, University of California Los Angeles, Los Angeles, California, United States of America

Abstract

Prostaglandin E$_2$ (PGE$_2$), a pleiotropic immunomodulatory molecule, and its free radical catalyzed isoform, iso-PGE$_2$, are frequently elevated in the context of cancer and chronic infection. Previous studies have documented the effects of PGE$_2$ on the various CD4+ T cell functions, but little is known about its impact on cytotoxic CD8+ T lymphocytes, the immune cells responsible for eliminating virally infected and tumor cells. Here we provide the first demonstration of the dramatic effects of PGE$_2$ on the progression of human CD8+ T cells toward replicative senescence, a terminal dysfunctional state associated multiple pathologies during aging and chronic HIV-1 infection. Our data show that exposure of chronically activated CD8+ T cells to physiological levels of PGE$_2$ and iso-PGE$_2$ promotes accelerated acquisition of markers of senescence, including loss of CD28 expression, increased expression of *p16* cell cycle inhibitor, reduced telomerase activity, telomere shortening and diminished production of key cytotoxic and survival cytokines. Moreover, the CD8+ T cells also produced higher levels of reactive oxygen species, suggesting that the resultant oxidative stress may have further enhanced telomere loss. Interestingly, we observed that even chronic activation *per se* resulted in increased CD8+ T cell production of PGE$_2$, mediated by higher COX-2 activity, thus inducing a negative feedback loop that further inhibits effector function. Collectively, our data suggest that the elevated levels of PGE$_2$ and iso-PGE$_2$, seen in various cancers and HIV-1 infection, may accelerate progression of CD8+ T cells towards replicative senescence *in vivo*. Inhibition of COX-2 activity may, therefore, provide a strategy to counteract this effect.

Editor: Derya Unutmaz, New York University, United States of America

Funding: R01AG032422 (Effros), U01 AI35040 (Detels). The funders had no role in study design, data collection and analysis, decision to publish, or preparation of the manuscript.

Competing Interests: The authors have declared that no competing interests exist.

* E-mail: reffros@mednet.ucla.edu

Introduction

Lipid mediators have long been recognized as key regulators of inflammation and homeostasis. Prostaglandins constitute one of the most important families of these mediators. In particular, prostaglandin E$_2$ (PGE$_2$), a common arachidonic acid-derived eicosanoid produced by cyclooxygenases (COX1 and COX2), is involved in a wide variety of physiological events. It is markedly increased during inflammatory processes, and it helps promote vasodilation; moreover, its chronic biological effects have been linked to the pathogenesis of certain malignancies and HIV disease. Within the immune system, PGE$_2$ modulates such critical processes as cytokine production, differentiation, proliferation, migration and antigen presentation [1,2].

Several pathologies suggest a role for PGE$_2$ in specifically modulating the function of T cells. For example, CD8+ T cells from HIV-infected persons have increased intracellular cyclic AMP (cAMP), a downstream target of the PGE$_2$ signaling cascade. Furthermore, elevated serum levels of prostaglandins correlate with worse clinical prognoses in HIV/AIDS [3,4]. In addition, T cells from patients with PGE$_2$-secreting cancers show decreased proliferation in response to anti-CD3 antibody stimulation [5]. Interestingly, aging in both mice and humans is associated with increased PGE$_2$ secretion by activated macrophages, which could

potentially impact responses of T cells in their proximity [6]. A great deal of the PGE$_2$/immunology research has been focused on the development and differentiation of the CD4+ T cell subset, particularly in regard to its role in facilitating expansion of Th1 and Th17 cells [7,8]. However, little is known about the effect of PGE$_2$ on CD8+ T cells, for example, with respect to their progression towards replicative (cellular) senescence, a state of functional dysregulation and irreversible cell cycle arrest considered to be a contributor to failed immune responses during chronic infection and aging.

Oxidative stress, previously documented to increase the levels of PGE$_2$ and its free-catalyzed isoform, iso-PGE$_2$ [9], is also known to accelerate the process of replicative senescence. In this study, we addressed the question of whether PGE$_2$ and iso-PGE$_2$ themselves might have effects on replicative senescence that are distinct from those caused by oxidative stress. To address this question, we used a well-established *in vitro* model of T cell replicative senescence to measure changes in CD8+ T cell proliferation, telomerase activity, production of key cytokines, and expression of costimulatory molecules during chronic activation in the presence of these immunomodulators. Our data show that exposure to exogenous PGE$_2$ and iso-PGE$_2$ accelerates the senescence trajectory and associated effector functions of CD8+ T cells. Importantly, persistent, chronic stimulation of T cells *per se* increases COX-2 activity in CD8+ T cells, leading to endogenous production of PGE_2. Our data suggest a mechanism by which cancer cells, aging and chronic infections may each contribute to T cell dysfunction and senescence.

Materials and Methods

Ethics Statement

All study participants for this study were recruited from the Los Angeles metropolitan area. This study was approved by the University of California, Los Angeles Medical Institutional Review Board and each participant provided written, informed consent per the approved protocol.

Cell Cultures

Human peripheral blood samples from self-reported healthy donors were acquired by venipuncture after informed consent, and in accordance with the UCLA IRB. After centrifugation, the layer of peripheral blood mononuclear cells (PBMC) was carefully removed and washed twice in complete RPMI (5% fetal bovine serum, 10 mM Hepes, 2 mM glutamine, 50 IU/mL penicillin/ streptomycin). The EasySep CD8+ enrichment kit (Miltenyi Biotec) was used to isolate CD8+ T cells by negative selection, and purity of the cells was verified by flow cytometry (routinely > 90% CD8+). Cultures of purified T cell were established as described previously [10]. Briefly, CD8+ T cells were exposed to diluent (DMSO) or to 100 nM–1 μM PGE_2, iso-PGE_2, the EP2 antagonist AH6809, EP4 antagonist CAY10598, or a COX-2 inhibitor CAY10404 (all from Cayman Chemical) for 30 minutes and then activated with anti-CD2/CD3/CD28 microbeads, used as surrogate antigen (Miltcnyi Biotec) with 10 μl microbead cocktail added for every 1×10^6 cells. Stimulation and the modulator pre-treatment were repeated every 14–17 days. In some experiments, 500 nM butaprost (EP2 agonist), 500 nM misoprostol (EP4, EP3> EP1> EP2 agonist; each from Cayman Chemical), 1 μM Forskolin or H89 dihydrochloride (both Tocris Bioscience) were added. Cultures were supplemented with recombinant IL-2 (20 U/mL). Every 3–4 days, viable cell concentration was determined by trypan blue exclusion, and when the concentration reached $\geq 8 \times 10^5$/ml, cells were sub-cultivated to a density of 5×10^5 cells/ml. Population doublings (PD) were determined according to the formula: PD = $\log_2$ (final cell concentration/initial cell concentration).

Quantitative PCR

Gene expression was evaluated by quantitative polymerase chain reaction (qPCR) analysis. In brief, after extraction by RNeasy Mini kit (Qiagen), 500 ng of RNA from T cells was reverse-transcribed with the iScript cDNA synthesis kit (Bio-Rad). The qPCR assays were performed using the Bioline SensiFAST SYBR Kit and CFX 96 (Bio-Rad). The housekeeping gene, *36B4*, was used as an internal control. The sequences of the primers were designed using Primer 3 software, listed below. Samples were run in triplicate in a 96-well plate using the settings of 95°C for 2 minutes, 95°C for 5 s and 60°C for 15 min (single fluorescence measurement) with the 2nd and 3rd step repeated for 39 cycles. Primer sequences are listed on Table 1.

Flow Cytometry

Surface expression of CD28, CD8, and CD3 was examined by immunostaining and flow cytometry. Cells were incubated with fluorescently labeled anti-CD3, -CD8, -CD28, -CD25, fluorophore conjugated antibodies (BD Biosciences) at 4°C for 20 min, washed, and fixed in PBS containing 1% paraformaldehyde.

Parallel samples were incubated with Ig isotype control antibody or secondary Abs (BD Biosciences). For intracellular staining, cells were stimulated for 5 hr with anti-CD2/CD3/CD28 microbeads with or without the immunomodulators, treated with Golgistop for 6 hours, permeabilized and stained with PE-anti-IFN-γ and FITC-anti-TNF-α antibodies using the Cytofix/Cytoperm Plus kit (BD Biosciences). All samples were analyzed on a FACSCalibur flow cytometer (Beckton Dickson). Fluorescence data from at least 25,000 cells were acquired. Analysis of data was performed using Cell Quest Pro (BD Biosciences).

Telomerase Activity Measurements

Telomerase activity was determined using a modified version of the Telomerase Repeat Amplification Protocol (TRAP) as previously described [11]. Briefly, for each sample 1×10^6 CD8+ cells were pelleted and washed twice with PBS. Cell pellets were lysed in 100 μL of M-PER Mammalian Protein Extraction Reagent (Pierce Biotechnology) and allowed to incubate on ice for 1 hour. To control for inter-sample cell number variance, samples were normalized according to nucleic acid concentration, which was determined using spectrophometric readings for dsDNA. The endogenous telomerase present in the cell extract adds telomeric repeats to the telomerase substrate (TS), a nontelomeric oligonucleotide. The extension products are then amplified several-fold by PCR carried out by Taq polymerase using a Cy-5-labeled forward primer (TS: 5′−/5Cy5/ AATCCGTCGACGCAGAGTT) as a substrate for telomerase-mediated addition of TTAGGG repeats, and an anchored reverse primer (ACX: 5′-GCGCCGCTTACCCTTACCCTTACCC-TAACC-3′). Each sample was mixed with 20 ul of Bromothenol Blue loading dye and 35 μl of sample+dye and was loaded and run at least twice using 10% non-denaturing PAGE in 1X TBE buffer. Gels were run first at 100V for 20 min, followed by approximately 250 V for 2 h. Gels were scanned on a STORM 865 (GE Healthcare,) and quantified using the software ImageQuant 5.2, which integrates signal intensity over the telomere length distribution on the gel as a function of molecular weight (GE Healthcare).

PGE_2 Measurements

Culture supernatants were harvested 72 h post-stimulation and analyzed for PGE_2 using the PGE_2 EIA ELISA kit (Enzo Life Sciences). All measurements were performed in triplicate wells and in accordance to manufacturer's recommendations. The sensitivity for this kit is 13.4–2,500 pg/ml.

Measurement of Telomere Length

Genomic DNA was extracted from CD8+ T cells using the DNeasy Tissue Kit according to manufacturer's instructions (Qiagen). Real-Time PCR was performed on a total of 5 ng of DNA per sample using IQ Sybr Green Supermix according to the manufacturer's instructions (Bio-Rad) and an established quantitative telomere PCR protocol [12]. The primers used for: Tel 1b: 3′-CGGTTTGTTTGGGTTTGGGTTTGGGTTTGGGTTT-GGGTT-5′ and Tel 2b: 3′-GGCTTGCCTTACCCTTACCCT-TACCCTTACCCTTACCCT-5′. HGB 1: 3′-GCTTCTGACA-CAACTGTGTTCACTAGC-5′ and HGB 2: 3′-CACCAACTT-CATCCACGTTCACC-5′. Genomic DNA extracted from SAOS cells (Human osteocarcinoma cell line; American Type Culture Collection) with known telomere length was included in each PCR reaction to control for inter-assay variation and for comparison among donors. A no-template control was included in all PCR reactions, and data from all samples were expressed as a

Table 1. List of primers.

36B4	F-5'-CAATCTGCAGACAGACACTGG-3'
	R-5'-TCTACAACCCTGAAGTGCTTGAT-3'
hTERT	F-5'-AAGTTCCTGCACTGGCTGATG-3'
	R-5'-GCTTTGCAACTTGCTCCAGAC-3'
CD28	F-5'-AGGCTCCTGCACAGTGACTA-3'
	R-5'-GAGCGATAGGCTGCGAAG-3'
IL-2	F-5'-TCACCAGGATGCTCACATTTAAGTTTT-3'
	R-5'-TTCCTCCAGAGGTTTGAGTTCTTCTTC-3'
CTLA-4	F-5'TGAGTTGACCTTCCTAGATGA-3'
	R-5'CTGGGTTCCGTTGCCTATGC-3'
IFN-G	F-5'TCTGAGACAATGAACGCTAC-3'
	R-5'GAGTAGGCTCACCAGGTG-3'
COX-2	F-5'TGCTTGTCTGGAACAACTGC-3'
	R-5'TGAGCATCTACGGTTTGCTG-3'
p16	F-5'ATATGCCTTCCCCCACTACC-3'
	R-5'CCCCTGAGCTTCCCTAGTTC-3'

percentage of the telomere length of the tumor cell line, SAOS (~23 kb), as described previously [13].

Intracellular cAMP Determination

CD8+ T cells were cultured as described, and at 72 h or 14 d post stimulation with anti-CD2/CD3/CD28 microbeads, the cells were pelleted and washed twice with 1xPBS. Cells were then lysed during incubation for 20 min with HCl (0.1 M). Cell debris was removed by centrifugation at 600×g for 10 min, and the level of cAMP in the supernatants was determined using a direct cAMP enzyme immunoassay kit (Enzo Life Sciences), following the manufacturer's protocol. Assays were performed in triplicate.

COX-2 Enzyme Activity Assay

Changes to the enzymatic activity of COX-2 were measured using a COX enzyme activity assay (Cayman Chemical), according to the manufacturer's protocol. This assay measures COX-2 activity by oxidation of the peroxidase cosubstrate TMPD (N,N,N1,N1-tetra-methyl-p-phenylenediamine) in 96-well plates and has been shown to accurately reflect the rate of conversion of arachidonic acid to PGH2. In brief, CD8+ T cells were collected 72 h or 14–17 d post Ab-bead activation. Cells were then rinsed twice in 1xPBS, lysed in ice-cold 0.1 M Tris (pH 7.8, 1 mM EDTA), and stored at −80C until the assay was performed. The assay mixture containing assay buffer, heme, sample (or protein standard prepared by boiling lysates), and the COX-1 inhibitor SC-560 to eliminate COX-1 activity (or as a control reaction the COX-2 inhibitor DuP-697 to eliminate COX-2 activity) was incubated for 5 min at 25°C, and TMPD was added. The reactions were initiated by adding arachidonic acid to all wells, and plates gently were shaken and incubated for 5 min at 25°C and the absorbance was read at 590 nM. COX-2 activity was then calculated using the following formula whereby 1 unit is defined as the amount of enzyme to oxidize 1 nmol of TMPD per min at 25°C: COX-2 activity = $[(\Delta 590/5 \text{ min}/0.00826 \text{ }\mu\text{M-1}) \times (0.21 \text{ ml}/0.01 \text{ ml})]/2$ (it takes two molecules of TMPD to reduce PGG2 to PGH2) = nanomoles per minute per milliliter (units per milliliter).

Intracellular ROS Measurement

Intracellular ROS were measured by flow cytometry using the fluorescent probe dichlorodihydrofluorescein diacetate (H2DCFDA, Molecular Probes), which is oxidized to highly fluorescent dichlorodihydrofluorescein (DCF) by hydroxides, hydrogen peroxides, and hydroxyl radicals. Briefly, T lymphocytes $(1 \times 10^6/\text{ml})$ were treated with PGE_2 and iso-PGE_2 for 24 h, and then incubated with DCFDA (2 μM) for 30 min at 37°C in the dark. At the end of incubation, cells were washed and resuspended in HBSS at 37°C. To determine the effects by mitochondrial ROS, MitoSOX Red–based flow cytometric detection of mitochondrial superoxide was used. Cells were incubated with MitoSOX Red superoxide indicator (Invitrogen) for 30 min and washed, and PGE_2 and iso-PGE_2 were added for 2 h. The cells were analyzed on a FACSCalibur (BD Biosciences). Analyses of data were performed using Cell Quest Pro (BD Biosciences).

Statistical Analysis

Mean values and standard deviation as well as medians and IQRs were calculated for each time-point. Significance was established by the Kruskall Wallis test for between group comparisons, a non-parametric test similar to ANOVA using SAS V. 9.2 (SAS Institute, Cary, NC). For data where each donor had a control sample and a treatment sample, differences were used so that each donor could serve as his or her own control. Differences for these data were assessed using the nonparametric permutation test for paired data; p values of <0.05 were considered significant.

Results

CD8+ T Cells Upregulate Prostaglandin Receptors upon Activation and are Sensitive to PGE_2 and iso-PGE_2

In order to initiate studies on the specific CD8+ T cell effects of PGE_2, it was first necessary to confirm that this subset expresses the same PGE_2-specific receptors previously reported for the total CD3+ T cell population, namely EP2 and EP4 [7]. Figure 1A shows that CD8+ T cells from peripheral blood of healthy donors upregulated *EP2* and *EP4* mRNA and protein upon activation with anti-CD2/CD3/CD28 microbeads, with no evidence of expression when tested immediately *ex vivo*. These observations suggest that T cell receptor (TCR) and CD28 engagement is required for the upregulation of the EP receptors. Consistent with previous reports, no transcripts of *EP1* and *EP3*, the other known EP receptors, were observed after activation (data not shown). Therefore, these results indicate that EP2 and EP4 constitute the major PGE_2 receptors on CD8+ T cells. If similarly enhanced receptor expression occurs *in vivo*, CD8+ T cells may show increased sensitivity to the effects of PGE_2 in immune-suppressed HIV+ persons.

PGE_2 has been reported to modulate function of murine T cells and the human Jurkat T cell tumor line via cAMP-PKA signaling [14,15]. The data in Figure 1B extend these findings to normal human CD8+ T cells, showing that inclusion of 500 nM PGE_2 and iso-PGE_2 in cell culture results in a significant increase in intracellular cAMP, which peaked shortly after exposure and remained elevated even after 72 hours. T cells treated with butaprost (500 nM) and misoprostal (500 nM), which are agonists for EP2 and EP2/EP4, respectively, also showed similar levels of intracellular cAMP (Fig. 1B). These results indicate that human CD8+ T cells are able to recognize and be affected by PGE_2 and its free-catalyzed isoform, iso-PGE_2.

PGE$_2$ and iso-PGE$_2$ Decrease Proliferative Potential and Increase the Transcription of the *p16* Cell Cycle Arrest Gene

The ability to rapidly expand *in vivo* upon TCR and CD28 engagement is central to T cell function and is crucial for an effective immune response. To assess the effects of PGE$_2$ and iso-PGE$_2$ on CD8+ T cell proliferative potential, we measured the total number of population doublings (PD) of CD8+ T cell cultures that are driven to the end stage of replicative senescence following multiple rounds of chronic activation, as described previously [16,17]. The end stage of replicative senescence is experimentally defined as the inability of CD8+ T cells to enter cell cycle in response to two rounds of stimulation, and coincides with several functional changes, such as loss of telomerase activity and surface expression of CD28, an important costimulatory molecule [18].

Using this cell culture protocol, we found that a 30-minute pre-treatment with physiological concentrations of the immunomodulators (0.05–1 μM PGE$_2$ or iso-PGE$_2$) prior to each round of activation decreased the total PD in a dose-dependent manner. PGE$_2$ and iso-PGE$_2$ treated T cells maximally reached a total PD 14–16 versus 20–24 observed in diluent (DMSO)-treated cultures (Fig. 2A). All donors followed a similar pattern of growth when treated with PGE$_2$ or iso-PGE$_2$, with observed PDs 35–60% less than control cultures. Furthermore, we tested the effects of PGE$_2$ and iso-PGE$_2$ on proliferation and metabolic activity of T cells using an MTT assay (data not shown), and found that a 4hr incubation with the immunomodulators decreased absorbance at 570 nm by an average of 31% among three donors.

Upregulation of the cyclin dependent kinase inhibitor, p16, is a major mediator of senescence in many cell types [17,19]. Our data demonstrate that CD2/CD3/CD28 activation in the presence of PGE$_2$ and iso-PGE$_2$ significantly increases *p16* transcripts during the later phases of the culture, i.e., 14–18 PD (p = 0.0315 for both PGE$_2$ and iso-PGE$_2$) (Fig. 2B). This upregulation of the cell-cycle

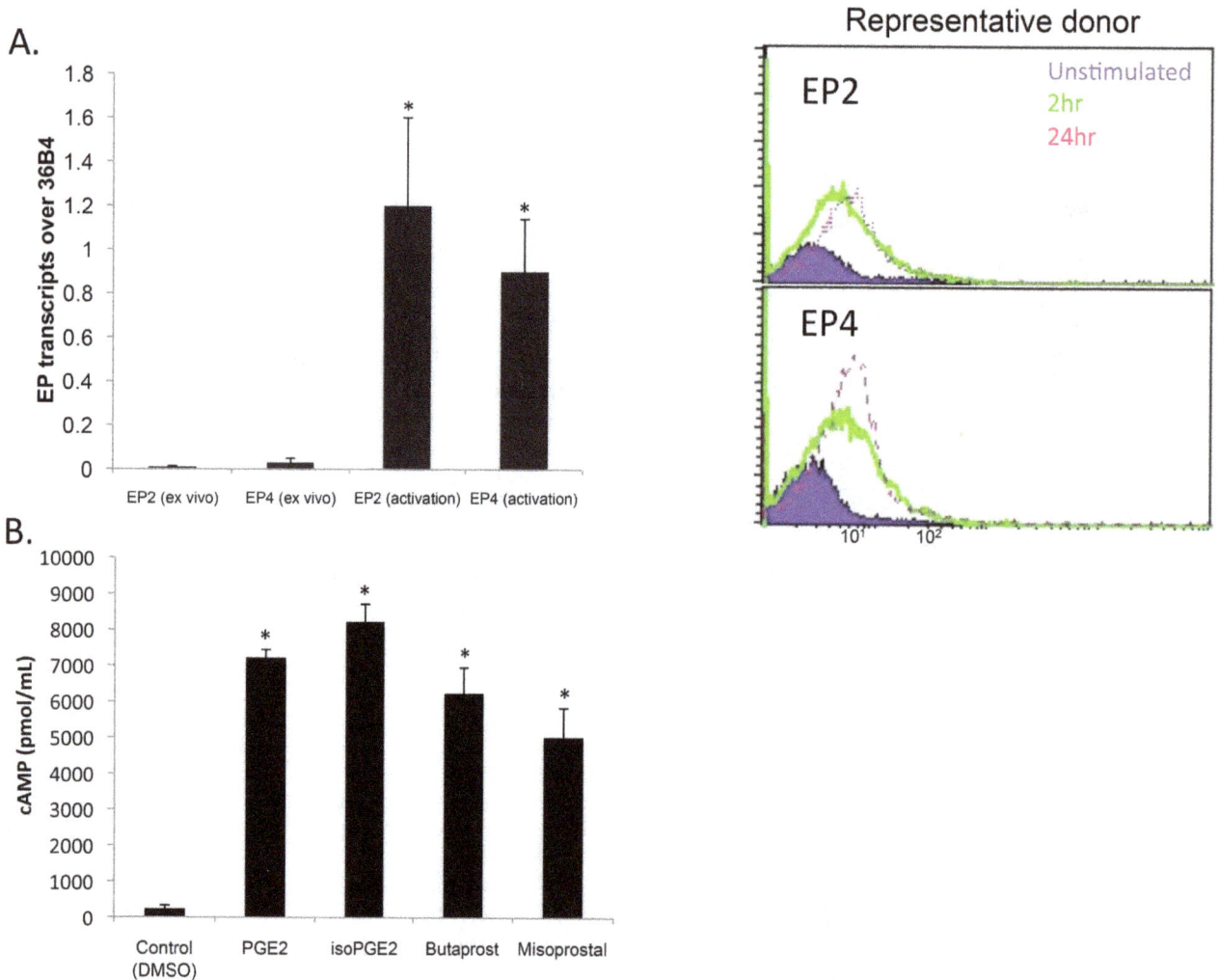

Figure 1. EP receptor expression and cAMP upregulation in CD8+ T cells. CD8+ T cells were freshly isolated from PBMC from whole blood derived from healthy donors or HIV+ persons. (A) (Left) *EP2* and *EP4* transcripts were evaluated by quantitative PCR in *ex vivo* samples and in T cells activated with anti-CD2/CD3/CD28 microbeads for 24 hours. *36B4* was used as the housekeeping gene and data represents 3 healthy donors performed on a single plate (*p = 0.05). (Right) EP2 and EP4 surface expression was also evaluated in healthy at 2 hours and 24 hours post activation, or with no Ab-coated bead activation. Flow cytometric histogram shows one representative donor from a healthy person stained with PE–anti-human EP2 or PE–anti-EP receptor antibodies (Cayman Chemical). (B) Intracellular cAMP was evaluated using a direct cAMP ELISA kit (Enzo Biosceinces) in T cells treated with PGE$_2$, isoPGE$_2$, and known EP agonists, misoprostol (EP2, EP3, and EP4) and butaprost (EP2) for 72 h (n = 3; p<0.005 by Kruskal Wallis for the comparison of all treatment groups to control).

arrest marker leading to premature induction of senescence-like characteristics, if occurring *in vivo*, would presumably reduce the ability of activated CD8+ T cells to expand and mount a vigorous offense against pathogens and tumor cells.

PGE$_2$ and iso-PGE$_2$ Induce Premature Replicative Senescence: Telomeres and Telomerase Activity

One of the signature features of T cell replicative senescence is the loss in activity of telomerase, a holoenzyme that extends the protective ends of chromosomes called telomeres [20]. The induction of telomerase is essential for T cell proliferation and memory T cell maintenance during infection. Loss of telomerase in CD8+ T cells is also predictive of more rapid pathogenesis and worse clinical outcomes in HIV disease, several cancers, age-related bone disorders, and a host of other pathologies [21,22]. We therefore evaluated the effects of PGE$_2$ and iso-PGE$_2$ on telomerase activity and telomere length of CD8+ T cells over time. The data in Figure 3A document that after the first two rounds of activation, there was a dose-dependent decrease in both transcription of *hTERT*, the telomerase catalytic subunit, and actual telomerase activity in cultures exposed to PGE$_2$ and iso-PGE$_2$. To elucidate the underlying mechanism for this downregulation, we treated the T cells with forskolin, a potent stimulator of the cAMP-PKA pathway, and observed a similar pattern of hTERT message reduction (Fig. 3A) and telomerase activity (data not shown). In addition, H89, an inhibitor of PKA, modestly restored some telomerase activity when pre-incubated with the cells prior to PGE$_2$ or iso-PGE$_2$ addition (Fig. 3B).

As expected, the reduction of telomerase activity was associated with telomere shortening in the PGE$_2$- and iso-PGE$_2$-treated cells. The shorter telomere lengths in the treated vs. control cultures were evident both after the same number of days in culture as well as after identical numbers of PD, illustrated in one representative donor (Fig. 3C). Critically short telomeres may cause the T cells to abruptly enter permanent cell-cycle arrest, consistent with the observed increase of *p16* transcripts (Fig. 2B). Given that increased oxidative stress is a known inducer of cellular senescence, we tested the possibility that PGE$_2$ and iso-PGE$_2$ may be contributing to accelerated telomere shortening in the T cells via induction of

reactive oxygen species (ROS). Indeed, increased mean fluorescence intensity of CD8+ T cells labeled with ROS-sensitive dye DCFDA was observed in the presence of both modulators, but not in the control cultures (Fig. 3D), reaching levels comparable to those caused by H_2O_2 treatment. The MitoSOX red dye was used to detect mitochondrial superoxide, another free radical species thought to contribute to DNA damage and senescence. Oxidation of MitoSOX red was observed to be modestly higher in PGE$_2$ and iso-PGE$_2$ CD8+ T cells (Fig. 3D), indicating that chronic exposure to these modulators can increase ROS production and contribute to the development of dysfunctional phenotypes in T cells.

Key Features of T Cell Function are Modulated by PGE$_2$ and iso-PGE$_2$

The T cell co-stimulatory receptor, CD28, provides an important second signal that is necessary for a robust activation through the T cell receptor, promoting cell expansion while preventing the induction of anergy or cell death [23]. Since loss of CD28 gene and surface expression is a key feature of replicative senescence, the effects of PGE$_2$ and its free-catalyzed isoform on CD28 were evaluated. We observed that CD28 surface expression and *CD28* transcripts were reduced in the presence of PGE$_2$ and iso-PGE$_2$, with pronounced effects after the third round of activation. In the representative experiment shown in Fig. 4A (left panel), compared to DMSO-controls, which were nearly 49% CD28+, the PGE$_2$- and iso-PGE$_2$-treated CD8+ T cells were only ~32% and ~28% CD28+, respectively. Representative time courses for three cultures show that loss of CD28 surface expression was more rapid in the treated cultures than in controls (Fig. 4A). These results may explain the reduced telomerase activity described above, since CD28 has been shown to play a direct regulatory role on gene expression of *TERT*, the catalytic subunit of telomerase, and telomerase activity [10].

Concomitant with this decline in CD28 expression was a detectable increase in gene expression of *CTLA-4*, a transiently expressed antigen that competes with CD28 for its binding partner, B7, on antigen-presenting cells (APCs). CTLA-4 delivers an inhibitory signal in activated T cells and thereby downregulates T cell function and expansion [23,24]. Even after 72 hours

A.

B.

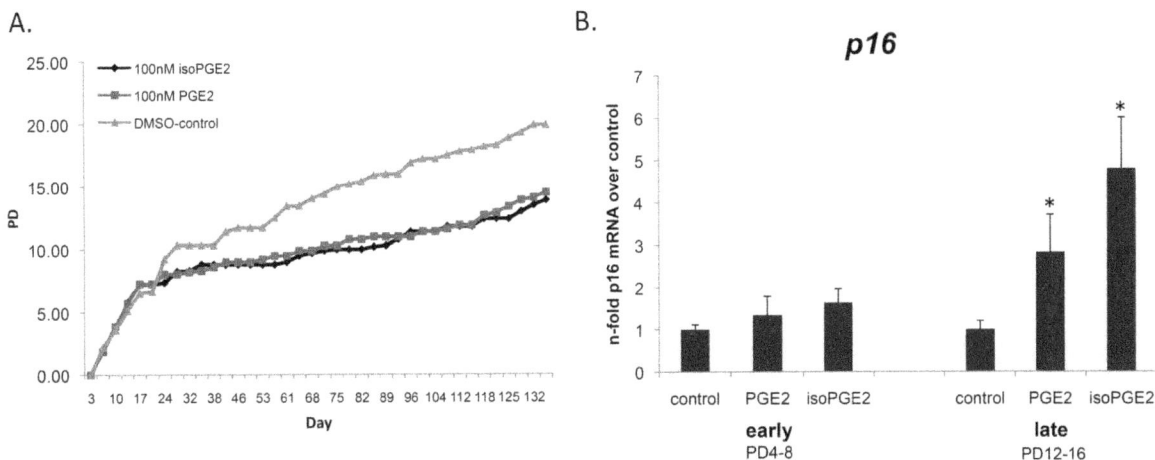

Figure 2. Proliferative potential decreases and *p16* transcripts increase in the presence of PGE$_2$ and iso-PGE$_2$. T cells were activated with anti-CD2/CD3/CD28 microbeads with or without PGE$_2$ or iso-PGE$_2$ and population doublings (PD) was calculated by the formula PD = log$_2$ (final cell concentration/initial cell concentration) (A) Long term culture of one representative donor. (B) *p16* transcripts were quantified by qPCR during early (PD4–8) and late (PD12–16) time points in the presence of PGE$_2$, iso-PGE$_2$ or diluent (n = 5; *p = 0.031 compared to control by the paired permutation test). *36B4* was used as the housekeeping gene.

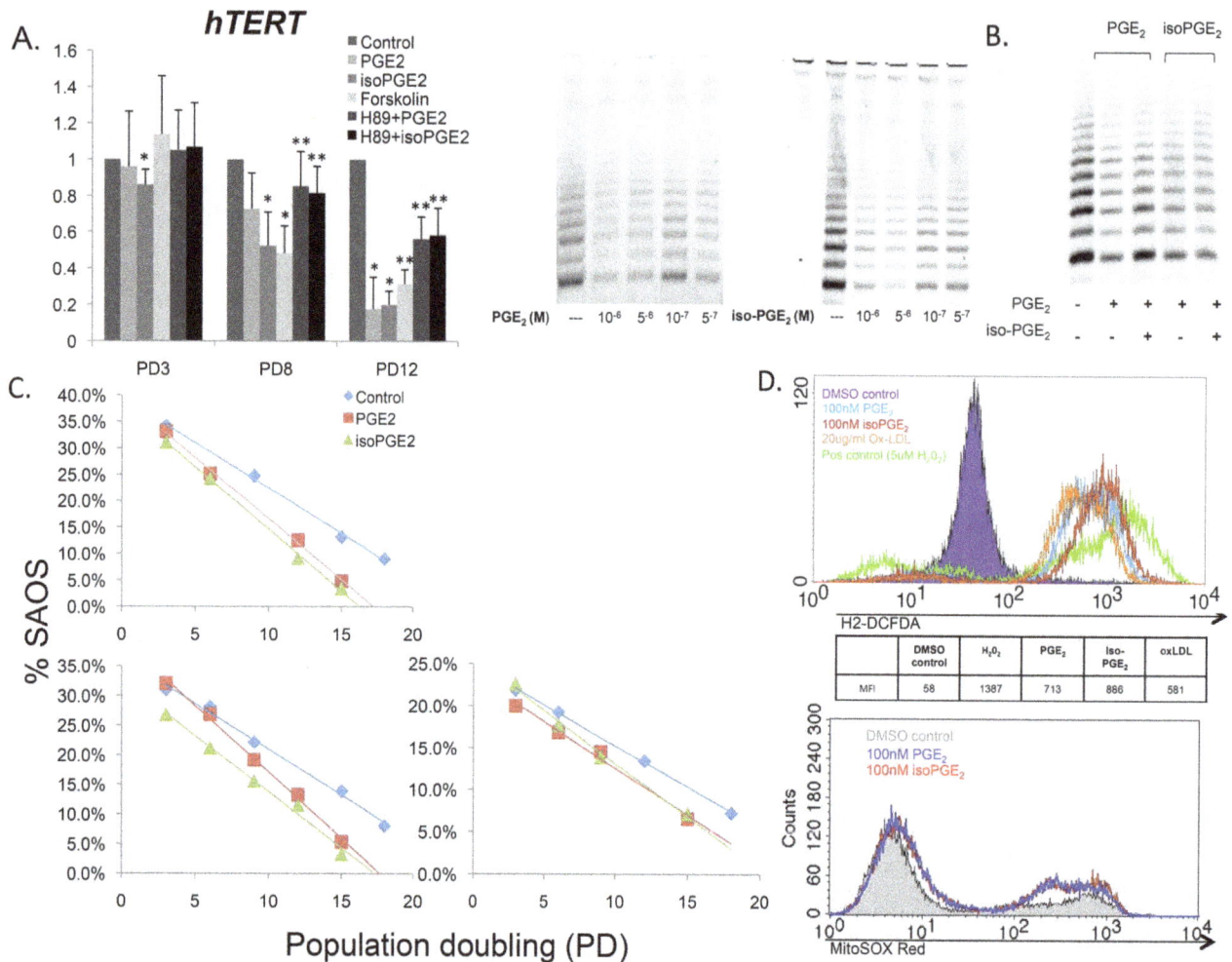

Figure 3. PGE$_2$ and iso-PGE$_2$ inhibit telomerase activity while increasing intracellular ROS. CD8+ T cells were negatively selected after 72 hours post activation with anti-CD2/CD3/CD28 microbeads with or without PGE$_2$ or iso-PGE$_2$, and inhibitors of PKA pathway. (A) (Top Left) hTERT expression was quantified at equivalent PDs by qPCR (n = 5; *p = 0.0312; **p = 0.031 using one-sided T test because of decreased sample size for these conditions only; n = 4). (Top Middle) Representative gel showing effects of PGE$_2$ (10^{-6} to 5^{-7}M) and iso-PGE$_2$ (10^{-6} to 5^{-7}M) on telomerase activity of CD8+ T cells. Band intensity per lane correlates with relative telomerase activity of 1,250 CD8+ T cells in each treatment group. (B) Telomerase activity was measured as described in (A) with PGE$_2$ or iso-PGE$_2$ in the presence of 1 μM of a PKA inhibitor, H89 dihydrochloride. (C) CD8+ T cell cultures were established and chronically activated as previously described in the presence of the immune modulators. Telomere lengths were evaluated by Real-Time PCR and expressed as a percentage of telomere length of a human tumor cell line, SAOS (~23Kb). Data represent telomere lengths over the lifetime from 3 representative donor cultures. (D) (Top) The relative amount of intracellular ROS was determined by the mean fluorescence intensity of DCFDA–stained, live CD8+ T cells after 24 h of culture with media alone or in the presence of PGE$_2$, isoPGE$_2$, ox-LDL, or H$_2$O$_2$ (pos control). (Bottom) Representative flow cytometry profile of MitoSOX red oxidation in PGE$_2$- and iso-PGE$_2$-treated T cells.

post-activation in the presence of PGE$_2$ or iso-PGE$_2$, *CTLA-4* transcripts remained significantly higher than controls by 1.5–2 fold for PGE$_2$ and 1.5–4 fold for iso-PGE$_2$ (Fig. 4A - top right).

Senescence is also marked by the loss of IL-2, a cytokine that promotes T cell survival and differentiation into effector T cells [17]. In HIV/AIDS, IL-2 production is frequently used to assess T cell immunity since IL-2 producing CD8+ T cells are found in very low frequencies in viremic individuals progressing rapidly to AIDS, compared to long-term non-progressors [13]. Furthermore, HIV-1-specific IFN-γ/IL-2-secreting CD8+ T cells support CD4-independent proliferation of HIV-1-specific CD8+ T cells [25]. Figure 4 illustrates the significant downregulation of *IL-2* mRNA in the presence of PGE$_2$ and iso-PGE$_2$ during the early and late phases of the cultures (Fig. 4B) and an observed downregulation of the IL-2 receptor, CD25 (Fig. 4A). Studies have indicated that dysfunctional HIV-specific T cells with features of senescence lack

responsiveness to exogenous IL-2 [26] and the downregulation of CD25 may contribute to their inability to actively expand *in vivo* [27,28].

Another important cytokine that is critical for effector function, and whose loss is associated with senescence, is IFN-γ, a potent and multifunctional anti-viral effector molecule that is readily secreted by CD8+ T cells upon recognition of foreign peptide presented on HLA class I molecules. In metastatic cancers and chronic HIV infection, loss of IFN-γ-producing T cells correlates with more rapid disease progression and worse clinical outcomes [29,30,31]. Consistent with reports on the role of prostaglandins on lymphocytes, PGE$_2$ and iso-PGE$_2$ significantly downregulated IFN-γ, measured both in the form of intracellular protein expression (Fig. 4C) and transcript abundance (data not shown). Also in accord with previous reports [8], TNF-α cytokine production was decreased in the presence of the modulators

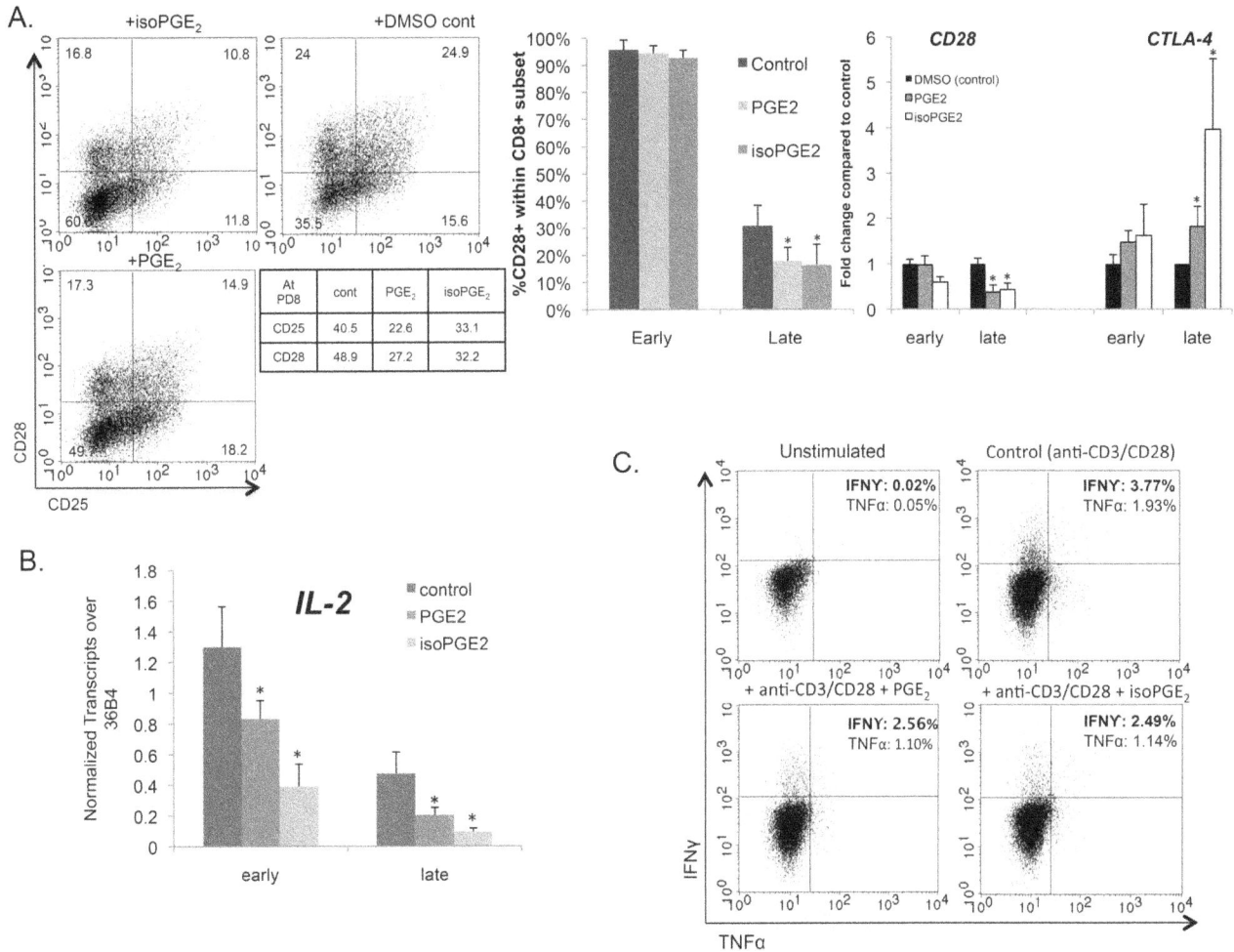

Figure 4. Key features of T cell function are modulated by PGE$_2$ and isoPGE$_2$. (A) (Top Left) CD8+ T cells treated with iso-PGE$_2$ (top) and PGE$_2$ (bottom) were immunostained with FITC–anti-CD25, PE–anti-CD28, and gated on PerCP–anti-CD8 and APC–anti-CD3+ T cells (all BD Biosciences). Samples were compared at the same PD. (Top Middle) The %CD28+cells from different treatment samples over the lifetime of the culture in five donors; *p = 0.031 (Top right) *CD28* and *CTLA-4* expression was determined by qPCR during both early (PD4–8) and late (PD12–16) culture stages in CD8+ T cells treated with the immunomodulators (n = 5; *p = 0.031). All samples were tested in triplicate and normalized to the housekeeping gene *36B4* (B) *IL-2* message was similarly quantified by qPCR as in (A) after treatment (n = 5; *p = 0.031) (C) CD8+ T cells were stimulated with Ab-coated microbeads for 72 h in the presence of PGE$_2$, iso-PGE$_2$, or were treated with diluent (DMSO). Intracellular IFN-γ and TNF-α was analyzed flow cytometrically using FITC–anti-TNF-α, PE–anti-IFN-γ, PerCP–anti-CD8 and APC–anti-CD3. The frequencies of the IFN-γ– and TNF-α producing cells in T-cell fractions gated on CD3+CD8+ are shown as percentages.

(Fig. 4C). These data demonstrate significant impairments in CD8+ T cell function caused by PGE$_2$ and iso-PGE$_2$, ranging from the cells' ability to express the costimulatory molecule CD28 to the secretion of important anti-viral cytokines. Taken together, these data suggest that PGE$_2$ and iso-PGE$_2$ promote the acquisition of multiple senescent features and may therefore play a key role in the accumulation of dysfunctional CD8+ T cells seen in chronic infections and cancer.

COX-2 Activity and EP4 Expression Increases in T cells during Chronic Activation

The data presented thus far have focused on the effects of exogenous PGE$_2$ and iso-PGE$_2$ on repeatedly activated CD8+ T cells. However, we wondered whether the chronic activation in itself might result in increased production of PGE$_2$, mediated by COX-2, which synthesizes PGE$_2$ from arachidonic acid released from the plasma membrane. This possibility would be consistent with a report documenting observed elevated intracellular cAMP and the fact that COX-2 inhibitor therapy reduces features of immune dysfunction and exhaustion in CD8+ T cells in HIV-infected persons [3]. We therefore examined *COX-2* gene expression and activity in chronically activated T cells.

Figure 5A shows that in cultures from healthy donors, there was a dramatic increase in *COX-2* transcripts 24 hours after CD2/CD3/CD28 engagement. Furthermore, repeated rounds of stimulation were associated with progressively increasing expression of *COX-2* and *EP4* transcripts, COX-2 activity and PGE$_2$ in culture supernatants (Fig. 5A). Elevated intracellular cAMP (Fig. 5B – control cultures) was also detected in these "older" T cell cultures, suggesting that the modulation of the cAMP-PKA signaling pathway by TCR and CD28 engagement may significantly change during chronic activation, as seen in cancer, HIV infection and aging.

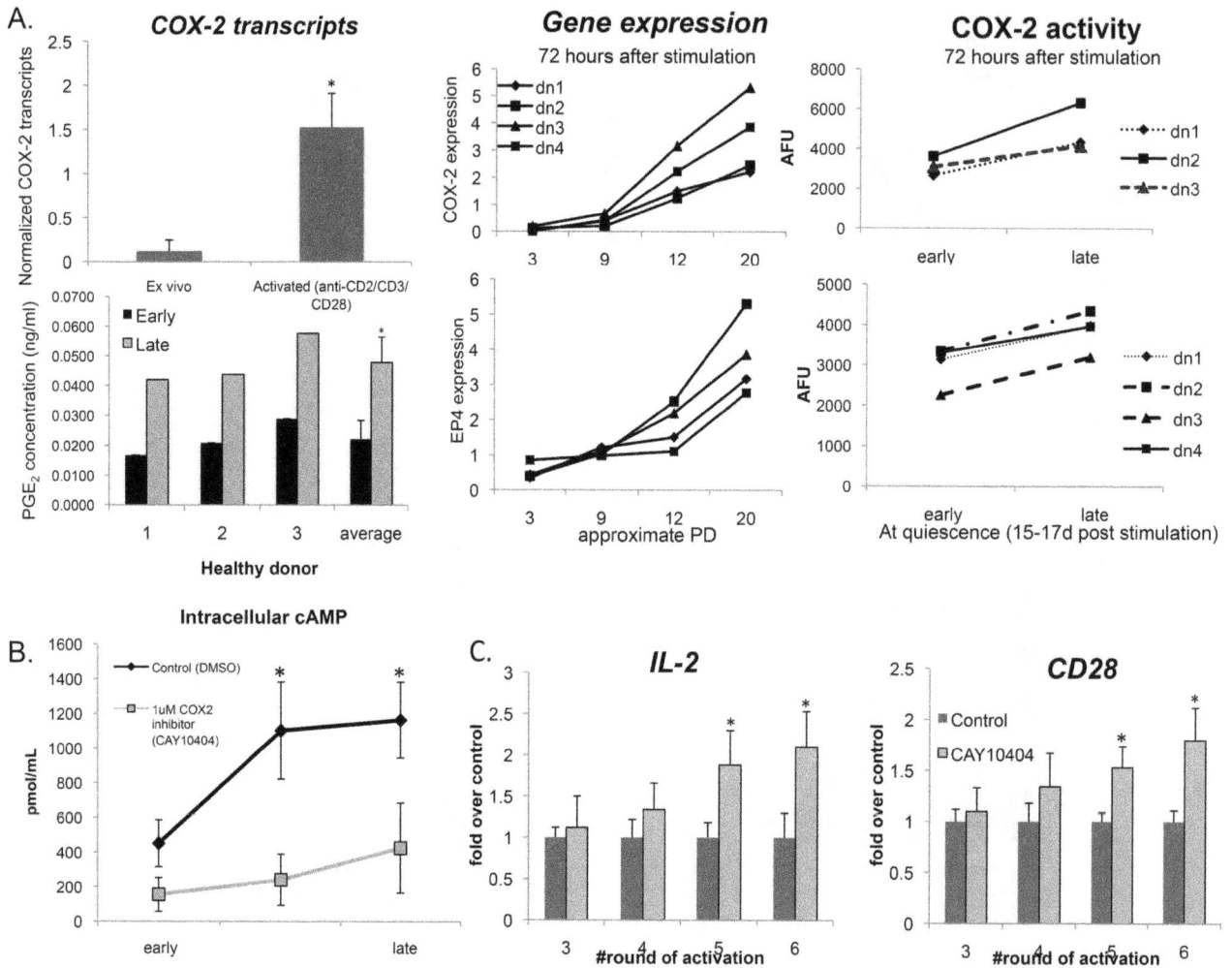

Figure 5. COX-2 activity and EP4 expression increases in T cells during chronic activation. (A) (Top left) *COX-2* transcripts were quantified by qPCR in *ex vivo* and activated (anti-CD2/CD3/CD28) CD8+ T cell samples from healthy donors. Each sample was tested in triplicate and normalized to the housekeeping gene $36B4$ (n = 5; *p = 0.031). Supernatants from early and late cultures from 3 donors were collected 72 h post activation with Ab-coated microbeads and their average PGE_2 concentration was calculated from triplicate wells, *p = 0.05. (Top Right) *COX-2* and *EP4* transcripts were quantified 72 h post each round of activation in four healthy donors. Each sample was tested in triplicate and normalized to the housekeeping gene, $36B4$. In addition, COX-2 activity was determined in CD8+ T cells at early and late time points 72 h post activation and at quiescence (15–17 d post stimulation) in three healthy donors using the COX Activity Assay (Cayman Chemical). (B) CD8+ T cells were pre-incubated with a highly specific COX-2 inhibitor CAY10404 (1 µM) (Cayman Chemical) or diluent (DMSO) for 30 min and then activated with Ab-coated microbeads as described. 1×10^6 CD8+ T cells were collected 24h post activation during early and late PDs and intracellular cAMP was measured in triplicate using a direct cAMP ELISA kit (Enzo Life Sciences) (n = 4; *p = 0.05). (C) CD8+ T cells were cultured in the presence of 1 µM CAY10404 or DMSO for 30 min, and then activated with Ab-coated microbeads. 72 h after each round of activation, cells were collected and *IL-2* and *CD28* transcripts were quantified by qPCR. Each sample was tested in triplicate and normalized to the housekeeping gene $36B4$ (n = 5; *p = 0.031).

COX2 Inhibition may Prevent the Development of Features of CD8+ T Cell Dysfunction

The data shown in Fig. 5A suggest that upregulation of COX-2 activity and subsequent increase in secreted PGE_2 during chronic T cell activation may contribute to the development of features of replicative senescence associated with persistent infections, cancer and aging. To address one potential therapeutic approach, we investigated whether COX-2 inhibition in mid-to-late culture (i.e. PD12–20) would retard some of the features of replicative senescence described above. T cells were activated as previously described after a 30 min pretreatment with the highly specific COX-2 inhibitor, CAY10404. The specificity and activity of the COX-2 inhibition was first validated by measuring intracellular cAMP in CD8+ T cells after TCR and CD28 engagement

(Fig. 5B). Pretreatment of CD8+ T cells with CAY10404 resulted in higher mean levels of *CD28* and *IL-2* transcripts (2-fold and 1.8-fold, respectively, over DMSO-control at the 6th round of stimulation) (Fig. 5C). The data suggest that endogenous COX-2 activity and production of PGE_2 may contribute to the development of immune senescence, and that reducing COX-2 activity may retard some of its features. Together, these results suggest potential therapeutic benefits of COX-2 inhibition in slowing the senescence trajectory of CD8+ T cells that arise during chronic activation.

Discussion

The current study represents the first report documenting the effects of PGE_2 and iso-PGE_2 on the senescence trajectory of human CD8+ T cells, in particular with regard to their CD28 expression, IL-2 transcription and telomerase activity. It provides a potential mechanism by which cancer cells, aged APCs, and HIV infection promote immune dysfunction and inefficient surveillance during chronic activation. To our knowledge, this is also the first documentation of the cAMP-PKA pathway in modulating telomerase and CD28 expression. One recent study found that this signaling cascade is a regulator of IL-2 expression [32], but it was unclear how the critical players of the cAMP-PKA pathway, which cross talks with such pathways as NFAT and MAPK/ERK, affect expression of hTERT and CD28. Interestingly, it has been reported that PKA increases phosphorylation of the Wilms tumor suppressor (WT1) protein, a potent transcriptional repressor that inhibits hTERT expression by direct binding to the hTERT promoter. This observation suggests that the effects of PGE_2 can also be a result of its ablation of IL-2 signaling via blockade of JAK3 activation [32], thereby suppressing the cell's ability to proliferate, which would then lead to the loss of telomerase.

In the course of these experiments, we also observed that pretreatment of CD8+ T cells with PGE_2 and iso-PGE_2 leads to a marked reduction of surface expression of IL-7R (CD127) during chronic activation (data not shown). The presence of CD127 on CD8+ T cells during the antiviral immune responses is thought to be a biomarker of effector T cells that successfully mature into highly proliferative protective memory T cells [33,34]. Thus, loss of CD127 expression would be detrimental to long-term memory T cell maintenance and immune surveillance. In addition, many of the PGE_2-associated inhibitory effects on CD8+ T cells including reductions in *hTERT* transcription, telomerase activity, and proliferative potential, were even more pronounced by its free-catalyzed isoform, iso-PGE_2. This highlights a potential avenue by which free radicals, which can directly induce the peroxidation of arachidonic acid in the lipid membrane to produce this isoprostane, may weaken effector T cell functions and proliferation.

An unexpected finding of our study was that chronic activation itself amplifies COX-2 activity and production of PGE_2. If this scenario occurs *in vivo*, the secreted PGE_2 could directly interact with cell populations–including those of the immune system–within the local microenvironment. Although other cell types, such as myeloid and stromal cells, secrete the major portion of PGE_2 *in vivo*, the production of this small-molecule derivative by T cells can affect other cells in a paracrine manner, possibly inducing maturation of dendritic cells and promoting active inflammation through its role as a vasodilator [8]. Indeed, the upregulation of COX-2 activity by T cells may enhance certain aspects of innate immune responses while dampening others; the autologously secreted PGE_2 may also function in a negative feedback fashion to inhibit normal CD8+ T cell effector functions [8,35]. Interestingly, increased PGE_2 was recently detected in cervical tissue samples from women who were HIV-1 positive [36], implicating a potential causative relationship between chronic activation and PGE_2 production by a variety of cell types. Clearly, COX-2 and PGE_2 play a complex, sometimes paradoxical role, in immunity. Future *in vivo* studies will clearly be required in order to define the role of PGE_2 secretion on and by T cells, and its effects on APCs and inflammation during chronic activation.

Finally, our study began to address possible therapeutic strategies to diminish the deleterious *in vivo* effects of PGE_2. Since COX-2 activity was found to increase with each round of T cell activation, it seemed that COX-2 inhibition might be a promising approach to enhance T cell function, while simultaneously inhibiting secretion of PGE_2 by certain tumor cells. Although our data (Fig. 5C) support this notion, clinical observations regarding the negative cardiac effects of the widely prescribed COX-2 inhibitor, celecoxib, suggest that other methods might be preferable for enhancing immunity. For example, blockade via knockdown or antagonists of alternative targets, including the major receptors, EP2 and EP4, or Microsomal prostaglandin E2 synthase-1 (mPGES-1), which catalyzes the formation of PGE_2 from PGH_2 downstream of COX-2, may be alternative therapeutic strategies to prevent accelerated acquisition of senescent features in T cells. Future *in vitro* and *in vivo* studies should clarify the utility and safety of the EP receptor or mPGES-1 blockade as therapeutic targets.

Author Contributions

Conceived and designed the experiments: JPC RBE. Performed the experiments: JPC DMR MPK. Analyzed the data: JPC CMR. Contributed reagents/materials/analysis tools: JPC RBE. Wrote the paper: JPC RBE.

References

1. Hammarstrom S (1983) Leukotrienes. Annu Rev Biochem 52: 355–377.
2. Samuelsson B, Goldyne M, Granstrom E, Hamberg M, Hammarstrom S, et al. (1978) Prostaglandins and thromboxanes. Annu Rev Biochem 47: 997–1029.
3. Pettersen FO, Torheim EA, Dahm AE, Aaberge IS, Lind A, et al. (2011) An exploratory trial of cyclooxygenase type 2 inhibitor in HIV-1 infection: downregulated immune activation and improved T cell-dependent vaccine responses. J Virol 85: 6557–6566.
4. Sarr D, Aldebert D, Marrama L, Frealle E, Gaye A, et al. (2010) Chronic infection during placental malaria is associated with up-regulation of cyclooxygenase-2. Malar J 9: 45.
5. Pockaj BA, Basu GD, Pathangey LB, Gray RJ, Hernandez JL, et al. (2004) Reduced T-cell and dendritic cell function is related to cyclooxygenase-2 overexpression and prostaglandin E2 secretion in patients with breast cancer. Ann Surg Oncol 11: 328–339.
6. Plowden J, Renshaw-Hoelscher M, Engleman C, Katz J, Sambhara S (2004) Innate immunity in aging: impact on macrophage function. Aging Cell 3: 161–167.
7. Boniface K, Bak-Jensen KS, Li Y, Blumenschein WM, McGeachy MJ, et al. (2009) Prostaglandin E2 regulates Th17 cell differentiation and function through cyclic AMP and EP2/EP4 receptor signaling. J Exp Med 206: 535–548.
8. Kalinski P (2012) Regulation of immune responses by prostaglandin E2. J Immunol 188: 21–28.
9. Brose SA, Thuen BT, Golovko MY (2011) LC/MS/MS method for analysis of E(2) series prostaglandins and isoprostanes. J Lipid Res 52: 850–859.
10. Parish ST, Wu JE, Effros RB (2010) Sustained CD28 expression delays multiple features of replicative senescence in human CD8 T lymphocytes. J Clin Immunol 30: 798–805.

11. Saldanha SN, Andrews LG, Tollefsbol TO (2003) Analysis of telomerase activity and detection of its catalytic subunit, hTERT. Anal Biochem 315: 1–21.
12. Cawthon RM (2002) Telomere measurement by quantitative PCR. Nucleic Acids Res 30: e47.
13. Kilpatrick RD, Rickabaugh T, Hultin LE, Hultin P, Hausner MA, et al. (2008) Homeostasis of the naive CD4+ T cell compartment during aging. J Immunol 180: 1499–1507.
14. Bauman GP, Bartik MM, Brooks WH, Roszman TL (1994) Induction of cAMP-dependent protein kinase (PKA) activity in T cells after stimulation of the prostaglandin E2 or the beta-adrenergic receptors: relationship between PKA activity and inhibition of anti-CD3 monoclonal antibody-induced T cell proliferation. Cell Immunol 158: 182–194.
15. Sreeramkumar V, Fresno M, Cuesta N (2012) Prostaglandin E2 and T cells: friends or foes? Immunol Cell Biol 90: 579–586.
16. Effros RB, Dagarag M, Valenzuela HF (2003) In vitro senescence of immune cells. Exp Gerontol 38: 1243–1249.
17. Stein GH, Drullinger LF, Soulard A, Dulic V (1999) Differential roles for cyclin-dependent kinase inhibitors p21 and p16 in the mechanisms of senescence and differentiation in human fibroblasts. Mol Cell Biol 19: 2109–2117.
18. Effros RB, Dagarag M, Spaulding C, Man J (2005) The role of CD8+ T-cell replicative senescence in human aging. Immunol Rev 205: 147–157.
19. Kong Y, Cui H, Ramkumar C, Zhang H (2011) Regulation of senescence in cancer and aging. J Aging Res 2011: 963172.
20. Valenzuela HF, Effros RB (2002) Divergent telomerase and CD28 expression patterns in human CD4 and CD8 T cells following repeated encounters with the same antigenic stimulus. Clin Immunol 105: 117–125.

21. Tosato M, Zamboni V, Ferrini A, Cesari M (2007) The aging process and potential interventions to extend life expectancy. Clinical Interventions in Aging 2: 401–412.

22. Chou JP, Effros RB (2013) T Cell Replicative Senescence in Human Aging. Current Pharmaceutical Design 19: 1680–1698.

23. Lenschow DJ, Walunas TL, Bluestone JA (1996) CD28/B7 system of T cell costimulation. Annu Rev Immunol 14: 233–258.

24. Bluestone JA (1997) Is CTLA-4 a master switch for peripheral T cell tolerance? J Immunol 158: 1989–1993.

25. Zimmerli SC, Harari A, Cellerai C, Vallelian F, Bart PA, et al. (2005) HIV-1-specific IFN-gamma/IL-2-secreting CD8 T cells support CD4-independent proliferation of HIV-1-specific CD8 T cells. Proc Natl Acad Sci U S A 102: 7239–7244.

26. Jin X, Wills M, Sissons JG, Carmichael A (1998) Progressive loss of IL-2-expandable HIV-1-specific cytotoxic T lymphocytes during asymptomatic HIV infection. Eur J Immunol 28: 3564–3576.

27. DosReis GA, Nobrega AF, de Carvalho RP (1986) Purinergic modulation of T-lymphocyte activation: differential susceptibility of distinct activation steps and correlation with intracellular 3′,5′-cyclic adenosine monophosphate accumulation. Cell Immunol 101: 213–231.

28. Perillo NL, Naeim F, Walford RL, Effros RB (1993) The in vitro senescence of human T lymphocytes: failure to divide is not associated with a loss of cytolytic activity or memory T cell phenotype. Mech Ageing Dev 67: 173–185.

29. Betts MR, Nason MC, West SM, De Rosa SC, Migueles SA, et al. (2006) HIV nonprogressors preferentially maintain highly functional HIV-specific CD8+ T cells. Blood 107: 4781–4789.

30. Migueles SA, Laborico AC, Shupert WL, Sabbaghian MS, Rabin R, et al. (2002) HIV-specific CD8+ T cell proliferation is coupled to perforin expression and is maintained in nonprogressors. Nat Immunol 3: 1061–1068.

31. Pantaleo G, Koup RA (2004) Correlates of immune protection in HIV-1 infection: what we know, what we don't know, what we should know. Nat Med 10: 806–810.

32. Rodriguez G, Ross JA, Nagy ZS, Kirken RA (2013) Forskolin-inducible cAMP pathway negatively regulates T-cell proliferation by uncoupling the interleukin-2 receptor complex. J Biol Chem 288: 7137–7146.

33. Lv G, Ying L, Ma WJ, Jin X, Zheng L, et al. (2010) Dynamic analysis of CD127 expression on memory CD8 T cells from patients with chronic hepatitis B during telbivudine treatment. Virol J 7: 207.

34. Huster KM, Busch V, Schiemann M, Linkemann K, Kerksiek KM, et al. (2004) Selective expression of IL-7 receptor on memory T cells identifies early CD40L-dependent generation of distinct CD8+ memory T cell subsets. Proc Natl Acad Sci U S A 101: 5610–5615.

35. Fabricius D, Neubauer M, Mandel B, Schutz C, Viardot A, et al. (2010) Prostaglandin E2 inhibits IFN-alpha secretion and Th1 costimulation by human plasmacytoid dendritic cells via E-prostanoid 2 and E-prostanoid 4 receptor engagement. J Immunol 184: 677–684.

36. Fitzgerald DW, Bezak K, Ocheretina O, Riviere C, Wright TC, et al. (2012) The effect of HIV and HPV coinfection on cervical COX-2 expression and systemic prostaglandin E2 levels. Cancer Prev Res (Phila) 5: 34–40.

7

The Role of Nibrin in Doxorubicin-Induced Apoptosis and Cell Senescence in Nijmegen Breakage Syndrome Patients Lymphocytes

Olga Alster[1], Anna Bielak-Zmijewska[1], Grazyna Mosieniak[1], Maria Moreno-Villanueva[2], Wioleta Dudka-Ruszkowska[3], Aleksandra Wojtala[1], Monika Kusio-Kobiałka[3], Zbigniew Korwek[1], Alexander Burkle[2], Katarzyna Piwocka[3], Jan K. Siwicki[4], Ewa Sikora[1]*

1 Laboratory of the Molecular Bases of Aging, Nencki Institute of Experimental Biology, Polish Academy of Sciences, Warsaw, Poland, 2 Molecular Toxicology Group, Department of Biology, University of Konstanz, Konstanz, Germany, 3 Laboratory of Cytometry, Nencki Institute of Experimental Biology, Polish Academy of Sciences, Warsaw, Poland, 4 Department of Immunology, Maria Sklodowska-Curie Memorial Cancer Center and Institute of Oncology, Warsaw, Poland

Abstract

Nibrin plays an important role in the DNA damage response (DDR) and DNA repair. DDR is a crucial signaling pathway in apoptosis and senescence. To verify whether truncated nibrin (p70), causing Nijmegen Breakage Syndrome (NBS), is involved in DDR and cell fate upon DNA damage, we used two (S4 and S3R) spontaneously immortalized T cell lines from NBS patients, with the founding mutation and a control cell line (L5). S4 and S3R cells have the same level of p70 nibrin, however p70 from S4 cells was able to form more complexes with ATM and BRCA1. Doxorubicin-induced DDR followed by cell senescence could only be observed in L5 and S4 cells, but not in the S3R ones. Furthermore the S3R cells only underwent cell death, but not senescence after doxorubicin treatment. In contrary to doxorubicin treatment, cells from all three cell lines were able to activate the DDR pathway after being exposed to γ-radiation. Downregulation of nibrin in normal human vascular smooth muscle cells (VSMCs) did not prevent the activation of DDR and induction of senescence. Our results indicate that a substantially reduced level of nibrin or its truncated p70 form is sufficient to induce DNA-damage dependent senescence in VSMCs and S4 cells, respectively. In doxorubicin-treated S3R cells DDR activation was severely impaired, thus preventing the induction of senescence.

Editor: Arianna L. Kim, Columbia University Medical Center, United States of America

Funding: This work was supported by National Center of Science in Poland (grants: 2011/01/M/NZ1/01597, UMO-2011/01/B/NZ3/02137 and 0728/B/P01/2011/40). The funders had no role in study design, data collection and analysis, decision to publish, or preparation of the manuscript.

Competing Interests: The authors have declared that no competing interests exist.

* Email: e.sikora@nencki.gov.pl

Introduction

Nijmegen Breakage Syndrome (NBS) is a rare autosomal recessive disorder characterized by genomic instability and increased risk of haematopoietic malignancies observed in more than 40% of the patients by the time they are 20 years old [1]. NBS is caused by mutations in the *NBN* gene (originally designated as *NBS1*) encoding nibrin. More than 90% of the patients are homozygous for the same mutation (c.657-661del5) what results in the formation of two truncated fragments of the 95 kDa nibrin: 26 kDa N-terminal fragment (p26-nibrin) and 70 kDa C-terminal fragment (p70-nibrin), which are produced by alternative initiation of translation at a cryptic upstream start codon. This mutation is actually hypomorphic as the truncated p70-nibrin is able to retain some of the vital cellular functions of the full-length protein. The truncated p70-nibrin can form the MRN (Mre11-Rad50-Nbs1) complex with two other proteins, Mre11 and Rad50 [2,3]. However, null mutation of the *Nbn* gene is lethal in mice [4].

Stress-induced premature senescence (SIPS) is a relatively fast, telomere erosion independent, process. Among its characteristic features we can distinguish irreversible growth arrest, altered cell morphology, DNA foci formation, activation of senescence-associated β-galactosidase (SA-β-Gal) and senescence associated secretory phenotype-SASP (reviewed in [5]). Recently, it was shown that double-strand DNA breaks (DSBs), after induction of the DNA damage response (DDR), are crucial for cellular senescence [6]. Briefly, upon DSB induction ataxia telangiectasia mutated (ATM) kinase is activated. The activated kinase phosphorylates nibrin at its Ser 343 residue and H2AX histone, at its Ser 139 residue (γH2AX). Phosphorylated nibrin forms a trimeric complex (MRN) along with Mre11 and Rad50, which is recruited to the vicinity of DSBs where nibrin interacts with γH2AX [7]. Ultimately, Chk1, Chk2 (checkpoint kinase 1 and 2, respectively) and p53 are activated. p53 promotes senescence (when DNA damage is irreparable) *via* transactivation of *CDKN1A*, which encodes the cyclin dependent kinase inhibitor p21 [5].

DDR activation, not only can lead to senescence but also to transient cell cycle arrest and DNA repair or apoptosis. Improperly functioning DDR often results in increased radiosensitivity, genomic instability and cancer development. Since NBS1 deficient cells are characterized by genomic instability and NBS patients suffer from haematopoietic malignancies, we hypothesized that the molecular pathways leading to DNA damage-induced senescence might be impaired in patients affected with this disease. Most cell lines derived from NBS patients were established following transformation with viral oncogenes, which inhibit key regulatory genes such as the tumor suppressor gene proteins p53 and pRb, thus allowing the cell to bypass the senescence program and become immortal [8]. Accordingly, spontaneously immortalized T cell lines, S3R and S4, carrying the same mutation within the *NBN* gene, but with a seemingly functional p53/p21 response after gamma irradiation [9], are a very useful cellular model in studying the mechanisms of DNA damage-induced senescence. Therefore we used two cell lines derived from NBS patients (S3R and S4) and the control, L5 cell line (spontaneously immortalized spleenocytes obtained from a healthy donor) to examine if they are prone to DNA damage-induced senescence. To induce DNA damage and DDR activation we used doxorubicin, which is a DNA damaging agent acting through different mechanisms. It can lead to the formation of direct and indirect DNA damage through: intercalation into DNA, DNA binding and alkylation, DNA cross-linking, interference with DNA unwinding or DNA strand separation, helicase activity as well as inhibition of topoisomerase II and generation of free radicals [10].

Materials and Methods

1. Cell lines

The spontaneously immortalized T cell lines: S3R and S4 were established from peripheral blood mononuclear cells (PBMC) derived from NBS patients homozygous for the 657del5 mutation of the *NBN* gene [9] and the L5 cell line was established from the spleen of a healthy donor as described previously [9,11]. All of the cell lines were cultured in the RPMI 1640 medium (Gibco, Life Technologies, Warsaw, Poland) supplemented with 10% FCS (Biochrom, Biomibo, Warsaw, Poland), 50 µg/ml gentamycin (Sigma, Poznan, Poland), 2 mM glutamine (Sigma, Poznan, Poland) and 20 U/ml of IL-2 (R&D, Biokom, Warsaw, Poland). Human vascular smooth muscle cells (VSMCs) were obtained from Lonza (Basel, Switzerland). hVSMC were grown in SmBM medium (Lonza, Basel, Switzerland). S3R, S4 and L5 cells were seeded at a density of 0.2×10^6/ml 24 h before doxorubicin (Sigma, Warsaw, Poland) treatment. VSMCs were seeded at a density of 2×10^3/cm^2 24 h before transfection.

2. DNA content and cell cycle analysis

For DNA analysis the cells were fixed in 70% ethanol and stained with PI solution (3,8 mM sodium citrate, 50 µg/ml RNAse A, 500 µg/ml PI in PBS). All of the used agents were purchased at Sigma Aldrich (Poznan, Poland). DNA content was assessed using flow cytometry and analyzed with the CellQuest Software. 10000 events were collected per sample (FACSCalibur, Becton Dickinson, Warsaw, Poland).

3. Immunoprecipitation

S3R and S4 cells were lysed with modified RIPA buffer [12]. Equal amounts of protein (750 µg) were taken for immunoprecipitation. The supernatants were precleared by adding Protein A/G PLUS-Agarose Immunoprecipitation Reagent (Santa Cruz Biotechnology, Inc., Dallas, Texas, USA) and incubated with IP antibody-IP matrix complexes overnight using NBS1 rabbit polyclonal antibody (Sigma Aldrich, Poznan, Poland), Mre11 rabbit monoclonal antibody (Cell Signaling, Lab-JOT Ltd.,

Warsaw, Poland), ATM rabbit monoclonal antibody (Epitomics, Burlingame, California, USA) according to the manufacturer' protocol (Santa Cruz Biotechnology, Inc., Dallas, Texas, USA). Beads were washed with PBS and immune complexes were eluted with sodium dodecyl sulphate (SDS)-containing buffer and boiled. Mre11, BRCA1, ATM and NBS1 were detected using the Western blotting technique with the following antibodies: BRCA1 mouse monoclonal (R&D, Biokom, Warsaw, Poland), ATM rabbit monoclonal antibody (Epitomics, Burlingame, California, USA), Mre11 rabbit monoclonal antibody (Cell Signaling, Lab-JOT Ltd., Warsaw, Poland), NBS1 rabbit polyclonal antibody (Sigma Aldrich, Poznan, Poland) and secondary rabbit polyclonal antibody conjugated with horseradish peroxidase (Dako, Poland).

4. Western blotting analysis

Whole cell protein extracts were prepared according to the Laemmli method [13]. Equal amounts of protein were separated electrophoretically in 8, 12 or 15% SDS-polyacrylamide gels and afterwards transferred to nitrocellulose membranes. Membranes were blocked in 5% non-fat milk dissolved in TBS containing 0,1% Tween-20 (Sigma Aldrich, Poznan, Poland) for 1 h at RT and incubated with one of the primary monoclonal or polyclonal antibodies: anti-ATM (1:500) (Millipore, Merck, Warsaw, Poland), anti-p-ATM Ser 1981 (1:1000), H2AX (1:500) and anti-γH2AX (1:1000) (Abcam, Cambridge, UK), anti-p16 (1:500), anti-p53 (DO-1) (1:500), anti-p21 (C-19) (1:500) (Santa Cruz Biotechnology Inc., Dallas, Texas, USA), anti-p-p53 Ser 15, anti-Chk1, anti-p-Chk1 Ser 317, anti-Chk2, anti-p-Chk2 Thr 68, anti-NBS1 Ser 343 (Cell Signaling, Lab-JOT Ltd., Warsaw, Poland), anti-PARP1 (1:1000) (Becton Dickinson, Diag-med, Warsaw, Poland) anti-NBS1 (1:500), anti-β-actin (1:50000) (Sigma Aldrich, Poznan, Poland) and anti-GAPDH (1:50000) (Millipore, Merck, Warsaw, Poland). The proteins were detected with appropriate secondary antibodies conjugated with horseradish peroxidase and ECL reagents (GE Healthcare, Buckinghamshire, UK), according to the manufacturer's protocol.

5. Gamma irradiation procedure

Asynchronously growing cells were treated with 4 Gy of γ-irradiation. Immediately after irradiation the cells were diluted to a concentration 0.25×10^6 cells/ml and cultured for 3 h. Cells were collected after 3 h (untreated and treated with 4 Gy of irradiation). Whole cell extracts were prepared for Western blotting analysis.

6. Silencing of the *NBN* gene

To downregulate *NBN* expression the cells were seeded in 6 or 12-well plates (2×10^4 or 8×10^3 cells per well, respectively) and transfected with 60 nM siRNA (*NBN* or negative) (Life Technologies, Warsaw, Poland) using Lipofectamine 2000 (Life Technologies, Warsaw, Poland). Transfection was performed according to the manufacturer's protocol. About 20 h after transfection medium was replaced with fresh one and cells were cultured for three days in the presence of doxorubicin (100 nM) (Sigma Aldrich, Poznan, Poland).

7. Detection of SA-β-Gal

Detection of SA-β-Gal was performed according to Dimri et al. (1995) [14]. Briefly, cells were fixed with 2% formaldehyde, 0,2% glutaraldehyde in PBS, washed and exposed overnight at 37°C to a solution containing: 1 mg/ml 5-bromo-4-chloro-3-indolyl-b-D-galactopyranoside, 5 mM potassium ferrocyanide, 5 mM potassium ferrycyanide, 150 mM NaCl, 2 mM MgCl$_2$ and 0,1 M phosphate buffer, pH 6,0. All of the used agents were purchased at

Sigma Aldrich (Poznan, Poland). Photos were taken using the Evolutions VF digital CCD camera (Media Cybernetics, Rockville, Maryland, USA).

8. Apoptosis detection

The level of apoptosis was measured by flow cytometry (FACSCalibur) using the annexin V/7-AAD assay (Becton Dickinson, Diag-med, Warsaw, Poland). Externalization of phosphatidylserine (PS) to the outer layer of the cell membrane was examined by binding of annexin V in the presence of 7-AAD, a dye which stains dead cells. Briefly, cells were washed with PBS, suspended in the annexin V binding buffer, stained for 15 min with annexin V conjugated with PE and 7-AAD. Analysis was performed with FACSCalibur using the CellQuest Software (BD Biosciences, Warsaw, Poland). 10000 events were collected per sample.

9. Bromodeoxyuridine labeling assay

To evaluate DNA synthesis BrdU (Sigma Aldrich, Poznan, Poland) was added to the medium (10 µM) and cells were cultured for 24 h. Afterwards the cells were fixed in ethanol. BrdU was detected using a primary antibody against BrdU (Becton Dickinson, Warsaw, Poland) and a secondary Alexa 488 antibody (Life Technology, Warsaw, Poland). The cells were observed under a fluorescence microscope (Nikon, Tokyo, Japan) with the use of 450–490 nm -excitation wavelength. Photos were taken using the Evolutions VF digital CCD camera (Media Cybernetics, Rockville, Maryland, USA).

10. Immunocytochemistry

For immunofluorescence the cells were fixed with 2% paraformaldehyde (Sigma Aldrich, Poznan, Poland) at RT for 20 minutes and afterwards were incubated on slides with the anti-53BP1 monoclonal antibody (Novus, Cambridge, USA). Secondary anti-rabbit Alexa 488-conjugated IgG antibody was used (Life Technology, Warsaw, Poland). Cells were observed under a fluorescence microscope (Nikon, Tokyo, Japan) and photos were taken using the Evolutions VF digital CCD camera (Media Cybernetics, Rockville, Maryland, USA).

11. Fluorimetric Detection of DNA unwinding (FADU) method

A modified and automated version of the FADU (Fluorimetric Detection of alkaline DNA Unwinding) method was used to measure the percentage of double-stranded DNA after treatment with doxorubicin (1 and 10 µM). The percentage of DNA damage was analyzed 30, 60 and 90 min after treatment with a DNA damaging agent as described previously by Moreno-Villanueva et al. [15,16]. The method is based on partial denaturation "unwinding" of double-stranded DNA under controlled alkaline and temperature conditions. DNA strand breaks are sites where DNA unwinding can start. Briefly, after infliction of DNA damage cell lysis was performed. DNA unwinding was terminated by adding a neutralization solution. SybrGreen, a commercially available dye, which only binds to double stranded DNA, was used to determine the amount of double-stranded DNA. The lower the fluorescence the less double-stranded DNA in the sample.

12. Statistical analysis

Student's T test was used to calculate statistical significance: *, p<0,05; **, p<0,01; ***, p<0,001.

Results

1. FADU analysis of L5, S3R and S4 cells treated with doxorubicin

Doxorubicin is a DNA-damaging agent which is widely used in chemotherapy. It has been shown that cytostatic doses of doxorubicin can lead to the induction of cellular senescence. Cells sensitivity to this agent can vary between different types of cells. Therefore the first step was to analyze the cells sensitivity to treatment with this agent. To do this we used the FADU method. FADU enables to measure, in an automatic way, the percentage of double-stranded DNA [15,16], which accounts for 100% in control cells (Fig. 1). SybrGreen, a fluorescent dye used in this method, binds only to double-stranded DNA. Therefore, the less intensive fluorescence the less double-stranded DNA can be observed. To this end we treated all of the cell lines: with the mutated form of nibrin (S3R and S4) and spontaneously immortalized cells from a healthy donor (L5) with two concentrations of doxorubicin (1 and 10 µM) and analyzed the percentage of double-stranded DNA, after short periods of time (30, 60 and 90 min). The most sensitive, to treatment with doxorubicin, were the S3R cells. In the case of this cell line, a significantly lower amount of double-stranded DNA could be found at all of the analyzed time points after treatment with both concentrations of doxorubicin, in comparison with the untreated cells. In the case of S4 cell line a statistically significant decrease of the percentage of double-stranded DNA, in comparison with control cells, could be observed 90 min after treatment with the lower (1 µM) concentration of doxorubicin and in all of the time points after treatment with the higher (10 µM) concentration of this agent. This shows that even though S3R and S4 cell lines possess the same NBN mutation their sensitivity to treatment with doxorubicin is different. Furthermore, it turned out that, the control (L5) cells are more sensitive to doxorubicin treatment than the S4 cells, however less sensitive than the S3R cells. The obtained results allowed us to speculate that different concentrations of doxorubicin could be cytostatic for particular cell lines and different doses could be needed for the induction of doxorubicin-induced senescence.

2. Cell cycle arrest and apoptosis in doxorubicin-treated L5, S3R and S4 cells

One of the hallmarks of senescence is cell cycle arrest. Cells undergoing senescence can be arrested in the G1/S or G2/M phases of the cell cycle, however stress-induced premature senescence (SIPS) is predominantly associated with cell cycle arrest in the G2/M phase of the cell cycle. We treated L5, S3R and S4 cells with various concentrations of doxorubicin, ranging from 10 to 250 nM and analyzed DNA content using flow cytometry. As it is shown in Figure 2A and in Table 1 treatment with doxorubicin arrested cells from all of the cell lines in the G2/M phase of the cell cycle. In case of the control (L5) cell line the majority of cells were arrested after treatment with 50 nM doxorubicin (approximately 30%). The largest fraction of S4 cells (almost 50%) arrested in the G2/M, was observed after treatment with 100 nM doxorubicin. In the S3R cell population the majority of cells were found in the G2/M phase of the cell cycle after treatment with 10 and 50 nM doxorubicin (about 35%). The subG1 fraction which represents apoptotic cells did not exceed 11% in the case of the L5 cell line and 12% in the case of S4 cells. S3R cells were much more prone to spontaneous apoptosis and about 30% of the cells were found in the subG1 fraction. A concentration dependent increase in the level of apoptosis could be observed after treatment with doxorubicin in all of the cell lines.

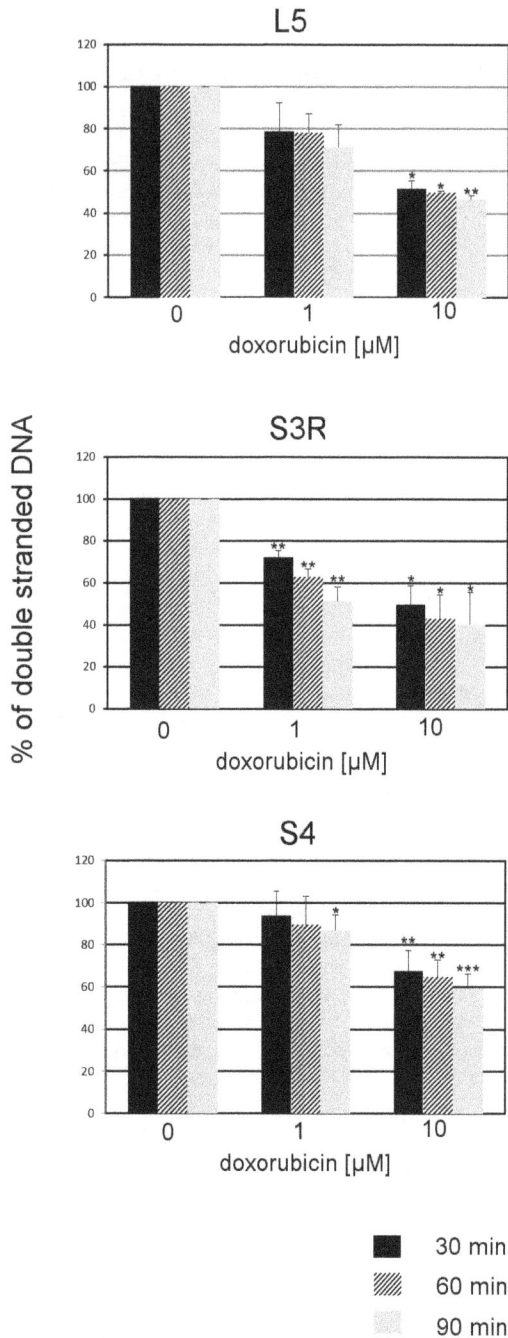

Figure 1. FADU analysis in L5, S3R and S4 cells treated with doxorubicin. The percentage of double-stranded DNA, was measured in all of the cell lines using the FADU method. All of the cell lines were treated with 1 and 10 μM doxorubicin and the measurements were performed 30, 60 and 90 min after treatment with this agent. Data is calculated as the percentage of control. The values are means ± SD obtained from three independent experiments. Statistical significance was estimated using the Student's T test.

The DNA content analysis can underestimate the level of apoptosis due to the fact that cells with 4C DNA undergoing apoptosis, may have ≥2C DNA and cannot be distinguished from the cells found in the S and G1 phases of the cell cycle. Therefore, to estimate more accurately the percentage of cells undergoing apoptosis, we performed the Annexin V/7-AAD cytometric

analysis. As expected this method revealed more apoptotic cells in all of the analyzed cell lines in comparison with the DNA content analysis. However, in the S4 cells, concentration dependence after treatment with doxorubicin still could not be observed. In the case of S3R cells about half of the cell population underwent cell death after treatment with 50 and 100 nM doxorubicin, i.e. significantly more than control cells (Fig. 2B). These results show that S3R cells are very prone to both spontaneous and doxorubicin induced apoptosis and generally more sensitive to the treatment than the S4 cells. Nonetheless, a substantial fraction of cells from all of the cell lines can be arrested in the G2/M phase of the cell cycle upon treatment with different concentrations of doxorubicin.

Since DNA-damage induced senescence is associated with persistant activation of the DNA-damage response (DDR) pathway, which can be observed 24–48 h after treating the cells with a DNA damage inducing agent, we decided to analyze the activation of this pathway after treating the cells with the selected concentrations of doxorubicin. Such concentrations of doxorubicin were selected which led to the accumulation of the most cells in the G2/M phase of the cell cycle and relatively low level of cell death. S3R cells were treated with 10 nM and S4 cells with 100 nM doxorubicin. For comparison we used spontaneously immortalized spleenocytes obtained from a healthy donor (L5), treated with 50 nM doxorubicin (Fig. 2C). In the case of the L5 cell line, we observed the presence of p-ATM (Ser 1981), p-p53 (Ser 15) and p-Chk1 (Ser 317), even in untreated cells. After treatment with doxorubicn (24 h) increased levels of these proteins and the presence of Chk2 and p-Chk2 (Thr 68) was observed proving the presence of an active DDR. In untreated S4 cells the phosphorylated form of Chk1 (Chk1 Ser 317) was detected. Interestingly, after treatment with doxorubicin we noticed a significant increase in the level of p-ATM (Ser 1981), p-Chk1 (Ser 317), p-Chk2 (Thr 68), p-p53 (Ser 15) and γH2AX. Our results show that upon treatment with doxorubicin the DDR pathway is only activated in the L5 and S4 cell lines, however this process can't be observed in the S3R cell line.

3. Doxorubicin-induced senescence of L5 and S4, but not S3R cells

There is data showing that immortalized and cancer cells retain the ability to undergo senescence including that induced by DNA damage [17,18]. We have previously shown [19] that treatment of human colon cancer HCT116 cells with a low dose of doxorubicin for one day, followed by culture in a drug-free medium, led to the induction of senescence. Therefore, we decided to use the same experimental approach and treated the L5, S3R and S4 cells with the chosen concentrations of doxorubicin (50 nM for L5, 10 nM for S3R and 100 nM for S4) for 24 hours and afterwards cultured the cells for four days in a drug free medium (1+4). We observed a time-dependent increase in the number of SA-β-Gal positive cells in L5 and S4, but not in S3R cell line (Fig. 3A, B). In case of the L5 cell line the majority of SA-β-Gal-positive cells (approximately 95%) were observed on day 1+4. In case of the S4 cell line the most SA-β-Gal positive cells were observed on day 1+3 (approximately 50%). The presence of SA-β-Gal positive cells was accompanied by an increase in the level of p53 (Ser 15) in both cell lines, however a time dependent increase in the level of p21 was only observed in the S4 cell line. Surprisingly, in the L5 cell line, a time dependent decrease in the level of this protein was found (Fig. 3C). Two crucial pathways play an important role in senescence: p53-p21 and p16-pRb. Sometimes these pathways overlap therefore we also decided to check the level of p16, which is a key protein in the p16-pRb pathway.

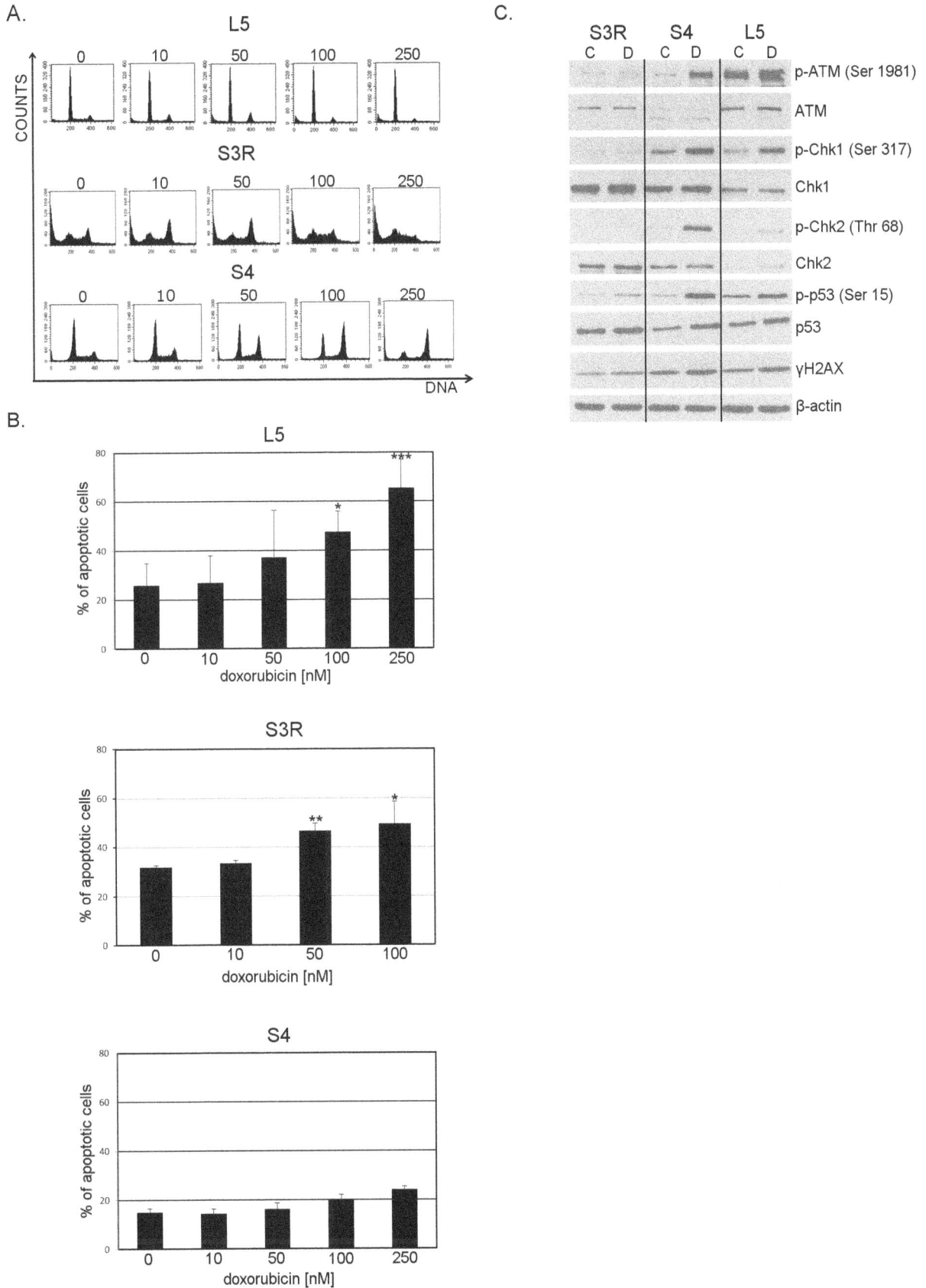

Figure 2. Dose-dependent influence of doxorubicin on cell cycle arrest, apoptosis and activation of the DNA damage response (DDR). A. DNA content, analyzed by flow cytometry, 24 h after treatment with different concentrations of doxorubicin (0–250 nM). Representative

histograms from one of three independent experiments. **B.** Concentration-dependent apoptosis measured 24 h after treatment with doxorubicin (0–250 nM). The percentage of apoptotic cells was estimated by the Annexin V/7-AAD flow cytometry assay in three independent experiments. The bars show means ± SD values. Data was analyzed using the CellQuest software. Statistical significance was estimated using the Student's T test. **C.** Expression of the DDR proteins analyzed by Western blotting in control (C) and treated with doxorubicin (D) S3R, S4 and L5 cells. Whole cell extracts were prepared 24 h after cell treatment with the following cytostatic concentrations of dox: 50 nM (L5), 10 nM (S3R), 100 nM (S4) and β-actin was used as a loading control.

The p16-mediated senescence acts mainly through the retinoblastoma (pRb) pathway by inhibiting the action of the cyclin dependent kinases and leads to G1 cell cycle arrest [20]. We did not observe any changes in the level of this protein in the S3R and S4 cell lines, however, a time dependent decrease in the level of p16 was observed in the L5 cell line (Fig. 3C). The observation made in the L5 cell line requires further elucidation. It seems that untreated S3R cells might have the p53/p21 pathway already active, which is further slightly activated after treatment with doxorubicin, but this is not accompanied by an increase in SA-β-Gal activity. In the L5 and S4 cells stronger activation of the p53/p21 pathway correlated with an increase in SA-β-Gal activity. This encouraged us to investigate whether the lack of induction of senescence in the S3R cell line was due to the fact that the cells underwent cell death. Using the annexin V/7-AAD assay, we measured the level of apoptosis a day after treatment with doxorubicin and on subsequent days after transferring the cells to fresh medium (Fig. 3D). In all of the cell lines we observed a time-dependent increase in the level of apoptosis. Three days after culturing the cells in drug free medium (1+3) approximately 55% of cells underwent apoptosis in all of the cell lines, however it should be underlined that the cells were treated with different concentrations of doxorubicin. The S4 cells were treated with a ten times higher concentration of doxorubicin (100 nM) than the S3R cells (10 nM). Moreover, in the case of the L5 and S3R cell lines a high basal level of apoptosis could be observed. Despite the high level of cell death, a fraction of S4 (more than 40% of SA-β-Gal positive cells on day 1+4) and L5 (about 95% of SA-β-Gal positive cells on day 1+4) of cells, that survived, were able to undergo senescence.

4. The level of p70-nibrin in S3R and S4 cells

We were interested whether the differences in the cells susceptibility to doxorubicin treatment and cell fate were due to a different level of the truncated form of nibrin (p70), which is present in the S3R and S4 cells. To elucidate this we performed an immunoprecipitation assay which showed the same level of p70-nibrin in both untreated and doxorubicin treated S3R and S4 cells (Fig. 4A). The p95 form of nibrin was not detected neither in S3R nor in S4 cells, however it was observed in VSMC cells, which were used as a positive control. To confirm the above observation and to exclude the possibility that the amount of immunoprecipitated protein was not equal, we verified the p70-nibrin level also after IP, using the anti-Mre11 antibody. In this case we checked the level of Mre11 by WB, as a loading control, and followed with analysis of nibrin. Also this time we did not detect any differences

Table 1. DNA content (%) in L5, S3R and S4 cells treated with different concentration of doxorubicin.

L5

%	untreated	10 nM	50 nM	100 nM	250 nM	
SubG1	11,47±5,32	7,18±5,85	**13,83±5,45**	20,48±5,42	24,64±9,37	
G1	59,57±5,61	65,19±3,24	**49,67±4,6**	57,49±10,15	59,28±5,42	
S	7,49±4,86	6,27±3,92	**3,92±0,21**	2,92±0,92	3,33±0,24	
G2/M	19,52±3,46	21,73±5,98	**30,1±11,14**	17,95±6,36	11,73±2,99	

S3R

%	untreated	10 nM	50 nM	100 nM	250 nM	
SubG1	27,93±4,14	**29,23±5,9**	31,64±5,49	33,63±5,23	32,64±1,28	
G1	25,83±4,1	**19,04±3,9**	17,18±4,01	19,77±4,56	25,87±2,45	
S	15,57±3,72	**12,53±1,12**	10,7±1,22	15,28±1,12	16,01±0,59	
G2/M	25,08±2,09	**34,84±4,49**	35,24±4,4	26,07±3,57	19±5,57	

S4

%	untreated	10 nM	50 nM	100 nM	250 nM	500 nM
SubG1	6,43±4,87	7,59±4,07	6,56±2,74	**6,72±1,57**	11,37±3,39	10,67±0,73
G1	42,01±15,9	40,37±12,17	31,63±9,31	**20,07±8,12**	18,15±2,18	35,53±1,49
S	17,13±5,69	16,67±5,85	14,12±5,28	**11±4,73**	7,68±3,56	20,78±4,08
G2/M	20,8±6,52	24,11±6,18	35,54±5,18	**48,48±5,64**	39,79±9,42	31,02±5,35

The cells were treated with doxorubicin for 24 h and DNA content was measured by flow cytometry. The percentage of DNA in all phases (including subG1) of the cell cycle is shown. Data obtained after treatment with the selected concentrations of doxorubicin, chosen for the induction of senescence, is shown in bold.

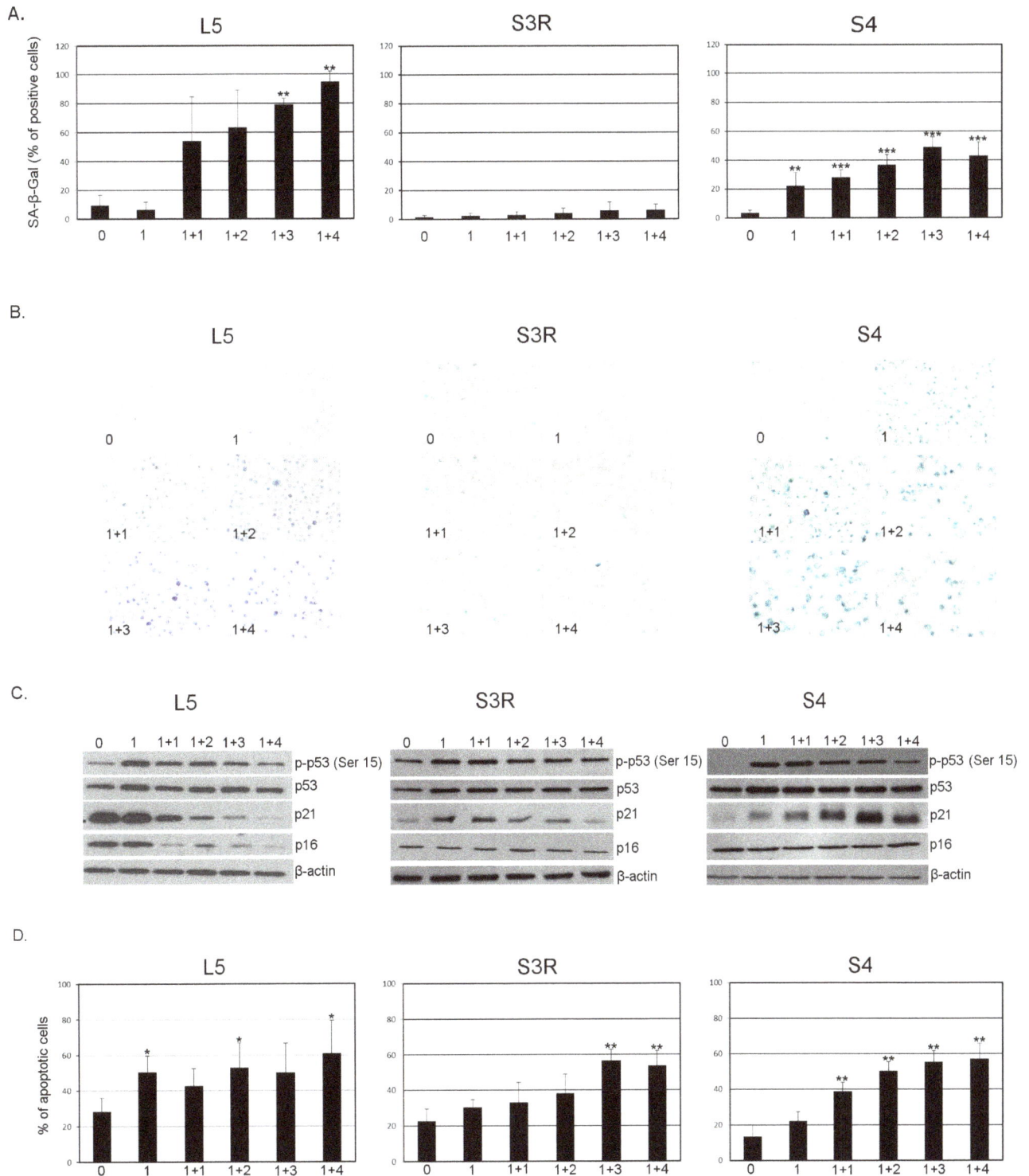

Figure 3. The induction of cellular senescence and apoptosis upon doxorubicin treatment. A. SA-β-Gal activity. Cells were treated for 1 day with doxorubicin (L5 - 50 nM, S3R - 10 nM and S4 - 100 nM) and then cultured in doxorubicin-free medium (1+n; n- are days of culture without doxorubicin). The bars show means ± SD. The percentage of SA-β-Gal positive cells from at least three independent experiments and representative images from one of three independent experiments. B. Magnification 200x. C. Expression of protein markers of senescence (p-p53, p53, p21 and p16) analyzed by Western blotting in untreated (0) cells and on the following days after culturing in doxorubicin-free medium (1+n), β-actin was used as a loading control. D. The percentage of apoptotic cells after treatment with doxorubicin estimated by the AnnexinV/7-AAD flow cytometry assay. The bars show means ± SD values. Data were obtained from three independent experiments. Statistical significance was estimated using the Student's T test.

in the level of p70-nibrin. To verify the functionality of the truncated nibrin we analyzed its binding to ATM. After immunoprecipitating either ATM or nibrin it was observed that p70-nibrin was able to form a complex with ATM in both NBS1 deficient cell lines (Fig. 4B). However, the IP revealed that more ATM immunoprecipitated with p70-nibrin in S4 than S3R cells. This may suggest that formation of DNA damage-induced ATM-nibrin complex is more efficient in S4 cells. This difference was already found in untreated cells and correlated with the observed higher phosphorylation of ATM in response to doxorubicin treatment of S4 cells (Fig. 2C). The possible better function of the DNA damage/repair response in S4 cells was confirmed by a further IP experiment showing that in these cells more BRCA1 was immunoprecipitated with ATM (Fig. 4C) suggesting that S4 are more efficient in DNA repair than the S3R cells.

5. Radiation induced activation of the DDR pathway in L5, S3R and S4 cells

Despite the fact that Nijmegen Breakage Syndrome was caused by the same mutation in the S3R and S4 cell lines their susceptibility to doxorubicin treatment differed. To verify whether this was a characteristic feature of only doxorubicin, we used a different DNA-damaging agent. Therefore the cells ability to activate the DDR pathway after being exposed to γ-radiation (4Gy and cultured for 3 h) was analyzed (Fig. 5). Interestingly, exposure to γ-radiation of both S4 and S3R as well as control (L5) cells led to an efficient induction of DDR. An increase in the level of the following proteins was observed in all of the analyzed cell lines: p-ATM (Ser 1981), p-Chk1 (Ser 317), p-p53 (Ser 15) and γH2AX. The phosphorylated form of Chk2 (Thr 68) was only noticed upon exposure to γ-radiation of the S4 cells. This indicated that these cells retain the capacity to upregulate the components of the DDR pathway, at least for a short period of time.

6. The role of nibrin in DNA damage induced senescence of human Vascular Smooth Muscle Cells

Since a relatively low level of the truncated nibrin (p70-nibrin) in S4 cells was sufficient for activation of the DDR signaling pathway followed by senescence, we asked whether downregulation of the NBS1 protein in normal cells would influence DDR activation and senescence upon treatment with doxorubicin. Transfection of L5 cells, using the nucleofection method, turned out to be unsuccessful. Only 25% of the transfected cells were viable 24 h after transfection. Therefore to analyze the effect of downregulation of nibrin on the induction of senescence, we used vascular smooth muscle cells (VSMCs) which were shown by us to undergo senescence after treatment with doxorubicin [21]. Before treatment with doxorubicin, the cells were transfected with negative siRNA or *NBN* siRNA with 85% transfection efficiency measured a day after transfection (not shown). As shown in Figure 6A the level of NBS1 in cells transfected with *NBN* siRNA and cultured in the presence of doxorubicin for three days was reduced from two to four times. Moreover the levels of p-NBS1 (Ser 343) and p-ATM (Ser 1981) were substantially reduced in these cells. However, there were no differences in the level of p53 and p21 proteins between cells transfected with negative siRNA and *NBN* siRNA (Fig. 6A). Next we decided to verify whether the downregulation of nibrin would affect the formation of 53BP1 foci, after treatment with doxorubicin. Recently 53BP1 has been recognized as a convenient marker of DSBs [22]. We observed that the formation of 53BP1 foci was not affected when the level of NBS1 was reduced (Fig. 6B, 6C). This could suggest that senescence was also not affected in cells with reduced level of

NBS1. Indeed, the percentage of SA-β-Gal positive cells was substantially increased already two days after treatment with doxorubicin in both types of cells and accounted for 100% on day 3 of treatment with doxorubicin (Fig. 6D, 6E). These results were confirmed using the BrdU incorporation assay, which showed complete inhibition of proliferation in cells which were transfected with negative siRNA and *NBN* siRNA and subsequently treated with doxorubicin (Fig. 6F).

Taken together, the obtained results performed on human VSMCs indicate that a substantially reduced level of NBS1 did not influence doxorubicin-induced DDR and senescence in these cells.

Discussion

The aim of our study was to investigate the role of nibrin in doxorubicininduced senescence.

Cellular senescence is associated withpermanent growth arrest. We can distinguish two types of cellular senescence: replicative which is telomere shortening dependent and stress-induced premature senescence, which is telomere shortening independent. Replicatively senescing cells are believed to activate the G1 restriction point. However, it was recently documented that replicative senescence can stop the cells in both the G1/S and G2/M phases of the cell cycle [23] while SIPS is mainly associated with cell cycle arrest cells in the G2/M phase of the cell cycle.

NBS1 deficient cells have improperly functioning cell cycle checkpoints [24], including a defect of the DNA damage induced intra-S-phase checkpoint which is responsible for the radio-resistant DNA synthesis (RDS)- a continuation of DNA synthesis despite the presence of radiation-induced DNA damage [25]. However, the reports concerning the status of cell cycle checkpoints in NBS deficient cells are discrepant, since both impaired and normal G1/S or G2/M arrest after cell irradiation have been reported (reviewed by [26]). Previously it was documented that S3R cells had a reduced capacity to undergo G1 arrest and showed a marked accumulation of cells in the G2/M phase of the cell cycle 24 h after 4Gy γ-irradiation, though to a lesser extent than the S4 cells [27]. We have shown that treatment with doxorubicin of L5, S3R and S4 cells led to an arrest in the G2/M phase of the cell cycle. However, we proved that S3R cells had a less efficient G2 checkpoint than S4 cells. Treatment of S3R cells with 100 nM doxorubicin, the concentration which halted most of the S4 cells in the G2/M phase of the cell cycle, led to massive cell death of S3R cells. Nevertheless the percentage of S3R cells which were arrested in the G2/M phase of the cell cycle, after treatment with the selected, cytostatic concentrations of doxorubicin, was comparable to the one observed in control L5 cells.

The higher propensity of S3R than S4 cells to undergo apoptosis was connected with a decrease in the level of double-stranded DNA as revealed using the FADU method. One should keep in mind that doxorubicin is a DNA-damaging agent which acts through different mechanisms. Amongst all, it induces the formation of cross-links which prevent DNA from unwinding. The FADU method enables to measure DNA susceptibility to unwind, which is a function of the number of chromatin modifications. Therefore the FADU method, in the context of this particular agent, can only be used as a screening method which enables to verify the cells susceptibility to treatment with different concentrations of doxorubicin. Nevertheless, the decrease in the amount of double-stranded DNA was observed with the increasing concentrations of doxorubicin and time of treatment in all of the three examined cell lines, proving that at least a portion of DNA acquires double strand breaks upon treatment with doxorubicin.

A. IP: Nibrin

WB: Nibrin

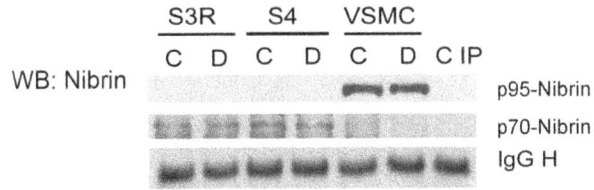

IP: Mre11

WB: Mre11

WB: Nibrin

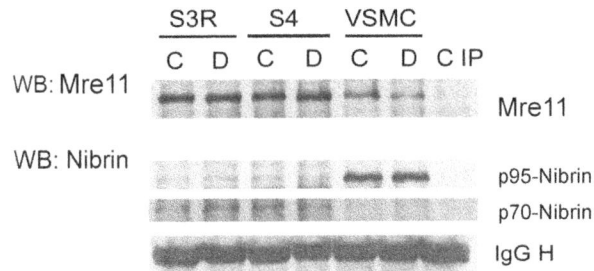

B.

IP: Nibrin

WB: Nibrin

WB: ATM

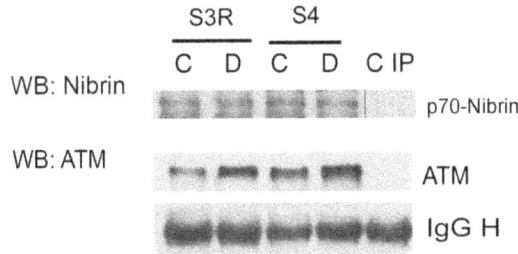

IP: ATM

WB: ATM

WB: Nibrin

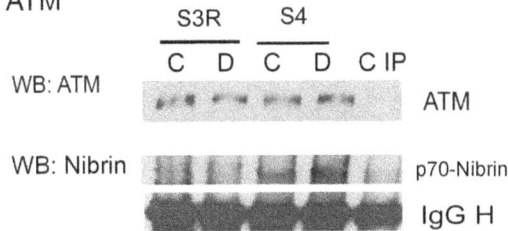

C.

IP: ATM

WB: ATM

WB: BRCA1

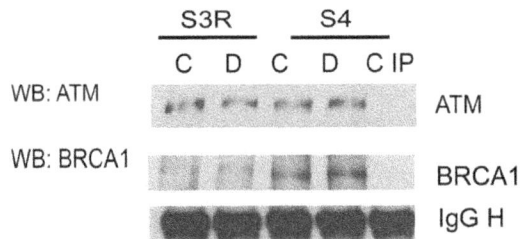

Figure 4. Levels of nibrin, p70-nibrin, MRE11, ATM and BRCA1 in the DDR complex estimated by immunoprecipitation assay. A. Level of nibrin: wild-type (p95) and the truncated form (p70) in control (C) and doxorubicin treated (D, 1 μM/1 h) S3R, S4 and VSMCs. Expression of nibrin was analyzed by immunoprecipitation using an anti-NBS1 antibody followed by Western blotting with anti-NBS1 (upper panel). Alternatively, IP using anti-MRE11 antibody was performed followed by WB with anti-NBS1 (lower panel). MRE11 was used as a loading control. The last lane (C IP) shows the negative IP control. Note that p95 is only present in VSMCs, in which there is no p70-nibrin. **B.** ATM binding to nibrin in control and doxorubicin-treated S3R and S4 cells analyzed by immunoprecipitation using anti-NBS1 antibody (upper panel) or anti-ATM antibody (lower panel). Levels of ATM and p70 were detected by WB. Loading controls were performed in both variants of IP. **C.** Expression of BRCA1 in control and dox-treated S3R and S4 cells was analyzed by immunoprecipitation using anti-ATM antibody followed by WB using an anti-BRCA1 antibody. Loading and negative IP controls were performed as above.

Generally, NBS1 deficient cells have impaired DNA repair. This process seems to be more severe in the S3R than in the S4 cells due to the lower level of the BRCA1 protein, which doesn't interact with ATM in the S3R cells. It was reported that downregulation of the NBS1 protein level by siRNA led to an increase in irradiation-induced mutation frequency in human lymphoblastoid cells [26]. Moreover, it is worth to note that null mutation of *Nbs* is lethal in mice [4].

Interestingly, the presence of less double-stranded DNA, after treatment with doxorubicin, in the S3R cells, than in the S4 and L5 cells, was not linked to ATM activation. However, we observed increased levels of p-ATM and its downstream targets such as p-Chk1, p-p53 and γH2AX 24 h after treatment with doxorubicin in control (L5) and S4 cells. Moreover in the S4 cells upon doxorubicin treatment, a substantial increase in the level of p-Chk2 (Thr 68) could be seen. Surprisingly all of the cell lines retained the ability to activate DDR upon exposure to γ-radiation. Several studies showed severe impairment of the DDR activation in NBS1 deficient cells. Namely, cells from NBS patients have been reported to be deficient in ATM phosphorylation of p53, Chk2 and other substrates following DNA damage. Other studies showed that the C-terminal fragment of nibrin was sufficient to stimulate ATM activation at early times after irradiation. In contrast, nuclear expression of a nibrin transgene lacking the C-terminal 100 amino acids was unable to stimulate ATM activation under the same conditions ([28] and literature there). This was most likely due to the lack of the ATM binding domain. We have

shown that despite the presence of the same *NBN* gene mutation, DDR is only activated in the S4 cells. Furthermore, this pathway was also activated in the L5 cells. In S3R cells some elements of the DDR (p-p53, p-Chk1 and p-Chk2) were already present in untreated cells and 24 h treatment with doxorubicin did not lead to an increase in the level of these proteins. It is tempting to speculate that the different response of the two NBS1 deficient cell lines to treatment with doxorubicin is caused by the presence of a lower level and/or nonfunctional truncated form of nibrin (p70-nibrin) in S3R cells. Indeed, it has been shown that the level of p70-nibrin can vary in cells obtained from NBS patients [2]. However, our results showed the same amount of p70-nibrin in S4 and S3R cells. Moreover, in both cell lines p70-nibrin co-immunoprecipitated with ATM. Nevertheless we observed that a higher level of p70-nibrin precipitated with ATM in S4 cells than in the S3R cells. In contrast to the results obtained using the S4 cells and the L5 cells with wild-type *NBN* gene, we did not observe ATM phosphorylation after treatment with doxorubicin in S3R cells. On the other hand, a low level of the phosphorylated form of p53 (p-p53 Ser 15) was detected in untreated, S3R cells and its level increased after treatment with doxorubicin. Others [29] showed impaired, but still detectable, ATM and p53 phosphorylation in doxorubicin-treated NBS fibroblasts. Interestingly, in NBS fibroblasts the p26 instead of the p70 fragment of nibrin could be found, which doesn't possess the ATM binding domain. This discrepancy could be explained by the fact that p53 can be phosphorylated on Ser 15 not only by ATM, but also by DNA-PK, which plays a vital role in DSB repair as well as in driving cells to apoptosis [30]. Nonetheless, the results obtained by Hou et al. [29] allowed to conclude that NBS1 is acting upstream of ATM. On the other hand, ATM phosphorylates nibrin at its Ser 343 residue [7]. We showed that nibrin can act both downstream and upstream of ATM, as downregulation of nibrin affected phosphorylation of both nibrin and ATM. These results suggested that DDR could be compromised in cells with a diminished level of nibrin. However, in VSMCs, in which the level of nibrin was substantially reduced, the p53/p21 pathway was practically not affected which suggests that in normal cells there must be a redundancy of this protein. Surprisingly, despite the presence of the same amount of p70-nibrin in both cell lines, the p53/p21 pathway was only activated in the S4 cells. This could imply a failure in DDR activation downstream of ATM in the S3R cells. However, these cells had much less ATM bound to nibrin in the IP assay.

Moreover, we detected a higher basal level of apoptosis in control S3R cells, but a substantially lower level of the BRCA1 protein in comparison with S4 cells in the IP assay. This indicates that S3R cells could have a limited capacity for DNA repair what could be reflected by a very high rate of spontaneous apoptosis in these cells. Indeed, also the basal level of p-p53 was higher in S3R than in S4 cells indicating p53-dependent apoptosis.

It seems that DDR can be a culprit of cell senescence, therefore we wondered whether S3R cells would be able to senesce after treatment with doxorubicin. Indeed, in both L5 and S4 cells we

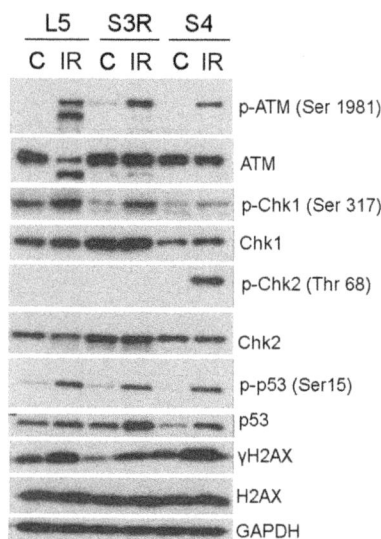

Figure 5. Activation of the DNA damage response pathway upon γ-irradiation. Expression of the DDR proteins analyzed by Western blotting in control (C) and exposed to radiation (IR) S3R, S4 and L5 cells. Whole cell extracts were prepared 3 h after exposure to 4 Gy of γ-radiation, β-actin was used as a loading control.

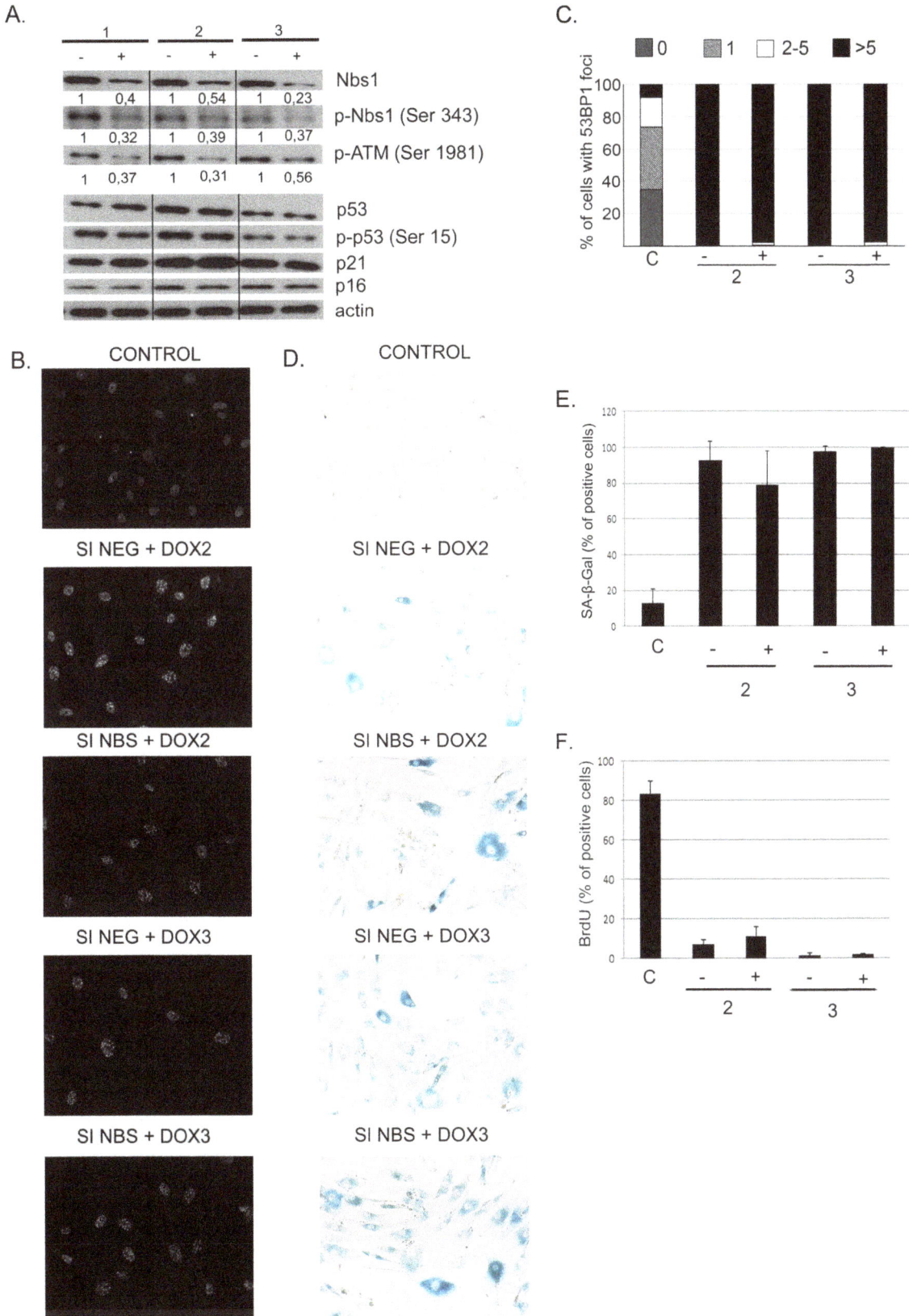

Figure 6. The role of nibrin in doxorubicin-induced senescence of human Vascular Smooth Muscle Cells (VSMCs). Cells were transfected with negative siRNA (−) or *NBN* siRNA (+) and afterwards cultured for three days in the presence of doxorubicin (100 nM). **A.** Downregulation of the NBS1 protein level in VSMCs using specific siRNA (60 nM). Whole cell extracts were prepared at indicated time points after treatment with doxorubicin. Expression of the indicated proteins was estimated by Western blotting, β-actin was used as a loading control. The amount of the protein in cells transfected with *NBN* siRNA was calculated by densitometry as a fraction of that present in cells transfected with

negative siRNA (1). **B.** 53BP1 staining in doxorubicin-treated control cells and cells with silenced nibrin. Representative images from one of three independent experiments. Magnification 100x. **C.** 53BP1 staining in doxorubicin treated control cells and cells with silenced nibrin. Cells with DNA damage were divided into four groups based on the number of 53BP1 foci: cells without 53BP1 foci, with one focus, with 2–5 foci, with more than 5 foci. Means from three independent experiments. **D.** SA-β-Gal activity in doxorubicin treated VSMC cells. Representative images from one of three independent experiments, magnification 100x. **E.** The percentage of SA-β-Gal positive cells (a mean ± SD) from three independent experiments. **F.** BrdU incorporation assay. Control cells and cells transfected with negative siRNA or *NBN* si RNA were cultured with BrdU for 24 h. Data presented as means ± SD from three independent experiments.

observed the appearance of the common and widely used marker of senescence, which is increased SA-β-Gal activity. The presence of this marker of senescence is common in adherent cells [5] however data concerning senescence of lymphoid cells and the presence of this hallmark is scarce [31]. Additionally increased activity of SA-β-Gal in the S4 cells was accompanied by a time-dependent increase in the level of p21, which is a cdk inhibitor. Thus, we can conclude that L5 and S4 cells, contrary to S3R cells, are able to activate the DDR and undergo senescence. Moreover VSMCs with a highly reduced level of nibrin were also able to undergo senescence just like cells with the proper level of this protein. We can speculate that there is a minimal amount of nibrin or its truncated p70 form which is indispensable for the activation of DDR and the subsequent induction of senescence. Interestingly, it has been shown very recently that doxorubicin treated ATM-deficient human fibroblasts underwent Akt-dependent SIPS without DDR activation [32]. It seems that S3R cells are unable to activate such a program and, most likely any senescence pathway.

We showed that S3R cells are generally more sensitive to doxorubicin treatment than the S4 and L5 cell lines. Also others showed extreme variations in the propensity to undergo DNA damage-induced apoptosis (40-fold) amongst lymphoid cells derived from the NBS patients [33]. The authors did not find a correlation between the propensity to undergo apoptosis and the level of the truncated form of nibrin-p70. The mechanisms of cell death in these cells is still awaiting elucidation.

It seems that, despite the presence of a similar level of p70-nibrin, in the S3R and S4 cell lines, the differences in ATM phosphorylation and its ability to bind nibrin were crucial for the efficient activation of DDR and the induction of senescence. We observed that some proteins which are involved in the DNA damage/repair pathway (ATM, BRCA1) were more efficiently recruited to the DNA damage-induced complex in S4 than in S3R cells what might explain the differences in the cell fate after treatment with doxorubicin.

Moreover it cannot be excluded that the described in this paper differences in the S3R and S4 cell phenotype, may result from genomic instability of patients with Nijmegen Breakage Syndrome or the immortalization process. It has also been previously shown that NBS patients with the same genotype may vary in the phenotypic expression [34]. It is worth to note that unsupervised clustering of whole genome gene expression arrays of S3R and S4 cells indicated that common gene expression changes, between the two lines, also exist [35].

Acknowledgments

Experiments using flow cytometry were performed at the Laboratory of Cytometry at the Nencki Institute of Experimental Biology. We would like to thank Mrs. Anna Leonowicz for her skillful technical assistance.

Author Contributions

Conceived and designed the experiments: OA ABZ GM ES. Performed the experiments: OA ABZ GM WDR AW MKK. Analyzed the data: OA ABZ GM MMV ZK KP ES. Contributed reagents/materials/analysis tools: MMV KP AB JKS. Contributed to the writing of the manuscript: OA ABZ GM ES.

References

1. Chrzanowska KH, Gregorek H, Dembowska-Baginska B, Kalina MA, Digweed M (2012) Nijmegen breakage syndrome (NBS). Orphanet J Rare Dis 7: 1–19.
2. Kruger L, Demuth J, Neitzel H, Varon R, Sperling K, et al. (2007) Cancer incidence in Nijmegen breakage syndrome is modulated by the amount of a variant NBS protein. Carcinogenesis 28: 107–111.
3. Maser RS, Wong KK, Sahin E, Xia H, Naylor M, et al. (2007) DNA-dependent protein kinase catalytic subunit is not required for dysfunctional telomere fusion and checkpoint response in the telomerase-deficient mouse. Mol Cell Biol 27: 2253–2265.
4. Zhu J, Petersen S, Tessarollo L, Nussenzweig A (2001) Targeted disruption of the Nijmegen breakage syndrome gene NBS1 leads to early embryonic lethality in mice. Curr Biol 11: 105–109.
5. Sikora E, Arendt T, Bennett M, Narita M (2011) Impact of cellular senescence signature on ageing research. Ageing Res Rev 10: 146–152.
6. d'Adda di Fagagna F (2008) Living on a break: cellular senescence as a DNA-damage response. Nat Rev Cancer 8: 512–522.
7. Kobayashi J, Tauchi H, Sakamoto S, Nakamura A, Morishima K, et al. (2002) NBS1 localizes to gamma-H2AX foci through interaction with the FHA/BRCT domain. Curr Biol 12: 1846–1851.
8. Freedman DA (2005) Senescence and its bypass in the vascular endothelium. Front Biosci 10: 940–950.
9. Siwicki JK, Degerman S, Chrzanowska KH, Roos G (2003) Telomere maintenance and cell cycle regulation in spontaneously immortalized T-cell lines from Nijmegen breakage syndrome patients. Exp Cell Res 287: 178–189.
10. Gewirtz DA (1999) A critical evaluation of the mechanisms of action proposed for the antitumor effects of the anthracycline antibiotics adriamycin and daunorubicin. Biochem Pharmacol 57: 727–741.
11. Siwicki JK, Hedberg Y, Nowak R, Loden M, Zhao J, et al. (2000) Long-term cultured IL-2-dependent T cell lines demonstrate p16(INK4a) overexpression, normal pRb/p53, and upregulation of cyclins E or D2. Exp Gerontol 35: 375–388.
12. Keeshan K, Mills K, Cotter TG, McKenna SL (2001) Elevated Bcr-Abl expression levels are sufficient for a haematopoietic cell line to acquire a drug-resistant phenotype. Leukemia 15: 1823–1833.
13. Laemmli UK (1970). Cleavage of structural proteins during the assembly of the head of bacteriophage T4. Nature. 227: 680–685.
14. Dimri GP, Lee X, Basile G, Acosta M, Scott G, et al. (1995). A biomarker that identifies senescence human cells in culture and in aging skin *in vivo*. Proc Natl Acad Sci USA 92: 9363–9367.
15. Moreno-Villanueva M, Eltze T, Dressler D, Bernhardt J, Hirsch C (2011) The automated FADU-assay, a potential high-throughput in vitro method for early screening of DNA breakage. Altex 28: 295–303.
16. Moreno-Villanueva M, Pfeiffer R, Sindlinger T, Leake A, Muller M (2009) A modified and automated version of the 'Fluorimetric Detection of Alkaline DNA Unwinding' method to quantify formation and repair of DNA strand breaks. BMC Biotechnol 9: 39.
17. Sherman MY, Meng L, Stampfer M, Gabai VL, Yaglom JA (2011) Oncogenes induce senescence with incomplete growth arrest and supress the DNA damage response in immortalized cells. Aging Cell 10(6): 949–961.
18. Shay JW, Roninson IB (2004) Hallmarks of senescence in carcinogenesis and cancer therapy. Oncogene 23: 2919–2933.
19. Sliwinska MA, Mosieniak G, Wolanin K, Babik A, Piwocka K, et al. (2009) Induction of senescence with doxorubicin leads to increased genomic instability of HCT116 cells. Mech Ageing Dev 130: 24–32.
20. Rayess H, Wang MB, Srivatsan ES (2012) Cellular senescence and tumor suppressor gene p16. Int J Cancer 130: 1715–1725.
21. Bielak-Zmijewska A, Wnuk M, Przybylska D, Grabowska W, Lewinska A, et al. (2014) A comparison of replicative senescence and doxorubicin-induced premature senescence of vascular smooth muscle cells isolated from human aorta. Biogerontology 15: 47–64.
22. Schultz LB, Chehab NH, Malikzay A, Halazonetis TD (2000) p53 binding protein 1 (53BP1) is an early participant in the cellular response to DNA double-strand breaks. J Cell Biol 151: 1381–1390.

23. Mao Z, Ke Z, Gorbunova V, Seluanov A (2012) Replicatively senescent cells are arrested in G1 and G2 phases. Aging 4: 431–435.
24. Shiloh Y (1997) Ataxia-telangiectasia and the Nijmegen breakage syndrome: related disorders but genes apart. Annu Rev Genet 31: 635–662.
25. Falck J, Petrini JH, Williams BR, Lukas J, Bartek J (2002) The DNA damage-dependent intra-S phase checkpoint is regulated by parallel pathways. Nat Genet 30: 290–294.
26. Zhang Y, Zhou J, Lim CU (2006) The role of NBS1 in DNA double strand break repair, telomere stability, and cell cycle checkpoint control. Cell Res 16: 45–54.
27. Siwicki JK, Berglund M, Rygier J, Pienkowska-Grela B, Grygalewicz B, et al. (2004) Spontaneously immortalized human T lymphocytes develop gain of chromosomal region 2p13–24 as an early and common genetic event. Genes Chromosomes Cancer 41: 133–144.
28. Cerosaletti K, Wright J, Concannon P (2006) Active role for nibrin in the kinetics of atm activation. Mol Cell Biol 26: 1691–1699.
29. Hou YY, Toh MT, Wang X (2012) NBS1 deficiency promotes genome instability by affecting DNA damage signaling pathway and impairing telomere integrity. Cell Biochem Funct 30: 233–242.
30. Hill R, Lee PW (2010) The DNA-dependent protein kinase (DNA-PK): More than just a case of making ends meet? Cell Cycle 9: 3460–3469.
31. Chebel A, Bauwens S, Gerland LM, Belleville A, Urbanowicz I, et al. (2009) Telomere uncapping during in vitro T-lymphocyte senescence. Aging Cell 8: 52–64.
32. Park J, Jo YH, Cho CH, Choe W, Kang I, et al. (2013) ATM-deficient human fibroblast cells are resistant to low levels of DNA double-strand break induced apoptosis and subsequently undergo drug-induced premature senescence. Biochem Biophys Res Commun 430: 429–435.
33. Thierfelder N, Demuth I, Burghardt N, Schmelz K, Sperling K, et al. (2008) Extreme variation in apoptosis capacity amongst lymphoid cells of Nijmegen breakage syndrome patients. Eur J Cell Biol 87: 111–121.
34. Nijmegen breakage syndrome (2000) The International Nijmegen Breakage Syndrome Study Group. Arch Dis Child. 82, 400–406.
35. Degerman S, Siwicki JK, Osterman P, Lafferty-Whyte K, Keith WN, et al. (2010) Telomerase upregulation is a postcrisis event during senescence bypass and immortalization of two Nijmegen breakage syndrome T cell cultures. Aging Cell 9: 220–235.

8

Ghrelin Protects against Renal Damages Induced by Angiotensin-II via an Antioxidative Stress Mechanism in Mice

Keiko Fujimura, Shu Wakino*, Hitoshi Minakuchi, Kazuhiro Hasegawa, Koji Hosoya, Motoaki Komatsu, Yuka Kaneko, Keisuke Shinozuka, Naoki Washida, Takeshi Kanda, Hirobumi Tokuyama, Koichi Hayashi, Hiroshi Itoh

Department of Internal Medicine, School of Medicine, Keio University, Tokyo, Japan

Abstract

We explored the renal protective effects by a gut peptide, Ghrelin. Daily peritoneal injection with Ghrelin ameliorated renal damages in continuously angiotensin II (AngII)-infused C57BL/6 mice as assessed by urinary excretion of protein and renal tubular markers. AngII-induced increase in reactive oxygen species (ROS) levels and senescent changes were attenuated by Ghrelin. Ghrelin also inhibited AngII-induced upregulations of transforming growth factor-β (TGF-β) and plasminogen activator inhibitor-1 (PAI-1), ameliorating renal fibrotic changes. These effects were accompanied by concomitant increase in mitochondria uncoupling protein, UCP2 as well as in a key regulator of mitochondria biosynthesis, PGC1α. In renal proximal cell line, HK-2 cells, Ghrelin reduced mitochondria membrane potential and mitochondria-derived ROS. The transfection of UCP2 siRNA abolished the decrease in mitochondria-derived ROS by Ghrelin. Ghrelin ameliorated AngII-induced renal tubular cell senescent changes and AngII-induced TGF-β and PAI-1 expressions. Finally, Ghrelin receptor, growth hormone secretagogue receptor (GHSR)-null mice exhibited an increase in tubular damages, renal ROS levels, renal senescent changes and fibrosis complicated with renal dysfunction. GHSR-null mice harbored elongated mitochondria in the proximal tubules. In conclusion, Ghrelin suppressed AngII-induced renal damages through its UCP2 dependent anti-oxidative stress effect and mitochondria maintenance. Ghrelin/GHSR pathway played an important role in the maintenance of ROS levels in the kidney.

Editor: Maria Cristina Vinci, Cardiological Center Monzino, Italy

Funding: This study was funded by the grant from Japanese Ministry of Health, Labor, Welfare. The funders had no role in study design, data collection and analysis, decision to publish, or preparation of the manuscript.

Competing Interests: The authors have declared that no competing interests exist.

* E-mail: shuwakino@z8.keio.jp

Introduction

Ghrelin is a 28-amino acid peptide containing an octanoyl modification isolated from the stomach and recognized as an endogenous ligand for the growth hormone (GH) secretagogue receptor (GHSR) [1,2]. In addition to its GH-releasing effects, various activities have been described so far that are consistent with the wide tissue distribution of GHSR including the kidney. A recent study demonstrated that the exogenous injection of Ghrelin protected against acute kidney injuries [3,4].

In chronic kidney damages, several humoral and hemodynamic factors have been shown to accelerate progression, including the activation of renin-angiotensin systems (RAS) [5]. AngII is the effector of RAS-induced renal tissue damage through multiple mechanisms, including pro-inflammatory or pro-fibrotic effects [6]. AngII has also been reported to provoke oxidative stress, mainly through the activation of NADPH-oxidase and accelerated tissue senescent changes [7,8]. This type of premature senescent reaction has been called stress-induced senescence, and it is accepted that premature renal senescence causes the deterioration of renal function and accelerates the progression of chronic kidney disease [9,10]. In diabetic nephropathy, renal tissues and tubular

cells are in a senescent state in comparison to the normal kidney [11,12], which is demonstrated by increased activity of β-galactosidase when assayed at pH 6. This type of β-galactosidase is known as senescence-associated (SA) β-gal, and it is often used as a marker for a senescent cell [13]. It has also been demonstrated that senescent cells express and produce various kinds of growth factors or cytokines, such as transforming growth factor-β (TGF-β) or plasminogen activator inhibitor-1 (PAI-1), which enhances tissue fibrosis and contributes to the functional decline [12].

Recent studies revealed that Ghrelin exerts its anti-oxidative function by reducing the production of reactive oxygen species (ROS) from mitochondria [14]. Ghrelin has been demonstrated to increase the expression of mitochondrial uncoupling protein UCP2 in neuronal cells [15], diminishing the mitochondrial membrane potential, reducing excessive oxidative phosphorylation reactions in mitochondria, and downregulating mitochondria ROS production [14]. Given the expression of Ghrelin and its receptor GHSR in the kidney [16], it is surmised that Ghrelin protects against the progression of chronic kidney damage and renal premature senescence.

In this study, the protective effects of Ghrelin on chronic renal damages induced by AngII infusion were investigated. We further

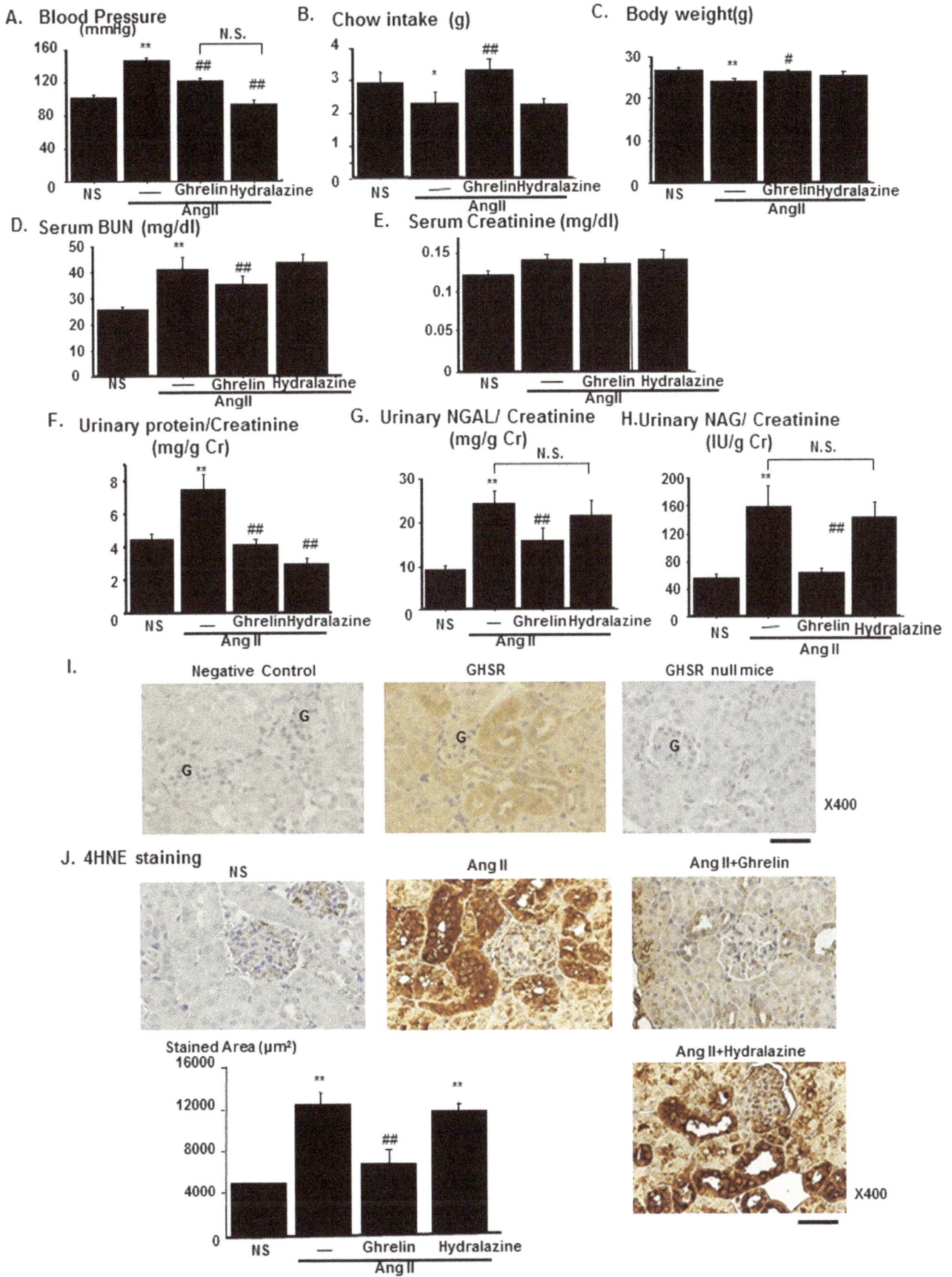

Figure 1. Amelioration of renal tubular damages and increased renal oxidative stress by Ghrelin in AngII-infused mice. The effects of Ghrelin treatment on the phenotypes of AngII-infused mice. Blood pressures (A), daily chow intake (B) and body weight (C) were compared among saline-infused mice (NS), AngII-infused mice (AngII), and AngII-infused mice treated with Ghrelin (AngII+Ghrelin) or Hydralazine (AngII+Hydralazine). Serum levels of blood urea nitrogen (BUN, D) and creatinine (E), urinary excretion of protein (F), neutrophil gelatinase-associated lipocalin (NGAL, G), n-acetyl-galactasaminase (NAG, H) were compared among the experimental groups. (I) Representative immunostaining for the Ghrelin receptor (Growth hormone secretagogue receptor, GHSR) is shown in the middle panel. Negative control without using anti-GHSR antibody is shown in the left panel. The staining of GHSR in the kidney of GHSR null mice is also shown in the right panel. Scale bar, 50 μm. G represents glomerulus. (J) Representative immunostaining for 4-Hydroxynonenal-2-nonenal (4HNE) of four experimental groups. Bar graphs represent the quantification of immunostained areas. Scale bar; 50 μm. **$p < 0.01$ vs. NS, *$p < 0.05$ vs. NS, ##$p < 0.01$ vs. AngII, #$p < 0.05$ vs. AngII, N.S. represents no significant difference. $n = 8$.

examined the role of endogenous Ghrelin/GHSR system in the kidney by using GHSR-null mice.

Results

Ghrelin attenuates renal tubular damages in AngII-infused mice models

Ghrelin treatment lowered the blood pressure of AngII-infused mice (AngII) as compared to that in saline-infused mice. To rule out the effects on blood pressure, the anti-hypertensive drug, hydralazine was given orally to AngII-infused mice. The treatment with hydralazine at the dose of 25 mg/kg/day [17] lowered blood pressure to levels similar to those with Ghrelin treatment (Figure 1A). Chow intake was decreased by AngII and this decrease was reversed by Ghrelin through its orexigenic effects (Figure 1B). Body weight was decreased in AngII-infused mice and this decrease was attenuated by Ghrelin (Figure 1C). Serum blood urea nitrogen (BUN) levels were increased in AngII-infused mice and this increase was attenuated by Ghrelin but not by hydralazine, although serum creatinine levels were not altered. (Figure 1D and 1E). Urinary protein excretion was increased in AngII-infused mice and this increase was attenuated both by Ghrelin and by hydralazine, indicating that the inhibitory effects by Ghrelin on urinary protein excretion were by blood pressure-dependent mechanism (Figure 1F). Urinary excretion of both neutrophil galatinase-associated lipocalin (NGAL) and n-acetyl-galactasaminase (NAG), markers for proximal tubular damages, increased in AngII-infused mice, and these increases were attenuated in Ghrelin-treated mice. However, hydralazine had no effects on urinary excretion of either NGAL or NAG (Figure 1G and 1H). In immunohistochemistry using antibody against GHSR, GHSR was expressed in the renal tubular area but not in the glomerular area (Figure 1I). Renal tissue oxidative stress levels were increased in the proximal tubular area in AngII-infused mice as assessed by the immunostaining for 4-Hydroxynonenal-2-nonenal (4HNE). This increase was abolished by Ghrelin treatment, although hydralazine had no effect (Figure 1J).

Ghrelin ameliorates renal senescence changes and fibrosis induced by AngII

Oxidative stress has been reported to induce cellular or tissue senescence, which is known as stress-induced premature senescence [9]. Anti-oxidative stress effects by Ghrelin in the kidney are suggested to cause renal anti-senescence effects, as previously reported in other tissues [18]. After AngII infusion, SA β-Gal staining revealed that staining levels were increased, particularly in tubular cells. This increase was attenuated by Ghrelin (Figure 2A). The cell cycle negative regulator p53 and its downstream target gene p21 were among the markers for cellular senescence. AngII infusion significantly increased the expression of both p53 and p21. These inductions were blocked by the treatment with Ghrelin (Figure 2B). The changes in the inflammatory cytokines characteristics of senescence reaction, including those in TGF-β and PAI-

1, were examined. AngII infusion to mice increased the expression of both TGF-β and PAI-1 in the kidney. These increases were significantly blocked by Ghrelin (Figure 2C, left and right panel, respectively). These cytokines contribute to the renal fibrotic changes [19] and we evaluated interstitial fibrosis by Masson-trichrome staining. AngII infusion increased perivascular fibrosis and this change was attenuated by the treatment with Ghrelin but not by the treatment with hydralazine (Figure 2D). Consistently, the expression levels of type I collagen in the kidney were increased in AngII-infused mice and this increase was attenuated by Ghrelin treatment (Figure 2E).

Ghrelin increased UCP2 expression and the number of mitochondria in the kidney

We examined the expression of various molecules related to oxidative stress. The expression levels of UCP2 were increased in Ghrelin-treated mice although AngII infusion failed to induce UCP2 expression (Figure 3A). The expression of catalase was not altered either by AngII or by Ghrelin (Figure 3B). The expressions of NADPH oxidase (NOX) contributing to the ROS production by AngII were examined and the expressions of two isoforms of NOX1 and NOX4 were increased by AngII (Figure 3C and 3D, respectively). The expression of the NOX subunit p22phox was also increased by AngII (Figure 3E). These molecules were downregulated by Ghrelin. The expression levels of peroxisome proliferator-activated receptor-γ coactivator 1α (PGC-1α), a key regulator of mitochondria number, increased by treatment with Ghrelin (Figure 3F). The number of mitochondria also increased in Ghrelin-treated mice (Figure 3G). These data suggested that Ghrelin not only attenuated AngII-induced ROS production, but also increased the number of mitochondria in the kidney through both inhibitory effect on AngII-dependent ROS production and its own anti-oxidative stress effects.

Ghrelin reduced mitochondria ROS through UCP2 dependent mechanism

By utilizing HK-2 cells, a human renal proximal tubular cell line, we further examined anti-oxidative stress effects of Ghrelin. HK-2 cells expressed both the mRNA and protein of GHSR (Figure S1A). Ghrelin increased the expression of UCP2 in a dose-dependent manner (Figure 4A). UCP2 reduces mitochondrial membrane potential and inhibits the excessive ATP production and mitochondrial ROS production [20]. Treatment with Ghrelin reduced membrane potential in a dose-dependent manner (Figure 4B). Due to the reduction of membrane potential, Ghrelin decreased mitochondria-derived ROS levels (Figure 4C). In addition, treatment with Ghrelin significantly increased the mitochondria number in a dose-dependent manner (Figure 4D). Ghrelin has been shown to activate AMP-kinase in central nervous systems [21]. The upregulation of UCP2 by Ghrelin was blocked by AMP-kinase inhibitor, Compound C in a dose-dependent manner (Figure 4E). These results implied that UCP2 was

A. SA-β Gal staining

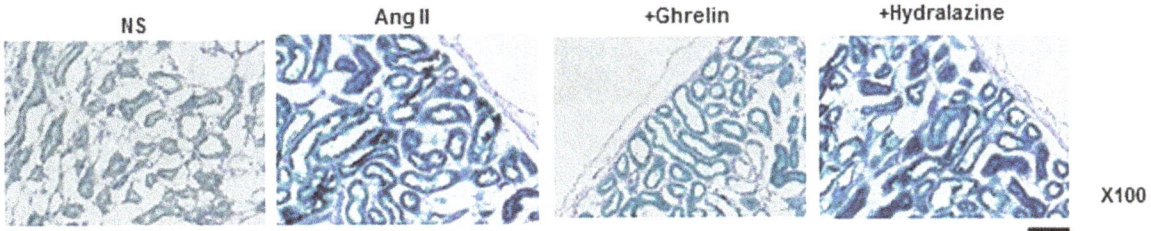

B.

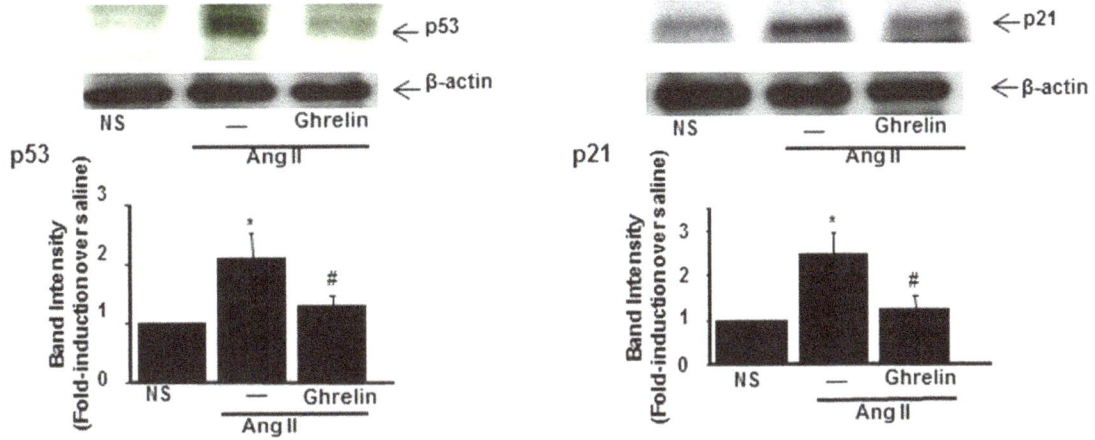

C.

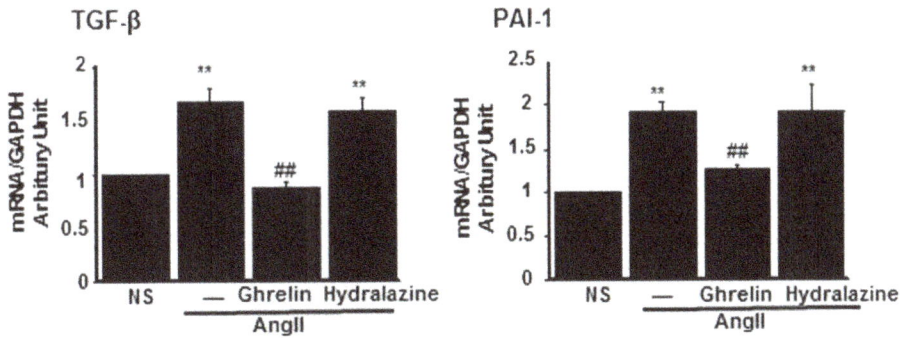

D.

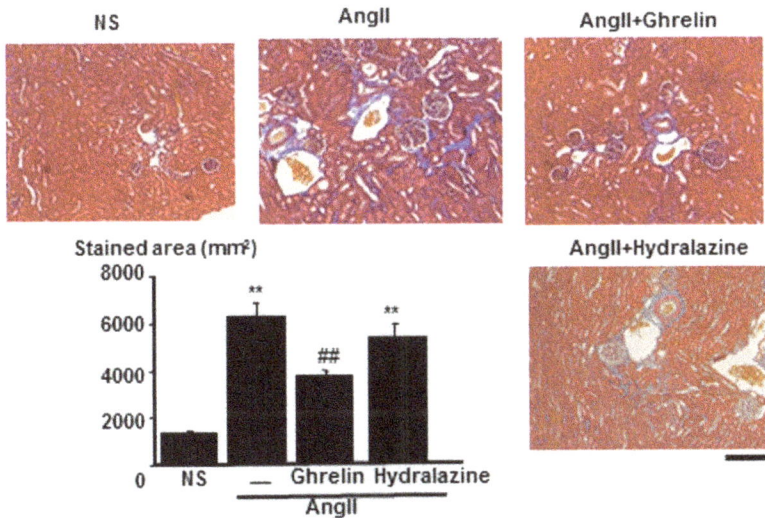

E. Type I Collagen expression

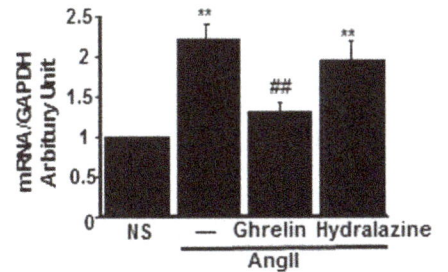

Figure 2. Amelioration of renal tissue senescent and fibrotic changes by Ghrelin in AngII-infused mice. (A) Representative staining of senescence-associated β-Galactosidase (SA β-Gal). Scale bar, 100 μm. NS represents normal saline. (B) The protein expressions of p53 (left) and p21 (right) in saline-infused mice (NS), AngII-infused mice (AngII), and AngII-infused mice treated with Ghrelin. The representative immunoblotting (upper panel) and the results of densitometry analysis (lower panel) are shown. (C) The expression of TGF-β (left) and PAI-1 (right) mRNA in mice of each group. (D) The representative results of Masson-Trichrome staining of each experimental group. Bar graphs represent the quantification of fibrotic areas. Scale bar; 100 μm. (E) The mRNA expression levels of type I collagen in the kidney of each group. **$p < 0.01$ vs. NS, *$p < 0.05$ vs. NS, ##$p < 0.01$ vs. AngII, #$p < 0.05$ vs. AngII, n = 8.

upregulated by Ghrelin through AMP kinase activation. We next designed siRNA for UCP2, which successfully knockdown both protein and mRNA expressions of UCP2 (Figure 4F, left and right panels, respectively). The expressions of other genes related to antioxidative stress or other isoforms of UCP were not affected by this siRNA, which confirmed the specificity of this siRNA (Figure S1B–S1E). Transfection of siRNA for UCP2 abolished the reduction of mitochondria-derived ROS production by Ghrelin (**Figure 4G**). UCP2 gene knockdown also abrogated the effects of Ghrelin on the production of ROS and superoxide from total cellular origin (Figure 4H and 4I, respectively). Ghrelin also reduced AngII-induced mitochondria-derived ROS production (Figure 4J).

Ghrelin attenuates AngII-induced renal proximal tubular cell senescence

The anti-senescence effects of Ghrelin in renal tubular cells were also investigated by using HK-2 cells. With AngII treatment, the population of senescent cells stained in the SA-β Gal assay was increased. This increase was inhibited by pretreatment with Ghrelin as well as with AngII receptor blockade, irbesartan but not with Des-acyl Ghrelin, the inactive form of Ghrelin (Figure 5A). AngII also increased the expressions of p53 and p21 in HK-2 cells. These increases were downregulated by the pretreatment with Ghrelin but not by Des-acyl Ghrelin (Figure 5B). The mRNA expression of TGF-β and the secretion of TGF-β in the medium were increased by AngII. These effects of AngII were inhibited by the pretreatment with Ghrelin (Figure 5C). Similar results were obtained for the expression and secretion of PAI-1 in HK-2 cells (Figure 5D).

Renal tubular damages were evident in GHSR-null mice

We further delineated the role of endogenous Ghrelin in the kidney by using GHSR-null mice [22]. Real-time PCR revealed that GHSR-null mice lacked expression of GHSR (Figure 6A). GHSR-null mice (KO) and wild-type (WT) littermates were infused with AngII or normal saline (NS). We compared various phenotype among the four group, WT mice infused with NS (WT+NS) or AngII (500 ng/kg/day, WT+AngII) and KO mice infused with NS (KO+NS) or AngII (KO+AngII). Systolic blood pressure was increased in KO+NS as compared with that in WT+NS and AngII further increased systolic blood pressure in KO mice (KO+NS vs. KO+AngII) (Figure 6C). Daily chow intake was reduced in KO mice and body weight was decreased in KO+NS as compared with those in WT. These changes were augmented by AngII infusion (Figure 6D and 6E, respectively). Serum BUN and creatinine levels were increased in KO+NS as compared to those in WT+NS, which were further aggravated by AngII infusion (Figure 6F and 6G, respectively). Urinary protein excretion (Figure 6H) as well as urinary excretion of renal tubular markers, NGAL (Figure 6I) and NAG (Figure 6J), were increased in KO+NS as compared with those in WT+NS. These increases were augmented by AngII infusion (KO+NS vs. KO+AngII). 4HNE staining showed that ROS levels in the kidney increased in KO+NS as compared with those in WT+NS. These increases

were enhanced by AngII infusion (KO+NS vs. KO+AngII) (Figure 6K). These data demonstrated that endogenous Ghrelin was involved in the regulation of renal ROS levels in the kidney and had a protective role against renal damages by ROS. We further treated AngII-infused GHSR-null mice with Ghrelin by daily intraperitoneal injection for 14 days. The treatment of Ghrelin failed to attenuate the AngII-induced increase in blood pressure, serum BUN concentration, serum creatinine concentration, urinary protein excretion, and urinary excretion of NAG and NGAL (Figure S2B–S2G, respectively). Similarly, Ghrelin had no effects on the expression of UCP2 and on AngII-induced oxidative stress increase in AngII-infused GHSR-null mice (Figure S2H and S2I, respectively). These data indicated that the effects of Ghrelin against AngII-induced renal damages were mediated by GHSR dependent mechanism.

GHSR-null mice exhibited renal senescence, fibrosis and mitochondrial loss

The increase in ROS levels in KO mice suggest that enhanced senescence changes and fibrotic changes in the kidney are evident in KO mice. SA-β Gal staining revealed that staining intensity increased in KO+NS as compared with that in WT+NS. AngII also increased SA-β Gal staining both in WT and in KO (Figure 7A). Masson-Tichrome staining revealed that fibrotic changes increased in KO+NS as compared with in WT+NS. AngII also enhanced fibrotic changes both in WT and in KO (Figure 7B). Similar results were obtained as regards the renal expression levels of type I collagen, the molecular marker for tissue fibrosis (Figure 7C). Our *in vitro* findings demonstrate that these changes were caused by the mitochondrial damages and increased mitochondrial ROS levels. In the electromicroscopic finding, the number of mitochondria was reduced in KO+NS as compared to that in WT+NS. This reduction of mitochondria number was enhanced by AngII infusion. In mitochondrial morphology, mitochondria were elongated in KO+NS, and this morphological alteration was enhanced in KO+AngII (Figure 7D).

Discussion

We demonstrated that the gut peptide Ghrelin exerts a renal protective effect by reducing oxidative stress levels and by retaining mitochondria, through the induction of mitochondria UCP2 expression and PGC1α expression. These effects contributed to the ameliorations of tissue senescent changes and fibrosis in AngII-induced renal damages (Figure 8). We also demonstrated that anti-oxidative effect by endogenous Ghrelin had also an important role in maintenance of redox state in the kidney.

UCP2 maintains the membrane potential and regulates mitochondrial ROS production during oxidative phosphorylation [20]. It has also been demonstrated that superoxide activates UCP2, and this regulatory mechanism functions as a feedback mechanism for excess oxidative stress [23]. In central nervous system [24] and human vascular smooth muscle cell [25], AngII-induced oxidative stress was silenced by the upregulation of UCP2 through the activation of p38 MAP kinase [24]. In our AngII-infusion kidney and also in AngII-stimulated HK-2 cells, the

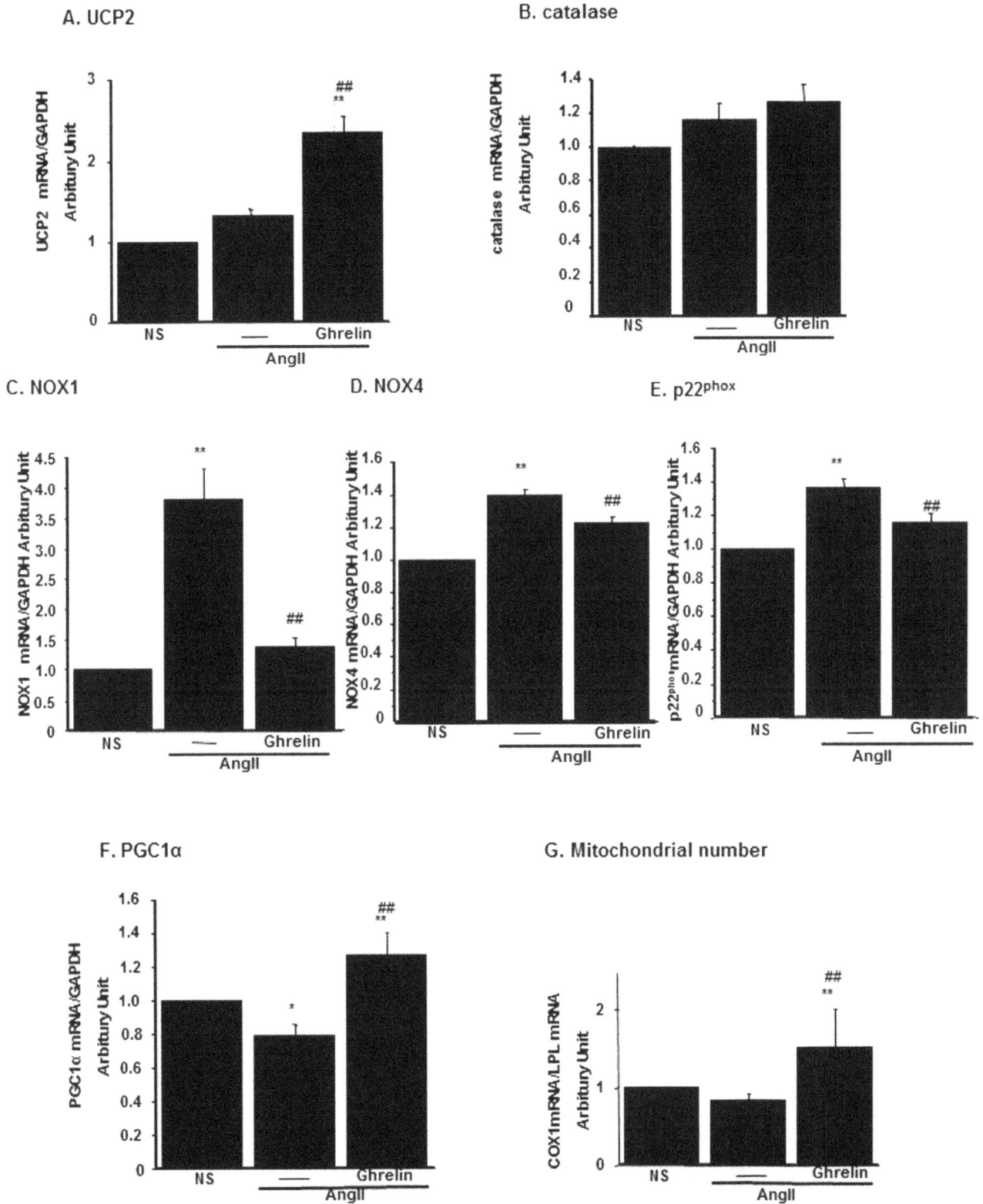

Figure 3. The mRNA expressions of anti-oxidative stress molecules and mitochondria number in the kidney. The mRNA expressions of UCP2 (A), catalase (B), NADPH oxidases, NOX1 (C), NOX4 (D), p22phox (E) and PGC1α (F) in saline-infused mice (NS), AngII-infused mice (AngII), and AngII-infused mice treated with Ghrelin were examined by real-time PCR. (G) The mitochondria number was assessed as real-time PCR for mitochondria-specific molecule, COX1 as described in Materials and Methods. $**p<0.01$ vs. NS, $*p<0.05$ vs. NS, $\#\#p<0.01$ vs. AngII, $\#p<0.05$ vs. AngII, n = 8.

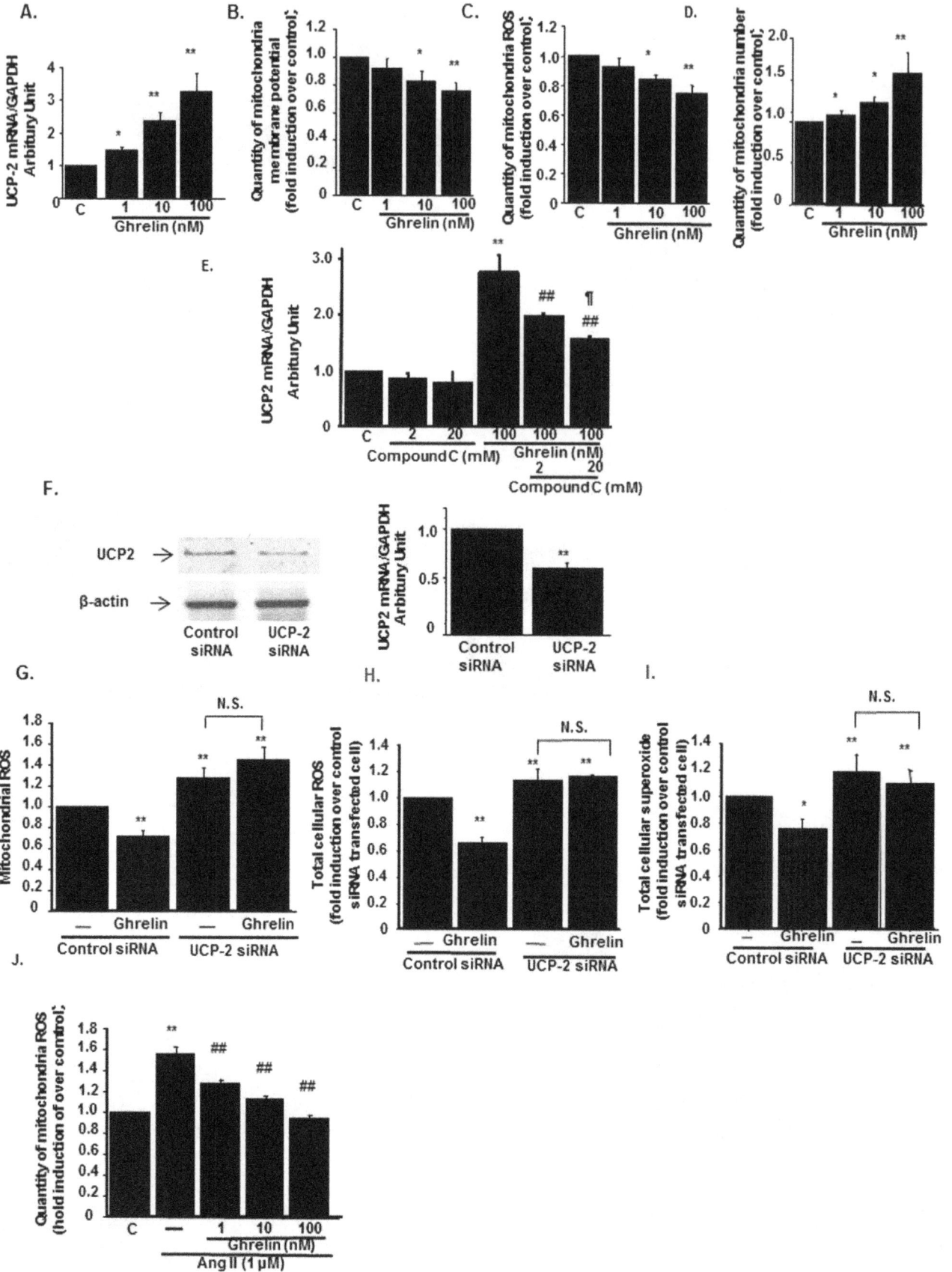

Figure 4. Mitochondria-derived ROS was reduced by Ghrelin through the induction of UCP2. (A) The effects of Ghrelin on mitochondria-derived UCP2 mRNA levels. (B) Mitochondrial membrane potential was measured by the specific dye as described in Materials and Methods. **p<0.01 vs. control cells, n = 8. (C, D) The effects of Ghrelin on mitochondria-derived ROS levels (C) and mitochondria number (D) in HK-2 cells. **p<0.01 vs. control HK-2 cells, *p<0.05 vs. control, n = 8. (E) The effects of AMP-kinase inhibitor on Ghrelin-induced UCP2 upregulation. Compound C, AMP-kinase inhibitor at the concentrations of 2 and 20 µM was pretreated 30 minutes before the Ghrelin administration to HK-2 cells. **p<0.01 vs. control HK-2 cells, ##p<0.01 vs. HK-2 cells treated with 100 nM of Ghrelin, ¶p<0.05 vs. Ghrelin-treated cell with 2 µM of Compound C administration, n = 8. (F) Knock-down of UCP2 protein and mRNA were shown in the representative immunoblotting (left panel) and real-time PCR (right panel), respectively. **p<0.01 vs. control siRNA-transfected cells, n = 6. (G–I) Mitochondria-derived ROS (G), total cellular ROS (H), and total cellular superoxide (I) were measured after the transfection of UCP2 siRNA or control siRNA. HK-2 cells were transfected with siRNA and treated with or without 100 nM of Ghrelin **p<0.01 vs. control siRNA-transfected cells without Ghrelin. N.S. represents no significant difference. n = 8. (J) The effects of Ghrelin on AngII-induced Mitochondrial ROS production. HK-2 cells were treated with 1 nM, 10 nM, and 100 nM of Ghrelin 30 minutes before the treatment with 1 mM of AngII. respectively. **p<0.01 vs. control cells, *p<0.05 vs. control cells, ##p<0.01 vs. AngII-treated HK-2 cells, #p<0.05 vs. AngII-treated HK-2 cells, n = 8.

upregulation of UCP2 was not observed (Figure 3A) and this deficiency of the compensatory mechanism in renal tubular cells might aggravate tissue damages by oxidative stress by AngII. However, this aggravation was ameliorated by Ghrelin-induced UCP2 upregulation by its action to mitochondria. In human vascular smooth muscle cells, adenovirus-mediated gene transfer of UCP2 ameliorated AngII-induced ROS production [25], which was consistent with our results in renal tubular cells. Previous reports demonstrated that UCP2 was upregulated by the AMP-kinase pathway [26]. AMP-kinase activation also resulted in the increased mitochondria number through the activation of PGC1α [27,28]. Ghrelin has been reported to activate AMP-kinase pathway in appetite regulation through the GHSR-dependent pathway [21]. The effects by Ghrelin on AMP-kinase activation would contribute to the UCP2 upregulation as shown in Figure 4E and also to the increase in the mitochondria number.

The production of ROS by AngII are main signal intermediates involved in renal pathophysiology [29,30]. AngII-induced ROS are important for renal inflammation and fibrosis [31]. In our AngII-infused model, AngII increased the expression of NOX1 and NOX4, major isoforms of NOX in the kidney. It has been found that AngII stimulates upregulation of various NADPH oxidase subunits, including NOX1, p47phox, p67phox, and p22phox in cytosolic fraction [29]. Ghrelin decreased the expression levels of NOX1 and p22phox. NOX expressions have been implicated to be regulated by the redox state [32,33]. Therefore, it can be surmised that Ghrelin partially downregulated AngII-induced NOXs increase through the potent reduction in oxidative stress [32,33] (Figure 3C–3E). However, these cytosolic ROS production was not completely ameliorated, which results were consistent with the results that AngII increased renal tissue oxidative stress levels and tissue damages even in the GHSR-null mice. A recent study also suggested AngII-stimulated mitochondrial ROS generation through the opening of mitochondrial K_{ATP} channels [34] and induced expression of mitochondrial NOX4 in renal tubular cells [35]. Our group previously demonstrated that AngII increased mitochondria-derived ROS and the number of mitochondria in muscle tissues [36]. The present data revealed that treatment with Ghrelin downregulated the increase in NOX4 expression in AngII-infused mice kidney. Therefore, Ghrelin reduced AngII-induced ROS production by mitochondria-dependent and/or independent mechanisms.

Mitochondria are sensitive to oxidative stress because its DNA lacks the histone protein and easily breaks down by ROS. Kidney proximal tubular cells possess large numbers of mitochondria and are highly dependent on mitochondrial energy production for their proper function [37]. Therefore, the damages of proximal tubular cells were dependent on the mitochondria damages or mitochondria loss evoked by tissue oxidative stress. Especially in acute kidney injuries such as ischemia-reperfusion injuries [38] or

cisplatin-induced kidney damages [39], mitochondria damages in proximal tubules contributed to the decline in renal function. We previously reported that the overexpression of NAD-dependent deacetylase Sirt1 in the proximal tubules reversed the decline in renal function by cisplatin-induced and ischemia-reperfusion renal damages by reducing oxidative stress and retaining mitochondria number [40]. In our AngII-infused models, the decreased number of mitochondria was induced presumably by the increased ROS production in the proximal renal tubules and renal proximal tubular damages were prominent as evaluated by urinary excretion of proximal tubular cell markers. Ghrelin treatment reduced mitochondria-derived ROS production, induced PGC1α and restored mitochondria number in the kidney of these mice. These effects by Ghrelin ameliorated renal tubular damages by AngII.

In the present study, we described the phenotype of GHSR-null mice. GHSR null mice already exhibited renal tubular damages, renal dysfunction and increase in oxidative stress levels. We also observed the increase in the number of elongated mitochondria and the decrease in total mitochondria number in proximal tubular cells in GHSR null mice. The elongated mitochondria indicated the accumulation of oxidative stress in mitochondria [41]. In addition, the elongated mitochondria develop due to the escape from the autophagy process [41]. Therefore, it is concluded that the damaged mitochondria were accumulated in the proximal tubules of GHSR-null mice. Moreover, GHSR-null mice exhibited the decline in renal function as indicated by increase in plasma creatinine levels. Our data demonstrated that Ghrelin/GHSR pathway stabilizes the ROS status and mitochondria quality and maintains renal function by the regulation of mitochondria oxidative stress levels.

In previous reports, Ghrelin mitigated acute renal damages induced by ischemia and reperfusion injuries [3]. These effects were mediated through the activation of the growth hormone-insulin-like growth factor 1 pathway. In another study, Ghrelin treatment protected against acute endotoxemia-induced kidney injury through the inhibition of multiple proinflammatory cytokines [4]. These studies did not demonstrated direct effects of Ghrelin on the kidney. Our study provides evidence for novel direct protective effects of Ghrelin on the tubular cells through anti-oxidative effects. The mRNA expressions of GHSR have been confirmed in the kidney, according to a recent study [16]. In the present study, immunostaining for GHSR was detected in the tubular area including in the proximal portion of tubules (Figure 1I). In addition, HK-2 cells of the proximal tubular cell line expressed both the mRNA and protein of GHSR (Figure 4A). The treatment with Ghrelin ameliorated the damages to proximal tubules as assessed by the proximal tubular marker, NAG and NGAL (Figure 1G and 1H). Our data indicates the possibility that GHSR is expressed in the proximal portion, and that Ghrelin

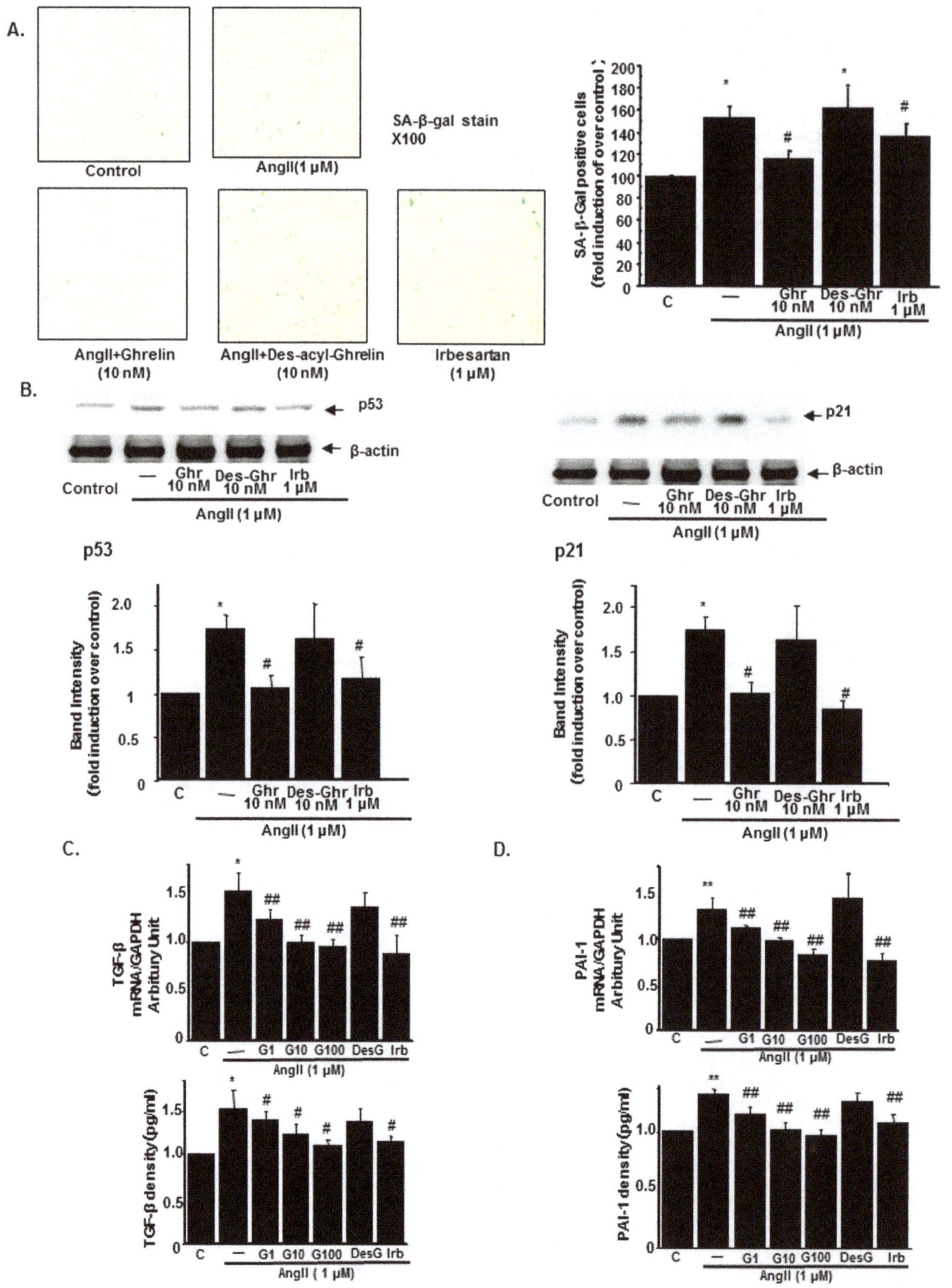
A.
Control
AngII(1 μM)
SA-β-gal stain
X100
AngII+Ghrelin
(10 nM)
AngII+Des-acyl-Ghrelin
(10 nM)
Irbesartan
(1 μM)
SA-β-Gal positive cells
(fold induction of over control)
C
Ghr 10 nM
Des-Ghr 10 nM
Irb 1 μM
AngII (1 μM)
B.
p53
β-actin
p21
Control
Ghr 10 nM
Des-Ghr 10 nM
Irb 1 μM
AngII (1 μM)
p53
p21
Band Intensity
(fold induction over control)
C.
D.
TGF-β
mRNA/GAPDH
Arbitury Unit
PAI-1
mRNA/GAPDH
Arbitury Unit
C
G1
G10
G100
DesG
Irb
AngII (1 μM)
TGF-β density (pg/ml)
PAI-1 density (pg/ml)

Figure 5. The amelioration of cellular senescent changes in AngII-treated HK-2 by Ghrelin. (A) Representative staining of senescence-associated β-Galactosidase (SA β-Gal) in untreated HK-2 cells (control), AngII-treated HK-2 cells (AngII, 1 μM), and AngII-treated with the pretreatment of 10 nM Ghrelin (AngII+Ghrelin), 10 nM Des-acyl-Ghrelin (AngII+Des-acy-Ghrelin), or 1 μM AngII type 1 receptor antagonist, irbesartan (left panel). Bar graphs represent the quantification of stained cells (right panel). (B) The protein expressions of p53 (left) and p21 (right) in HK-2 cells. The representative immunoblotting (upper panel) and the results of densitometry analysis (lower panel) were shown. (C) The expression of TGF-β mRNA in HK-2 cells (upper panel) and the concentration of TGF-β in the medium of HK-2 cells (lower panel). (D) The expression of PAI-1 mRNA in HK-2 cells (upper panel) and the concentration of PAI-1 in the medium of HK-2 cells (lower panel). C; control cells, AngII; HK-2 cells treated with 1 μM of AngII, G1, G10, G100; HK-2 cells treated with 1 nM, 10 nM, and 100 nM of Ghrelin, respectively, Des-G; HK-2 cells treated with 10 nM of Des-acyl-Ghrelin, Irb; HK-2 cells treated with 1 μM of irbesartan **$p<0.01$ vs. control HK-2 cells, *$p<0.05$ vs. control HK-2 cells, ##$p<0.01$ vs. AngII-treated HK-2 cells, #$p<0.05$ vs. AngII-treated HK-2 cells, $n=8$.

exerts its renal protective effect directly through GHSR in the kidney.

In conclusion, we demonstrated that Ghrelin ameliorated AngII-induced renal damages through the reduction of oxidative stress in the renal tissues through the induction of the mitochondria uncoupling protein UCP2. GHSR-null mice exhibited renal dysfunction with an increase in oxidative stress, fibrosis and senescent changes as compared to WT littermates, indicating that endogenous Ghrelin/GHSR systems were essential for the regulation of ROS levels of the kidney. Our data provide compelling evidence for a novel strategy against the progression of renal insufficiency.

Materials and Methods

Ethics Statement

This study was performed in accordance with the institutional guidelines of the Animal Care and Experimentation Committee at Keio University. The experimental protocols were approved by the Animal Care and Experimentation Committee at Keio University (No. 09119). All surgery was performed under sodium pentobarbital anesthesia, and all efforts were made to minimize suffering. At the end of the experiments, the mice were euthanized by intraperitoneal injection of sodium pentobarbital.

Animal experimental protocol

Sixteen-week-old male C57/BL6J mice (Nippon Clea, Tokyo, Japan) were divided into four groups ($n=8$ per group). Three groups were treated with continuous AngII (1500 ng/kg/day, Peptide Institute Inc., Osaka, Japan) infusion during 28 days by using an Alzet micro-osmotic pump (Model 1004D; Durect Co., Cupertino, CA). The dose of 1500 ng/kg/min AngII is most commonly used in rodents and causes relevant elevations of blood pressure. One group received Ghrelin (100 μg/kg/day) by daily intraperitoneal injection for 14 days. One group was administered hydralazine orally at the dose of 25 mg/kg/day [14]. Blood pressure was measured weekly by tail-cuff plethysmography (TSE 209000; TSE Systems) as previously described [40]. Body weight and chow intake were monitored every week. Five days before sacrifice, animals were housed in metabolic cages over 24 hours for urine collection. Daily urinary excretion of protein, NAG (beta-N-acetylglucosaminidase) and neutrophil-associated lipocalin (NGAL) were measured by ELISA (Quantikine, R&D Systems, Minneapolis) and expressed as normalized by urinary excretion of creatinine.

Histomorphology and Immunohistochemistry

Kidney tissues were fixed with PBS containing 4% paraformaldehyde and embedded in paraffin. Sections were cut 5 μm and used in immunohistochemical staining. Immunohistochemical staining was performed using primary antibody against 4-Hydroxynonenal-2-nonenal (4HNE) (NIKKEN SEIL Co.,Fukuroi, Japan) and GHSR (Sigma-Aldrich Co., St. Louis, MO).

Horseradish peroxidase-conjugated anti-mouse and anti-rabbit IgG antibodies (Dako, Glostrup, Denmark) were used for secondary antibody.

Electromicroscopic analysis

The samples were fixed with 2% paraformaldehyde (PFA), 2% glutaraldehyde (Distilled EM grade, Electron Microscopy Sciences, Hatfield, PA) in 0.1 M PBS pH 7.4 at 4°C overnight. After the fixation, the samples were rinsed three times with 0.1 M PBS for 30 minutes, followed by post-fixation with 2% osmium tetroxide(OsO$_4$) in PBS at 4°C for two hours. The samples were then infiltrated with propylene oxide (PO) twice for 15 min and put them into a mixture of PO and resin (Quetol-812; Nisshin EM Co.,Tokyo, Japan) for one hour, followed by keeping the cap of tube open, and PO was volatilized overnight. The samples was transferred to a fresh 100% resin, and polymerized at 60°C for 48 hours. The blocks were ultra-thin sectioned at 70 nm with a diamond knife using a ultramicrotome (ULTRACUT UCT; Leica, Wetzlar, Germany) and sections were placed on copper grids. They were stained with 2% uranyl acetate at room temparature for 15 min. and then rinsed with distilled water followed by being secondary-stained with Lead stain solution (Sigma-Aldrich) at room temparature for three minutes. The grids were observed by a transmission electron microscope (JEM-1200EM; JEOL Ltd., Akishima, Japan) at an acceleration voltage of 80 kv. Digital images (2048×2048pixels) were taken with a CCD camera (VELETA; Olympus Soft Imaging Solutions GmbH, Münster, Germany).

Cell culture and experimental protocols

The human renal proximal tubular cell line HK-2 was purchased from American Type Culture Collection (Rockville, MD, USA) and cultured in Dulbecco's Modified Eagle Medium Nutrient Mixture F-12 (DMEM/F12; GIBCO Life Technologies, Foster City, CA) with 10% bovine serum (FBS), penicillin and streptomycin in a humidified 5% CO$_2$ incubator at 37°C. The cells were seeded at a density of 1×10^6 cells per well. After HK-2 cells were grown to 80% confluence and made quiescent by serum starvation for 24 hours. Ghrelin at three different concentrations of 1, 10 and 100 nM, Des-acyl Ghrelin (Peptide Institute Inc., Osaka, Japan), inactive form of Ghrelin [1] at 10 nM and Irbesartan at 1 μM were added 30 minutes before the treatment with AngII at 1 μM (Sigma-Aldrich). Forty-eight hours after stimulation, cell lysates and culture supernatants were obtained. AMP-kinase inhibitor, Compound C was purchased from Calbiochem (San Diego, CA). The concentrations of TGF-β and PAI-1 were measured with the quantitative sandwich enzyme immunoassay technique (R&D Systems).

Senescence-associated β-galactosidase staining

Renal tubular cells (HK-2 cell) and kidney tissues were washed with PBS and fixed in 4% paraformaldehyde in PBS for 30 minutes, followed by three washes with PBS. The degree of

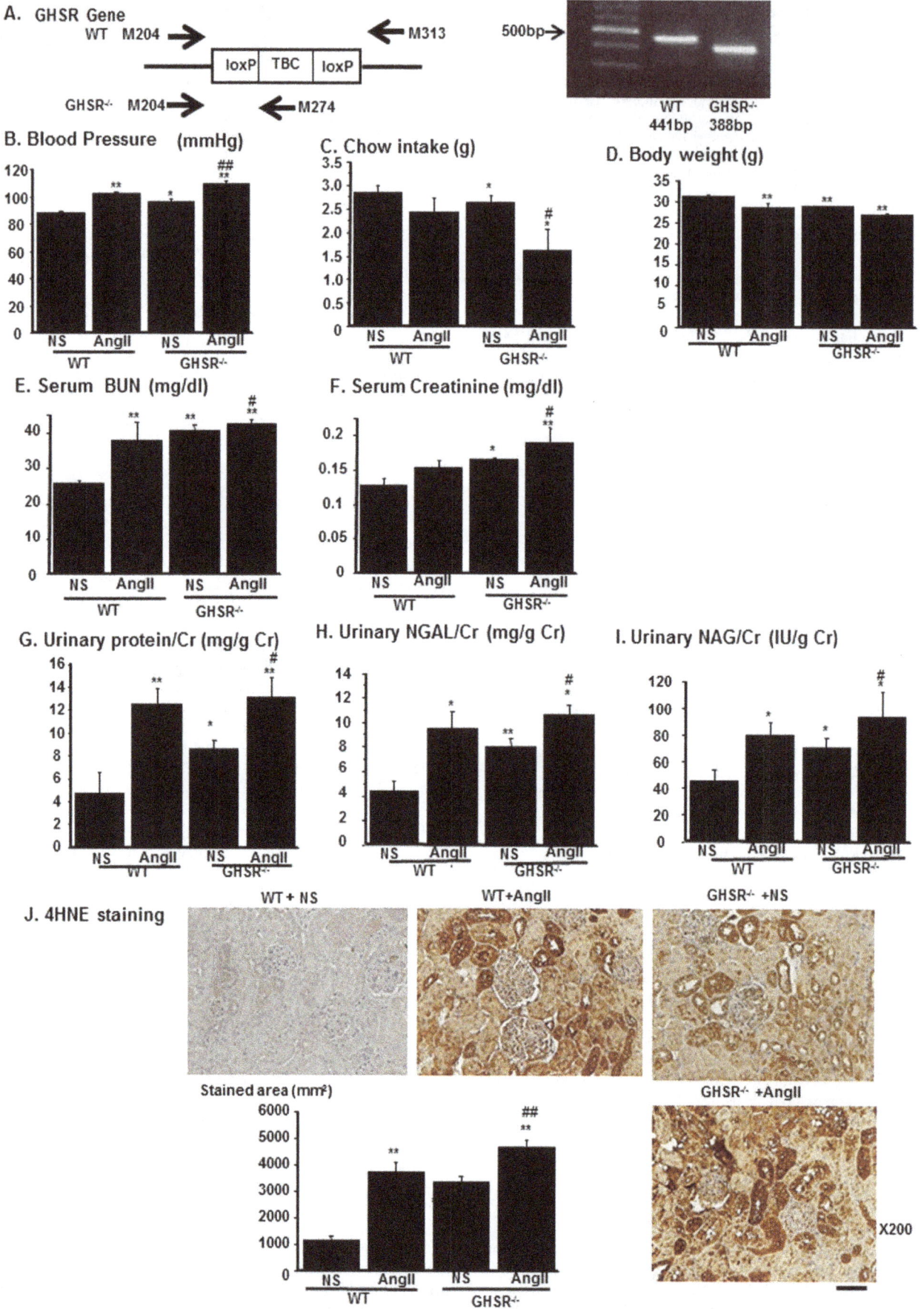

A. GHSR Gene

B. Blood Pressure (mmHg)

C. Chow intake (g)

D. Body weight (g)

E. Serum BUN (mg/dl)

F. Serum Creatinine (mg/dl)

G. Urinary protein/Cr (mg/g Cr)

H. Urinary NGAL/Cr (mg/g Cr)

I. Urinary NAG/Cr (IU/g Cr)

J. 4HNE staining

WT + NS   WT+AngII   GHSR-/- +NS

GHSR-/- +AngII

Stained area (mm²)

Figure 6. Phenotype of GHSR-null mice. (A) The primers used for the genotyping in the PCR (left) and representative results of genotyping (right). The primers used are indicated as arrows. TBC, transcription blocking cassette. (B–J) The phenotype differences among the four experimental groups: WT or GHSR$^{-/-}$ mice infused with normal saline (NS) or AngII. Blood pressure (B), daily chow intake (C), body weight (D) were compared among the four groups. Serum levels of blood urea nitrogen (BUN, E) and creatinine (F) and urinary excretion of protein (G), neutrophil gelatinase-associated lipocalin (NGAL, H), and n-acetyl-galactasaminase (NAG, I) were compared among the four experimental groups. Urinary excretion of each marker was normalized by that of creatinine. (J) Representative immunostaining for 4-Hydroxynonenal-2-nonenal (4HNE) of four experimental groups. Bar graph represents the quantification of immunostained areas. Scale bar; 50 µm. **p<0.01 vs. WT+NS, *p<0.05 vs. WT+NS, ##p<0.01 vs. GHSR$^{-/-}$+NS, #p<0.05 vs. GHSR$^{-/-}$+NS, n=8.

senescence in renal tubular cells and the kidney tissues were evaluated using the senescence-associated β-galactosidase (SA β-gal) staining kit (Sigma-Aldrich) according to manufacturer's instructions. The samples were incubated for 24 hours at 37°C β-gal staining solutions (pH 6.0) containing 1 mg/ml 5-bromo-4-chrolo-3-indlyl β-D-galavtopylanoside (X-gal), 5 mM potassium fericynide, 150 mM NaCl, 2 mM MgCl$_2$, 0.01% Nonidet-40.

After the stained kidney tissues were photographed, the samples were immersed in OCT compounds (Miles Inc., Monrovia, CA) and snap-frozen in liquid nitrogen to prepare cryostat sections. The frozen sections (5 µm) were subjected to immunohistochemistry. Senescent renal tubular cells (stained blue) were observed with microscope and digitally photographed.

UCP2 siRNA experiments

Small interfering RNAs (siRNAs) for UCP2 were prepared by Dharmacon (Lafayette, CO). The targeted sequences to silence the transcription of human UCP2 were 5′-GCAUCGGCCUGUAU-GAUUC-3′. We used siGENOME Non-Targeting siRNA with at least four mismatches to any human, mouse or rat gene as the negative control siRNA. The siRNA molecules (final concentration at 25 nM) were transfected into HK-2 cells at 60% confluence using Lipofectamine 2000 (Invitrogen, Carlsbad,CA) according to manufacturer's instructions. Forty-eight hours after transfection, we administered Ghrelin 100 nM and incubated the cells for 24 h.

Quantification of mitochondrial DNA copy number

Total DNA was extracted with the aid of a Qiamp DNA mini kit (Qiagen, Valencia, CA) from the HK-2 cells. The mitochondrial DNA copy number was determined by means of quantitative PCR analysis (ABI7500 Real-Time PCR System, Applied Biosystems, Foster City, CA), using specific primers for the mitochondrial DNA encoded COX 1 gene and the nuclear DNA encoded lipoprotein lipase (LPL) gene, as follows; the COX1 gene, 5′-TCG CCA TCA TAT TCG TAG GAG-3′ and 5′-GTA GCG TCG TGG TAT TCC TGA-3′; and the LPL gene,5′-CGAGTCGTCTTTCTCCT GATGAT-3′ and 5′-TTCTGGA-TTCCA ATGCTTCGA-3′ [42]. Samples were assayed in triplicate.

Quantification of mitochondrial mass, ROS production and membrane potential

Mitochondrial mass, mitochondrial ROS (Mit ROS) production, and membrane potential of the HK-2 cells were determined with the aid of the fluorescent dyes MitoTracker Green FM and MitoSOX Red, which can selectively detect superoxide derived from mitochondria and Rhodamine 123 (Molecular Probes, Eugene, OR), respectively, with the same procedures as described elsewhere [43,44]. To normalize the data, we used Hoechst 33342 (Molecular Probes, Wako, Osaka, Japan) for nuclear staining. The value for mitochondrial mass was normalized by that for nuclei, and the value for mitochondrial ROS and membrane potential was normalized by that for mitochondrial density. After the cells were cultured with the aforementioned agents for 24 hours, they

were treated with the dyes for 10 min, and washed twice with warm PBS. The fluorescent intensity was measured with a Wallac ARVO SX multiplate reader (Perkin-Elmer, Norwalk, CT).

Quantification of total cellular ROS and superoxide production

Total oxidative stress and superoxide derived from HK-2 cells were measured by total ROS/Superoxide Detection Kit (Enzo Life Science, Farmingdale, NY) as manufacturer's directions. This kit enables detection of comparative levels of total ROS and also allows determination of superoxide production using two specific fluorescent probes.

GHSR-null mice

GHSR-null mice were kindly provided from Professor Jeffrey M. Zigman (The University of Texas Southwestern Medical Center). These mice were generated on C57BL/6 background as described previously [21]. We crossed GHSR null mice onto C57BL/6 mice (Clea Japan Inc., Tokyo, Japan) to obtain the F1 generation. We further crossed these F1 mice for two generations to get homozygous null mice for GHSR and wild type littermates. We used these mice of two genotypes for the experiment. Genomic DNA was isolated from tail biopsies at four weeks of age using a DNeasy kit (Qiagen Inc., Valencia, CA) and screening of genomic DNA samples was done by polymerase chain reaction using transgene-specific oligonucleotide primers, GHSR-null genotype primers; Primer M204: CGGTCTCCACCCTTCATTACTTTA and Primer M274: CAGATGTAGCTAAAAGGCCTATCAC-AAACT. WT genotype; Primer M204: CGGTCTCCACCCTT-CATTACTTTA and Primer M313: GATGCTTGGGGAA GA-GAGAAGTGA. These groups were treated with continuous AngII (500 ng/kg/day, Peptide Institute Inc., Osaka, Japan) infusion during 28 days by using an Alzet micro-osmotic pump (Model 1004D; Durect Co., Cupertino, CA).

RNA extraction and real-time PCR fast SYBR green master mix

Total RNA was extracted from renal proximal tubular cells (HK-2) and the mouse kidney tissues using TRIzol reagent. Equal amounts (1 µg) of total RNA from each sample were converted to cDNA by PrimeScript RT reagent Kit with gDNA Eraser (TaKaRa, Ohtsu, Japan) in a 20 µl reaction volume. Real-time PCR was performed using an ABI Step One Plus sequence detector (PE Applied Biosystems, Tokyo, Japan).

Amplification products were analyzed by a melting curve, which confirmed the presence of a single PCR product in all reactions. Levels of mRNA were normalized to those of GAPDH. The primer sequences were as follows: TGF-β, sense 5′-GCACGTG-GAGCTCTACCA-3′ and antisense 5′-CAGCCGGTTGCTGA-GGTA -3′; PAI-1, sense5′-CTCTCTCTGCCCTCACCAAC-3′ and antisense 5′-GTGGAGAGG CTCTTGGTCTG-3′; GAP-DH, sense 5′-GCACCGTCAAGGCTGAGAAC-3′and antisense 5′-TGGTGAAGACGCCAGTGGA-3′ for HK-2cells. TGF-β, sense 5′-GTGTGGAGCAACATGTGGAACTCTA-3′ and anti-

A. SA-β Gal staining

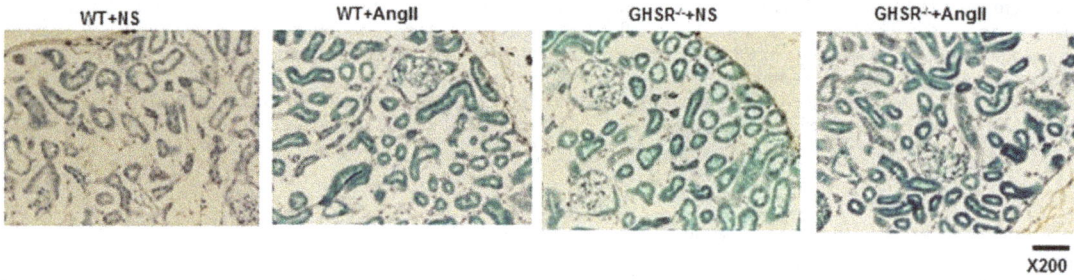

X200

B. Masson Trichrome staining

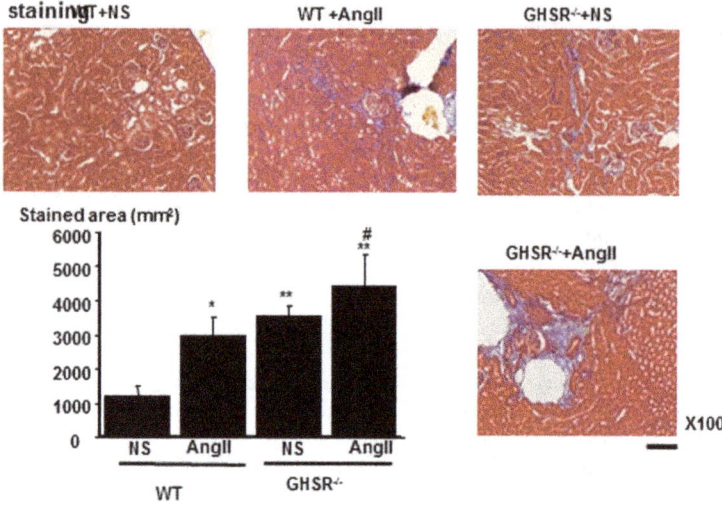

C. Type I Collagen expression

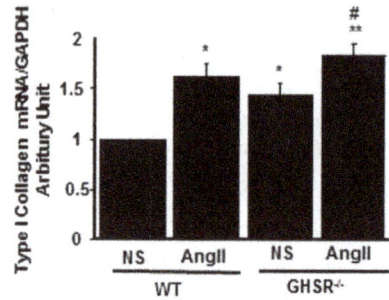

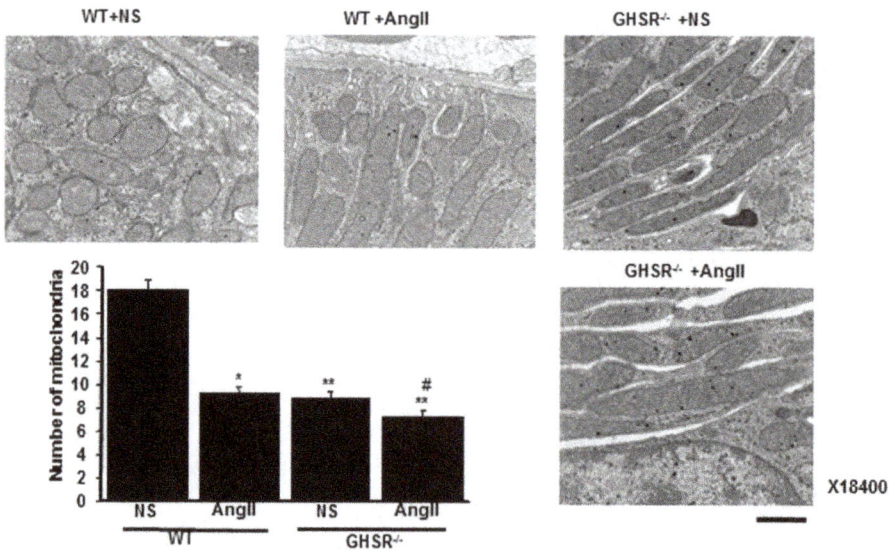

Figure 7. Tissue senescent, fibrotic changes and electromicroscopic findings in GHSR-null mice. (A) Representative staining of senescence-associated β-Galactosidase (SA β-Gal) in WT wild type mice (WT) or GHSR-null mice (GHSR$^{-/-}$) infused with normal saline (NS) or AngII. Scale bar, 50 μm. (B) The representative results of Masson-Trichrome staining of each experimental group. Bar graphs represent the quantification of fibrotic areas. Scale bar, 100 μm. (C) The mRNA expression levels of type I collagen of each experimental group. (D) Electron microscopic findings of mitochondria show that the number of mitochondria was reduced and that morphology of mitochondria was altered in GHSR-null mice (GHSR$^{-/-}$) with NS in comparison to that in WT+NS. Bar graph represents the result of number of mitochondria in the field of electron microscope in each mice group. Scale bar; 1 μm. **p<0.01 vs. WT+NS, *p<0.05 vs. WT+NS, #p<0.01 vs. GHSR$^{-/-}$+NS, n=6.

Mechanism for anti-senescence and anti-fibrotic effects of ghrelin through the reduction of ROS

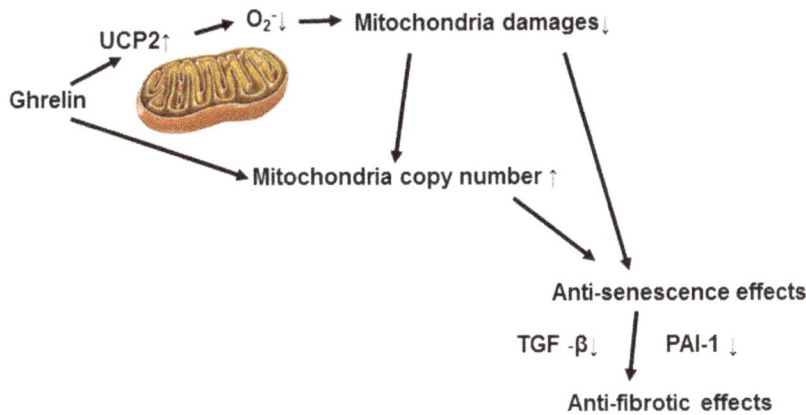

Figure 8. Schema depicting the renal protective effects by Ghrelin. Ghrelin upregulated UCP2 and decreased mitochondria-derived oxidative stress levels. These effects mitigated mitochondria damages and retained the mitochondria number, contributory to its anti-senescent effects. Anti-senescent effects by ghrelin was related to the downregulation of TGF-β and PAI-1, pro-fibrotic genes and inhibited the tissue fibrotic changes.

sense 5'-TTGGTTCAG CCACTGCCGTA-3'; PAI-1, sense 5'-GAGTGGCCTGCTA GGAAATCCATTC-3' and antisense 5'-GACCTTGCCAAGGTGATGCTTGGCAAC-3'; GAPDH, sense 5'-ATGTTCCAGTATGACTCCACTCACG-3' and antisense 5'-GAAGACACCA GTAGACTCCACGACA -3' for mouse. The amplification program was 95°C for three minutes, and then 40 cycles consisting of 95°C for 10 seconds, 62°C for 10 seconds, and 72°C for 10 seconds.

Immunoblotting

Kidney tissues were removed at the sacrifice and snap frozen. Tissues were lysed and sonicated in lysis buffer and centrifuged at 15,000 g for 15 minutes. Supernatant aliquots were subject to immunoblotting using primary antibody against p53, p21 (Cell Signaling Technology, Frankfurt, Germany), and UCP2 (Calbiochem, Darmstadt, Germany). After blots were incubated with secondary antibody (HRP-linked whole body anti-rabbit or -mouse IgG, GE healthcare, Backhamshire, England), immunoreactive bands were detected using an ECL detection kit (Amersham Biosciences, Uppsala, Sweden).

Statistical Analysis

Data are expressed as mean±SEM. One-way analysis of variance was used to determine significant differences among groups. In the overall analysis of variance, Kruskal-Wallis test for multiple comparisons was used to assess individual group differences. $P < 0.05$ was considered statistically significant.

Supporting Information

Figure S1   Expression of GHSR and the effects of siRNA for UCP2 in HK-2 cells. (A) Real-time PCR (left panel) and immunoblotting (right panel) revealed the expressions of GHSR in HK-2 cells. RT$^-$ represents the results of real-time PCR without reverse transcription. Control; control cells, AngII; HK-2 cells treated with 1 μM of AngII, AngII+Ghr; HK-2 cells treated with

AngII plus 10 nM of Ghrelin. AngII+Des-Ghr; HK-2 cells treated with AngII plus 10 nM of desacyl-Ghrelin. B, After the transfection of siRNA for UCP2, expressions of MnSOD (B), Zn/Cu SOD (C), UCP1 (D), and UCP3 (E) were examined by real-time PCR.

Figure S2   Effects of Ghrelin on the phenotype of AngII-infused GHSR-null mice. (A) Real-time PCR analysis using specific primers shows the mRNA expression of GHSR in the kidney. WT, wild type mice. GHSR$^{-/-}$, GHSR-null mice. n = 6. (B–I) The effects of Ghrelin on the phenotype of GHSR$^{-/-}$ mice infused with AngII. Fourteen-weeks treatment with Ghrelin did not affect blood pressure (B), serum levels of blood urea nitrogen (BUN, C) and creatinine (D) and urinary excretion of protein (E), neutrophil gelatinase-associated lipocalin (NGAL, F), and n-acetyl-galactasaminase (NAG, G). Urinary excretion of each marker was normalized by that of creatinine. (H) The expression of UCP2 was also unaffected by Ghrelin in AngII-infused GHSR-null mice. (I) Representative immunostaining for 4-Hydroxynonenal-2-nonenal (4HNE) of four experimental groups. Bar graph represents the quantification of immunostained areas. Scale bar; 50 μm. (B–I) **p<0.01 vs. GHSR$^{-/-}$+NS, *p<0.05 vs. GHSR$^{-/-}$+NS, n = 8.

Acknowledgments

We acknowledge Professor Jeffrey M. Zigman (The University of Texas Southwestern Medical Center) for his kind gift of the GHSR-null mice.

Author Contributions

Conceived and designed the experiments: SW K. Hayashi HI. Performed the experiments: KF SW HM K. Hasegawa K.Hosoya TK HT. Analyzed the data: KF SW KS MK YK NW. Contributed reagents/materials/analysis tools: KF SW. Wrote the paper: KF SW HI.

References

1. Kojima M, Hosoda H, Date Y, Nakazato M, Matsuo H, et al. (1999) Ghrelin is a growth-hormone-releasing acylated peptide from stomach. Nature 402: 656–660.
2. Date Y, Kojima M, Hosoda H, Sawaguchi A, Mondal MS, et al. (2000) Ghrelin, a Novel Growth Hormone-Releasing Acylated Peptide is Synthesized in a Distinct Endocrine Cell Type in the Gastrointestinal Tracts of Rats and Humans. Endocrinology 141: 4255–4261.
3. Takeda R, Nishimatsu H, Suzuki E, Satonaka H, Nagata D, et al. (2006) Ghrelin improves renal function in mice with ischemic acute renal failure. J Am Soc Nephrol 17: 113–121.
4. Wang W, Bansal S, Falk S, Ljubanovic D, Schrier R (2009) Ghrelin protects mice against endotoxemia-induced acute kidney injury. Am J Physiol Renal Physiol 297: 1032–1037.
5. Mezzano S, Ruiz-Ortega M, Egido J (2001) Angiotensin II and Renal Fibrosis. Hypertension 38: 635–638.
6. Ruiz-Ortega M, Rupérez M, Esteban V, Rodríguez-Vita J, Sánchez-López E, et al. (2006) Angiotensin II, A key factor in the inflammatory and fibrotic response in kidney diseases. Nephrol Dial Transplant 21: 16–20.
7. Benigni A, Cassis P, Remuzzi G (2010) Angiotensin II revisited: new roles in inflammation, immunology and aging. EMBO Mol Med 2: 247–257.
8. Krause KH (2007) Aging: a revisited theory based on free radicals generated by NOX family NADPH oxidases. Exp Gerontol 42: 256–262.
9. Yang H, Fogo AB (2010) Cell senescence in the aging kidney. J Am Soc Nephrol 21: 1436–1439.
10. Melk A (2003) Senescence of renal cells: molecular basis and clinical implications. Nephrol Dial Transplant 18: 2474–2478.
11. Verzola D, Gandolfo MT, Gaetani G, Ferraris A, Mangerini R, et al. (2008) Accelerated senescence in the kidneys of patients with type 2 diabetic nephropathy. Am J Physiol Renal Physiol 295: 1563–1573.
12. Satriano J, Mansoury H, Deng A, Sharma K, Vallon V, et al. (2010) Transition of kidney tubule cells to a senescent phenotype in early experimental diabetes. Am J Physiol Cell Physiol 299: 374–380.
13. Sikora E, Arendt T, Bennett M, Narita M (2011) Impact of cellular senescence signature on ageing research. Ageing Res Rev 10: 146–152.
14. Andrews ZB, Liu ZW, Walllingford N, Erion DM, Borok E, et al. (2008) UCP2 mediates ghrelin's action on NPY/AgRP neurons by lowering free radicals. Nature 454: 846–851.
15. Andrews ZB, Erion DM, Beiler R, Choi CS, Shulman GI, et al. (2010) Uncoupling protein-2 decreases the lipogenic actions of ghrelin. Endocrinology 151: 2078–2086.
16. Els S, Beck-Sickinger AG, Chollet C (2010) Ghrelin receptor: high constitutive activity and methods for developing inverse agonists. Methods Enzymol 485: 103–121.
17. Diep QN, El Mabrouk M, Cohn JS, Endemann D, Amiri F, et al. (2002) Structure, Endothelial Function, Cell Growth, and Inflammation in Blood Vessels of Angiotensin II–Infused Rats:Role of Peroxisome Proliferator-Activated Receptor-γ. Circulation 105: 2296–2302.
18. Rizk DE, Hassan HA, Ramadan GA, Shafiullah M, Fahim MA (2005) Estrogen and ghrelin increase number of submucosal urethral and anal canal blood vessels in ovariectomized rats. Urology 66: 1343–1348.
19. Kagami S, Border WA, Miller DE, Noble NA (1994) Angiotensin II Stimulates Extracellular Matrix Protein Synthesis through Induction of Transforming Growth Factor-β Expression in Rat Glumerular Mesangial Cells. J Clin Invest 93: 2431–2437.
20. Andrews ZB (2010) Uncopling Protein-2 and the Potential Link Between Metabolism and Longevity. Current Aging Science 3: 102–112.
21. Verhulst PJ, Janssen S, Tack J, Depoortere I (2012) Role of the AMP-activated protein kinase (AMPK) signaling pathway in the orexigenic effects of endogenous ghrelin. Regul Pept 173: 27–35.
22. Zigman JM, Nakano Y, Coppari R, Balthasar N, Marcus JN, et al. (2005) Mice lacking ghrelin receptors resist the development of diet-induced obesity. J Clin Invest 115: 3564–3572.
23. Echtay KS, Roussel D, St-Pierre J, Jekabsons MB, Cadenas S, et al. (2002) Superoxide activates mitochondrial uncoupling proteins. Nature 415: 96–99.
24. Chan SH, Wu CA, Wu KL, Ho YH, Chang AY, et al. (2009) Transcriptional upregulation of mitochondrial uncoupling protein 2 protects against oxidative stress-associated neurogenic hypertension. Circ Res 105: 886–896.
25. Park JY, Park KG, Kim HJ, Kang HG, Ahn JD, et al. (2005) The effects of the overexpression of recombinant uncoupling protein 2 on proliferation, migration and plasminogen activator inhibitor 1 expression in human vascular smooth muscle cells. Diabetologia 48:1022–8.
26. Thompson MP, Kim D (2004) Links between fatty acids and expression of UCP2 and UCP3 mRNAs. FEBS Lett 568: 4–9.
27. Bergeron R, Ren JM, Cadman KS, Moore IK, Perret P, et al. (2001) Chronic activation of AMP kinase results in NRF-1 activation and mitochondrial biogenesis. Am J Physiol Endocrinol Metab 281: 1340–1346.
28. Reznick RM, Shulman GI (2006) The role of AMP-activated protein kinase in mitochondrial biogenesis. J Physiol 574: 33–39.
29. Sachse A, Wolf G (2007) Angiotensin II-induced reactive oxygen species and the kidney. J Am Soc Nephrol 18: 2439–2446.
30. Paravicini TM, Touyz RM (2006) Redox signaling in hypertension. Cardiovasc Res 71: 247–258.
31. Shah SV, Baliga R, Rajapurkar M, Fonseca VA (2007) Oxidants in chronic kidney disease. J Am Soc Nephrol 18: 16–28.
32. Sen CK, Packer L (1996) Antioxidant and redox regulation of gene transcription. FASEB J 10: 709–720.
33. Pendyala S, Natarajan V (2010) Redox regulation of Nox proteins. Respir Physiol Neurobiol 174: 265–271.
34. Kimura S, Zhang GX, Nishiyama A, Shokoji T, Yao L, et al. (2005) Role of NAD(P)H oxidase- and mitochondria-derived reactive oxygen species in cardioprotection of ischemic reperfusion injury by angiotensin II. Hypertension 45: 860–866.
35. Kim SM, Kim YG, Jeong KH, Lee SH, Lee TW, et al. (2012) Angiotensin II-induced mitochondrial Nox4 is a major endogenous source of oxidative stress in kidney tubular cells. PLoS One 7:e39739.
36. Mitsuishi M, Miyashita K, Muraki A, Itoh H (2009) Angiotensin II reduces mitochondrial content in skeletal muscle and affects glycemic control. Diabetes 58: 710–717.
37. de Cavanagh EM, Piotrkowski B, Basso N, Stella I, Inserra F, et al. (2003) Enalapril and losartan attenuate mitochondrial dysfunction in aged rats. FASEB J 17: 1096–1098.
38. Feldkamp T, Kribben A, Roeser NF, Senter RA, Kemner S, et al. (2004) Preservation of complex I function during hypoxia-reoxygenation-induced mitochondrial injury in proximal tubules. Am J Physiol Renal Physiol 286: F749–759.
39. Brooks C, Wei Q, Cho SG, Dong Z (2009) Regulation of mitochondrial dynamics in acute kidney injury in cell culture and rodent models. J Clin Invest 119: 1275–1285.
40. Hasegawa K, Wakino S, Yoshioka K, Tatematsu S, Hara Y, et al. (2010) Kidney-specific overexpression of Sirt1 protects against acute kidney injury by retaining peroxisome function. J Biol Chem 285: 13045–13056.
41. Rambold AS, Kostelecky B, Elia N, Lippincott-Schwartz J (2011) Tubular network formation protects mitochondria from autophagosomal degradation during nutrient starvation. Proc Natl Acad Sci U S A 108: 10190–10195.
42. Balakrishnan VS, Rao M, Menon V, Gordon PL, Pilichowska M, et al. (2010) Resistance Training Increases Muscle Mitochondrial Biogenesis in Patients with Chronic Kidney Disease. Clin J Am Soc Nephrol 5: 996–1002.
43. López-Lluch G, Hunt N, Jones B, Zhu M, Jamieson H, et al. (2006) Calorie restriction induces mitochondrial biogenesis and bioenergetic efficiency. Proc Natl Acad Sci U S A 103: 1768–1773.
44. Civitarese AE, Ukropcova B, Carling S, Hulver M, DeFronzo RA, et al. (2006) Role of adiponectin in human skeletal muscle bioenergetics. Cell Metab 4: 75–87.

9

Circulating MicroRNAs as Easy-to-Measure Aging Biomarkers in Older Breast Cancer Patients: Correlation with Chronological Age but Not with Fitness/Frailty Status

Sigrid Hatse[1]*, **Barbara Brouwers**[1], **Bruna Dalmasso**[1,2], **Annouschka Laenen**[3], **Cindy Kenis**[1,4], **Patrick Schöffski**[1], **Hans Wildiers**[1]

1 Laboratory of Experimental Oncology (LEO), Department of Oncology, KU Leuven, and Department of General Medical Oncology, University Hospitals Leuven, Leuven Cancer Institute, Leuven, Belgium, 2 Department of Internal Medicine, Istituto di Ricerca a Carattere Clinico e Scientifico (IRCCS), Azienda Ospedaliera Universitaria (AOU) San Martino Istituto Nazionale Tumori (IST), Genoa, Italy, 3 Interuniversity Centre for Biostatistics and Statistical Bioinformatics, Leuven, Belgium, 4 Department of Geriatric Medicine, University Hospitals Leuven, Leuven, Belgium

Abstract

Circulating microRNAs (miRNAs) hold great promise as easily accessible biomarkers for diverse (patho)physiological processes, including aging. We have compared miRNA expression profiles in cell-free blood from older versus young breast cancer patients, in order to identify "aging miRNAs" that can be used in the future to monitor the impact of chemotherapy on the patient's biological age. First, we assessed 175 miRNAs that may possibly be present in serum/plasma in an exploratory screening in 10 young and 10 older patients. The top-15 ranking miRNAs showing differential expression between young and older subjects were further investigated in an independent cohort consisting of another 10 young and 20 older subjects. Plasma levels of miR-20a-3p, miR-30b-5p, miR106b, miR191 and miR-301a were confirmed to show significant age-related decreases (all p≤0.004). The remaining miRNAs included in the validation study (miR-21, miR-210, miR-320b, miR-378, miR-423-5p, let-7d, miR-140-5p, miR-200c, miR-374a, miR376a) all showed similar trends as observed in the exploratory screening but these differences did not reach statistical significance. Interestingly, the age-associated miRNAs did not show differential expression between fit/healthy and non-fit/frail subjects within the older breast cancer cohort of the validation study and thus merit further investigation as true aging markers that not merely reflect frailty.

Editor: Consuelo Borras, University of Valencia, Spain

Funding: HW is a recipient of the 'Fonds voor Wetenschappelijk Onderzoek – Vlaanderen (FWO).' BB is a recipient of the 'Vlaamse Liga tegen Kanker (VLK).' The funders had no role in study design, data collection and analysis, decision to publish, or preparation of the manuscript.

Competing Interests: The authors have declared that no competing interests exist.

* Email: sigrid.hatse@med.kuleuven.be

Introduction

Given the increasing proportion of older people in the general population, oncologists nowadays encounter the great challenge of proper cancer management in older patients. A major problem is the heterogeneous health condition among older cancer patients, making it difficult to rely on standard treatment guidelines established for distinct cancer types and, hence, demanding a more individualized approach. Secondly, long-term impact of chemotherapy on the patient's global health condition may be more pronounced and, at the same time, less predictable in older individuals.

Body aging is a complex phenomenon involving several, partly overlapping, molecular mechanisms. Among others, these include the accumulation of oxidative stress [1] and DNA damage [2], the shortening of telomeres [3,4] and neuroendocrine and immunologic changes [5,6].

It is generally assumed that chemotherapy may accelerate the aging process through interference at the level of one or several of these aging driving forces [7]. For example, free radical intermediates are generated during the metabolism anthracyclines, alkylating agents directly cause DNA damage, while topoisomerase inhibitors, such as epirubicin, inhibit DNA repair enzymes. Also, chemotherapy may accelerate leukocyte telomere attrition, due to telomerase inhibition [8] and/or repeated cycles of intense hematological repopulation [9–11]. Moreover, chemoradiotherapy may have more severe effects on the replicative capacity of blood cells in older as compared to younger patients [12]. Finally, neuroendocrine and immune functions can also be affected by chemotherapeutic agents and by corticosteroids that are often incorporated in chemotherapeutic regimens [7].

At the cellular level, aging is intimately linked with tumorigenesis through the mechanism of cellular senescence [13], a cancer-protective stress response that causes irreversible growth arrest in order to prevent further proliferation of damaged, potentially harmful cells. While being a potent anti-tumor mechanism early in life, cellular senescence is at the same time responsible for tissue aging at older age, through accumulation of non-proliferative cells [13], finally resulting in tissue dysfunction and age-related diseases. Standard chemotherapy and radiotherapy might function in part by inducing senescence within the tumor mass [14,15], but might concurrently cause increased senescence induction in healthy, proliferating tissues as well.

Taken together, chemotherapeutic treatment may potentially lead to accelerated aging and/or premature onset of frailty in older cancer patients [7]. Therefore, the patient's biological aging profile is of particular relevance in geriatric oncology and may aid in oncological decision making and individual treatment optimization. Several aging biomarkers have already been described, most particularly mean leukocyte telomere length and $p16^{INK4a}$ mRNA expression in T lymphocytes [16–18]. However, none of these so far made its way into routine clinical practice and the search for robust and easy-to-measure aging biomarkers is still ongoing.

MicroRNA's (miRNAs) are short (20–24 nt), non-coding and highly stable RNA's that are involved in post-transcriptional regulation of gene expression. They are known as fine-tuning mediators of a wide variety of normal physiological pathways, developmental processes and pathological conditions; it is thus plausible that they also play a role in cellular senescenceand tissue/body aging [19,20]. Several miRNAs involved in DNA damage response, cellular senescence and cell death (such as let-7, miR-34 and miR-43), were indeed identified in the widely used *C. elegans* aging model and turned out to be highly conserved among species [21]. In aging mice, miR-34a was shown to be upregulated, concomitantly with a decreased mRNA expression of its primary target gene SIRT1, in brain tissue but also in peripheral blood mononuclear cells and plasma [22]. Therefore, it was suggested that circulatory miR-34a may hold great promise as an accessible biomarker for brain aging.

Circulating miRNAs actually are attractive candidate biomarkers for clinical use, because of their easy accessibility and outstanding stability in serum/plasma [23]. Here, we describe the potential use of microRNA signatures expressed in serum/plasma for the assessment of biological age in breast cancer patients. We compared a panel of 175 different microRNAs, known to be among the most relevant in serum/plasma, between older and young breast cancer patients and validated the findings of this initial exploratory screening in an independent breast cancer cohort. At least 5 circulating microRNAs emerged from this study that are worth to be further explored as potential aging biomarkers in larger cohorts of young *versus* old fit *versus* old frail individuals, both within and beyond a cancer background.

Results

The experimental design of our study is shown in Fig. 1. In the first stage, the expression profiles of 175 miRNAs were analyzed in serum samples of 10 young (mean age 34.5 years) and 10 older (mean age 82.8 years) breast cancer patients. Distinct breast cancer subtypes were equally represented in both groups (see Table 1). From this initial screening experiment, the 15 top-ranking miRNAs (showing the highest significance for differential expression between both groups) were selected, together with 4 candidate reference miRNAs (showing stable expression among all samples). In the second stage, the selected potential aging miRNAs and candidate reference miRNAs were re-evaluated by individual RT-qPCR in plasma samples from a new, independent study cohort consisting of 10 young (mean age 41 years) and 20 older (mean age 78 years) breast cancer

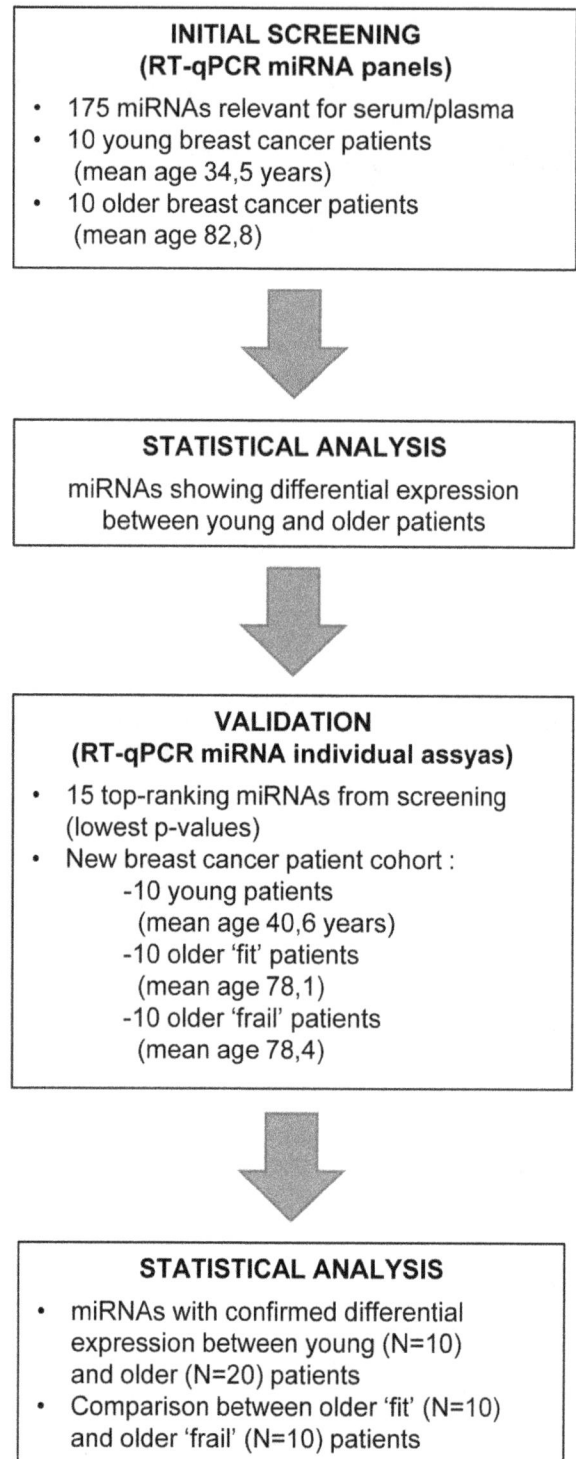

Figure 1. Experimental study design.

patients, all diagnosed with lymph node negative, luminal A (grade 1–2, ER-positive, PR-positive, HER2-negative) tumors (see Table 2). Geriatric assessment in the older cohort was performed as described by Kenis *et al.* [24].

Table 1. Patient and tumor characteristics of the pilot study cohort.

	Young group	Older group
	N = 10	N = 10
Age at diagnosis		
Mean (years)	34,5	82,8
Range (years)	28–38	80–89
Breast cancer subtype		
Luminal A-like phenotype	7	7
Luminal B-like phenotype	1	1
Triple negative-like phenotype	2	2
Tumor grade		
I	2	2
II	7	5
III	1	3
Histological subtype		
Invasive ductal carcinoma	9	7
Invasive lobular carcinoma	1	1
Other	0	2
Estrogen receptor status		
Positive	8	8
Negative	2	2
Progesteron receptor status		
Positive	7	8
Negative	3	2
HER-2 receptor status		
Positive	0	0
Negative	10	10
Pathological staging (pT)		
pT1a	1	0
pT1b	0	1
pT1c	4	1
pT2	4	8
x	1	0
Nodal status		
pN0	10	10

Exploratory screening for differentially expressed miRNAs in older versus young breast cancer patients

Profiles of circulating miRNAs were analyzed in the 10 young and 10 older breast cancer patients of the exploratory cohort using the Exiqon miRNA serum/plasma focus panels, including 175 different miRNAs (refer to File S2 for a complete list of included miRNAs). Plate-to-plate variations in qPCR efficiency were small: the standard deviation of Cp values obtained for the individual interplate calibrator wells was 0.33 cycles, and no outliers (deviation of 4 times the standard deviation or more) were detected. Comparable RNA extraction and reverse transcription efficiency across all samples of the cohort was ascertained by the UniSp6 spike-in control : standard deviation of the UniSp6 PCR Cp values (after interplate calibration) was 0.55 cycles (mean Cp was 25,99) and no outliers were detected, indicating that no inhibitors of reverse transcription and/or PCR reactions were present. The average signal of all miRNAs was comparable in both age categories : the global mean Cp of the young patient group was 33.80 ± 2.01, compared to 33.90 ± 1.67 for the old group. Thus, there were no significant age-related changes in total miRNA content of the serum samples.

After global mean normalisation (i.e. normalisation to the average signal of all miRNAs included in the panel) [25], statistical analysis of the results revealed 37 miRNAs with significantly different ($p < 0.05$) expression in serum samples from the older compared to the young patient group. The first 50 miRNAs of the t-test p-value ranking are listed in Table 3. Interestingly, older and young patients clustered in two relatively distinct groups in a principal component analysis incorporating these top 50-ranking miRNAs (Fig. 2A), whereas patients were randomly scattered when PCA analysis was performed with the bottom 50-ranking miRNAs (Fig. 2B). The dendrogram in Fig. 3 also clearly demonstrates a high degree of clustering of the patients from both age groups. This indicates that there are indeed important

Table 2. Patient and tumor characteristics of the validation study cohort.

	Young group	Older 'fit' group	Older 'non-fit' group
	(N = 10)	(N = 10)	(N = 10)
Age at diagnosis			
Mean (years)	41	78	78
Range (years)	37–43	71–83	73–91
Frailty status (Balducci)			
Frail	N/A	0	9
Vulnerable	N/A	4	1
Fit	N/A	6	0
Frailty status (LOFS[a])			
0–2 (severely frail)	N/A [b]	0	1
3–4 (frail)	N/A	0	1
5–6 (vulnerable)	N/A	0	8
7–8 (slightly vulnerable)	N/A	0	0
9–10 (fit)	N/A	10	0
Breast cancer subtype			
Luminal A-like	10	10	10[c]
Tumor grade			
I	4	2	2
II	6	8	8
III	0	0	1[c]
Histological subtype			
Invasive ductal carcinoma	8	6	5
Invasive lobular carcinoma	2	3	2
Other	0	1	3
Estrogen receptor status			
Positive	10	10	10
Negative	0	0	0
Progesteron receptor status			
Positive	10	10	10
Negative	0	0	0
HER-2 receptor status			
Positive	0	0	0
Negative	10	10	10
Pathological staging (pT)			
pT1a	0	0	0
pT1b	4	1	2
pT1c	2	3	1
pT2	4	5	7
pT3	0	1	0
Nodal staging (pN)			
pN0	10	10	10

[a]Leuven Oncology Frailty Score : refer to File S1 for more details.
[b]N/A : not applicable.
[c]One patient had a mixed luminal A (grade II)/luminal B (grade III) tumor.

age-related differences in circulating miRNA profiles. Some miRNAs showed an age-related increase in abundance, while others were found to be down-regulated in older, as compared to young, patients. When considering the 15 miRNAs exhibiting the most pronounced age-related changes (lowest p-values), increased abundance in serum of older *versus* young patients was noted for miR-21, miR-210, miR-320b, miR-378 and miR-423-5p (Fig. 4). Conversely, circulating levels of let-7d, miR-20a-3p, miR-301a, miR-374a, miR-376a, miR-191, miR-200c, miR-30b-5p, miR-

Table 3. Exploratory serum/plasma miRNA panel screening of circulating miRNAs in older (N = 10) *versus* young (N = 10) breast cancer patients.

miRNA[a]	Age-related change[b]	Fold change	t-test P value
hsa-miR-320b	up	2.10	0.0003
hsa-miR-301a	down	3.34	0.0012
hsa-miR-210	up	2.48	0.0024
hsa-miR-21	up	2.32	0.0025
hsa-miR-376a	down	3.24	0.0036
hsa-miR-378	up	2.87	0.0037
hsa-miR-374a	down	2.13	0.0038
hsa-miR-423-5p	up	1.66	0.0044
hsa-miR-20a-3p	down	8.64	0.0049
hsa-let-7d	down	2.33	0.0052
hsa-miR-191	down	1.49	0.0061
hsa-miR-200c	down	4.88	0.0063
hsa-miR-30b-5p	down	1.78	0.0063
hsa-miR-140-5p	down	2.00	0.0064
hsa-miR-106b-5p	down	2.17	0.0097
hsa-miR-382	down	2.66	0.0109
hsa-miR-495	down	2.81	0.0132
hsa-miR-199a-3p	down	1.80	0.0141
hsa-miR-146a	up	1.83	0.0203
hsa-miR-15b*	down	2.31	0.0213
hsa-miR-320a	up	5.17	0.0218
hsa-miR-551b	down	7.10	0.0227
hsa-miR-766	up	2.24	0.0244
hsa-miR-409-3p	down	4.82	0.0261
hsa-miR-543	down	3.75	0.0308
hsa-miR-10b	up	2.06	0.0328
hsa-miR-34a	up	2.36	0.0367
hsa-miR-331-3p	down	2.37	0.0368
hsa-miR-423-5p	up	5.41	0.0383
hsa-miR-222	up	2.43	0.0410
hsa-miR-199a-5p	down	2.13	0.0436
hsa-miR-33a	up	2.09	0.0451
hsa-miR-92a	up	2.06	0.0470
hsa-miR-324-5p	down	1.51	0.0471
hsa-miR-130a	down	1.44	0.0474
hsa-miR-151-5p	down	1.39	0.0484
hsa-miR-486-5p	up	2.50	0.0489
hsa-miR-150	up	2.16	0.0511
hsa-miR-126	up	2.38	0.0568
hsa-miR-342-3p	up	1.94	0.0703
hsa-miR-15a	up	1.60	0.0759
hsa-miR-30e	up	1.29	0.0823
hsa-miR-424	up	3.15	0.0825
hsa-miR-660	up	1.53	0.0899
hsa-miR-10a	up	1.69	0.0924
hsa-miR-885-5p	down	2.44	0.0943
hsa-miR-30c	down	1.53	0.0948
hsa-miR-324-3p	up	2.07	0.0963
hsa-miR-152	up	1.58	0.1003

Table 3. Cont.

miRNA[a]	Age-related change[b]	Fold change	t-test P value
hsa-miR-326	down	1.83	0.1055

[a]This table only shows the top-50 ranking miRNAs for differential expression according to t-test. A list of all miRNAs included in the entire panel is shown in File S2.
[b]up : higher plasma levels found in older compared to young subjects; down : lower plasma levels found in older compared to young subjects.

140b-5p and miR-106b were decreased in older compared to young patients (Fig. 4).

Identification of candidate reference miRNAs via miRNA serum/plasma panel screening

A second purpose of the initial screening experiment was the identification of stably expressed miRNAs that could serve as valuable references for normalisation in future validation experiments. As subsequent experiments will probably only include a limited number of selected miRNAs, global mean normalisation, requiring at least 50 genes, will not be possible anymore. To this end, the 10 miRNAs most resembling the behaviour of the global mean, i.e. the miRNAs having least variation after global mean normalisation, were selected as candidate reference miRNAs (Table 4). From these selected candidates, miR-191 was excluded since it ranged within the top 15 of age-related differential expression in the panel screening (see Table 3). The remaining 9 miRNAs, i.e. let-7i, miR-484, miR-29a, miR-29c, miR-140-3p, miR-30e, miR-30d, miR-29b and miR-590-5p, were further evaluated by the use of Normfinder [26] and GeNorm [27], two popular algorithms to select the most stably expressed reference genes from a set of tested candidate genes in a given sample panel. Normfinder, which basically calculates for each candidate reference gene the standard deviation from the global average expression (and thus mirrors the variance after global mean normalisation), yielded the following stability order: let-7i>miR-140-3p> miR-29c>miR-29a>miR-484> miR-30e>miR-29b>miR-30d>miR-590-5p. The respective stability values ranged between 0.27 for let-7i and 0.56 for miR-590-5p, with superior stability indicated by the lowest value (Table 4). Normfinder analysis also indicated that 4 is a reasonable number of normalisation genes: accumulated standard deviation values were 0.27, 0.21, 0.18, 0.16, 0.16, 0.15, 0.15, 0.14 and 014 when the number of normalizing genes was increased from just 1 to 9. Thus, the inclusion of a fourth reference gene still afforded a substantial reduction of variation retained in the dataset, while additional reference genes only contributed a minor further improvement. GeNorm analysis, which is based on a different mathematical approach, resulted in a slightly different stability ranking: miR-29a = miR-29c>miR-140-3p>let-7i>miR-29b>miR-484> miR-30e>miR-30d>miR-590-5p. The corresponding M-values (gene stability measure) increased from 0.31 for let-7i to 0.59 for miR-590-5p, again with the most stably expressed genes having the lowest M-values (Table 4). Taken together, both algorithms pointed at let-7i, miR-29a, miR-29c and miR-140-3p as the common best reference miRNAs for normalisation, which all had GeNorm and Normfinder stability values below the 0.50 cut-off for suitable reference genes [26,27]. However, we decided not to retain let-7i since it was previously reported to be involved in genome-wide miRNA signatures of human longevity [28] and might thus be somehow age-related, which would not be desirable for the current study. Based on the above-described results, we instead selected miR-484 as the fourth reference gene.

Validation of age-associated miRNAs

To further examine potential aging miRNAs, we focussed on the 15 miRNAs that emerged from the pilot study as those showing the most significantly different expression levels in young versus older individuals. For this validation study, a new independent breast cancer patient cohort was selected that basically consisted of a young group (<45 years, N = 10) and an older group (>70 years, N = 20). The latter comprised a subgroup (N = 10) of 'fit' older breast cancer patients and a second subgroup (N = 10) of 'frail' patients. These two subcategories were included to investigate whether the observed age-associated differences in plasma miRNA levels were truly related to the aging process itself (i.e. pure "aging biomarkers"), or were caused by age-related pathologies and functional decline (i.e. "frailty biomarkers").

Individual PCR assays were carried out for each of the selected candidate aging miRNAs (i.e. miR-320b, miR-301a, miR-210, miR-21, miR-376a, miR-378, miR-374a, miR-423-5p, miR-20a-3p, let-7d, miR-191, miR-200c, miR-30b-5p, miR-140-5p and miR-106b), along with the 4 selected normalisation miRNAs (i.e. miR-29a, miR-29c, miR-140-3p and miR-484). In addition, miR-451 and miR-23a-3p were also included for hemolysis control (see Materials and Methods section). Comparable RNA extraction and reverse transcription efficiency across all 30 samples of the validation cohort was ascertained by the UniSp6 spike-in control: standard deviation of the UniSp6 PCR Cp values (after interplate calibration) was ≤0.37 cycles (mean Cp value was 20.48 cycles).

Analysis of the data first confirmed miR-29a, miR-29c, miR-140-3p and miR-484 as reliable normalisation references, all GeNorm M-values being lower than 0.5 (data not shown). However, miR-23a-3p was additionally identified as an excellent reference miRNA. This is not surprising; miR-23a-3p is incorporated in the hemolysis control test because of its stable expression in serum/plasma samples and is often used as a suitable reference miRNA for normalisation. Hence, we decided to add it to our reference miRNA panel, which thus finally consisted of 5 miRNAs.

When comparing older (N = 20) with young (N = 10) patients, significantly decreased miRNA plasma levels were confirmed for miR-20a-3p, miR-301a, miR-374a, miR-30b-5p, miR-106b-5p and miR-191, whereas let-7d, miR-140-5p, miR-200c and miR-376a did not reach statistical significance at the 5% significance level (Table 5). When applying Bonferroni correction for multiple testing, p-values for miR-20a-3p, miR-30b-5p, miR-106b-5p, miR-191 and miR301a were still below the corrected significance threshold of 0.00341 (Table 5).

Increased expression in older compared to young subjects was only confirmed for miR-378 (p = 0.0077) and was close to the 5% significance threshold for miR-320b (p = 0.0585) and miR-423-5p (p = 0.0566), while miR-21 and miR-210 were not close to statistical significance in the validation experiment. However, none of these miRNAs showing apparently increased expression in older subjects remained significant after Bonferroni correction for multiple testing (Table 5). An overview of upregulated and

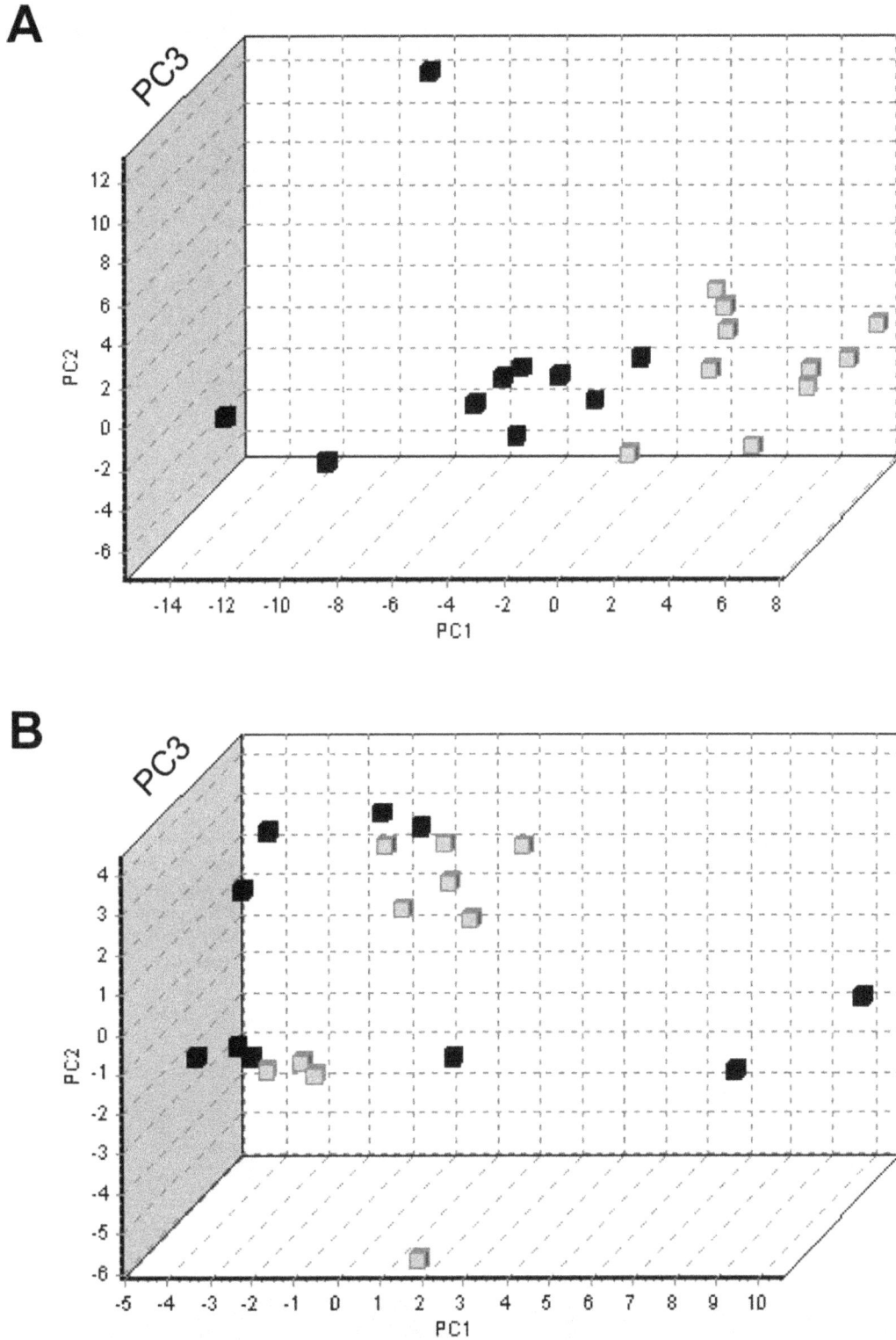

Figure 2. Principal component analysis (PCA) of the panel screening results. (A) PCA analysis of the top-50 ranking (lowest P-values in t-test) miRNAs of the panel screening; **(B)** PCA analysis of the bottom-50 ranking miRNAs (highest P-values in t-test). Black symbols represent young patients; grey symbols represent older, frail patients. PC1, PC2 and PC3 on X, Y and Z-axis represent the 3 principal components generated by this statistical algorithm.

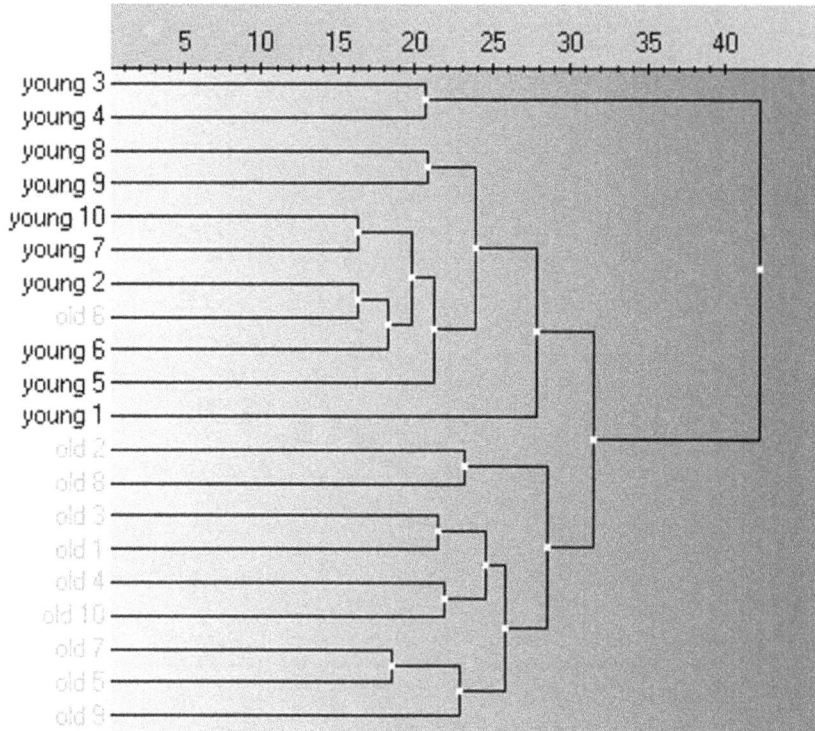

Figure 3. Dendrogram showing hierarchical clustering of patients according to the exploratory miRNA screening panel results. Young patients are shown in black, older patients are shown in grey. The clustering was performed on all 20 patients of the exploratory cohort and on the entire miRNA screening panel, applying complete linkage as the clustering method and Euclidean distance as the distance measure.

downregulated miRNAs in the exploratory screening and the validation study is shown in Fig. 5.

Interestingly, no significant differences were revealed in a subanalysis comparing the 'fit' and 'non-fit' subgroups of the older cohort for any of the microRNAs included in this validation study (all p>0.1) (Table 5). These results indicate that the observed differences in plasma miRNA levels between young and older breast cancer patients reflect a pure aging effect and do not result from age-associated changes in the patient's global health status.

Discussion

MicroRNA's circulating in plasma are particularly interesting as easily accessible biomarkers for aging and age-related diseases. However, relatively little data are presently available on age-related changes in miRNA expression that can directly be monitored in human plasma. A previous study in humans has compared the miRNA expression profile in peripheral blood mononuclear cells from older versus young individuals and revealed significant age-associated down-regulation of miR-24,

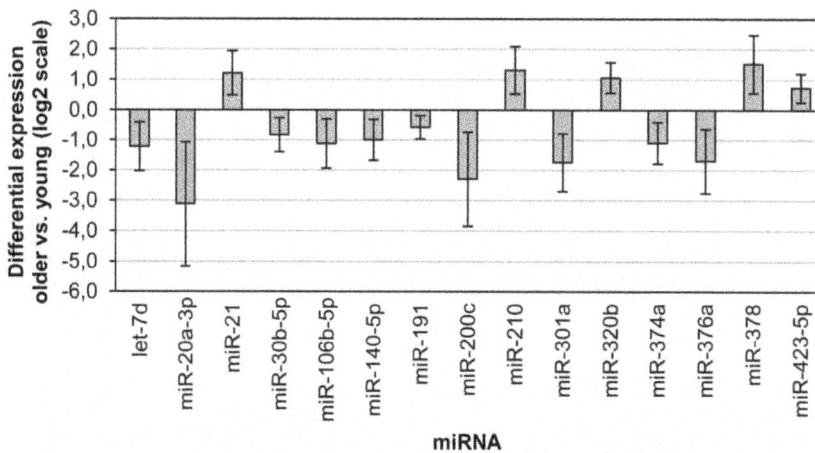

Figure 4. Differential expression of the top-15 ranking miRNAs from the panel screening. The selected miRNAs are displayed in numerical order. Bars represent the difference in expression in older compared to young patients on a 2-logarithmic scale, with indication of the 95% confidence interval (based on t-test).

Table 4. Candidate reference miRNAs identified by exploratory serum/plasma miRNA panel screening.

miRNA	Variance[a] after GMN	Normfinder SD[b]	GeNorm M-value[c]
hsa-let-7i	0.09	0.27	0.40
hsa-miR-484	0.10	0.44	0.49
hsa-miR-29a	0.18	0.36	0.31
hsa-miR-29c	0.20	0.34	0.31
hsa-miR-140-3p	0.22	0.32	0.35
hsa-miR-30e	0.23	0.46	0.53
hsa-miR-30d	0.24	0.51	0.56
hsa-miR-191	0.25	–	–
hsa-miR-29b	0.26	0.50	0.45
hsa-miR-590-5p	0.28	0.57	0.59

[a]Variance after global mean normalisation (GMN) : reflects the deviation of a specific miRNA from the behavior of the global mean (i.e. average signal of all miRNAs included).
[b]Standard deviation returned by NormFinder algorithm.
[c]Expression stability measure (M) returned by GeNorm algorithm (the lower, the more stable the expression).

miR-103, miR-107, miR-128, miR-130a, miR-155, miR-221, miR-496 and miR-1538 [29], but Hunter et al. reported marked differences in miRNA expression between the peripheral blood mononuclear cells and plasma fractions of human blood [30]. In order to identify plasma microRNAs implicated in the aging process, we have compared circulating microRNA's between young and older subjects, by applying a comprehensive RT-qPCR platform for focused microRNA profiling on serum/plasma, using samples from the large blood bank of breast cancer patients that has been established at our institution. We have chosen to perform this search for aging miRNAs in a female breast cancer population, on the plasma samples readily available from our biorepositories, in view of our eventual aim to investigate the

Table 5. Validation of differentially expressed miRNAs in older (N = 10) *versus* young (N = 20) breast cancer patients and comparison between older 'fit' (N = 10) and older 'frail' (N = 10) subjects.

miRNA	Older vs. young P-value[a]	Fold change[b]	Older 'fit' vs. 'frail' P-value[a]
Decreased expression			
hsa-let-7d	*0.1083*	1.59	0.7861
hsa-miR-20a-3p	**0.0004***	**2.48**	0.7405
hsa-miR-30b-5p	**<0.0001***	**2.47**	0.8428
hsa-miR-106b-5p	**0.0001***	**1.56**	0.8784
hsa-miR-140-5p	*0.8431*	1.06	*0.2413*
hsa-miR-191	**0.0010***	**2.23**	0.5611
hsa-miR-200c	*0.5235*	1.21	0.5097
hsa-miR-301a	**0.0024***	**2.34**	0.6111
hsa-miR-374a	**0.0109**	**2.36**	0.6765
hsa-miR-376a	*0.4679*	1.23	0.4195
Increased expression			
hsa-miR-21	0.4133	1.12	0.8749
hsa-miR-210	*0.1528*	1.29	*0.3447*
hsa-miR-320b	0.0585	1.25	0.6679
hsa-miR-378	**0.0077**	**1.71**	0.2817
hsa-miR-423-5p	0.0566	1.34	0.7050

[a]P-values are derived from parametric t-test (unpaired, 2-tail, C.I = 95%), unless data are not normally distributed (values indicated *in italic*). In such cases, P-value derived from Mann-Whitney test is displayed. **Bold values** indicate significant values according to the 5% significance threshold. Values indicated with an asterisk (*) remained significant after correction for multiple testing.
[b]Negative values indicate x-fold *decreased* expression, positive values indicate x-fold *increased* expression.

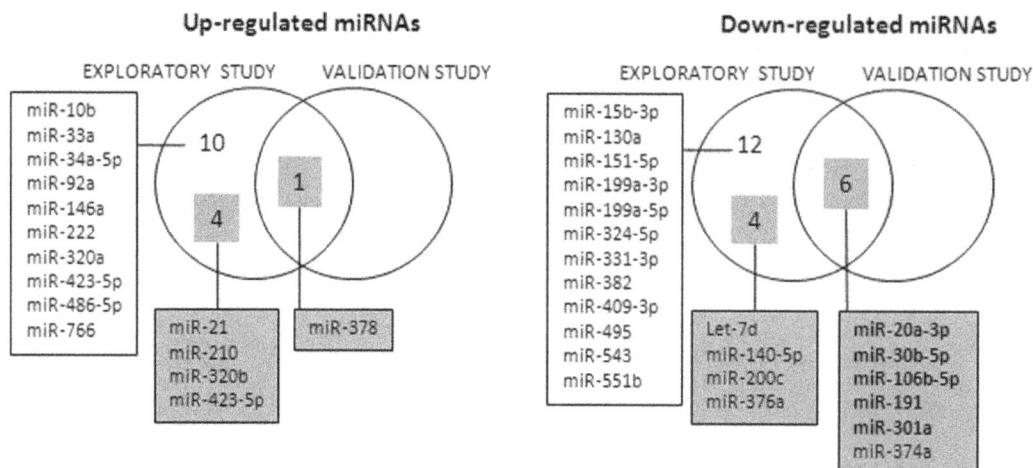

Figure 5. Venn diagram showing up-regulated and down-regulated miRNAs in the exploratory screening and the validation study. In the exploratory screening, there were in total 37 circulating miRNAs exhibiting age-related expression (p<0.05). Of those, only the top-15 miRNAs with the lowest p-values (shown in grey boxes) were further investigated in the validation study. Seven age-related miRNAs were confirmed in the validation study (p<0.05), of which 5 (all showing decreased expression) remained significant after correction for multiple testing; these are indicated in bold. Obviously, the right-hand zone (i.e. miRNAs showing altered expression in the validation study but not the exploratory screening) cannot contain any miRNAs, since the validation study only included those miRNAs that emerged from the exploratory study as the most significantly age-related ones.

impact of chemotherapeutic treatments on the biological age of older breast cancer patients.

For 5 miRNAs, i.e. miR-301a, miR-20a-3p, miR-106b-5p, miR-191 and miR-30b-5p, plasma expression levels were convincingly confirmed to significantly correlate with chronological age. Six other miRNAs that were selected from the intial screening (i.e. let-7d, miR-21, miR-140, miR200c, miR-210 and miR-376a) showed no significant differences between young and older patients in the validation experiment, two (i.e. miR-320b and miR-423-5p) were close to the 5% significance level and two (i.e. miR-374a and miR-378) actually reached statistical significance, but were not retained after correction for multiple testing. Nevertheless, each of the miRNAs included in the validation study consistently showed the same trend, regarding decreased or increased expression in older *versus* young subjects, as observed in the exploratory screening. It should be kept in mind that patient numbers were rather small in both the initial screening and the validation. This might explain why several miRNAs, emerging as candidate aging miRNAs from the exploratory experiment, did not reach statistical significance in the subsequent validation step. On the other hand, we neither can exclude the possibility that for these miRNAs, the 'differences' initially observed in the screening study did not reflect 'real' differential expression but were merely coincidental findings due to multiple testing. Another aspect that may explain inconsistencies between the screening and validation steps is the use of different specimens : because of sample availability issues, the validation study was done on plasma, while serum was used in the initial screening. Nevertheless, one can argue that if the same five miRNA were found to be differentially expressed between age categories in both serum and plasma, regardless of the preparation procedure, these can be considered as particularly strong biomarkers.

It is well possible that we 'missed' significant aging-related miRNAs, either because they are not included in the initial screening panel (which contains a selection of the 175 most commonly detected circulating miRNAs out of the ~300–400 miRNAs that have ever been annotated to serum/plasma), or because they were not among the top-15 ranking differentially

expressed miRNAs in the pilot study and were thus not selected for further investigation, future studies will not exclusively be limited to the five aging miRNAs identified here. For instance, we have observed significantly increased expression of miR-34a in older compared to young subjects in our exploratory screening, which is in line with previous findings [22]. However, miR-34a was not included in our validation experiment because for the present study, we have chosen for an unbiased, straight-forward selection of the top 15 differentially expressed miRNAs to be included in the validation study. We are currently starting a miRNA profiling study including miR-34a in older breast cancer patients receiving chemotherapy.

Interestingly, of the 15 potential aging-related miRNAs selected from the initial screening, 8 miRNAs (i.e. let-7d, miR-106b-5p, miR-20a-3p, miR-21, miR-301a, miR-320b, miR-374a and miR-423-5p) were previously reported to be associated with healthy longevity in a recent study by El Sharawy et al. on genome-wide miRNA signatures [28]. In line with our current findings, this study also revealed age-related down-regulation of let-7d, miR-106b-5p, miR-20a-3p, miR-301a and miR-374a, while miR-320b and miR-423-5p were shown to be upregulated with increasing age. The 7 other potential aging miRNAs that were selected from our initial screening, i.e. miR-140-5p, miR-200c, miR-210, miR-376a, miR-378, miR-191, miR-30b-5p, were not reported to show age-related changes in the longevity study, although the latter two miRNAs were definitely confirmed in our validation study. On the other hand, several miRNAs showing age-related differential expression in the longevity study were also included in our initial screening panel but did not show significant differences between young and older patients and were therefore not further investigated. However, the different context of both studies must be underscored : while the study by El Sharawy and coworkers refers to healthy aging and longevity, the age-related miRNAs reported here are found in a breast cancer background. Moreover, both studies were conducted on relatively small patient cohorts, each containing only ≤20 older patients. Thus, it is well possible that they both lacked sufficient statistical power to detect subtle differences between young and older patients. This, together with the use of different experimental methodology and statistical thresholds, may account for the partial discrepancies. Nonetheless, it is quite remarkable that such highly significant age-related changes in circulating miRNAs, as observed in our study for miR-301a, miR-20a-3p, miR-106b-5p, miR-191 and miR-30b-5p, can be evidenced with as little as 10 patients per age group, suggesting that these miRNAs can be considered as robust and reliable aging biomarkers.

Several of the top-ranking miRNAs for age-related differences between young and older breast cancer patients in our exploratory study have already been linked with cellular senescence in previous reports. A study using diverse human cellular as well as organismal aging models revealed miR-17, miR-19b, miR-20a and miR-106a as biomarkers of aging [31]. These miRNAs, which all belong to the oncogenic miR-17~92 cluster [32,33], prevent cellular senescence by down-regulating the cell cycle inhibitor p21/CDKN1A. Likewise, family members of the paralog miR-106b~25 cluster also promote cell cycle progression — and thus inhibit senescence — by directly targeting p21/CDKN1A [34]. Consistent with these findings, we observed a highly significant age-related decrease in plasma levels of miR-20a and miR-106b, which might thus correspond to an increased level of senescence. Notably, these two miRNAs have previously also been reported to be down-regulated in peripheral blood mononuclear cells from octogenarians *versus* young people, whereas centenarians exhibiting a healthy aging phenotype seemed capable of maintaining high levels of these senescence inhibitors [35]. We found no evidence, however, pointing to miR-17, miR-19b or miR-106a as circulating aging markers, although these miRNAs were also included in the serum/plasma screening panel used in our exploratory study. Neither did we find age-related changes in plasma expression of miR-24, which has been shown to suppress the expression of the senescence gene p16^{INK4A} in human diploid fibroblasts [36]. As opposed to the senescence inhibiting miRNAs miR20a and miR-106b, 6 other miRNAs that were identified as candidate circulating aging miRNAs in our initial exploratory study (i.e. miR-21, miR-191, miR-200c, miR-210, miR-376a and let-7d) have been reported to *trigger* cellular senescence in specific cell types [20,37–40]; miR-21 has even been described as a new circulating marker of inflammaging [41]. Yet, only miR-191 was convincingly confirmed in our validation study; its significant age-associated down-regulation in serum/plasma is in agreement with earlier findings in mononuclear cells [35]. The remaining 7 candidate aging miRNAs miR-320b, miR-301a, miR-378, miR-374a, miR-423, miR-30b, miR-140 that emerged from our initial screening and of which two (i.e. miR-301a and miR-30b) were convincingly confirmed in the validation study, have previously not been linked with cellular senescence and are now for the first time directly associated with aging in humans. It should be mentioned, though, that one of the target genes of miR-320 family members is IGFBP5 (insulin-like growth factor binding protein 5), an important modulator of the aging-related insulin/IGF-1 signaling pathway. IGFBP5 and miR-320 are expressed in a wide variety of overlapping tissues (e.g. liver, brain, lung, kidney, heart, colon ...) and are secreted into the circulation. Serum IGFBP5 concentrations have been reported to decline with age and to show a significant positive correlation with circulating levels of IGF-1 [42]. Thus, the age-associated increase in circulating miR-320b observed in our present study – albeit not statistically significant in the validation experiment – might possibly be linked with our previous finding that plasma IGF-1 levels are decreased in older compared to younger patients (our own data, manuscript in preparation). Therefore, miR-320b will still be considered as a potential miRNA of interest in our future aging biomarker studies.

For reasons outlined above, we are not studying aging miRNAs in a healthy population but in a breast cancer context. In order to minimize cancer-related confounding effects, we have selected highly homogeneous cohorts with regard to tumor characteristics. Nevertheless, it cannot be excluded that the organismal response to breast cancer disease might override otherwise regulated miRNAs. Small age-related changes in plasma miRNA expression might possibly be masked by substantial cancer-related under- or overexpression of particular miRNAs in older breast cancer patients. The processes of aging and carcinogenesis are indeed intimately linked, since cellular senescence constitutes an intrinsic tumor suppressor mechanism *in vivo* but, at the same time, is the major driving force in age-related tissue degeneration and dysfunction [43]. It is thus conceivable that miRNAs implicated in aging are also modulated in human cancers and *vice versa*. Several miRNAs that emerged from our exploratory screening as candidate aging miRNAs have actually been reported as "oncomirs" or "tumor suppressor miRNAs". For instance, let-7d is considered a tumor suppressor microRNA, as it is strongly down-regulated in poorly differentiated lung and breast tumor cells [44]. Also, miR-376a is downregulated in several tumors and makes part of a miRNA cluster frequently silenced in malignant melanoma [45]. In contrast, miR-20a, miR-21, miR-378, miR-106b and miR-191 were found to exert oncogenic activity and are overexpressed in several types of cancer [20,31,34,46,47]. Moreover, high (tumor) expression of miR-210 has been associated with higher risk of recurrence in breast cancer [48]. Serum miR-200c was reported as a novel prognostic and metastasis-predictive biomarker in colorectal cancer [49], while miR-423-5p was found to be upregulated in serum from patients with gastric cancer [50]. Therefore, it should be kept in mind when interpreting our data that certain miRNAs exert their action at the interface between cancer and aging. To our knowledge, this is the first miRNA study comparing "fit" and "non-fit/frail" older individuals. We did not observe any significant differences between those two subgroups, at least not with regard to the miRNAs investigated in the validation study. This is somewhat surprising, since several of these miRNAs have also been implicated in age-related diseases. For instance, let-7d, miR-191 and miR-301a make part of a unique circulating 7-miRNA signature that can distinguish patients with Alzheimer's disease from normal controls [51], and miR-20a and miR-106b are both implicated in transcriptional inhibition of Alzheimer's amyloid precursor protein (APP) [52]. Also, miR-320 was shown to be upregulated in neurodegeneration in mice [53]. Furthermore, miR-21 expression has been reported to be higher in patients suffering from cardiovascular disease [41] and loss of miR-140 contributes to the development of age-related osteoarthritis-like changes in mice [54]. However, other miRNAs than those included in our validation study have been more consistently associated with age-related physical and mental decline: e.g. the miRNA most clearly associated with age-related neurodegeneration in the aging *Drosophila* brain is miR-34 [55]. Our data indicate that the observed age-related differential expression of the 5 validated aging miRNAs represents a direct effect of physiological aging and is not merely associated to the age-related frailty syndrome. Yet, the newly identified aging miRNAs should be further validated in larger cohorts of frail *verus* non-frail older persons that are not affected by cancer, in order to ultimately sustain this conclusion. A search for "frailty miRNAs" is another issue of clinical interest, which would, however, demand a different experimental set-up, such as exploratory screening and subsequent validation in healthy *versus* frail subjects of comparable age.

In conclusion, we have discovered five miRNAs (miR-301a, miR-20a-3p, miR-106b-5p, miR-191 and miR-30b-5p) that can be used as aging biomarkers in future research projects. Since we have chosen for a straight-forward selection of 15 miRNAs from the initial screening, certain potentially interesting miRNAs, most particularly miR-34a, were not further investigated in this study. These, together with several miRNAs that remained inconclusive because of borderline statistical significance (e.g. miR-320b, miR-374a, miR-378, miR-423), might yet merit further attention in future studies. The newly identified aging miRNAs will now be examined in a prospective study that has recently been conducted in our institution with the aim to investigate the impact of chemotherapy on the biological age of older breast cancer patients. While common acute adverse events of chemotherapy, such as neutropenia and mucosal degeneration, are well-known and may be tolerated/accepted by the patient, the long term impact of cytotoxic treatments (and perhaps other anti-cancer therapies such as hormonal drugs, monoclonal antibiodies and oral targeted agents) on healthy tissues is actually poorly documented. For instance, premature telomere shortening due to DNA-targeting chemotherapeutic drugs may impact on the long-term replicative potential of regenerative tissues like hair follicles, the hematopoietic and gastrointestinal system, and germline and skin cells [56]. To learn more about such delayed aging-related side effects in long-term survivors of cancer, a better insight into aging mechanisms and associated biomarkers is mandatory, along with detailed investigation of the impact of common chemotherapeutic regimens on these aging biomarkers.

Materials and Methods

Ethics statement

This study was performed in compliance with the Helsinki Declaration and national law. All patients included in the study gave written informed consent for future translational research. Blood sampling, collection of patient data and genetic analysis were approved by the ethics committee of our institution (Ethics Committee of the University Hospitals Leuven, study number S53608; Approval number : ML7994).

Patients

Since 2003, the Leuven Multidisciplinary Breast Center (University Hospitals Leuven) has systematically collected plasma and serum from all consenting (i.e. ±75%) breast cancer patients at the time of diagnosis, before initiation of any local or systemic therapy. All breast cancer patients are also included in a clinical database, containing extensive general and tumor-related information, as well as clinical follow-up. In addition, most older (70+) breast cancer patients diagnosed since 2009 are also included in one of the large-scale geriatric cancer projects running in our institution: geriatric assessment (GA) − integrating two geriatric screening tools G8 and Flemish version of the Triage Risk Screening Tool (fTRST), Activities of Daily Living (ADL), instrumental Activities of Daily Living (iADL), Geriatric Depression Scale, Mini Mental State Examination, and Mini Nutritional Assessment − is systematically performed prior to initiation of any chemotherapy, radiotherapy or surgery [24]. Furthermore, the Charlson Comorbidity Index (at the time of diagnosis) can easily be calculated retrospectively using the patient's electronic file.

Selection of the exploratory cohort

For an initial exploratory pilot experiment, eligible subjects were selected from the clinical breast cancer database based on the following inclusion criteria: (i) diagnosed with primary (i.e. non-

relapse) early (i.e. non-locally advanced, non-metastatic) invasive breast cancer *without* lymph node involvement; (ii) received primary surgery and pathological confirmation in our institution; (iii) serum collected at the time of diagnosis (i.e. before initiation of any treatment); (iv) all pathological parameters available to identify histological subtype according to recent guidelines [57,58]. A study group of 10 young (<45 years) patients and 10 older (>70 years) patients (all female), the latter with GA performed at the time of diagnosis (i.e. before initiation of any treatment), was selected and both age groups were matched in order to contain an equal distribution of different breast cancer subtypes: 7 so-called luminal A, 1 luminal B, 2 triple negative [58]. Tumor characteristics are summarized in Table 1. Determination of tumor grading and estrogen receptor (ER), progesterone receptor (PR), and HER2/*neu* status was done according to standard procedures. ER and PR were considered positive if >1% of cells stained positive on immunohistochemistry. HER2 was considered positive if the fluorescent in situ hybridization (FISH) test, systematically performed in all immunohistochemistry (IHC) 2+ tumors, showed HER2 genomic amplification or, in the absence of FISH, if IHC was 3+.

Selection of the validation study cohort

For the subsequent validation experiment, an independent cohort of early breast cancer patients (all with primary invasive, node-negative luminal A tumors) was selected consisting of 10 young (<45 years) female patients and 20 older (>70 years) female patients, from whom 10 were 'fit' while 10 others were classified as 'non-fit'. Fitness/frailty status was estimated based on the results of the GA, which were condensed into (i) the generally used Balducci score [59] and (ii) the novel Leuven Oncogeriatric Frailty Score (LOFS), a final score from 0 (severly frail) to 10 (entirely fit), described in File S1. Patients of the older 'fit' group had LOFS = 9–10, whereas patients of the older 'non-fit' group had LOFS ≤5. Clinical characteristics of patients from the validation study cohort are summarized in Table 2.

Serum and plasma collection

Peripheral blood was routinely sampled in 4-mL BD Vacutainer SST II Advance tubes (for serum collection) and in 4-mL BD Vacutainer EDTA K2E tubes (for plasma collection). The blood samples were incubated at room temperature for 20 to 60 min. After centrifugation at 1600xg for 10 min at 4°C, the supernatant (serum/plasma) was isolated and stored in aliquots at −80°C. Because of sample availability issues, the validation study was done on plasma specimens, whereas the exploratory screening was done on serum.

MicroRNA isolation

After spinning down thawed serum/plasma to remove debris, the absorbance spectrum of the sample was recorded on a NanoDrop ND-1000 in order to detect hemolysis, which may cause severe perturbation of serum/plasma miRNA profiles due to cell-derived microRNA contamination. Samples showing a clear absorption peak at 415 nm (i.e. absorbance maximum of hemoglobin) were excluded from the experiment. Absence of hemolysis in the included samples was further verified after qPCR (see below). RNA was purified from non-hemolysed serum/plasma samples using the miRNeasy Mini kit (Qiagen) following the manufacturer's protocol with slight modifications in order to achieve optimal microRNA extraction from serum/plasma samples, which typically contain very low amounts of RNA. Briefly, to 200 µL of serum/plasma, 1 µg of carrier MS2 RNA (Roche) was added, together with 750 µL of QIAzol (Qiagen).

Subsequently, 1 μL of a synthetic RNA spike-in (UniSp6 at 10^8 copies/μL, Exiqon) was added to allow evaluation of the efficiency and uniformity of the entire RNA extraction/cDNA synthesis procedure. After 5 min of incubation, 200 μL chloroform was added. After incubation and centrifugation according to the normal procedure, the upper aqueous phase was isolated, 1.5 volumes of ethanol was added and the sample was loaded onto the spin column. The column was washed once with RWT buffer and three times with RPE buffer (both included in the kit). After air-drying of the column, the RNA sample was eluted with 50 μL of nuclease-free water and immediately frozen at $-80°C$ until further analysis. In both the pilot and the validation experiment, duplicate RNA extractions were performed in parallel from each plasma sample.

cDNA synthesis

Because of the very low amounts of RNA in serum/plasma and, therefore, the use of an RNA carrier during the extraction procedure, standard spectrophotometric measurement of RNA yield and quality is not suitable for serum/plasma RNA extracts. Therefore, RNA input in the reverse transcription (RT) reaction was based on sample volume and not RNA quantity. Preliminary test experiments with several commonly used control miRNAs (i.e. miR-103, miR-191, miR-423-3p and miR-451) were carried out to determine the optimal amount of RNA template to be used in the RT reaction; these titration experiments showed that an RNA input of 4 μL mostly resulted in good RT efficiency and subsequent PCR amplification without significant interference by RT and/or PCR inhibitors, which are frequently present in RNA preparations from serum/plasma. Thus, cDNA was synthesized from each of both duplicate RNA extracts using 4 μL of RNA in a 20-μL reaction by use of the Universal cDNA synthesis kit II (Exiqon) according to the manufacturer's instructions. cDNA samples were stored frozen until PCR analysis was performed.

RT-qPCR-based miRNA assays

In the initial experiment, a broad exploratory miRNA screening was performed using the 96-well Serum/Plasma Focus microRNA PCR Panel (Exiqon) that comprises microRNA PCR assays for 175 different microRNAs that are commonly found in serum/plasma. Since individual samples are assessed on separate plates, the panel assay also includes triplicate wells of an interplate calibrator (UniSp3) to account for technical run-to-run differences in amplification signal. Data from different plates were normalized using the Cp-values of the interplate calibrator. For each serum sample, both duplicate cDNA samples were pooled before running the miRNA panel assay. Assays were carried out following the manufacturer's protocol. Briefly, pooled cDNA was diluted 50x in nuclease-free water and mixed with an equal volume of 2x SYBR Green master mix (Exiqon). Final reaction volume was 10 μL. Plates were run on a LightCycler 480 (LC480, Roche) instrument applying the following thermal cycling protocol : activation step (10 min at 95°C); 45 amplification cycles (10 s at 95°C, 1 min at 60°C, ramp rate 1,6°C/s); melting curve analysis.

In the subsequent validation study on plasma samples from a different, independent patient cohort, 21 selected miRNAs were assessed by the use of individual PCR assays (MicroRNA LNA PCR primer sets, Exiqon). These included the 15 top-ranking candidate aging miRNAs, showing the most pronounced age-related differences in the pilot screening experiment. In addition, 4 miRNAs that were identified as good reference candidates in the pilot experiment and 2 additonal quality control miRNAs were also included. For each plasma sample, duplicate RNA extracts were prepared and reverse transcribed and separate PCR assays

were run on each of both duplicate cDNA samples. All PCR assays were done in triplicate microplate wells (96-well format). Reaction mixtures were prepared according to the provided assay protocol and contained 4 μL of 40-fold diluted cDNA (20-fold diluted for miR-20a-3p) in a final volume of 10 μL. For each miRNA, all samples were run together on the same plate to avoid bias introduced by plate-to-plate variations in qPCR efficiency. Plates were run on the LC480 instrument using the same thermal cycling protocol as described above for the panel assays.

Data analysis

RT-qPCR Cp values were determined by the LC480 instrument software using the second derivative method and were subsequently imported and further processed by GenEx Pro software (MultiID Analyses). The absence of hemolysis in the initial serum/plasma samples was verified by means of the miR-451/miR-23a-3p hemolysis test: ΔCp values between miR-23a-3p, known to be stably expressed in serum/plasma samples, and miR-451a, known to show highly increased expression in hemolysed samples, were below 5 for all samples.

Data of the initial screening experiment were normalized using the global mean of the entire miRNA panel [25]. Candidate reference miRNAs were then identified by variance analysis of the normalized dataset and were further examined using the specified algorithms GeNorm [27] and Normfinder [26], which are both incorporated in the GenEx Pro software package (MultiID Analyses). Five miRNAs with superior expression stability among all samples were used for data normalisation in the subsequent validation study.

Statistical tools incorporated in the GenEx software package were applied to assess differences in serum/plasma miRNA expression between the different patient groups. These included parametric t-test (unpaired, two-tailed) for normally distributed miRNA results and Mann-Whitney test (unpaired, two-tailed) for cases where the data were not normally distributed. Normality was assessed with the Kolmogorov-Smirnov test. In the exploratory study, principal component analysis and hierarchical clustering were additionally applied to reveal sample grouping patterns in the multivariate dataset. In the validation study, the age effect was first assessed by comparing the young patient group (N = 10) with the total older patient group (N = 20), combining both 'fit' (N = 10) and 'frail' (N = 10) subgroups. Subsequently, a comparison between 'fit' and 'frail' patients was done within the older cohort. Correction for multiple testing was done according to the Dunn-Bonferroni method.

Supporting Information

File S1 Leuven Oncogeriatric Frailty Score (LOFS). Description and illustration of the composition of the new, refined scoring system that was used to evaluate the fitness/frailty status of the patients.

File S2 List of all microRNAs included in the exploratory screening panel.

File S3 Data set of the exploratory screening study.

File S4 Data set of the validation study.

Acknowledgments

We thank Kathleen Corthouts for excellent technical assistance.

References

1. Balaban RS, Nemoto S, Finkel T (2005) Mitochondria, oxidants, and aging. Cell 120: 483–495.
2. Lombard DB, Chua KF, Mostoslavsky R, Franco S, Gostissa M, et al. (2005) DNA repair, genome stability, and aging. Cell 120: 497–512.
3. Blasco MA (2007) Telomere length, stem cells and aging. Nat Chem Biol 3: 640–649.
4. Campisi J, Kim SH, Lim CS, Rubio M (2001) Cellular senescence, cancer and aging: the telomere connection. Exp Gerontol 36: 1619–1637.
5. Zhang G, Li J, Purkayastha S, Tang Y, Zhang H, et al. (2013) Hypothalamic programming of systemic ageing involving IKK-beta, NF-kappaB and GnRH. Nature 497: 211–216.
6. Alcedo J, Flatt T, Pasyukova EG (2013) Neuronal inputs and outputs of aging and longevity. Front Genet 4: 71.
7. Maccormick RE (2006) Possible acceleration of aging by adjuvant chemotherapy: a cause of early onset frailty? Med Hypotheses 67: 212–215.
8. Li P, Hou M, Lou F, Bjorkholm M, Xu D (2012) Telomere dysfunction induced by chemotherapeutic agents and radiation in normal human cells. Int J Biochem Cell Biol 44: 1531–1540.
9. Franco S, Ozkaynak MF, Sandoval C, Tugal O, Jayabose S, et al. (2003) Telomere dynamics in childhood leukemia and solid tumors: a follow-up study. Leukemia 17: 401–410.
10. Schroder CP, Wisman GB, de Jong S, van der Graaf WT, Ruiters MH, et al. (2001) Telomere length in breast cancer patients before and after chemotherapy with or without stem cell transplantation. Br J Cancer 84: 1348–1353.
11. Wynn RF, Cross MA, Hatton C, Will AM, Lashford LS, et al. (1998) Accelerated telomere shortening in young recipients of allogeneic bone-marrow transplants. Lancet 351: 178–181.
12. Unryn BM, Hao D, Gluck S, Riabowol KT (2006) Acceleration of telomere loss by chemotherapy is greater in older patients with locally advanced head and neck cancer. Clin Cancer Res 12: 6345–6350.
13. Serrano M, Blasco MA (2007) Cancer and ageing: convergent and divergent mechanisms. Nat Rev Mol Cell Biol 8: 715–722.
14. Roninson IB (2003) Tumor cell senescence in cancer treatment. Cancer Res 63: 2705–2715.
15. Chang BD, Swift ME, Shen M, Fang J, Broude EV, et al. (2002) Molecular determinants of terminal growth arrest induced in tumor cells by a chemotherapeutic agent. Proc Natl Acad Sci U S A 99: 389–394.
16. Liu Y, Sanoff HK, Cho H, Burd CE, Torrice C, et al. (2009) Expression of p16(INK4a) in peripheral blood T-cells is a biomarker of human aging. Aging Cell 8: 439–448.
17. Vandenberk B, Brouwers B, Hatse S, Wildiers H (2011) p16(INK4a): A central player in cellular senescence and a promising aging biomarker in elderly cancer patients. Journal of Geriatric Oncology 2: 259–269.
18. Pallis AG, Hatse S, Brouwers B, Pawelec G, Falandry C, et al. (2013) Evaluating the physiological reserves of older patients with cancer: The value of potential biomarkers of aging? Journal of Geriatric Oncology in press.
19. Grillari J, Grillari-Voglauer R (2010) Novel modulators of senescence, aging, and longevity: Small non-coding RNAs enter the stage. Exp Gerontol 45: 302–311.
20. Olivieri F, Rippo MR, Monsurro V, Salvioli S, Capri M, et al. (2013) MicroRNAs linking inflamm-aging, cellular senescence and cancer. Ageing Res Rev.
21. Inukai S, Slack F (2013) MicroRNAs and the genetic network in aging. J Mol Biol 425: 3601–3608.
22. Li X, Khanna A, Li N, Wang E (2011) Circulatory miR34a as an RNAbased, noninvasive biomarker for brain aging. Aging (Albany NY) 3: 985–1002.
23. Mitchell PS, Parkin RK, Kroh EM, Fritz BR, Wyman SK, et al. (2008) Circulating microRNAs as stable blood-based markers for cancer detection. Proc Natl Acad Sci U S A 105: 10513–10518.
24. Kenis C, Bron D, Libert Y, Decoster L, Van Puyvelde K, et al. (2013) Relevance of a systematic geriatric screening and assessment in older patients with cancer: results of a prospective multicentric study. Ann Oncol 24: 1306–1312.
25. Mestdagh P, Van Vlierberghe P, De Weer A, Muth D, Westermann F, et al. (2009) A novel and universal method for microRNA RT-qPCR data normalization. Genome Biol 10: R64.
26. Andersen CL, Jensen JL, Orntoft TF (2004) Normalization of real-time quantitative reverse transcription-PCR data: a model-based variance estimation approach to identify genes suited for normalization, applied to bladder and colon cancer data sets. Cancer Res 64: 5245–5250.
27. Vandesompele J, De Preter K, Pattyn F, Poppe B, Van Roy N, et al. (2002) Accurate normalization of real-time quantitative RT-PCR data by geometric averaging of multiple internal control genes. Genome Biol 3: RESEARCH0034.
28. ElSharawy A, Keller A, Flachsbart F, Wendschlag A, Jacobs G, et al. (2012) Genome-wide miRNA signatures of human longevity. Aging Cell 11: 607–616.

Author Contributions

Conceived and designed the experiments: SH BB CK HW. Performed the experiments: SH. Analyzed the data: SH BD AL PS HW. Contributed reagents/materials/analysis tools: SH BB CK AL. Contributed to the writing of the manuscript: SH BB BD AL CK PS HW.

29. Noren Hooten N, Abdelmohsen K, Gorospe M, Ejiogu N, Zonderman AB, et al. (2010) microRNA expression patterns reveal differential expression of target genes with age. PLoS One 5: e10724.
30. Hunter MP, Ismail N, Zhang X, Aguda BD, Lee EJ, et al. (2008) Detection of microRNA expression in human peripheral blood microvesicles. PLoS One 3: e3694.
31. Hackl M, Brunner S, Fortschegger K, Schreiner C, Micutkova L, et al. (2010) miR-17, miR-19b, miR-20a, and miR-106a are down-regulated in human aging. Aging Cell 9: 291–296.
32. Grillari J, Hackl M, Grillari-Voglauer R (2010) miR-17-92 cluster: ups and downs in cancer and aging. Biogerontology 11: 501–506.
33. He L, Thomson JM, Hemann MT, Hernando-Monge E, Mu D, et al. (2005) A microRNA polycistron as a potential human oncogene. Nature 435: 828–833.
34. Ivanovska I, Ball AS, Diaz RL, Magnus JF, Kibukawa M, et al. (2008) MicroRNAs in the miR-106b family regulate p21/CDKN1A and promote cell cycle progression. Mol Cell Biol 28: 2167–2174.
35. Serna E, Gambini J, Borras C, Abdelaziz KM, Belenguer A, et al. (2012) Centenarians, but not octogenarians, up-regulate the expression of microRNAs. Sci Rep 2: 961.
36. Lal A, Kim HH, Abdelmohsen K, Kuwano Y, Pullmann R, Jr., et al. (2008) p16(INK4a) translation suppressed by miR-24. PLoS One 3: e1864.
37. Dellago H, Preschitz-Kammerhofer B, Terlecki-Zaniewicz L, Schreiner C, Fortschegger K, et al. (2013) High levels of oncomiR-21 contribute to the senescence-induced growth arrest in normal human cells and its knock-down increases the replicative lifespan. Aging Cell 12: 446–458.
38. Lena AM, Mancini M, Rivetti di Val Cervo P, Saintigny G, Mahe C, et al. (2012) MicroRNA-191 triggers keratinocytes senescence by SATB1 and CDK6 downregulation. Biochem Biophys Res Commun 423: 509–514.
39. Magenta A, Cencioni C, Fasanaro P, Zaccagnini G, Greco S, et al. (2011) miR-200c is upregulated by oxidative stress and induces endothelial cell apoptosis and senescence via ZEB1 inhibition. Cell Death Differ 18: 1628–1639.
40. Faraonio R, Salerno P, Passaro F, Sedia C, Iaccio A, et al. (2012) A set of miRNAs participates in the cellular senescence program in human diploid fibroblasts. Cell Death Differ 19: 713–721.
41. Olivieri F, Spazzafumo L, Santini G, Lazzarini R, Albertini MC, et al. (2012) Age-related differences in the expression of circulating microRNAs: miR-21 as a new circulating marker of inflammaging. Mech Ageing Dev 133: 675–685.
42. Mohan S, Farley JR, Baylink DJ (1995) Age-related changes in IGFBP-4 and IGFBP-5 levels in human serum and bone: implications for bone loss with aging. Prog Growth Factor Res 6: 465–473.
43. Finkel T, Serrano M, Blasco MA (2007) The common biology of cancer and ageing. Nature 448: 767–774.
44. Yu F, Yao H, Zhu P, Zhang X, Pan Q, et al. (2007) let-7 regulates self renewal and tumorigenicity of breast cancer cells. Cell 131: 1109–1123.
45. Zehavi L, Avraham R, Barzilai A, Bar-Ilan D, Navon R, et al. (2012) Silencing of a large microRNA cluster on human chromosome 14q32 in melanoma: biological effects of mir-376a and mir-376c on insulin growth factor 1 receptor. Mol Cancer 11: 44.
46. Lee DY, Deng Z, Wang CH, Yang BB (2007) MicroRNA-378 promotes cell survival, tumor growth, and angiogenesis by targeting SuFu and Fus-1 expression. Proc Natl Acad Sci U S A 104: 20350–20355.
47. Volinia S, Calin GA, Liu CG, Ambs S, Cimmino A, et al. (2006) A microRNA expression signature of human solid tumors defines cancer gene targets. Proc Natl Acad Sci U S A 103: 2257–2261.
48. Camps C, Buffa FM, Colella S, Moore J, Sotiriou C, et al. (2008) hsa-miR-210 Is induced by hypoxia and is an independent prognostic factor in breast cancer. Clin Cancer Res 14: 1340–1348.
49. Toiyama Y, Hur K, Tanaka K, Inoue Y, Kusunoki M, et al. (2013) Serum miR-200c Is a Novel Prognostic and Metastasis-Predictive Biomarker in Patients With Colorectal Cancer. Ann Surg.
50. Liu R, Zhang C, Hu Z, Li G, Wang C, et al. (2011) A five-microRNA signature identified from genome-wide serum microRNA expression profiling serves as a fingerprint for gastric cancer diagnosis. Eur J Cancer 47: 784–791.
51. Kumar P, Dezso Z, MacKenzie C, Oestreicher J, Agoulnik S, et al. (2013) Circulating miRNA biomarkers for Alzheimer's disease. PLoS One 8: e69807.
52. Hebert SS, Horre K, Nicolai L, Bergmans B, Papadopoulou AS, et al. (2009) MicroRNA regulation of Alzheimer's Amyloid precursor protein expression. Neurobiol Dis 33: 422–428.
53. Saba R, Goodman CD, Huzarewich RL, Robertson C, Booth SA (2008) A miRNA signature of prion induced neurodegeneration. PLoS One 3: e3652.
54. Miyaki S, Sato T, Inoue A, Otsuki S, Ito Y, et al. (2010) MicroRNA-140 plays dual roles in both cartilage development and homeostasis. Genes Dev 24: 1173–1185.

55. Aw S, Cohen SM (2012) Time is of the essence: microRNAs and age-associated neurodegeneration. Cell Res 22: 1218–1220.
56. Beeharry N, Broccoli D (2005) Telomere dynamics in response to chemotherapy. Curr Mol Med 5: 187–196.
57. Brouckaert O, Schoneveld A, Truyers C, Kellen E, Van Ongeval C, et al. (2013) Breast cancer phenotype, nodal status and palpability may be useful in the detection of overdiagnosed screening-detected breast cancers. Ann Oncol 24: 1847–1852.
58. Goldhirsch A, Winer EP, Coates AS, Gelber RD, Piccart-Gebhart M, et al. (2013) Personalizing the treatment of women with early breast cancer: highlights of the St Gallen International Expert Consensus on the Primary Therapy of Early Breast Cancer 2013. Ann Oncol 24: 2206–2223.
59. Balducci L, Extermann M (2000) Management of the frail person with advanced cancer. Crit Rev Oncol Hematol 33: 143–148.

10

Expression of the Genetic Suppressor Element 24.2 (GSE24.2) Decreases DNA Damage and Oxidative Stress in X-Linked Dyskeratosis Congenita Cells

Cristina Manguan-Garcia[1,2], Laura Pintado-Berninches[1], Jaime Carrillo[1], Rosario Machado-Pinilla[1,2], Leandro Sastre[1,2], Carme Pérez-Quilis[3,4], Isabel Esmoris[3,4], Amparo Gimeno[3,4], Jose Luis García-Giménez[2,3,4], Federico V. Pallardó[2,3,4], Rosario Perona[1,2]*

1 Instituto de Investigaciones Biomédicas CSIC/UAM, Madrid, Spain, 2 CIBER de Enfermedades Raras, Valencia, Spain, 3 Biomedical Research Institute INCLIVA, Valencia, Spain, 4 Department of Physiology, Faculty of Medicine and Dentistry, University of Valencia, Valencia, Spain

Abstract

The predominant X-linked form of Dyskeratosis congenita results from mutations in *DKC1*, which encodes dyskerin, a protein required for ribosomal RNA modification that is also a component of the telomerase complex. We have previously found that expression of an internal fragment of dyskerin (GSE24.2) rescues telomerase activity in X-linked dyskeratosis congenita (X-DC) patient cells. Here we have found that an increased basal and induced DNA damage response occurred in X-DC cells in comparison with normal cells. DNA damage that is also localized in telomeres results in increased heterochromatin formation and senescence. Expression of a cDNA coding for GSE24.2 rescues both global and telomeric DNA damage. Furthermore, transfection of bacterial purified or a chemically synthesized GSE24.2 peptide is able to rescue basal DNA damage in X-DC cells. We have also observed an increase in oxidative stress in X-DC cells and expression of GSE24.2 was able to diminish it. Altogether our data indicated that supplying GSE24.2, either from a cDNA vector or as a peptide reduces the pathogenic effects of Dkc1 mutations and suggests a novel therapeutic approach.

Editor: Gabriele Saretzki, University of Newcastle, United Kingdom

Funding: This work was supported by grants: PI11-0949 and PI12/02263 FIS, SAF2008-01338 from the Ministerio de Ciencia e Innovación. Grants, PROMETEO2010/074 from Generalitat Valenciana and Fundación Salud 2000 to FVP. CMG, JLGG and CPQ are supported by CIBER de Enfermedades Raras. The funders had no role in study design, data collection and analysis, decision to publish, or preparation of the manuscript.

Competing Interests: The authors have declared that no competing interests exist.

* Email: RPerona@iib.uam.es

Introduction

Telomeres are nucleoprotein complexes located at the ends of linear chromosomes and consist of tandem repeats of simple DNA sequences (TTAGGG in humans) and proteins that interact directly or indirectly with these sequences [1]. Sequence erosion of terminal repeats is inherent to each round of genome replication. The replenishment of the telomeric repeats is accomplished by the extension of their 3′ ends, through a reaction mediated by the telomerase complex [2]. In humans, the active telomerase complex consists of a minimum of three essential components: hTERT, hTR and dyskerin [3]. Besides forming part of the telomerase complex, dyskerin is a pseudouridine synthase component of H/ACA small nuclear RNPs [4], complexes that mediate the conversion of specific uridines (U) to pseudouridine in newly synthesized ribosomal RNAs [5] [6] [7]. Point mutations in dyskerin cause a rare disease named X-linked dyskeratosis congenita (X-DC) [8]. Individuals with X-DC display features of premature ageing, as well as nail dystrophy, mucosal leukoplakia, interstitial fibrosis of the lung and increased susceptibility to cancer [9]. The tissues affected by X-DC, such as bone marrow and skin, are characterized by the high rate of turnover of their progenitor cells.

Telomere shortening prevents the formation of the loop-like structure maintained by a nucleoprotein structure consisting of telomeric DNA and 6 proteins that are together known as shelterin [1]. This capping structure prevents the otherwise exposed ends of different chromosomes from being recognized as double strand breaks (DSBs) by the cell's DNA repair machinery which would result in telomere fusion. When telomeres become critically short or unprotected because of shelterin deficiency, they trigger a DNA damage response (DDR), leading to the activation of an ataxia telangiectasia mutated (ATM) or ataxia telangiectasia and Rad3 related (ATR)-dependent DNA damage response at chromosome ends [10] [11] [12] [13]. 53BP1 is a C-non-homologous-end-joining (C-NHEJ) component and an ATM target that accumulates at DSBs and uncapped telomeres [14] [15]. The binding of 53BP1 close to DNA breaks impacts the dynamic behavior of the local chromatin and facilitates the non-homologous-end-joining (NHEJ) repair reactions that involve distant sites [16]. ATM phosphorylates Chk2 leading to activation of cell cycle checkpoints. Chk2 acts as a signal distributor, dispersing checkpoint signal to downstream targets such as p53, Cdc25A, Cdc25C, BRCA1 and E2F1 [17].

Senescence, initially described as stable cell proliferation arrest, can be induced by telomere shortening and also by activated oncogenes, DNA damage and drug-like inhibitors of specific enzymatic activities [18]. Senescent cells are typically characterized by a large flat morphology and the expression of a senescence-associated-β-galactosidase (SA-β-gal) activity of unknown function. In the nucleus of senescent cells chromatin undergoes dramatic remodeling through the formation of domains of heterochromatin called senescence-associated heterochromatin-foci (SAHF). SAHF contain histone modifications and proteins characteristic of silent heterochromatin such as methylated lysine 9 of histone H3 (H3K9me), heterochromatin protein 1 (HP1), and the histone H2A variant macroH2A.1 [18] [19]. Proliferation-promoting genes such as E2F-target genes (e.g. cyclin A) are recruited into SAHF, dependent on the pRB suppressor protein, thereby irreversibly silencing expression of those genes.

In cultured cells and animal models, telomere erosion promotes chromosomal instability via breakage-fusion-bridge cycles, contributing to the early stages of tumorigenesis. Telomere shortening in Dyskeratosis congenita is associated with a higher risk of some types of cancer such as head and neck squamous cell carcinoma (HNSCC) (mostly tongue), skin squamous cell carcinoma (SCC), anogenital, stomach, esophagus, and lymphomas, as well as myelodysplastic syndrome (MDS) [20] [21] [22] [23]. Altogether, these findings provide direct clinical evidence that short telomeres in hematopoietic cells are dysfunctional, mediate chromosomal instability and predispose to malignant transformation in a human disease.

We previously isolated the peptide GSE24.2, in a screen of cDNAs for those that confer survival ability on cells treated with cisplatin [24]. Intriguingly GSE24.2 turned out to be a short dyskerin fragment containing two highly conserved motifs implicated in pseudouridine synthase catalytic activity. GSE24.2 prevents telomerase inhibition mediated by different chemotherapeutic agents, including cisplatin and telomerase inhibitors. In X-DC cells and WI-38-VA13 cells, GSE24.2 induces an increase in hTERT mRNA levels and the recovery of telomerase activity [24]. Mutations in DKC1 lead to severe destabilization of telomerase RNA (TR), a reduction in telomerase activity and a significant continuous loss of telomere length during growth [25]. When a peptide encoding GSE24.2, was introduced into mutant cells, it rescued telomerase activity and prevented the decrease in TR levels induced by the Dkc1 mutation [26] GSE24.2 was recently approved as an orphan drug for the treatment of Dyskeratosis congenita (EU/3/12/1070 - EMA/OD/136/11).

To obtain more information on the biological activity of this dyskerin fragment we studied its effect on the DNA damage pathway in patient derived X-DC cells and a mouse F9 cell line carrying the A353V mutation in the *Dkc1* gene [26]. This is the mutation most frequently found in patients with X-DC (about 40% of patients) [27] [28] and is localized in the PUA RNA binding domain, the putative site for interaction with hTR. Recently, it has been described that mouse ES cells expressing a small dyskerin deletion, removing exon 15 of *Dkc1*, additionally showed decreased proliferative rate and increased sensitivity to DNA damage [29] that was independent on telomere length suggesting that decreased telomerase activity induced by the mutation in *Dkc1* resulted in induction of DNA damage probably by extratelomeric activity of *Dkc1* gene. Therefore the use of a mouse F9A353V model would allow study the effect of GSE24.2 directly on DNA damage, independently of telomeric elongation. Here we show that human X-DC cells showed both basal DNA damage foci and phosphorylation of ATM and CHK2 together with increased content of heterochromatin. Expression of the GSE24.2 was able to reduce DNA damage in X-DC patient and F9 X-DC mouse cell line models, by decreasing the formation of DNA damage foci. Finally, we also report that expression of

GSE24.2 decreases oxidative stress in X-DC patient cells and that may result in reduced DNA damage. These data support the contention that expression of GSE24.2, or related products, could prolong the lifespan of dyskeratosis congenita cells.

Materials and Methods

Cell lines and constructs

Dermal fibroblasts from a control proband (X-DC-1787-C) and two X-DC patients (X-DC-1774-P and X-DC3) were obtained from Coriell Cell Repository. GSE24.2, DKC, motif I and motif II were cloned as previously described in the pLXCN vector [24]. PGATEV protein expression plasmid [30] was obtained from Dr. G. Montoya. PGATEV-GSE24.2 was obtained by subcloning the GSE24.2 fragment into the NdeI/XhoI sites of the pGATEV plasmid as previously described [24].

F9 cells and F9 cells transfected with A353V targeting vector were previously described [31] [26]. F9A353V cells were cultured in Dulbecco modified Eagle medium (DMEM) 10% fetal bovine serum, 2 mM glutamine (Gibco) and Sodium bicarbonate (1,5 gr/ml).

Cell transfection and analysis of gene expression

F9 cells were transfected with 16 µg of DNA/10^6 cells, using lipofectamine plus (Invitrogen, Carlsbad, USA), according to the manufacturer's instructions. Peptides transfection was performed by using the Transport Protein Delivery Reagent (50568; Lonza, Walkersville, USA) transfection kit. Routinely from 6 to 15 µg were used per 30 mm dish.

Antibodies. The source of antibodies was as follow: phospho-Histone H2A.X Ser139 (2577; Cell Signaling), phospho-Histone H2A.X Ser139 clone JBW301 (05-636; Millipore), macroH2A.1 (ab37264; abcam), 53BP1 (4937; Cell Signaling), anti-ATM Protein Kinase S1981P (200-301-400; Rockland), phospho-Chk2-Thr68 (2661; Cell Signaling), Monoclonal Anti-α-tubulin (T9026; Sigma-Aldrich), Anti-8-Oxoguanine Antibody, clone 483.15 (MAB3560, Merck-Millipore). Fluorescent antibodies were conjugated with Alexa fluor 488 (A11029 and A11034, Molecular Probes) and Alexa fluor 647 (A21236, Molecular Probes, Carlsbad, USA)).

Immunofluorescence and Fluorescence in situ hybridization (FISH) for telomeres

Protein localization was carried out by fluorescence microscopy. For this purpose, cells were grown on coverslips, transfected and fixed in 3.7% formaldehyde solution (47608; Fluka, Sigma, St. Louis, USA) at room temperature for 15 min. After washing with 1x PBS, cells were permeabilized with 0.2% Triton X-100 in PBS and blocked with 10% horse serum before overnight incubation with γ-H2A.X, 53BP1, p-ATM, p-CHK2 antibodies. Finally, cells were washed and incubated with secondary antibodies coupled to fluorescent dyes (alexa fluor 488 or/and alexa fluor 647).

For immuno-FISH, immunostaining of 53BP1 was performed as described above and followed by incubation in PBS 0,1% Triton X-100, fixation 5 min in 2% paraformaldehyde (PFA), dehydration with ethanol and air-dried. Cells were hybridized with the telomeric PNA-Cy3 probe (PNA Bio) using standard PNA-FISH procedures. Imaging was carried out at room temperature in Vectashield, mounting medium for fluorescence (Vector Laboratories, Burlingame, USA). Images were acquired with a Confocal Spectral Leica TCS SP5. Using a HCX PL APO Lambda blue 63×1.40 OIL UV, zoom 2.3 lens. Images were acquired using LAS-AF 1.8.1 Leica software and processed using LAS-AF 1.8.1

Leica software and Adobe Photoshop CS. Colocalization of 53BP1 foci and the PNA FISH probe was quantified in at least 200 cells.

Telomeric repeat amplification protocol (TRAP) assay

Telomerase activity was measured using the TRAPeze kit [32] (Millipore, Billerica, MA USA) according to the manufacturer's recommendations. TRAP assay activity was normalized with the internal control [24].

Real-time quantitative PCR

RNA isolation and cDNA synthesis. Total cellular RNA was extracted using Trizol (Invitrogen, Carlsbad, USA) according to the manufacturer's instructions. For reverse transcription reactions (RT), 1 µg of the purified RNA was reverse transcribed using random hexamers with the High-Capacity cDNA Archive kit (Applied Biosystems, P/N: 4322171; Foster City, CA) according to the manufacturer's instructions. RT conditions comprised an initial incubation step at 25°C for 10 min. to allow random hexamers annealing, followed by cDNA synthesis at 37°C for 120 min, and a final inactivation step for 5 min. at 95°C.

Measurement of mRNA Levels. The mRNA levels were determined by quantitative real-time PCR analysis using an ABI Prism 7900 HT Fast Real-Time PCR System (Applied Biosystems, Foster City, CA). Gene-specific primer pairs and probes for *SOD1* (*SOD Cu/Zn*), *SOD2* (*SOD Mn*), *GPX1* (*Glutathione peroxidase 1*) and *CAT* (*Catalase*) (Assay-on-demand, Applied Biosystems), were used together with TaqMan Universal PCR Master Mix (Applied Biosystems, Foster City, USA) and 2 µl of reverse transcribed sample RNA in 20 µl reaction volumes. PCR conditions were 10 min. at 95°C for enzyme activation, followed by 40 two-step cycles (15 sec at 95°C; 1 min at 60°C). The levels of glyceraldehyde-3-phosphate dehydrogenase (*GAPDH*) expression were measured in all samples to normalize gene expression for sample-to-sample differences in RNA input, RNA quality and reverse transcription efficiency. Each sample was analyzed in triplicate, and the expression was calculated according to the $2^{-\Delta\Delta Ct}$ method.

GSE24.2 peptide production and purification

E. Coli DH5a cells were transformed with pGATEV GSE24.2 and lysates prepared as described [30]. The fusion protein was purified with glutathione-sepharose and purity analyzed by gel electrophoresis. GSE24.2 was obtained from the purified fusion protein by TEV protease digestion according to the manufacturer's recommendations. Typically, over 90% of the fusion protein was cleaved, as determined by SDS-PAGE. The protein was passed twice over a 5 ml Hi-Trap Ni-NTA column to remove the polyhistidine tags, un-cleaved protein, TEV protease and impurities. Synthetic GSE24.2 was obtained from Peptide 2.0 Inc (Chantilly, USA) and purified by HPLC

Western Blot

Whole-cell extracts were prepared essentially as described previously [33]. Nuclear extracts were obtained as previously reported [24]. Western blotting was performed using standard methods [33]. Protein concentration was measured by using the Bio-Rad protein assay.

Senescence analysis

Control and X-DC fibroblasts (1×10^4 cells) were plated onto 6 well plates and fixed after four days to assay the SA-β-gal (Senescence Detection Kit, BioVision, Milpitas, USA). The percentage of senescent cells was calculated in 6 images per

sample taken in the bright field microscopy at 100× magnification (Nikon Eclipse TS100 Microscopy, Melville, NY, USA).

Determination of reactive oxygen species (ROS) content with dihydroethidium

Cells were cultured in 12 chamber plates for 4 days (at confluence). Afterwards cells were washed 2 times with prewarmed PBS medium, 2 µL/mL of diluted dihydroethidium (Dihydroethidium, D7008-Sigma, St. Louis, USA) was added to the plate. Cells were incubated at 37°C for 20 min. After washing the plate with PBS, medium was replaced, and cells cultured for an additional 1 hour at 37°C. The fluorescence was measured using spectraMAX GEMINIS (Molecular Device, Sunnyvale, USA), with 530 nm of excitation wavelength and 610 nm of emission wavelength. Mean fluorescence intensity (MFI) for each cell line, was normalized by the cellular protein content.

Measurement of CuZnSOD and MnSOD activity

To determine MnSOD and CuZnSOD activity the cells were treated as described in the Cayman "Superoxide Dismutase Assay kit" (Ann Arbor, USA). After centrifugation at 10,000 g for 10 min, supernatant was used to measure CuZnSOD activity. The mitochondrial pellet was lysed using a lysis buffer compatible with the manufacturer's instructions (10 mM HEPES, pH7.9, 420 mM NaCl, 1,5 mM $MgCl_2$, 0,5 mM EDTA, 0.1% Triton X-100) for 20 min on ice. After centrifugation at 12,000 g for 5 min, the supernatant was collected for MnSOD activity assay. Measurements of CuZnSOD and MnSOD activities were performed in a 96 well plate prepared using 3–4 replicates from different cellular extracts for each sample. The final absorbance was measured at 450 nm using a spectrophotometer spectraMAXPLUS 384 (Molecular Devices, Sunnyvale, USA).

Measurement of catalase activity

The method for measuring the catalase enzymatic activity was based on the reaction of the enzyme with methanol in the presence of hydrogen peroxide to produce formaldehyde. Cells were lysed using freeze (liquid N_2, 10 s) and thaw (ice, 15 min) procedure repeated three times. After centrifugation of the cell lysate at 13,000 g, for 10 min. at 4°C, supernatants were recovered and quantified using Lowry method. A 96 well plate was prepared using at least 4 replicates for each sample, obtained from different cellular extracts.

Assay reaction consisted in mixing on a 96 well plate: 100 µL of phosphate buffer 100 mM pH 7.0; 30 µL methanol and 20 µL of the sample with the same protein concentration. Then, the reaction was started with 20 µL of 85 mM H_2O_2, maintained during 20 min at room temperature and finally stopped using 30 µL of KOH 10 M. The formaldehyde produced reacts with 35 mM purpald reagent dissolved in 0,5 M HCl during 10 min at room temperature. Finally, 10 µL of 0.5% KIO_4 in KOH 0.5 M were added and the absorbance at the wavelength of 540 nm was measured with spectrophotometer spectra MAXPLUS 384 (Molecular Devices, Sunnyvale, USA).

Measurement of glutathione peroxidase activity

Gpx activity was measured by using a glutathione peroxidase assay kit (Cayman (Ann Arbor, USA). Briefly, cells were collected and lysed using cold buffer (50 mM Tris-HCl, pH 7.5, 5 mM EDTA and 1 mM DTT) and two freeze-thaw cycles as described above. The lysates were centrifuged at 10,000 g for 15 min at 4°C and the supernatants recovered in fresh tubes. A 96 well plate was prepared using at least 3 replicates for each sample from different

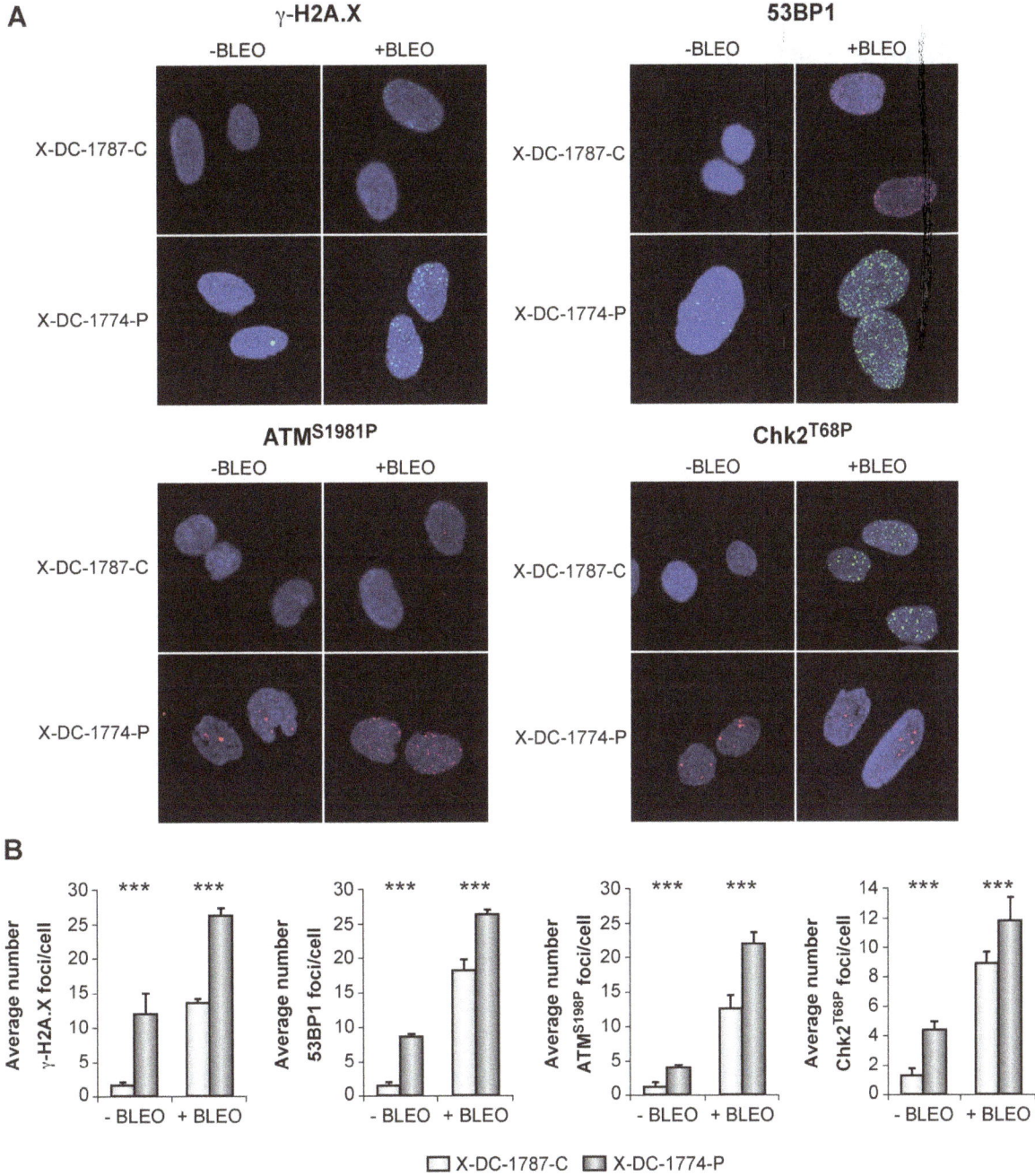

Figure 1. DNA damage signaling in X-DC patient cells. (A) Immunofluorescence staining of DNA damage proteins. Control X-DC-1787-C and patient X-DC-1774-P cells were, either not treated (-Bleo) or treated (+Bleo) with bleomycin (10 μg/ml) for 24 hours, fixed and incubated with antibodies against γ-H2AX, 53BP1, p-ATM or p-CHK1 and secondary fluorescent antibodies. Nuclear DNA was counterstained with DAPI (blue). (B). Quantification of γ-H2A.X foci, pATM, 53BP1 and pCHK2 associated foci in X-DC-1787-C and X-DC-1774-P cells. More than 200 cells were analyzed in each cell line and indicated as the average number of foci/cell. Asterisks indicate significant differences in relation to control cells lines or to untreated cells. Average values and standard deviations of two independent experiments are shown. Experiments were repeated 3 times with similar results.

cellular extracts. After protein quantification by Lowry method, samples containing 20 μg of total proteins were added to the 96 well plate containing a solution with 1 mM GSH, 0.4 U/mL of glutathione reductase, 0.2 mM NADPH. The reaction was initiated by adding 0.22 mM of cumene hydroperoxide and the reduction of the absorbance was recorded at 340 nm each 1 min during 8 min. The Gpx activity was determined by the rate of

decrease in absorbance at 340 nm (1 mU/mL Gpx). Molar coefficient extinction for NADPH was 0.00622 mM^{-1} cm^{-1}.

Statistical analysis

For the statistical analysis of the results, the mean was taken as the measurement of the main tendency, while standard deviation was taken as the dispersion measurement. T-Student was performed. The significance has been considered at *p<0.05, **

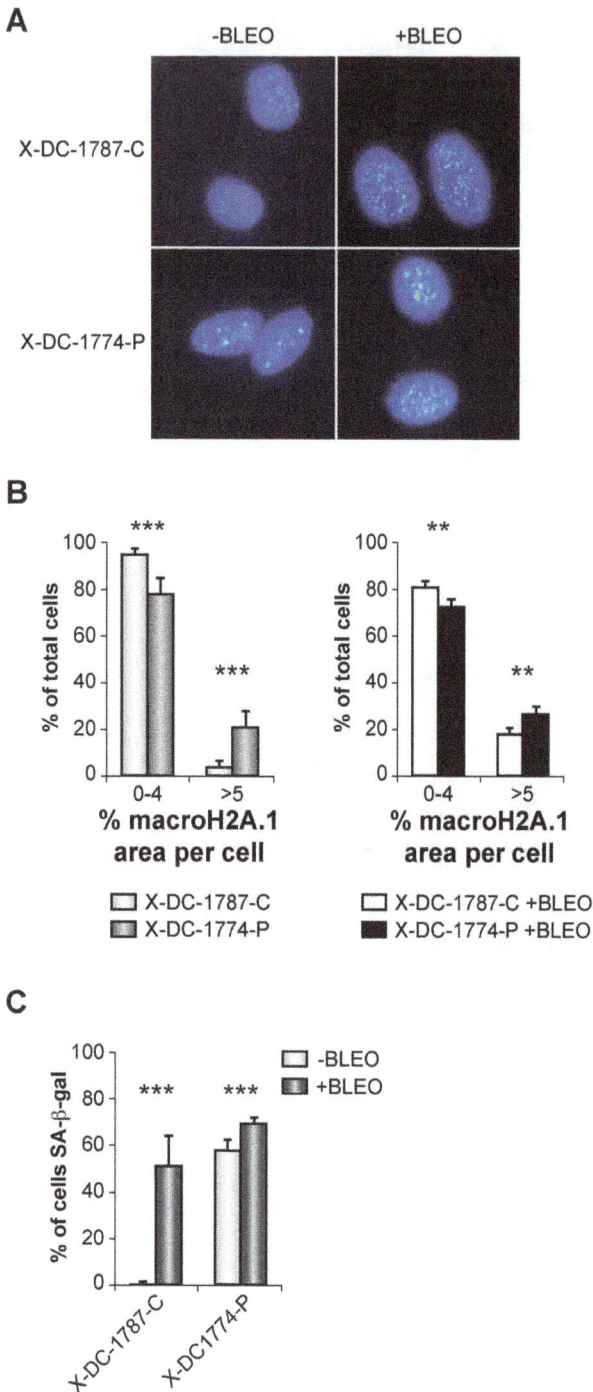

for p<0.01 and *** for p<0.001. GraphPad Software v5.0 was used for statistical analysis and graphic representations.

Results

1-Basal and induced DNA damage response in X-DC cells involves 53BP1, ATM and CHK2 and results in increased heterochromatin formation and senescence

It has been previously demonstrated [29] that a pathogenic mutation in murine *Dkc1* causes growth impairment and the enhancement of DNA damage responses after treatment with the chemotherapeutic agent etoposide. In the context of telomeres of normal length, cells with the dyskerin mutation $Dkc1^{\Delta15}$ (deletion of exon 15) showed increased number of DNA damage foci as observed by detection of p-H2A.X^{Ser139} (γ-H2A.X) foci and activation of the ATM/p53 pathway.

We have used paired human cell lines (heterozygous carrier and patient) harboring the same mutation in *DKC* gene, responsible for X-DC and studied the DNA damage response pathway. Telomere length of the control cell line (healthy carrier grandmother from X-DC-1774-P patient) was the right length for the age of this control (60 year old and 10.7 kpb). Both basal DNA damage and that produced in response to the DNA damaging agent bleomycin were studied. Our results show that the number of γ-H2A.X-associated foci/cell was dramatically higher in cells obtained from the X-DC-1774-P patient than in the carrier cell line X-DC-1787-C (Fig. 1A and B). When cells were treated with bleomycin, which induces double strand breaks, we found an increase in the number of γ-H2A.X associated foci/cell in both X-DC-1774-P and X-DC-1787-C cells. Although basal DNA damage in X-DC-1774-P was already much higher than that of control cells the increase was similar or even lower to that observed in control cells. We also investigated the presence of 53BP1 foci in these cell lines, since 53BP1 is recruited to DNA-damage associated foci. We found the average number of foci/cell was similar to that observed for γ-H2A.X, higher to that observed in control cells but even if there is an increase after bleomycin treatment, the increase in the number of foci/cell was smaller than control cells ATM protein is also recruited to DNA-damage sites at the chromatin and phosphorylated, we found that X-DC-1774-P cells showed higher number of foci/cell with phosphorylated ATM compared to carrier cells. In bleomycin treated cells both patient and carrier cells showed increased response to DNA damage although similar to what happen with the other indicators of DNA damage the increase observed in X-DC-1774-P was lower than control cells. CHK2 is a protein, substrate of ATM-kinase. We studied the number of cells with phosphorylated CHK2 at Thr68 and found a higher number of foci/cells in X-DC-1774-P in untreated cells, which increases after bleomycin treatment, but such increase is lower than control cells. Altogether these results indicate that basal DNA damage is higher in X-DC patient cells that in mutation carrier cells, in response to bleomycin this increase is not higher in X-DC cells probably due to the high basal damage observed in these cells. Furthermore we have found that the signaling pathway associated with this DNA damage, include at least 53BP1, ATM and CHK2, although we cannot exclude the participation of other proteins.

In order to verify if X-DC cells harbor an increased heterochromatin content we studied the nuclear distribution of histone-macroH2A.1-associated heterochromatin in X-DC-1774-P and X-DC-1787-C cells, both in basal conditions and after bleomycin treatment (Fig. 2A). X-DC-1774-P cells already showed an average of 20% of the nuclear area with positive expression for macroH2A.1, and after bleomycin treatment we detected an increase up to 30% (Fig. 2B). X-DC-1787-C cells showed a very

Figure 2. Determination of Histone-macroH2A.1-associated heterochromatin and senescence in X-DC cells. (A) Histone-macroH2A.1-associated heterochromatin detection in X-DC cells. X-DC-1787-C and X-DC-1774-P cells were either not treated (-Bleo) or treated (+Bleo) with bleomycin (10 mg/ml) for 24 hours, fixed and incubated with an antibody against Histone-macroH2A.1 followed by a secondary fluorescence labeled antibody. (B) Quantification of Histone-macroH2A.1-associated heterochromatin. More than 200 cells were analyzed in each cell line and grouped to the area presenting Macro H2A.1 foci per cell. Asterisks indicate significant differences between cells lines. Average values and standard deviations of two independent experiments are shown. (C) SA-β-gal activity in X-DC-1787-C and X-DC-1774-P cells either untreated (-Bleo) or treated (+Bleo) with bleomycin (10 µg/ml). Senescent cells were quantified in 6 images of random regions. Experiments were repeated 3 times with similar results. Asterisks indicate significant differences in response to bleomycin.

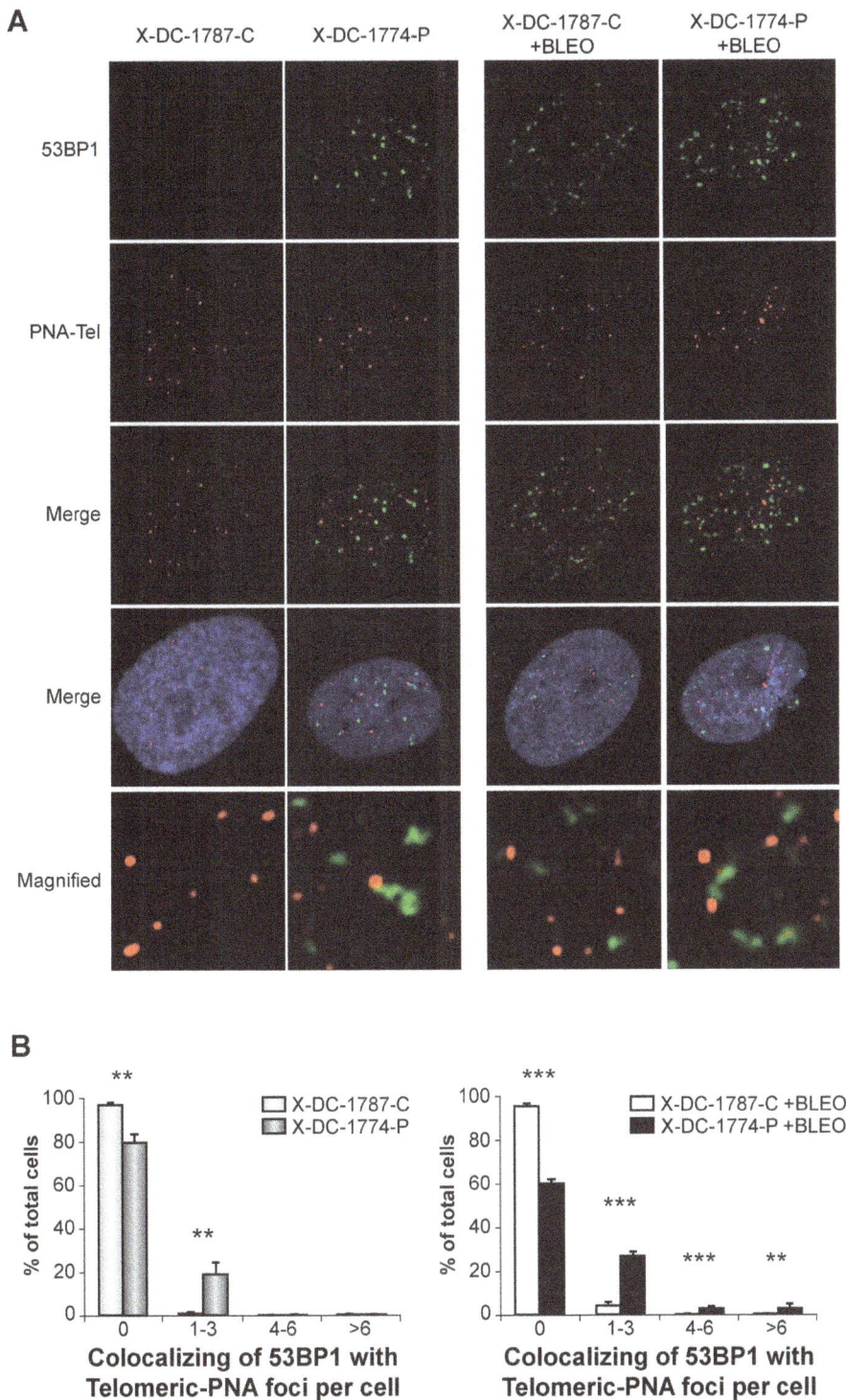

Figure 3. Localization of 53BP1 foci to telomeres in X-DC patient cells. X-DC-1787-C and X-DC-1774-P cells untreated (-Bleo) or treated (+ Bleo) with bleomycin (10 μg/ml) and incubated with γ-H2A.X and PNA-FISH probe. (A) Colocalization of 53BP1 foci (green) and telomeres as identified by hybridizing with a PNA-FISH probe (red). DNA was counterstained with DAPI (blue). Magnified views of merged images showing details of the colocalization are shown in the two lower series of panels (B) Colocalized 53BP1 foci and PNA-FISH probe at telomeres was quantified. More than 200 cells were analyzed in each cell line in an experiment performed three times with similar results. Asterisks indicate significant differences in relation to different cell lines.

low expression in basal conditions that increases to almost 20% after bleomycin treatment (Fig. 2C). These data indicated that X-DC patient cells show extensive areas of heterochromatin that further increased in response to bleomycin. Thus, both basal and induced DNA damage may trigger a relevant silencing of gene expression in these cells. Almost 60% of X-DC-1774-P cells were

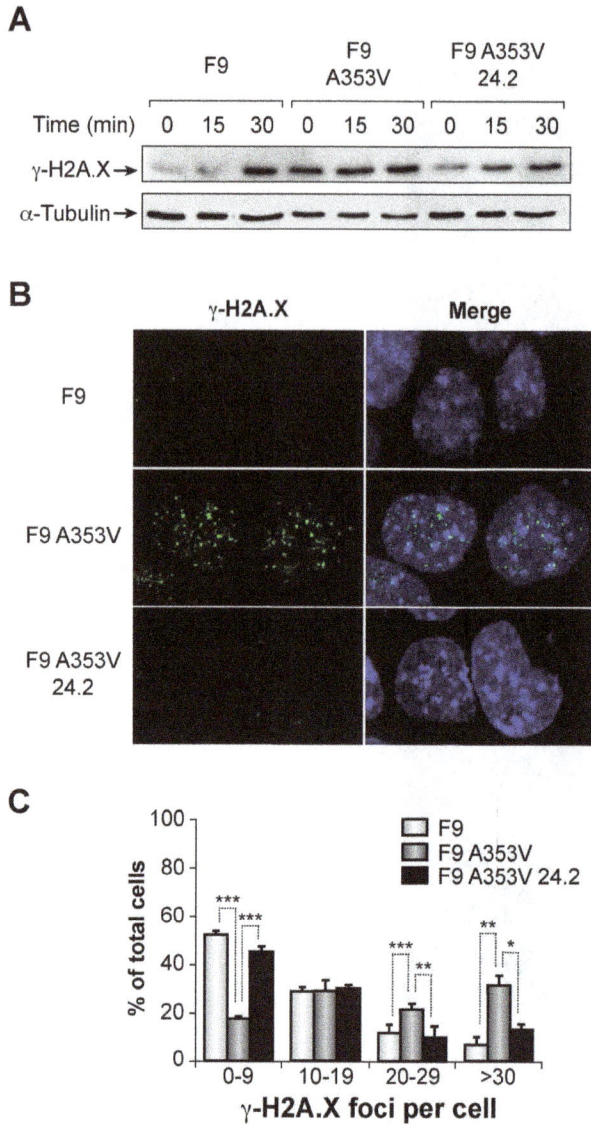

Figure 4. F9A353V cells show enhanced, basal and bleomycin induced, DNA damage response. (A) F9, F9A353V and F9A353V cells transfected with GSE24.2 (10 µg DNA per million cells). F9A353V 24.2 cells were treated with bleomycin (10 µg/ml). After 0, 15 or 30 minutes of treatment cells were lysed and the experiment analyzed by western blot with antibodies against γ-H2A.X or α-tubulin as a loading control. (B) Immunofluorescence staining of γ-H2A.X (green) in F9, F9A353V and F9A353V 24.2 cells (10 µg DNA per million cells). Nuclear DNA was counterstained with DAPI (blue). (C) Quantification of γ-H2AX foci in F9, F9A353V or F9A353V 24.2 cells. More than 200 cells were analyzed in each cell line and grouped to the number of γ-H2A.X foci observed per cell. Experiments were repeated 3 times with similar results. Asterisks indicate significant differences in relation to different cell lines.

positive for the senescence SA-β-gal activity that increases to almost 70% after bleomycin treatment. X-DC-1787-C cells showed low expression of SA-β-gal that also increases further after bleomycin treatment.

2- DNA damage is localized in telomeres in X-DC cells

Since telomere length is greatly diminished in X-DC patient cells we investigated if DNA damage was enriched at telomeres,

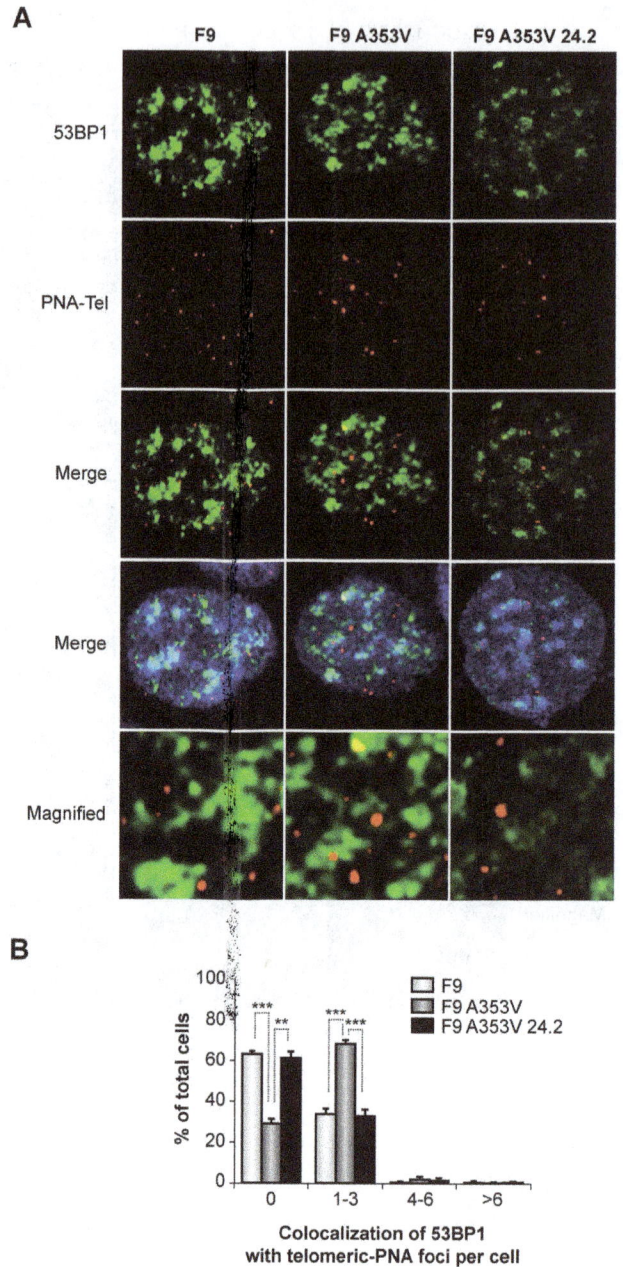

Figure 5. Localization of 53BP1 foci to telomeres in F9A353V cells. F9, F9A353V and F9A353V cells transfected with GSE24.2 (F9A353V 24.2) (F9 cells were treated with bleomycin,10 µg/ml for 24 hours) and incubated with 53BP1 antibodies and with a PNA-FISH probe. (A) Colocalization of 53BP1 foci (green) and PNA-FISH probe that identified telomeres (PNA-Tel, red). DNA was counterstained with DAPI (blue). Magnified views of merged images showing details of the colocalization are shown in the lower panels. (B) Quantification of the colocalization of 53BP1 foci and telomere signals shown in panel A. More than 200 cells were analyzed in each cell line and grouped to the number of 53BP1 foci associated to telomeres (PNA-Tel) per cell. Experiments were repeated 3 times with similar results. Asterisks indicate significant differences in relation to different cell lines.

both in basal conditions and after DNA damage induction. In order to investigate this, we combined a PNA FISH probe as a telomere marker, and 53BP1 for DNA damage detection. The results showed that there was a high association of damaged DNA

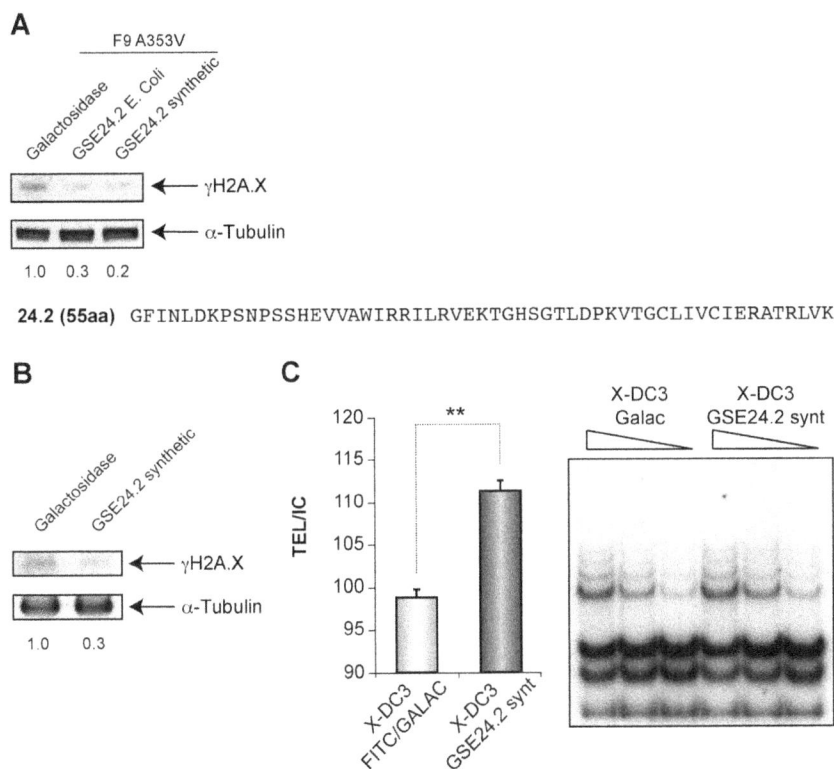

24.2 (55aa) GFINLDKPSNPSSHEVVAWIRRILRVEKTGHSGTLDPKVTGCLIVCIERATRLVK

Figure 6. Activity of the GSE24.2 peptide expressed in bacteria or chemically-synthesized. (A) F9A353V cells were transfected with 15 µg of β-galactosidase as a control (galactosidase), or GSE24.2 purified from E. Coli (GSE24.2E.coli) or obtained by chemical synthesis (GSE24.2 synthetic). After 24 hours cells were lysed and the levels of γ-H2AX and α-tubulin determined by western blot. The values at the bottom were obtained after quantification of the blot and show the ration between expression levels of γ-H2AX and α-tubulin in each line and referred to those found in β-galactosidase transfected cells. (B) Same experiment described in A, performed in X-DC3 cells transfected with β-galactosidase or chemically synthesized GSE24.2. (C) Reactivation of telomerase activity by chemically synthesized GSE24.2. X-DC3cells were transfected with β-galactosidase or chemically synthesized GSE24.2 and telomerase activity determined by TRAP assay (right). Different amounts extract were used for each TRAP assay as indicated. The activity was quantified by evaluating the intensity of the bands in relation with the internal control (TEL/IC) (left panel). The values for GSE24.2 transfected cells were referred to the β-galactosidase transfected cells. The experiments were repeated at least three times with similar results. Asterisks indicate significant differences between the two different transfected peptides.

at the telomeres in X-DC-1774-P cells that was not found in carrier X-DC-1787-C cells (Fig. 3A). Furthermore the increase in DNA damage observed after bleomycin treatment (Fig. 1B) was strongly associated with telomeres in X-DC-1774-P cells in contrast to X-DC-1787-C cells (Fig. 3) indicating the relevance of telomere shortening in the response to DNA damage in X-DC patient cells.

3-Expression of GSE24.2 impairs the induction of γ-H2A.X foci after DNA damage

Since F9 cells represent a good model system to study DNA damage responses as previously demonstrated (29), we used them in order to investigate if the expression of GSE24.2 could modify the activation of the DNA damage response. Therefore, we transfected F9A353V and control F9 cells [26] with the GSE24.2 expression plasmid and treated them either with bleomycin or etoposide, a topoisomerase inhibitor known to induce DNA double-stranded breaks. We found that, as expected, bleomycin treatment induced γ-H2A.X in both cell lines (Fig. 4A). However, the basal level of γ-H2A.X was much higher in F9A353V cells than in F9 cells expressing the WT dyskerin, indicating that the mutation renders the cells more susceptible to DNA damage. In the presence of the GSE24.2 F9A353V, γ-H2A.X decreased to values very similar to those observed in F9 cells in both, basal and

bleomycin-induced levels. Similar results were obtained in etoposide-treated cells (data not shown). We next investigated the presence of γ-H2A.X containing foci in basal conditions and the results confirmed those obtained in the western blot studies (Fig. 4B and 4C). Most F9 cells showed very few foci; the number increased in F9A353V cells but was reduced at similar level to those of F9 cells when the mutant cells were transfected with GSE24.2. Altogether, the results indicated that the expression of GSE24.2 decreases the DNA damage produced by the dyskerin mutation.

Afterwards, we investigated if the increased DNA damage in F9A353V cells was enriched at the telomeres (as already found in X-DC patient cells, Fig. 3) and also whether the protection from DNA damage induced by GSE24.2 also applies to damage at the telomeres. We use combined immunological detection of 53BP1 and PNA-FISH probe. The results (Fig. 5A and 5B) indicated that F9A353V cells have a stronger association of 53BP1 to the telomeres than in F9 cells treated with bleomycin, up to 60%. However in F9A353V cells transfected with the GSE24.2 there is little association of 53BP1 foci at the telomeres (30% 1–3 53BP1 foci per cell). These results indicate that the elevated DNA damage response found in F9A353V cells is probably caused by defects at the telomeres induced by the *Dkc1* mutation, in agreement with the results obtained in *Dkc1*^{Δ15} MEF cells. Interestingly, expression

A

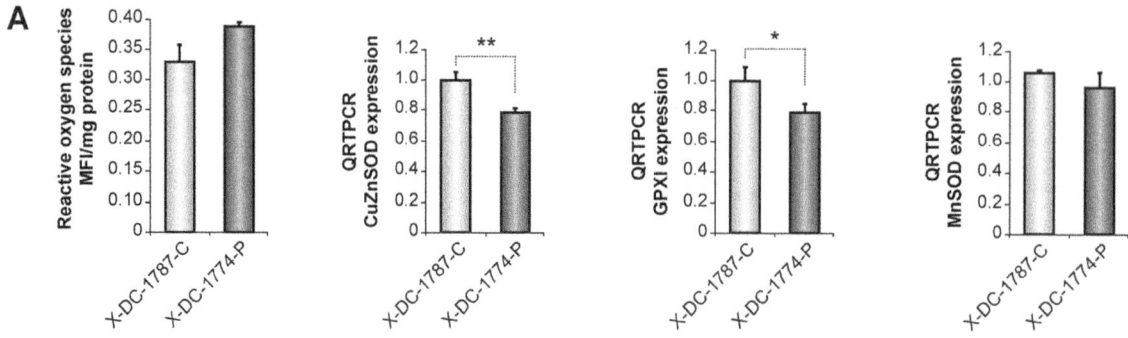

B

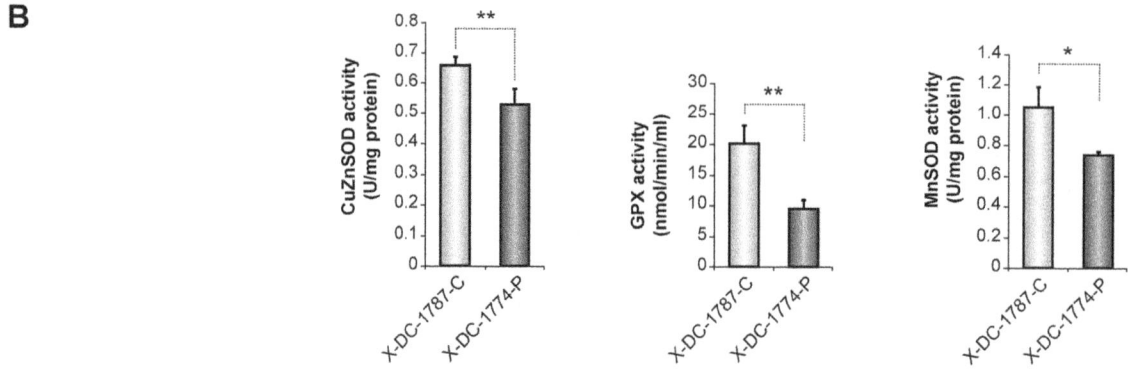

C

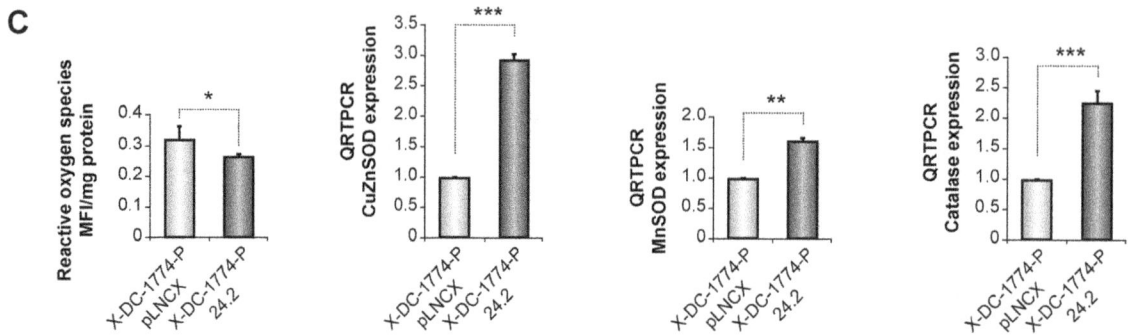

D

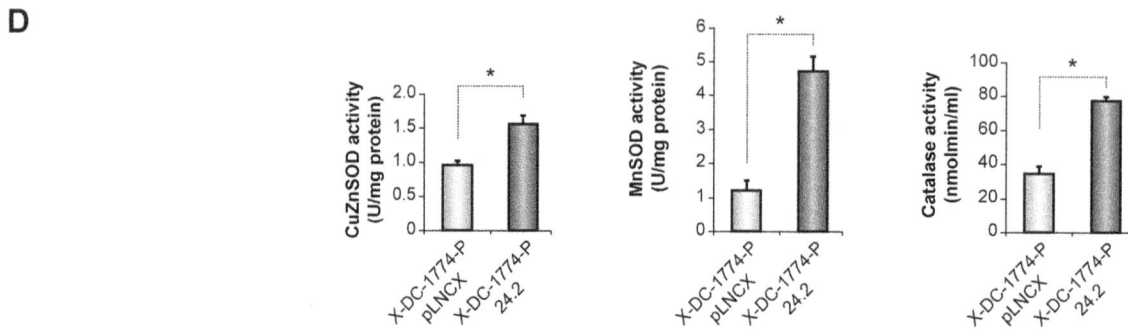

E

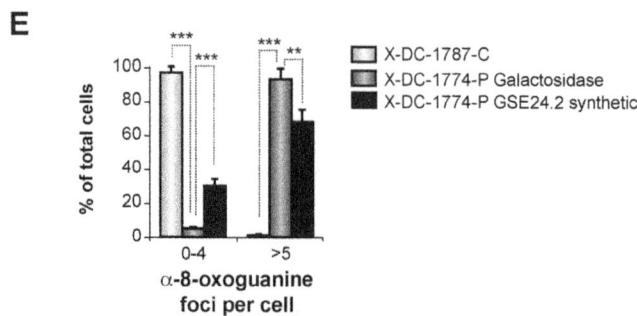

Figure 7. Oxidative stress analysis in X-DC fibroblasts after GSE24.2 transfection. (A) ROS levels were determined in fibroblasts from the carrier DC1787, and fibroblasts from the patient X-DC1774-P. Levels were determined using the fluorescent probe dihydroethidium in confluent cells (left panel). RNA expression was determined for CuZnSOD, MnSOD, and GPX1 by qRT-PCR (A right panels). B) Enzymatic activities of CuZnSOD,MnSOD, and Glutathione peroxidase 1 were also determined. C) ROS levels were studied in X-DC1774-P fibroblasts (expressing pLNCX vector) and X-DC-1774-P cells expressing GSE24.2 (X-DC1774-PGSE24.2, left panel). Cu/ZnSOD, MnSOD, and catalase expression levels were determined by qRT-PCR. D) Cu/ZnSOD, MnSOD, and catalase activities in confluent pLNCX and 24.2 cells are shown in left panels. E) X-DC1774-P and X-DC1774-PGSE24.2, cells were transfected with GSE24.2 synthetic peptide and levels of 8-oxoguanine studied by immunofluorescence. The 8-oxoguanine foci signal was expressed as the average number of foci/cell in 200 cells. Results are expressed as mean ± standard deviation from three independent experiments. Statistical significance is expressed as (*) p<0.05.

of GSE24.2 reverted the telomere damage in F9A353V cells, indicating its biological importance in the reversion of the mutant *Dkc1* phenotype.

4-Treatment of X-DC cells with GSE24.2 peptide rescues DNA damage

We have previously reported that the GSE24.2 peptide purified from bacteria was able to increase telomerase activity in F9A353V cells [26] therefore we next tested if the activity of the GSE24.2 peptide either purified from E-coli or chemically synthesized reduced the DNA damage. We found that the levels of γ-H2A.X in F9A353V cells decreased after transfecting this peptide (Fig. 6A) either obtained from bacteria or chemically synthesized to 30 and 20%, respectively. Moreover the synthetic peptide also decreased the DNA damage in X-DC3 cells (DKC1 mutated lymphocytes) by 30% (Fig. 6B). This decrease in DNA damage correlated well with the ability of the synthetic peptide to increase telomerase activity in these cells (Fig. 6C).

5- Oxidative stress in X-DC cells is decreased by expression of GSE24.2

Oxidative stress is one of the causes of DNA damage producing both single-strand breaks (SSBs) and double-strand breaks (DSBs). SSBs are the result from the interaction of hydroxyl radicals with deoxyribose and subsequent generation of peroxyl-radicals. These reactive oxygen species (ROS) are then responsible for nicking phosphodiester bonds that form the backbone of each helical strand of DNA [34]. To clarify the presence of higher oxidation levels in X-DC cells we have studied ROS levels, and the expression of antioxidant enzymes CuZn (SOD1) and Mn (SOD2) superoxide dismutase, glutathione peroxidase 1 (GPX1) and their corresponding enzymatic activities in X-DC-1787-C and X-DC-1774-P cell lines. Levels of ROS were elevated in X-DC-1774-P cells compared with X-DC-1787-C carrier cells and also higher than in GM03348, an age-matched cell line from a healthy subject (data not shown). In agreement with this result we found a decrease in gene expression levels of the antioxidant enzymes CuZnSOD and MnSOD and GPX1 when compared the X-DC-1774-P to the carrier cell line (Fig. 7A). We also determined the activity of the three enzymes with decreased expression in the X-DC-1774-P cells that also showed decreased activity in agreement with the gene expression data (Fig. 7B).

In order to investigate if expression of GSE24.2 was able to overcome the increased oxidative stress found in X-DC-1774-P cells, we expressed in this cell line either pLNCX-GSE24.2 or the empty vector (pLNCX). The results indicated that X-DC-1774-P cells expressing GSE24.2 showed lower levels of ROS. We also studied the expression levels of CuZnSOD, MnSOD and catalase in both cell lines and found that expression levels of these antioxidant enzymes were higher in X-DC-1774-P-24.2. When the corresponding protein activities were analyzed, we observed an increase in CuZnSOD, MnSOD and catalase activities (Fig. 7C) in X-DC-1774-P-24.2 when compared with the empty vector

transfected cells. Altogether, the data indicated that the observed decrease in oxidative stress in X-DC cells expressing GSE24.2 should contribute to protect these cells from DNA damage. We finally investigated if treatment with the GSE24.2 synthetic peptide was also able to induce a decrease in oxidative DNA damage. We transfected X-DC-1774-P cells with the GSE24.2 synthetic peptide and evaluated the levels of 8-oxoguanine by immunofluorescence (Fig 7E). The results showed that indeed the synthetic GSE24.4 reduced the signal obtained with 8-oxoguanine-antibody.

Discussion

We have previously reported that expression of a *dyskerin* internal peptide (GSE24.2) reactivates telomerase activity in cells that are deficient in this activity by increasing TERT and TERC levels [24] We have also reported that expression of GSE24.2 increases TR levels by stabilizing this RNA [26]. Because of this activity GSE24.2 has been recently approved as an orphan drug by EMA for the treatment of Dyskeratosis congenita. We have now studied the role of GSE24.2 in the DNA damage response of X-DC patient cells in an effort to better understand the mechanism of GSE24.2 action in X-DC. We studied several proteins involved in the DNA-damage response and found, as other authors have [35] [36], that X-DC patient cells presented higher levels of DNA damage associated foci detected by γ-H2A.X and 53BP1 and to a lesser extent p-ATM and p-CHK2. We also found increased levels of DNA damage in response to bleomycin that was more evident when we studied -H2A.X, p-ATM and p-CHK2 associated foci as previously described in mice (29) but this increase was not higher than that obtained in control cells probably because X-DC cells already have massive damage in basal conditions. Previous reports described increased levels of DNA damage in DC cells harboring mutations in *DKC1*, *TERC* or *TERT*. However in fibroblasts and lymphocytes from these patients the response to induced DNA-damage was not increased [35] in contrast to another study [29]. We have here used X-DC patient cells which exhibited short telomeres, p53 activation and senescence [37]. Indeed, a high level of DNA damage, both at basal and induced by bleomycin, was observed at telomeres suggesting that the shortening of telomeres in these cells induces further damage by preventing repair. Dysfunctional telomeres trigger a DNA damage response most likely because they are too short to adopt the normal t-loop structure needed to form the telomere with correctly ordered shelterin components. Recruitment of histone-macroH2A.1 has been associated to heterochromatin and senescent associated foci (SAHF) [18] [19]. We found that both senescence and macroH2A.1 associated-foci are increased in X-DC patient cells and also that bleomycin treatment increases these values, suggesting that the impairment in the repair of DNA lesions in X-DC cells likely contributes to the senescent phenotype.

Using the *in vitro* generated *Dkc1* mutant F9A353V cells we have found, in agreement with our previous results (and also [29]), that

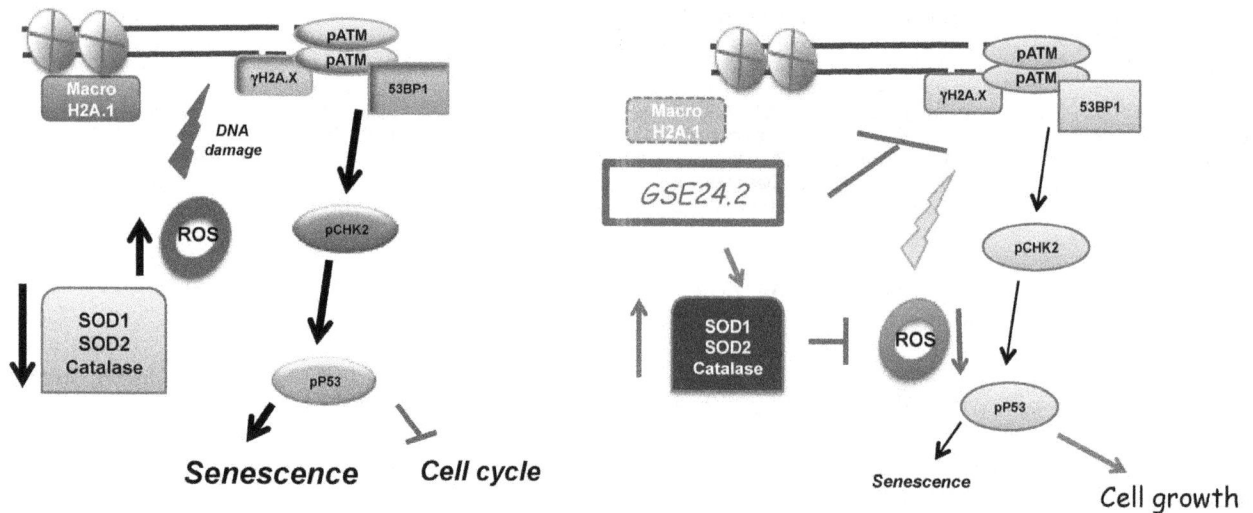

Figure 8. Proposed biological activity of GSE24.2 on DNA damage and oxidative stress. Dyskeratosis congenita cells display high basal DNA damage detected by increased γH2AX, p-ATM, p-CHK2 and 53BP1 foci. Additionally there are increased levels of ROS, and decreased expression and activity of antioxidant enzymes resulting in higher oxidative damage and senescence (left panel). GSE24.2 peptide increases expression of antioxidant enzymes and as a consequence decreased ROS levels (right panel). In parallel there is increased telomerase activity that may help to decrease global and telomeric DNA damage. Globally these two activities of GSE24.2 might result in increased viability and growth of DC cells (26).

these cells showed increased DDR compared with F9 cells, both in the steady state and when treated with bleomycin or etoposide. Other *Dkc1* mutations such as *Dkc1*$^{\Delta 15}$ have been shown to accumulate DNA damage indicating that DC cells have cellular defects even in the context of long telomeres [29]. We previously reported that an internal fragment of Dyskerin, the peptide GSE24.2 induces an increase in telomerase activity in X-DC cells [24]. Now we are showing that expression of GSE24.2 is able to induce protection against DNA damage. Furthermore, the repair of pre-existing DNA lesions should also take place at telomeres in F9A353V cells as shown by the decrease in 53BP1 and PNA-FISH telomeric colocalization (Fig. 5B). Interestingly, the observed decrease in DNA damage mediated by GSE24.2 expression in F9A353V cells, also occurs when we used either bacterially produced or chemically synthesized peptide, reinforcing the idea that GSE24.2 reactivates telomerase activity, by acting directly at the telomeric DNA [26] and/or changing telomere folding. According with these results the transfection of the GSE24.2 synthetic peptide into X-DC3 human patient lymphocytes resulted in both increased telomerase activity and decreased DNA damage. On the other hand the consequences of A353V-X-DC mutation on DNA damage resemble to those found in cells with mutations in *Tin2* and *Pot1*, which are structural components of telomeres [38] [39].

Diseases with telomerase deficiency are linked to oxidative stress. Elevated levels of the lipoperoxide malondialdehyde (MDA) [40], and MDA-DNA adducts have been reported in rare degenerative diseases [41] and in aging [42]. In addition, oxidative stress conditions caused by H_2O_2 increased the rate of telomere shortening in fibroblasts from ataxia-telangiectasia patients [43]. Furthermore, increased accumulation of ROS is involved in decreased cell growth in a *DKC*$^{\Delta 15}$ mouse model [36], though there is very little information about oxidative stress in human X-DC cells. Interestingly, the existence of oxidative stress in lymphocytes from patients with an autosomal dominant form of DC with mutations in *TERC* has been recently reported [44]. To further increase the characterization of the oxidative stress profile in X-DC we characterize the levels of ROS and the expression

and activity of the main antioxidant enzymes. We found in X-DC-1774-P an increase in ROS levels and a decrease in the expression and activity of antioxidant enzymes in patient cells when compared to carrier cells. Interestingly expression of GSE24.2 results in an increase in SOD1, SOD2 and catalase expression that might decrease ROS levels in X-DC-1774-P 24.2 cells. Different groups [45] [46] [47] [48] have reported decreased cellular ROS levels in stressed hTERT over-expressing cells, demonstrating that telomerase re-expression contributes to decrease oxidative stress [49]. The work by Westin et al. demonstrated that the reduction of the levels of superoxide in DC cells was not dependent of the localization of TERT in the mitochondria, but also p53/p21$^{WAF/CIP}$-dependent process in the context of telomere shortening in cells from DC patients. Therefore, our findings reinforce the notion that increased telomerase activity [24] and repair of DNA damage at telomeres induced by GSE24.2 is concomitant with a decrease in oxidative stress in X-DC cells. Alternatively the decreased DNA damage detected by γ-H2A.X, might corresponds to decreased oxidative damage, in agreement of our results evaluating the levels of 8-oxoguanine that decreased after transfection of the GSE24.2 synthetic peptide.

In summary our results show that, GSE24.2 attenuates the impact of the *DKC1* mutations on DNA damage and its incidence on telomeres (Fig. 8). Furthermore, oxidative stress decreases in GSE24.2 expressing cells, and this should contribute to decrease the rate of DNA damage and therefore enable restoration of cell cycle progression. Indeed, we have previously shown that expression of GSE24.2 X-DC fibroblasts restores proliferation [26].

Since GSE24.2 has been approved as an orphan drug for the treatment of DC, the results presented here indicate that expression of GSE24.2 may form the basis of a useful and safe therapeutic strategy for X-DC patients either by using it as a permanent or as a temporal telomerase activator. These results indicate that GSE24.2 expression has a broad effect on DC cells, reducing oxidative stress and DNA damage in addition to reactivating telomerase activity. All these protective effects could cooperatively contribute to increase DC cells survival and proliferation [26] and give further support to the recent approval of GSE24.2 as an orphan drug for DC treatment.

Acknowledgments

We thank to P. Mason for the F9 cell mouse model and for the critical review of the manuscript.

Author Contributions

Conceived and designed the experiments: CMG LPB JC RMP LS CPQ IE AG JLGG FVP RP. Performed the experiments: CMG LPB JC RMP LS CPQ IE AG JLGG FVP RP. Analyzed the data: CMG LPB JC RMP LS CPQ IE AG JLGG FVP RP. Contributed reagents/materials/analysis tools: CMG LPB JC RMP LS CPQ IE AG JLGG FVP RP. Wrote the paper: CMG RMP LS JLGG FVP RP.

References

1. Palm W, de Lange T (2008) How shelterin protects mammalian telomeres. Annu Rev Genet 42: 301–334.
2. Osterhage JL, Friedman KL (2009) Chromosome end maintenance by telomerase. J Biol Chem 284: 16061–16065.
3. Cohen SB, Graham ME, Lovrecz GO, Bache N, Robinson PJ, et al. (2007) Protein composition of catalytically active human telomerase from immortal cells. Science 315: 1850–1853.
4. Meier UT, Blobel G (1994) NAP57, a mammalian nucleolar protein with a putative homolog in yeast and bacteria. J Cell Biol 127: 1505–1514.
5. Ni J, Tien AL, Fournier MJ (1997) Small nucleolar RNAs direct site-specific synthesis of pseudouridine in ribosomal RNA. Cell 89: 565–573.
6. Yang Y, Isaac C, Wang C, Dragon F, Pogacic V, et al. (2000) Conserved composition of mammalian box H/ACA and box C/D small nucleolar ribonucleoprotein particles and their interaction with the common factor Nopp140. Mol Biol Cell 11: 567–577.
7. Decatur WA, Fournier MJ (2002) rRNA modifications and ribosome function. Trends Biochem Sci 27: 344–351.
8. Heiss NS, Knight SW, Vulliamy TJ, Klauck SM, Wiemann S, et al. (1998) X-linked dyskeratosis congenita is caused by mutations in a highly conserved gene with putative nucleolar functions. Nat Genet 19: 32–38.
9. Kirwan M, Dokal I (2008) Dyskeratosis congenita: a genetic disorder of many faces. Clin Genet 73: 103–112.
10. de Lange T (2009) How telomeres solve the end-protection problem. Science 326: 948–952.
11. Martinez P, Blasco MA (2010). Role of shelterin in cancer and aging. Aging Cell 9: 653–666.
12. Tejera AM, Stagno d'Alcontres M, Thanasoula M, Marion RM, Martinez P, et al. (2010).TPP1 is required for TERT recruitment, telomere elongation during nuclear reprogramming, and normal skin development in mice. Dev Cell 18: 775–789.
13. Martinez P, Flores JM, Blasco MA (2012) 53BP1 deficiency combined with telomere dysfunction activates ATR-dependent DNA damage response. J Cell Biol 197: 283–300.
14. Rappold I, Iwabuchi K, Date T, Chen J (2001) Tumor suppressor p53 binding protein 1 (53BP1) is involved in DNA damage-signaling pathways. J Cell Biol 153: 613–620.
15. Fernandez-Capetillo O, Chen HT, Celeste A, Ward I, Romanienko PJ, et al. (2002) DNA damage-induced G2-M checkpoint activation by histone H2AX and 53BP1. Nat Cell Biol 4: 993–997.
16. Dimitrova N, Chen YC, Spector DL, de Lange T (2008) 53BP1 promotes non-homologous end joining of telomeres by increasing chromatin mobility. Nature 456: 524–528.
17. Perona R, Moncho-Amor V, Machado-Pinilla R, Belda-Iniesta C, Sanchez Perez I (2008) Role of CHK2 in cancer development. Clin Transl Oncol 10: 538–542.
18. Zhang R, Chen W, Adams PD (2007) Molecular dissection of formation of senescence-associated heterochromatin foci. Mol Cell Biol 27: 2343–2358.
19. Xu C, Xu Y, Gursoy-Yuzugullu O, Price BD (2012).The histone variant macroH2A1.1 is recruited to DSBs through a mechanism involving PARP1. FEBS Lett 586: 3920–3925.
20. Hartwig FP, Collares T (2013). Telomere dysfunction and tumor suppression responses in dyskeratosis congenita: balancing cancer and tissue renewal impairment. Ageing Res Rev 12: 642–652.
21. Young NS (2012). Bone marrow failure and the new telomere diseases: practice and research. Hematology 17 Suppl 1: S18–21.
22. Stewart JA, Chaiken MF, Wang F, Price CM (2012). Maintaining the end: roles of telomere proteins in end-protection, telomere replication and length regulation. Mutat Res 730: 12–19.
23. Alter BP, Giri N, Savage SA, Rosenberg PS (2009) Cancer in dyskeratosis congenita. Blood 113: 6549–6557.
24. Machado-Pinilla R, Sanchez-Perez I, Murguia JR, Sastre L, Perona R (2008) A dyskerin motif reactivates telomerase activity in X-linked dyskeratosis congenita and in telomerase-deficient human cells. Blood 111: 2606–2614.
25. Zeng XL, Thumati NR, Fleisig HB, Hukezalie KR, Savage SA, et al. (2012).The accumulation and not the specific activity of telomerase ribonucleoprotein determines telomere maintenance deficiency in X-linked dyskeratosis congenita. Hum Mol Genet 21: 721–729.
26. Machado-Pinilla R, Carrillo J, Manguan-Garcia C, Sastre L, Mentzer A, et al. (2012). Defects in mTR stability and telomerase activity produced by the Dkc1 A353V mutation in dyskeratosis congenita are rescued by a peptide from the dyskerin TruB domain. Clin Transl Oncol 14: 755–763.
27. Knight SW, Heiss NS, Vulliamy TJ, Greschner S, Stavrides G, et al. (1999) X-linked dyskeratosis congenita is predominantly caused by missense mutations in the DKC1 gene. Am J Hum Genet 65: 50–58.
28. Vulliamy TJ, Marrone A, Knight SW, Walne A, Mason PJ, et al. (2006) Mutations in dyskeratosis congenita: their impact on telomere length and the diversity of clinical presentation. Blood 107: 2680–2685.
29. Gu BW, Bessler M, Mason PJ (2008) A pathogenic dyskerin mutation impairs proliferation and activates a DNA damage response independent of telomere length in mice. Proc Natl Acad Sci U S A 105: 10173–10178.
30. Kalinin A, Thoma NH, Iakovenko A, Heinemann I, Rostkova E, et al. (2001) Expression of mammalian geranylgeranyltransferase type-II in Escherichia coli and its application for in vitro prenylation of Rab proteins. Protein Expr Purif 22: 84–91.
31. Mochizuki Y, He J, Kulkarni S, Bessler M, Mason PJ (2004) Mouse dyskerin mutations affect accumulation of telomerase RNA and small nucleolar RNA, telomerase activity, and ribosomal RNA processing. Proc Natl Acad Sci U S A 101: 10756–10761.
32. Wright WE, Shay JW, Piatyszek MA (1995) Modifications of a telomeric repeat amplification protocol (TRAP) result in increased reliability, linearity and sensitivity. Nucleic Acids Res 23: 3794–3795.
33. Sanchez-Perez I, Murguia JR, Perona R (1998) Cisplatin induces a persistent activation of JNK that is related to cell death. Oncogene 16: 533–540.
34. Taghizadeh K, McFaline JL, Pang B, Sullivan M, Dong M, et al. (2008) Quantification of DNA damage products resulting from deamination, oxidation and reaction with products of lipid peroxidation by liquid chromatography isotope dilution tandem mass spectrometry. Nat Protoc 3: 1287–1298.
35. Kirwan M, Beswick R, Walne AJ, Hossain U, Casimir C, et al. (2011). Dyskeratosis congenita and the DNA damage response. Br J Haematol 153: 634–643.
36. Gu BW, Fan JM, Bessler M, Mason PJ (2011) Accelerated hematopoietic stem cell aging in a mouse model of dyskeratosis congenita responds to antioxidant treatment. Aging Cell 10: 338–348.
37. Carrillo J, Gonzalez A, Manguan-Garcia C, Pintado-Berninches L, Perona R (2013). p53 pathway activation by telomere attrition in X-DC primary fibroblasts occurs in the absence of ribosome biogenesis failure and as a consequence of DNA damage. Clin Transl Oncol. [Epub ahead of print]
38. Walne AJ, Vulliamy T, Beswick R, Kirwan M, Dokal I (2008) TINF2 mutations result in very short telomeres: analysis of a large cohort of patients with dyskeratosis congenita and related bone marrow failure syndromes. Blood 112: 3594–3600.
39. Hockemeyer D, Palm W, Wang RC, Couto SS, de Lange T (2008) Engineered telomere degradation models dyskeratosis congenita. Genes Dev 22: 1773–1785.
40. Ahamed M, Kumar A, Siddiqui MK (2006) Lipid peroxidation and antioxidant status in the blood of children with aplastic anemia. Clin Chim Acta 374: 176–177.
41. Patel KJ, Joenje H (2007) Fanconi anemia and DNA replication repair. DNA Repair (Amst) 6: 885–890.
42. Voss P, Siems W (2006) Free Radic Res. 40(12):1339–49
43. Tchirkov A, Lansdorp PM (2003) Role of oxidative stress in telomere shortening in cultured fibroblasts from normal individuals and patients with ataxia-telangiectasia. Hum Mol Genet 12: 227–232.
44. Pereboeva L, Westin E, Patel T, Flanikin L, Lamb L, et al. (2013). DNA damage responses and oxidative stress in dyskeratosis congenita. PLoS One 8: e76473.
45. Ahmed S, Passos JF, Birket MJ, Beckmann T, Brings S, et al. (2008) Telomerase does not counteract telomere shortening but protects mitochondrial function under oxidative stress. J Cell Sci 121: 1046–1053.
46. Kang HJ, Choi YS, Hong SB, Kim KW, Woo RS, et al. (2004) Ectopic expression of the catalytic subunit of telomerase protects against brain injury resulting from ischemia and NMDA-induced neurotoxicity. J Neurosci 24: 1280–1287.
47. Saretzki G (2009) Telomerase, mitochondria and oxidative stress. Exp Gerontol 44: 485–492.
48. Saretzki G, Murphy MP, von Zglinicki T (2003) MitoQ counteracts telomere shortening and elongates lifespan of fibroblasts under mild oxidative stress. Aging Cell 2: 141–143.
49. Westin ER, Aykin-Burns N, Buckingham EM, Spitz DR, Goldman FD, et al. (2011) The p53/p21(WAF/CIP) pathway mediates oxidative stress and senescence in dyskeratosis congenita cells with telomerase insufficiency. Antioxid Redox Signal;14(6):985–97.

11

Comparative Analysis of Gene Expression Data Reveals Novel Targets of Senescence-Associated microRNAs

Marco Napolitano[1], Marika Comegna[2,3], Mariangela Succoio[2,3], Eleonora Leggiero[3], Lucio Pastore[2,3], Raffaella Faraonio[2,3], Filiberto Cimino[1,2,3]*, Fabiana Passaro[2,3]*

1 IRCCS SDN Foundation, Naples, Italy, 2 Department of Molecular Medicine and Medical Biotechnologies, University of Naples Federico II, Naples, Italy, 3 CEINGE – Advanced Biotechnologies, Naples, Italy

Abstract

In the last decades, cellular senescence is viewed as a complex mechanism involved in different processes, ranging from tumor suppression to induction of age-related degenerative alterations. Senescence-inducing stimuli are myriad and, recently, we and others have demonstrated the role exerted by microRNAs in the induction and maintenance of senescence, by the identification of a subset of Senescence-Associated microRNAs (SAmiRs) up-regulated during replicative or stress-induced senescence and able to induce a premature senescent phenotype when over-expressed in human primary cells. With the intent to find novel direct targets of two specific SAmiRs, SAmiR-494 and -486-5p, and cellular pathways which they are involved in, we performed a comparative analysis of gene expression profiles available in literature to select genes down-regulated upon replicative senescence of human primary fibroblasts. Among them, we searched for SAmiR's candidate targets by analyzing with different target prediction algorithms their 3'UTR for the presence of SAmiR-binding sites. The expression profiles of selected candidates have been validated on replicative and stress-induced senescence and the targeting of the 3'UTRs was assessed by luciferase assay. Results allowed us to identify Cell Division Cycle Associated 2 (CDCA2) and Inhibitor of DNA binding/differentiation type 4 (ID4) as novel targets of SAmiR-494 and SAmiR-486-5p, respectively. Furthermore, we demonstrated that the over-expression of CDCA2 in human primary fibroblasts was able to partially counteract etoposide-induced senescence by mitigating the activation of DNA Damage Response.

Editor: Gianfranco Pintus, University of Sassari, Italy

Funding: This study was supported by the Ministero dell'Università e della Ricerca Scientifica e Tecnologica (MIUR PRIN 2007, MIUR MERIT RBNE08HWLZ_004) and POR Campania FESR 2007-2013 Project BIOFRAME. The funders had no role in study design, data collection and analysis, decision to publish or preparation of the manuscript.

Competing Interests: The authors have declared that no competing interests exist.

* E-mail: cimino@dbbm.unina.it (FC); fabiana.passaro@unina.it (FP)

Introduction

Described for the first time in 1961 by Hayflick and Moorhead [1] as a process that limited the proliferation of normal human cells in culture, cellular senescence currently refers to the essentially irreversible growth arrest that occurs when proliferating cells encounter a genotoxic stress and reveals a complex phenomenon incorporating both genetic and environmental components acting through convergent pathways. With the possible exception of embryonic stem cells [2], most division-competent cells, including adult stem cells and some tumor cells, can undergo senescence [3].

Cellular senescence is thought to have evolved as a mechanism to prevent that damaged DNA could be replicated and passed on to future generations of cells, thus being considered a tumor suppressor mechanism [3]. Nevertheless, despite their inability to replicate, senescent cells are metabolically active and develop an aberrant gene expression profile with proinflammatory behaviour, the so-called Senescence Associated Secretory Phenotype (SASP), that can induce or accelerate changes in normal surrounding tissues, explaining the possible implication in tumor promotion, aging and age-related pathologies [4]. Very recently, it has been reported that cellular senescence contributes also to embryonic development, both in mice and humans [5–6].

Distinctive features of senescent cells include enlarged and flattened morphology, the appearance of senescence-associated heterochromatin foci (SAHF), accumulation of senescence-associated DNA-damage foci (SDFs) and expression of Senescence-Associated β-galactosidase (SA-β-gal) [4].

Many senescence-inducing stimuli cause epigenomic disruption or genomic damage, like the gradual attrition of telomeres with each S phase [7], that generates a persistent DNA damage response (DDR), which initiates and maintains the senescence growth arrest of human cells both in culture and *in vivo* [8–9]. Persistent DDR signaling generated at nontelomeric sites also leads to the senescence growth arrest, such as that derived by strong mitogenic signals delivered by certain oncogenes or highly expressed pro-proliferative genes, that cause misfired replication origins and replication fork collapse [10–12]. Treatments with cytotoxic chemotherapeutic agents, such as etoposide, that cause DNA double strand breaks, also induce premature senescence via the p53 pathway [13]. Senescence can also occur, however, without detectable DDR signaling. These stresses could include inappropriate substrates or serum or oxidative stress, as the Reactive Oxygen Species (ROS) production after treatment with oxidative stress agents, such as the glutathione depletor Diethyl-maleate (DEM) [14–15].

In the last years microRNAs (miRs) have added a new layer of complexity to the comprehension of molecular mechanisms underlying senescence. Each miR can recognize up to hundred different targets, thus influencing a large variety of cellular processes [16]. We and others have recently demonstrated that some miRs are involved in the process of cellular senescence [17–20]. In particular, we have found a subset of five Senescence-Associated miRs (SAmiRs) up-regulated during Human Diploid Fibroblasts (HDFs) replicative senescence, whose ectopic expression in young cells promoted the premature senescence program by inducing DNA damage and ROS accumulation.

The main aim of this study has been the identification of novel mRNA targets of two selected SAmiRs, SAmiR-486-5p and SAmiR-494. We chose SAmiR-486-5p, as we previously showed that this miR was the most robust up-regulated upon replicative senescence and significantly up-regulated upon Etoposide-Induced Senescence (EIS) of HDFs and in human primary skin fibroblasts from old donors [17]. Furthermore, Kim and colleagues demonstrated that the over-expression of SAmiR-486-5p was able to induce premature senescence also in human adipose tissue-derived stem cells, by inhibiting SIRT1 [21]. We also chose SAmiR-494, as its over-expression seemed to better recapitulate all the features of a senescent phenotype, including reduced cell proliferation, induction of SA-β-gal, SAHFs, DNA damage, SDFs and ROS accumulation. Moreover, it resulted up-regulated also in DEM - Induced Senescence (DIS) [17] and its over-expression was able to induce senescence not only in HDFs, but also in cancer cells [22].

Our strategy has been to look for new SAmiR targets among the mRNAs down-regulated in HDF senescent cells, comparing six different gene expression profiles available in literature, selecting genes whose expression was reduced in at least three different arrays and searching for SAmiR's responsive elements into their 3'UTR by the use of different target prediction algorithms.

This approach allowed us to identify Cell Division Cycle Associated 2 (CDCA2) and Inhibitor of DNA binding/differentiation type 4 (ID4) as novel targets of SAmiR-494 and SAmiR-486-5p, respectively. Moreover, we have also demonstrated that the transient over-expression of CDCA2 in HDFs is able to partially counteract the premature senescent phenotype induced by etoposide treatment.

Materials and Methods

Bioinformatics analysis

We took advantage of available data reporting gene expression profiles in replicative senescent HDFs. Normalized data from 6 microarrays [23–28] have been crossed in order to select a list of common genes down-regulated in senescence, with a fold variation ≥ 1.5. We obtained a list of 139 genes down-regulated upon HDFs replicative senescence (Table S1). Functional annotations were obtained on *PubMed.gov*. For the identification of putative targets of SAmiR-494 or SAmiR-486-5p, the genes in the list have been analyzed with four different target prediction algorithms (Target Scan v6.2, miRDB, Diana, miRanda) and putative targets predicted by at least two algorithms have been selected for further studies.

Real time PCR

Total RNA was extracted with TRIzol Reagent (Life Technologies) and quantified by Nanodrop (Thermo Scientific, Wilmington, DE). The first-strand cDNA was synthesized according to the manufacturer's instructions (SS VILO Mastermix- Life Technologies). Real-time RT-PCR was carried out on an iCycler (BioRad) using Express Greener QPCR Master mix (Life Technologies).

The housekeeping beta-actin (ACTB) mRNA was used as an internal reference gene for normalization. PCR reactions were performed on biological duplicates or triplicates and in experimental triplicate. Fold changes were calculated using $2^{-\Delta\Delta Ct}$ method, by the formula: $2^{-(\text{sample }\Delta Ct\ -\ \text{calibrator }\Delta Ct)}$, comparing results from experimental samples (Replicative senescent cells, Etoposide-induced senescent cells or DEM-induced senescent cells) with both a calibrator (young PDL 33 cells for RS; DMSO treated cells for EIS and DIS) and the reference gene ACTB. ΔCt is the difference between the amplification fluorescent thresholds of the gene of interest and ACTB. The list of the primers used is reported in Table S2.

TaqMan MiRNA Assay Kit (Applied Bio-systems, Foster City, CA) was used to detect the expression of mature miRNAs. Briefly, 100 ng of total RNA was reversely transcribed (RT) at 16 °C for 30 min, 42 °C for 30 min and 85 °C for 5 min in 15 µl reaction volume. Two µl of RT product were used for PCR reaction in a final volume of 20 µl. The PCR reaction started with an initial denaturation step at 90 °C for 10 min, followed by 40 cycles of 95 °C for 15 sec and 60 °C for 1 min. Small nucleolar RNA RNU6 (Applied Biosystems, Foster City, CA) was used for normalization. PCR reactions were performed in triplicate and fold changes were calculated using $2^{-\Delta\Delta Ct}$ method, where ΔCt is the difference between the amplification fluorescent thresholds of the miRNA of interest and the RNA of RNU6.

Cell cultures, treatments and transfections

Normal human primary fibroblasts IMR90 and human embryonic kidney HEK-293 cells were obtained from American Type Culture Collection (Manassas, VA). Cells were cultured in Dulbecco's modified Eagle's medium (DMEM) supplemented with 10% (v/v) fetal bovine serum and 1% penicillin/streptomycin (Gibco). Cultures were maintained at 37 °C in a 5% CO_2-humidified atmosphere.

The IMR90 population doubling level (PDL) was calculated by using the formula: $\Delta PDL = \log(n_h/n_i)/\log 2$, where n_i is the initial number of cells and n_h is the final number of cells at each passage. The cells were used at 33 PDL (young) or 58 PDL (senescent) (Fig.S1).

To induce premature senescence, IMR90 at PDL 33 were treated with 150 µM DEM on alternate days for 10 days or with 20 µM etoposide (both from SIGMA-ALDRICH) for 24 h and then subcultured for 10 days more (Fig.S1).

Transfection of IMR90 cells at PDL 33 with synthetic pre-miR precursors (Ambion), miR inhibitors (Exiqon) or siRNAs (Dharmacon) were performed using Lipofectamine RNAiMAX Transfection Reagent (Life Technologies) with the reverse protocol following the manufacturer's instructions. Pre-miRs, miR inhibitors and siRNAs were used at 100 nM.

Transfection of IMR90 cells at PDL 33 with CMV-CDCA2 and CMV-ID4, as well as co-transfection of HEK-293 with both luciferase constructs and pre-miRs were performed using Lipofectamine 2000 (Life Technologies) following the manufacturer's instructions.

Plasmid construction

With the exception of ID4, for which it has been cloned a portion of 300 bp containing the putative SAmiR-486-5p binding site, the whole 3'UTRs sequences of CDCA2, FOXM1, NUSAP1 and BUB1b have been cloned by PCR amplification on human genomic DNA, using primer pairs with XhoI and SalI restriction enzyme sites in the forward primers and XbaI in the reverse primers. A 430 bp portion of the 3'UTR of human OLFM4, containing the validated SAmiR-486-5p binding site [29], was cloned as positive control using primer pairs with SalI restriction enzyme sites in the forward primers and XbaI in the reverse primers. All PCR products were cloned into the pMIR-GLO vector (Promega) between the XhoI and the XbaI site, downstream the Firefly luciferase (Normal clones). The inverted 3'UTR of CDCA2, ID4 and OLFM4 (Reverse clones) were cloned by digestion of Forward clones with SalI, that allowed the excision of the 3'UTR, and by recloning digested fragment in SalI unique site. The orientation of the inserted fragments were established by digestions and confirmed with sequencing. The 3'UTRs of CDCA2 and ID4 containing point mutations in the SAmiR seed region (Mutated clones) were obtained by PCR using the Quik Change II XL site direct mutagenesis kit (Agilent), following the manufacturer's instructions. Mutations were confirmed by sequencing.

The coding sequences of CDCA2 and ID4 were amplified by PCR from ULTIMATEHORF CLONE ID IOH44066 and ULTIMATEHORF CLONE ID IOH12413 (Life Technologies), respectively, and cloned into the pEGFPN1 vector, in place of the GFP coding sequence, between the AgeI and NotI sites. The obtained vectors were named CMV-CDCA2 and CMV-ID4. All primers used for plasmids construction and the oligos containing the mutated SAmiR seed regions are reported in Table S3.

Luciferase Reporter Assay

For luciferase assays, human HEK-293 cells were plated at 8×10^4 cells per well on 48 well plates (BD Falcon) 12 h before transfection. The Normal, Reverse or Mutated luciferase constructs (100 ng) were co-transfected with 50 nM pre-miRs. All transfection experiments were done in triplicate and each experiment was repeated three times. The Renilla luciferase reporter, contained into the pMIR-GLO vector, was used as an internal control. The luciferase activity was measured 48 hours after transfection using a Dual Luciferase Reporter Assay System (Promega) according to manufacturer's instructions, on a $20/20^n$ Luminometer instrument (Turner BioSystems). The data generated were expressed as relative to control-miR transfected cells, after normalization to Renilla luciferase reading.

SA-β-gal assay and BrdU assay

SA-β-gal was assayed according to Dimri et al. [30]. Briefly, cells were washed twice with PBS, fixed with 2% formaldehyde and 0.2% glutaraldehyde in PBS, and washed twice in PBS. Then, cells were stained overnight in X-gal staining solution [1 mg/ml X-gal, 40 mM citric acid/sodium phosphate (pH 6.0), 5 mM potassium ferricyanide, 5 mM potassium ferrocyanide, 150 mM NaCl, 2 mM MgCl$_2$] at 37°C.

For BrdU (5-bromo-2-deoxyuridine) incorporation assay (ROCHE), cells were seeded on glass coverslips and transfected with siRNAs to induce the knock-down of SAmiR targets, or transfected with CMV-CDCA2, CMV-ID4 or CMV-NEO (as control plasmid) and treated with 20 μM etoposide to induce EIS or with 150 μM DEM to induce DIS. 72 h after transfection (siRNAs) or 24 h after treatments (48 h after plasmids overexpression), cells were incubated for 4 h with BrdU (10 μM) and fixed following the kit instructions. Coverslips were incubated with a primary anti-BrdU and a secondary fluorescein-conjugated antibodies and then counterstained with Hoechst 33258, rinsed and mounted in Moviol on glass slides. The fluorescent signal was visualized with an epifluorescent microscope Leica DM IL LED FLUO (Leica Microsystems). At least 300 cells were counted in triplicate experiments.

Immunofluorescence

To perform γ-H2AX staining, IMR90 at PDL33 were plated on glass coverslips, transfected with CMV-NEO control vector or CMV-CDCA2 for 24 h and, then, treated with 20 μM etoposide. Coverslips were collected at 0 h, 6 h and 18 h after treatment, fixed with 4% paraformaldehyde in PBS for 30 minutes at RT, permeabilized with 10% FBS, 1% BSA, 0,2% Triton in PBS for 15 minutes at RT and incubated with Anti-phospho-Histone H2A.X Ser 139 primary antibody (Millipore) for 2 h at RT. After 4 washes of 5 minutes each, coverslips were incubated with an Alexa-488 goat anti-mouse antibody (Life Technologies) for 1 h at RT, counterstained with DAPI and mounted in Moviol on glass slides. Samples were observed with an epifluorescent microscope Leica DM IL LED FLUO (Leica Microsystems) and at least 300 cells were counted in triplicate experiments.

Western blotting

IMR90 cells were harvested following washing with PBS. Cells were lysed in a buffer containing 0.02M HEPES (pH 7.9), 0.4M NaCl, 0.1% NP-40, 10% (v/v) glycerol, 1 mM NaF, 1 mM sodium orthovanadate and a protease inhibitory cocktail (Sigma Chemical Co. St. Louis, MO). Extracts were subjected to Sodium Dodecyl Sulfate (SDS)-polyacrylamide gel electrophoresis, followed by blotting to PVDF. The blots were probed with antibodies from Santa Cruz to human CDCA2, ID4, p53, p21, β-actin and α-tubulin; from Cell Signaling to human phospho-ATM (Ser 1981) and phospho-p53 (Ser 15) ; from Sigma-Aldrich to human ATM.

Statistical analysis

Statistical analysis were carried out using the Student's t test and data were considered significant at a value of $p<0.05$.

Results

A set of mRNAs is down-regulated in human senescent fibroblasts

To select candidate targets of SAmiR-494 or SAmiR-486-5p, we speculated that SAmiRs induced upon Replicative Senescence (RS) of HDFs could contribute to the suppression of genes that must be kept down-regulated on the induction of RS. Thus, we generated a list of mRNAs down-regulated on HDFs senescence by comparing the normalized data of six different microarray gene expression profiles available on public databases [23–28]. This analysis allowed to select 139 mRNAs down-regulated($\geq$1.5 folds) in at least 3 out of 6 different arrays (Table S1). As summarized in Fig. 1A, we analyzed the 139 mRNAs for the presence of consensus motifs for SAmiR-494 and/or for SAmiR-486-5p, by using four different target prediction algorithms (Target Scan v6.2, miRDB, Diana, miRanda) and focusing on the results common to at least two algorithms. This screening led to the generation of the list of candidate targets shown in Fig. 1B, with 20 putative targets of SAmiR-494, 7 of SAmiR-486-5p and 3 common to both SAmiRs (in grey). Among them, there are many mRNAs encoding proteins involved in cell cycle regulation (e.g. CCNE2, NUSAP1, ZWINT) and DDR (e.g. RAD51, RAD51AP1, DEK), two biological processes modified by ectopic expression of SAmiRs [17] (see also Table S1 for functional annotations). Interestingly, some of the candidates are members of the same protein family (e.g. BUB3 and BUB1b; CDCA2, CDCA4 and CDCA7; RFC2 and RFC3). We excluded BIRC5 (survivin) from further investigation, as it was already validated by others [31].

To validate the results of our comparative analysis, we investigated in IMR90 cells the expression profile of putative

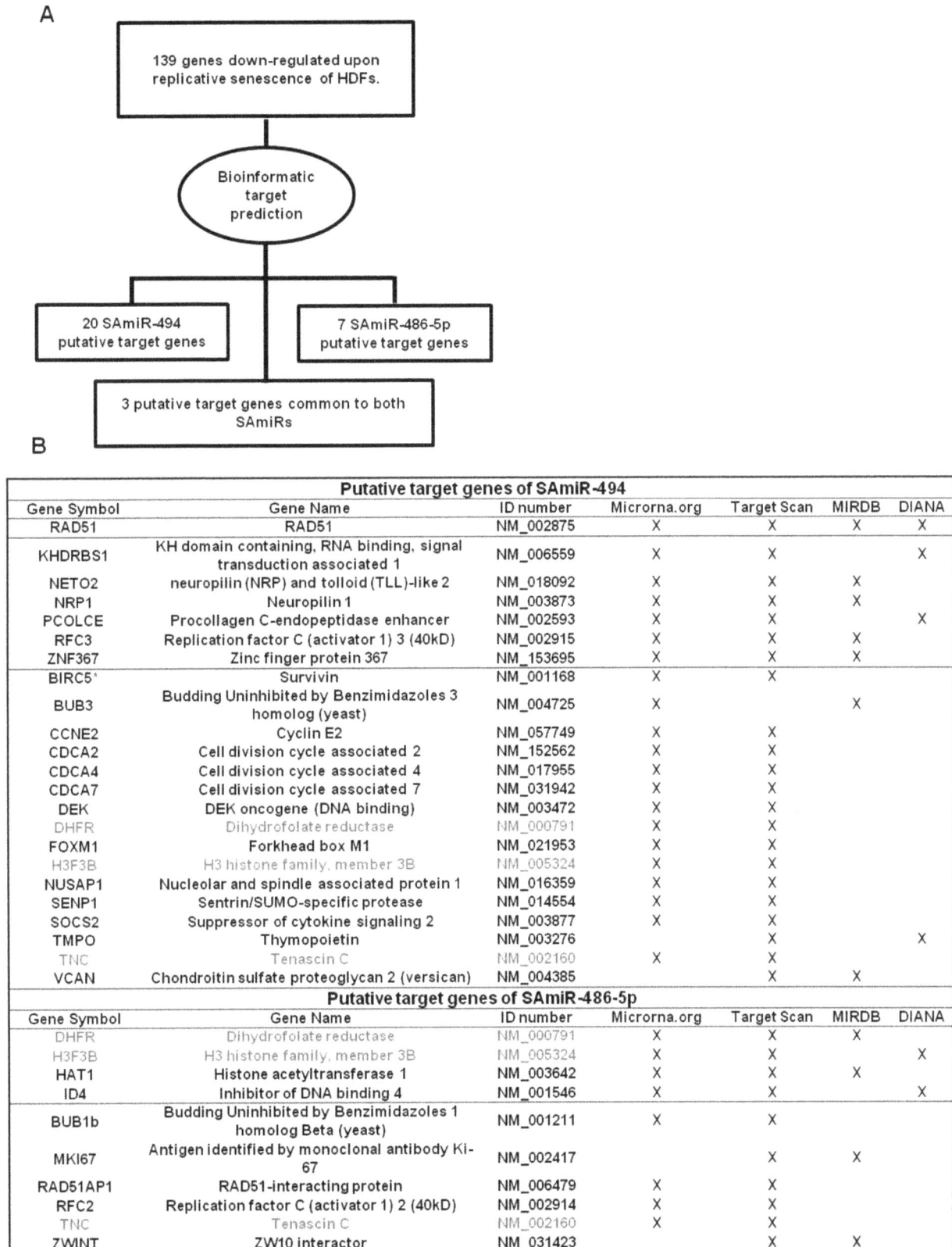

Figure 1. Strategy to identify putative targets of SAmiRs. A) The 3'UTR sequences of the 139 mRNAs down-regulated in replicative senescent fibroblasts and reported in Table S1 were analyzed with four different target prediction algorithms. This *in silico* analysis revealed 30 putative SAmiR targets: 20 of SAmiR-494, 7 of SAmiR-486-5p and 3 common to both SAmiRs. B) List of the 30 predicted target genes of both SAmiR-494 or SAmiR-486-5p. In grey, the three putative targets common to both SAmiRs.

targets upon induction of RS, EIS and DIS (Fig. 2). With the exception of CDCA7, SOCS2 and ZNF367, whose expression in IMR90 was undetectable (not shown), the results obtained by Real Time PCR demonstrated a common signature of gene expression in replicative and stress-induced senescence, with 17 out of 26 putative target genes that resulted significantly ($p<0.05$) down-regulated, with a fold variation$\geq$2, upon RS, 14 out of 26 upon EIS and 7 out of 26 upon DIS. These results prompted us to select for further investigation the 7 candidates, highlighted in Fig. 2 by a star, whose expression resulted down-regulated in all the examined conditions (RS, EIS and DIS).

A subset of putative targets are down-regulated upon SAmiR over-expression in human fibroblasts

In order to identify direct targets of SAmiRs, considering that mRNAs targeted by a miR are generally degraded [32–33], we analyzed by Real Time PCR the mRNA levels of BUB1b, CDCA2, FOXM1, ID4, MKI67, NUSAP1 and PCOLCE at day 2 after the transfection of the cognate synthetic SAmiR precursor (pre-miRs). As shown in Fig. 3A, CDCA2, FOXM1 and NUSAP1 resulted significantly ($p<0.01$) down-regulated 2 days after SAmiR-494 pre-miR transfection, whereas, among SAmiR-486-5p putative targets, ID4 and, at a lower extent, BUB1b, showed a significant reduction upon pre-miR transfection.

CDCA2 and ID4 are direct target of SAmiR-494 and SAmiR-486-5p, respectively

To address whether CDCA2, FOXM1, NUSAP1, ID4 and BUB1b, whose mRNAs resulted reduced after SAmiR over-expression, were direct targets, luciferase constructs containing their 3' UTR sequences were generated. As shown in Fig. 3B, in the case of CDCA2 and ID4 the reporter gene expression was significantly reduced by SAmiR-494 or SAmiR-486-5p pre-miR transfection, respectively, with a variation of relative luciferase expression similar to the positive control OLFM4 (N). In contrast, the co-transfection of FOXM1, NUSAP1 or BUB1b luciferase constructs with the cognate SAmiR didn't show any change in

luciferase expression compared to unrelated pre-miR transfected cells (Fig. S3A).

To further characterize the functionality of predicted target sites in the 3'UTRs of CDCA2 and ID4, the corresponding reverse fragments or the fragments mutated at the seed region of putative target sites were also generated. As shown in Fig. 3B, the luc-reverse constructs (R), as well as the constructs bearing mutated UTRs (M) were unaffected by the cognate SAmiR transfection (see also Fig. 3C for point mutations into SAmiRs seed regions), thus strongly suggesting that CDCA2 and ID4 were direct targets of selected SAmiRs.

We also investigated the expression profiles of the two targets by Western blot analysis, upon SAmiRs over-expression or down-regulation in PDL 33 IMR90 cells. As shown in Fig. 3D and 3E, the decrease in CDCA2 and ID4 endogenous expression levels was well detectable at protein level. Noteworthy, the transfection of miR inhibitors caused the increase of target expression levels.

All together, these data demonstrated that CDCA2 and ID4 are direct targets of SAmiRs-494 and SAmiR-486-5p, respectively.

Knock-down of CDCA2 or ID4 in young human primary fibroblasts does not induce senescence

To analyze the role of CDCA2 and ID4 in senescence, we asked whether their knock-down by RNAi in young cells was able to induce premature senescence, as the up-regulation of the cognate SAmiRs does. To this aim, we transfected siRNAs designed to silence CDCA2 or ID4 in young IMR90 at PDL 33 individually or as a mixture (Fig. S3B), and then we analyzed the cells until ten days after transfection, in order to detect any signs of senescence, as the decreasing of cell proliferation by BrdU incorporation, the change in cell morphology or the appearance of SA-β-gal. As showed in Fig. 4A, the knock-down of these genes seemed to be unable to affect cell proliferation, although a weak but significant decrease in BrdU incorporation was detected in siCDCA2 cells. Accordingly, knock-down cells did not senesce prematurely, as demonstrated by the absence of SA-β-gal staining 10 days after siRNA transfection (Fig. 4B). Probably, neither the transient

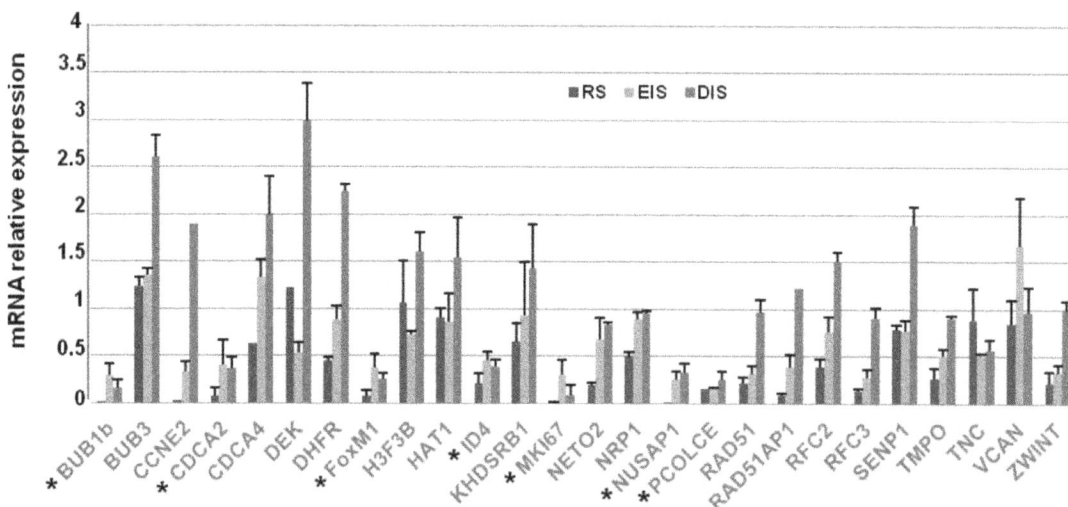

Figure 2. Expression profile of putative targets upon the induction of replicative or stress-induced senescence. The expression levels of the 26 candidates were measured by Real Time PCR in replicative (**RS**: IMR90 cells at PDL 58), etoposide- (**EIS**: PDL 33 IMR90 cells treated with 20 μM etoposide for 24 h and then subcultivated for additional 10 days) and DEM-induced (**DIS**: PDL 33 IMR90 cells treated with 150 μM DEM on alternate days for 10 days) senescent cells. The mRNA relative expression was calculated by assigning the arbitrary value 1 to the amount found in young or DMSO-treated cells. SD is used to refer to the values obtained in 2 different experiments. Results showed that 7 mRNAs, highlighted by a star, resulted significantly ($p<0.05$) down-regulated, with a cut-off$\geq$2 folds, in all conditions.

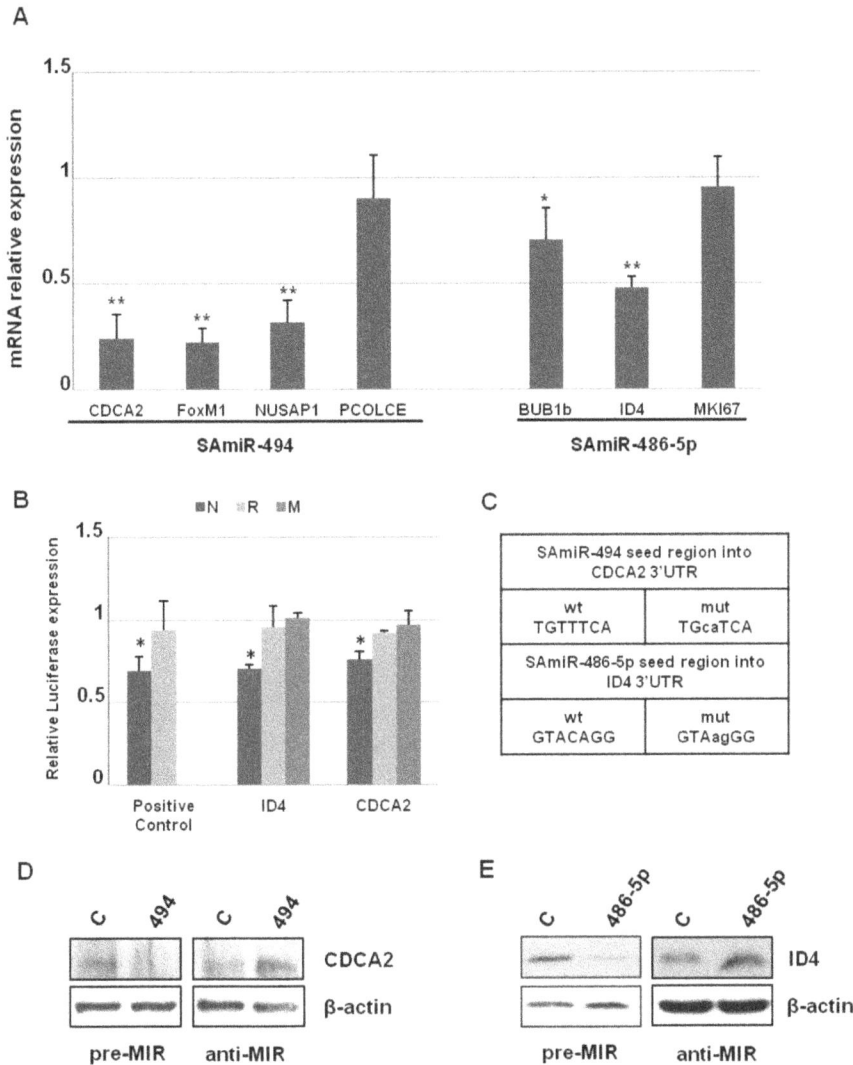

Figure 3. Expression profile of putative targets upon SAmiRs ectopic expression and validation of CDCA2 and ID4. A) Expression levels of SAmiR-494 and SAmiR-486-5p putative targets 2 days after the transfection of the cognate SAmiR pre-miR in PDL 33 IMR90 cells. mRNA levels were measured by Real Time PCR and mRNA relative expression was calculated by assigning the arbitrary value 1 to the amount found in control cells transfected with a scramble pre-miR. SD refers to the values obtained in 3 different experiments and the difference was significant (** p< 0.01; * p<0.05). The quantification of the expression levels of SAmiRs after their ectopic over-expression is reported in Panel A of Figure S2. B) Luciferase constructs bearing the normal 3'UTRs (N), reverse 3'UTRs (R) or mutated 3'UTRs (M) of CDCA2 and ID4 were transfected in HEK293 cells together with the cognate pre-miR or control pre-miR. The normal and reverse 3'UTR of OLFM4 were used as positive control. Luciferase levels were reported as fold changes compared to the values measured in control pre-miR transfected cells, after normalization with Renilla luciferase activity. SD refers to the values obtained in 3 different experiments (* p<0.01). C) Wild type seed regions of SAmiR-494 and SAmiR-486-5p, respectively present into the 3'UTRs of CDCA2 and ID4, compared to the mutated seed regions used for luciferase assays. D) Western blot analysis of CDCA2 in IMR90 cells over-expressing SAmiR-494 (pre-miR) or a specific SAmiR-494 inhibitor (anti-miR). E) Western blot analysis of ID4 in IMR90 cells over-expressing SAmiR-486-5p (pre-miR) or a specific SAmiR-486-5p inhibitor (anti-miR). In both cases, the proteins resulted suppressed by the SAmiR over-expression, as well as they resulted up-regulated by the anti-miR transfection, if compared to the control scramble transfected cells. The quantification of the expression levels of SAmiRs after their ectopic over-expression in D and E is reported in Panel B of Figure S2.

down-regulation of individual SAmiR target, nor the knock-down of both targets have the "strength" to switching-on the senescence program, as the contemporaneous reduction of many targets exerted by SAmiR's over-expression do.

Nevertheless, the down-regulation of CDCA2 or ID4 caused by the up-regulation of cognate SAmiRs could contribute to the acquisition of the final senescence phenotype. Thus, we investigated the possible role of CDCA2 or ID4 in cellular senescence by determining the effects of their over-expression.

Adoptive expression of CDCA2 promotes cell cycle progression in EIS

We transfected CDCA2 or ID4 in young PDL 33 IMR90 cells, one day before the induction of EIS or DIS. Then, we monitored the progression of senescence by checking for BrdU incorporation, cell morphology changes and appearance of SA-β-gal.

While DIS program seemed to be unaffected, the transient over-expression of CDCA2, but not ID4, was able to counteract the EIS program, promoting cell cycle progression (Fig. 5A), despite the DNA damage induced by etoposide (Fig. S4A). However, this is a

A

B

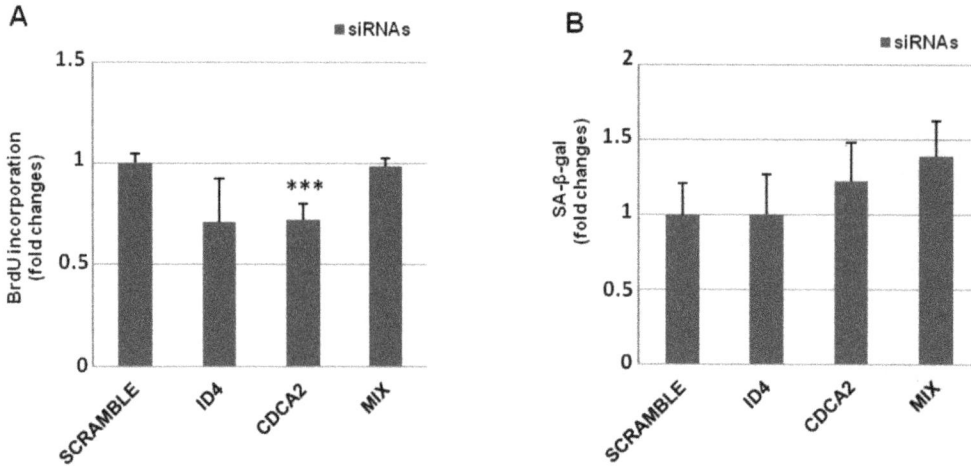

Figure 4. Knock-down of CDCA2, ID4 or both does not induce premature senescence in PDL 33 IMR90 cells. A) siRNAs designed to target the coding sequence of CDCA2 or ID4 were transfected, individually or as a mix, in PDL 33 IMR90 cells to knock-down the expression levels of target genes. After 72 h, transfected cells were incubated with BrdU for 4 h, then coverslips were fixed, incubated with a primary anti-BrdU antibody, washed and incubated with a secondary fluorescein-conjugated antibody, counterstained with Hoechst-33258 and counted by immunofluorescence. Counts of at least 1,000 cells were averaged and expressed as fold changes±SD, with respect to scrambled transfected cells (*** p<0.001). B) siRNA transfected cells were subcultivated for 10 days and stained for SA-β-gal. Counts of at least 300 cells were averaged and expressed as fold changes±SD, with respect to scrambled transfected cells.

temporary effect, as CDCA2 over-expressing cells finally arrested their growth and showed SA-β-gal accumulation, just like control cells (Fig. S4B).

Etoposide provokes DNA strand breaks that induce senescence through the activation of the p53 pathway [13]. Furthermore, it has been demonstrated that, in human non-tumorigenic cells (MCF10A), the over-expression of CDCA2 attenuates DDR

activation induced by etoposide treatment by recruiting PP1γ phosphatase to chromatin at damaged sites and causing the dephosphorylation of activated ATM [34]. This phenomenon could also explain the resistance to EIS showed by IMR90 cells over-expressing CDCA2. Therefore, we measured ATM activation in CDCA2 over-expressing cells 24 h after EIS induction.

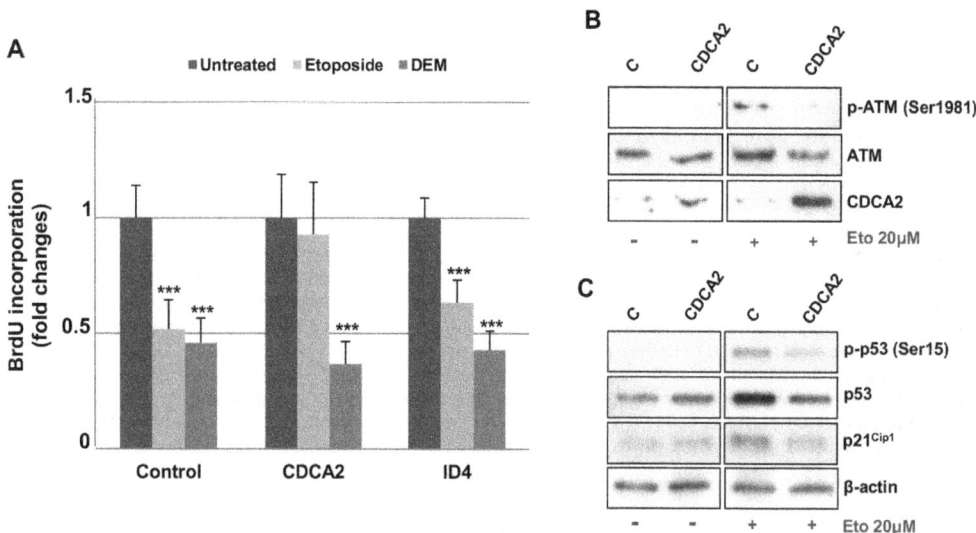

A

B

C

Figure 5. Adoptive expression of CDCA2 promotes cell cycle progression in Etoposide-Induced Senescence. A) CDCA2 and ID4 coding sequences were transfected in PDL 33 IMR90 cells. Cells transfected with CMV-NEO plasmid were used as control. After 24 h, transfected cells were treated with 20 μM etoposide or 150 μM DEM for 24 h and then incubated with BrdU for 4 h. Coverslips were then fixed, incubated with primary anti-BrdU and secondary fluorescein-conjugated antibodies, counterstained with Hoechst-33258 and counted by immunofluorescence. Counts of at least 800 cells were averaged and expressed as fold changes±SD, with respect to control transfected cells (***p<0.01). B) and C) PDL 33 IMR90 cells were transfected with the coding sequence of CDCA2. After 24 h, transfected cells were treated with 20 μM etoposide for 24 h and then were collected to obtain protein extracts. Cell extracts from CMV-neo over-expressing cells served as control. Western Blot analysis was used to detect the levels of phosphorylated ATM (p-ATM Ser1981), ATM, phosphorylated p53 (p-p53 Ser15), p53, p21Cip1 and CDCA2 in the cell lysates. β-actin was used as a loading control.

As shown in Fig. 5B and 5C, the over-expression of CDCA2 is accompanied by a reduction of ATM activation. This results in a reduced activation of p53 and a consequent weak expression of the cyclin-dependent kinase inhibitor p21Cip1, which can explain the sustained cell proliferation observed despite etoposide treatment.

All these data demonstrate that also in primary human cells CDCA2 over-expression is able to antagonize the activation of ATM-dependent signal transduction modulating DDR sensitivity, thus preventing the arrest of cell-cycle progression of premature senescence via decreased expression of CDKIs.

Discussion

In this study, with the intent to find novel direct targets of two specific SAmiRs previously associated to the induction and maintenance of cellular senescence [17], we took advantage of gene expression data available in literature to select by a comparative analysis and validate a subset of genes, whose expression was strongly reduced in replicative and stress-induced senescent cells. Among these genes we found that CDCA2, a specific nuclear regulatory subunit of protein phosphatase 1 γ (PP1γ), and ID4, a member of a family of helix-loop-helix transcription factors, are direct targets of SAmiR-494 and SAmiR-486-5p, respectively.

In our study, the down-regulation in HDFs of CDCA2, ID4 or both fails to cause a massive cell cycle arrest typical of premature senescence, that instead occurs after the over-expression of their negative regulators, SAmiR-494 or SAmiR-486-5p. Nevertheless, the ectopic expression of CDCA2, but not of ID4, was able to partially counteract the progression of EIS by the reduction of ATM activation, thus avoiding the cell cycle arrest caused by the activation of p53 and of DNA damage checkpoints after etoposide treatment. This would make cells less sensitive to DNA damage. Thus, it can be speculated that the down-regulation of CDCA2 expression that occurs in HDFs during cellular senescence could contribute to the accumulation of DNA damage that, in turn, sustains, rather than provokes, the senescence program.

CDCA2, also known as Repo-Man, is involved in cell cycle regulation [35–38], as well as in PP1γ-dependent essential DDR regulation [34]. Our data are in accordance with previous findings from Peng and colleagues, reporting that CDCA2 recruits PP1γ to chromatin to antagonize activation of ATM-dependent signal transduction in pre-malignant (not cancerous) cells [34].

Moreover, CDCA2-dependent DDR regulation is strengthened by CDCA2 over-expression during cancer progression, resulting in reduced DDR sensitivity. CDCA2 is frequently over-expressed in many tumor cells, as neuroblastoma, melanoma, breast cancer and in oral squamous cell carcinoma [39]. In particular, experiments on oral cancer cell lines showed that suppression of CDCA2 expression with shRNA significantly inhibits cellular proliferation, by arresting cell-cycle progression at the G1 phase through activation of the DDR in vitro, thus suggesting that up-regulation of CDCA2 in tumor cells might prevent the arrest of cell-cycle progression, via decreased expression of CDKIs and regulation of the DDR.

However, in our study CDCA2 over-expressing cells finally encounter a senescent growth arrest. This behavior might be explained by the fact that the reduction of p53 and p21 activation is only partial. Other mechanisms, parallel to ATM activation, may be involved in supporting the phosphorylation of p53.

Concerning ID4, it is an helix-loop-helix transcription factor that, having lost the basic DNA-binding domain, acts as dominant-negative regulator by forming inactive heterodimeric complexes with other helix-loop-helix transcription factors [40]. It performs different regulatory functions mainly during embryogenesis, being involved in the neural stem cell, oligodendrocyte and astrocyte differentiation.

Like CDCA2, ID4 is expressed in several tumors where it seems to play a key role in cellular transformation, immortalization, invasion, and in the metastatic process [41–42]. Thus, a decrease in ID4 expression levels could be one of the mechanisms adopted by cellular senescence to antagonize the tumor development in pre-cancerous cells. Nevertheless, the expression of ID4 is epigenetically silenced in prostate cancer and, very recently, it has been demonstrated that ectopic over-expression of ID4 promotes cellular senescence in prostate cancer cell line DU145 by increasing the expression of p16, p21, p27, E-cadherin and vimentin, but down-regulating E2F1 expression. ID4 also potentiated the effect of doxorubicin induced senescence and apoptosis [43]. These findings suggest that the role of ID4 in cellular senescence could be strictly dependent on tissue or cell types.

In conclusion, we have identified CDCA2 and ID4 as new direct targets of two different miRs, whose up-regulation in HDFs is correlated to the induction of cellular senescence. As expected, both targets are down-regulated during replicative- or stress-induced senescence, but cannot induce senescence when silenced in young HDFs. Nevertheless, for CDCA2, our results are in accordance with previous findings in pre-malignant (not cancerous) or tumor cells, in which the levels of CDCA2 determine the activation threshold of the DNA damage checkpoint. Thus, our results indicate that CDCA2 sets the threshold for checkpoint activation also in HDFs.

Supporting Information

Figure S1   Characterization of senescent IMR90 cells. A) Characterization of replicative senescent IMR90 cells. Primary human fibroblasts IMR90 were grown in DMEM supplemented with 10% (v/v) fetal bovine serum and 1% penicillin/streptomycin for some months, until PDL 58. B) Characterization of cellular senescence induced by etoposide treatment. PDL 33 IMR90 cells were exposed to etoposide 20 μM for 24 h and then cultured for 10 days before harvesting. C) Characterization of cellular senescence induced by DEM treatment. PDL 33 IMR90 cells were chronically exposed to DEM 150 μM on alternate days for 10 days before harvesting. In all cases, cellular senescence was assessed by SA-β-gal staining and gene expression profile [4]. For SA-β-gal staining, representative images of control and senescent cells are reported. For each experiment, at least 300 cells were counted. For gene expression profiling, quantitative Real-Time PCR analysis of cyclin A (CyclA), thymidylate synthase (THY), cyclin-selective ubiquitin carrier protein (UBI), interleukin-6 (IL6), cyclin-dependent kinase inhibitors p21Cip1 (p21) and p16INK4A (p16) mRNAs are showed. Results are the mean of triplicate determinations.

Figure S2   Quantification of SAmiR expression levels after their ectopic over-expression. The expression levels of SAmiR-494 and SAmiR-486-5p were measured by Real Time PCR in PDL 33 IMR90 cells transfected with 100 nM pre-miR. The microRNA relative expression was calculated by assigning the arbitrary value 1 to the amount found in control pre-miR transfected cells. SD is used to refer to the values obtained in 3 different experiments. In all cases, the difference was significant (p < 0.01). A) Data refers to SAmiR's over-expression of Figure 3A; B) data refers to SAmiR's over-expression of Figure 3D and 3E.

Figure S3 A) Luciferase assay of unvalidated SAmiR predicted target genes. Luciferase constructs bearing the normal 3'UTRs of FOXM1, NUSAP1 (predicted targets of SAmiR-494) and BUB1b (predicted target of SAmiR-486-5p) were transfected in HEK293 cells, together with the specific SAmiR pre-miR, control pre-miR or an unrelated pre-miR. Luciferase levels were reported as fold changes compared to the values measured in control pre-miR transfected cells, after normalization with Renilla luciferase activity. **B) SAmiR's target knock-down by siRNAs.** The expression levels of CDCA2 and ID4 were measured by Real Time PCR in PDL 33 IMR90 cells transfected with 100 nM siRNAs, individually or as a mix. The mRNA relative expression was calculated by assigning the arbitrary value 1 to the amount found in scramble-transfected cells. SD is used to refer to the values obtained in 3 different experiments. In all cases, the difference was significant ($p < 0.05$).

Figure S4 A) Etoposide treatment of IMR90 cells over-expressing CDCA2 induces γH2AX foci. PDL 33 IMR90 cells were transfected with control CMV-NEO vector or with CMV-CDCA2. After 24 h, transfected cells were treated with 20 μM etoposide. Cells were fixed and examined by immunofluorescence for a-H2AX phosphorylated on Ser139 (γH2AX) at 0, 6 or 18 hours after treatment. Coverslips were washed and incubated with Alexa-488 Goat anti-rabbit antibody and counterstained with DAPI. Counts of at least 300 cells were averaged and expressed as percent of cells positive to the presence of γH2AX foci ± SD. **B) Etoposide treatment of IMR90 cells over-expressing CDCA2 induces premature senescence.** PDL33 IMR90 cells were transfected with control vector or a vector containing the coding sequence of human CDCA2 gene. After 24 h, transfected cells were treated with 20 μM etoposide for 24 h and then were subcultivated for 10 days before harvesting. Cellular senescence was assessed by SA-β-gal staining. At least 300 cells were counted. Representative images of control and senescent cells are showed.

Table S1   Genes whose expression is down-regulated during senescence of human diploid fibroblasts.

Table S2   Primer pairs for Real Time PCR.

Table S3   Primer pairs for plasmid construction.

Acknowledgments

We thank Prof. Tommaso Russo for critical reading of the manuscript and for helpful discussions.

Author Contributions

Conceived and designed the experiments: MN FP FC. Performed the experiments: MN MC MS EL FP. Analyzed the data: MN FP LP RF FC. Wrote the paper: FP FC.

References

1. Hayflick L, Moorhead PS (1961) The serial cultivation of human diploid cell strains. Exp Cell Res 25: 585–621.
2. Miura T, Mattson MP, Rao MS (2004) Cellular lifespan and senescence signaling in embryonic stem cells. Aging Cell 3: 333–343.
3. Campisi J, d'Adda di Fagagna F (2007) Cellular senescence: when bad things happen to good cells. Nat Rev Mol Cell Biol 8: 729–740.
4. Rodier F, Campisi J (2011) Four faces of cellular senescence. J Cell Biol 192 (4): 547–556.
5. Muñoz-Espín D, Cañamero M, Maraver A, Gómez-López G, Contreras J, et al. (2013) Programmed cell senescence during mammalian embryonic development. Cell 155 (5): 1104–1118.
6. Storer M, Mas A, Robert-Moreno A, Pecoraro M, Ortells MC, et al. (2013) Senescence is a developmental mechanism that contributes to embryonic growth and patterning. Cell 155 (5): 1119–1130.
7. Bodnar AG, Ouellette M, Frolkis M, Holt SE, Chiu CP, et al. (1998) Extension of life-span by introduction of telomerase into normal human cells. Science 279: 349–352.
8. Rodier F, Coppe JP, Patil CK, Hoeijmakers WAM, Munoz DP, et al. (2009) Persistent DNA damage signaling triggers senescence-associated inflammatory cytokine secretion. Nat Cell Biol 11: 973–979.
9. d'Adda di Fagagna F, Reaper PM, Clay-Farrace L, Fiegler H, Carr P, et al. (2003) A DNA damage checkpoint response in telomere-initiated senescence. Nature 426: 194–198.
10. Serrano M, Lin AW, McCurrach ME, Beach D, Lowe SW (1997) Oncogenic ras provokes premature cell senescence associated with accumulation of p53 and p16INK4a. Cell 88: 593–602.
11. Lin AW, Barradas M, Stone JC, van Aelst L, Serrano M, et al. (1998) Premature senescence involving p53 and p16 is activated in response to constitutive MEK/MAPK mitogenic signaling. Genes Dev 12: 3008–3019.
12. Bartkova J, Rezaei N, Liontos M, Karakaidos P, Kletsas D, et al. (2006) Oncogene-induced senescence is part of the tumorigenesis barrier imposed by DNA damage checkpoints. Nature 444: 633–637.
13. Poele Te RH, Okorokov AL, Jardine L, Cunnings J, Joel SP (2002) DNA damage is able to induce senescence in tumor cells in vitro and in vivo. Cancer Res 62: 1876–83.
14. Faraonio R, Pane F, Intrieri M, Russo T, Cimino F (2002) In vitro acquired cellular senescence and aging-specific phenotype can be distinguished on the basis of specific mRNA expression. Cell Death Differ 9: 862–864.
15. Parrinello S, Samper E, Krtolica A, Goldstein J, Melov S, et al. (2003) Oxygen sensitivity severely limits the replicative lifespan of murine fibroblasts. Nat Cell Biol 5: 741–747.
16. Bartel DP (2009) MicroRNAs: target recognition and regulatory functions. Cell 136: 215–33.
17. Faraonio R, Salerno P, Passaro F, Sedia C, Iaccio A, et al. (2012) A set of miRNAs participates in the cellular senescence program in human diploid fibroblasts. Cell Death Differ 19 (4): 713–721.
18. Gorospe M, Abdelmohsen K (2011) MicroRegulators come of age in senescence. Trends Genet 27: 233–41.
19. Mancini M, Saintigny G, Mahé C, Annicchiarico-Petruzzelli M, Melino G, et al. (2012) MicroRNA-152 and -181a participate in human dermal fibroblasts senescence acting on cell adhesion and remodeling of the extra-cellular matrix. Aging (Albany) 4: 843–53.
20. Smith-Vikos T, Slack FJ (2012) MicroRNAs and their roles in aging. J Cell Sci 125: 7–17.
21. Kim YJ, Hwang SH, Lee SY, Shin KK, Cho HH, et al. (2012) miR-486-5p induces replicative senescence of human adipose tissue-derived mesenchymal stem cells and its expression is controlled by high glucose. Stem Cells Dev 21: 1749–1760.
22. Ohdaira H, Sekiguchi M, Miyata K, Yoshida K (2012) MicroRNA-494 suppresses cell proliferation and induces senescence in A549 lung cancer cells. Cell Prolif 45 (1): 32–38.
23. Binet R, Ythier D, Robles AI, Collado M, Larrieu D, et al. (2009) WNT16B is a new marker of cellular senescence that regulates p53 activity and the phosphoinositide 3-kinase/AKT pathway. Cancer Res 69 (24): 9183–91.
24. Zhang H, Pan KH, Cohen SN (2003) Senescence-specific gene expression fingerprints reveal cell-type-dependent physical clustering of up-regulated chromosomal loci. Proc Natl Acad Sci U S A 100 (6): 3251–6.
25. Hardy K, Mansfield L, Mackay A, Benvenuti S, Ismail S, et al. (2005) Transcriptional networks and cellular senescence in human mammary fibroblasts. Mol Biol Cell 16 (2): 943–53.
26. Zhang H, Herbert BS, Pan KH, Shay JW, Cohen SN (2004) Disparate effects of telomere attrition on gene expression during replicative senescence of human mammary epithelial cells cultured under different conditions. Oncogene 23 (37): 6193–8.
27. Schwarze SR, DePrimo SE, Grabert LM, Fu VX, Brooks JD, et al. (2002) Novel pathways associated with bypassing cellular senescence in human prostate epithelial cells. J Biol Chem 277 (17): 14877–83.
28. Johung K, Goodwin EC, Di Maio D (2007) Human papillomavirus E7 repression in cervical carcinoma cells initiates transcriptional cascade driven by the retinoblastoma family, resulting in senescence. J Virol 81 (5): 2102–16.
29. Oh HK, Tan AL-K, Das K, Ooi CH, Deng NT, et al. (2011) Genomic loss of miR-486 regulates tumor progression and the OLFM4 antiapoptotic factor in gastric cancer. Clin Cancer Res 17: 2657–2667.
30. Dimri GP, Lee X, Basile G, Acosta M, Scott G, et al. (1995) A biomarker that identifies senescent human cells in culture and in aging skin in vivo. Proc Natl Acad Sci U S A 92: 9363–9367.

31. Diakos C, Zhong S, Xiao Y, Zhou M, Vasconcelos GM, et al. (2010) TEL-AML1 regulation of survivin and apoptosis via miRNA-494 and miRNA-320a. Blood 116 (23): 4885–93.
32. Visvanathan J, Lee S, Lee B, Lee JW, Lee SK (2007) The microRNA miR-124 antagonizes the anti-neural REST/SCP1 pathway during embryonic CNS development. Genes Dev 21: 744–749.
33. Ziegelbauer JM, Sullivan CS, Ganem D (2009) Tandem array-based expression screens identify host mRNA targets of virus-encoded microRNAs. Nat Genet 41: 130–134.
34. Peng A, Lewellyn AL, Schiemann WP, Maller JL (2010) Repo-Man controls a protein phosphatase 1-dependent threshold for DNA damage checkpoint activation. Curr Biol 20 (5): 387–396.
35. Trinkle-Mulcahy L, Andersen J, Lam YW, Moorhead G, Mann M, et al. (2006) Repo-Man recruits PP1 gamma to chromatin and is essential for cell viability. J Cell Biol 172: 679–692.
36. Vagnarelli P, Hudson DF, Ribeiro SA, Trinkle-Mulcahy L, Spence JM, et al. (2006) Condensin and Repo-Man-PP1 co-operate in the regulation of chromosome architecture during mitosis. Nat Cell Biol 8: 1133–1142.
37. Qian J, Lesage B, Beullens M, Van Eynde A, Bollen M (2011) PP1/Repo-man dephosphorylates mitotic histone H3 at T3 and regulates chromosomal aurora B targeting. Curr Biol 21: 766–773.
38. Vagnarelli P, Ribeiro S, Sennels L, Sanchez-Pulido L, de Lima Alves F, et al. (2011) Repo-Man Coordinates Chromosomal Reorganization with Nuclear Envelope Reassembly during Mitotic Exit. Dev Cell 21: 328–342.
39. Uchida F, Uzawa K, Kasamatsu A, Takatori H, Sakamoto Y, et al. (2013) Overexpression of CDCA2 in Human Squamous Cell Carcinoma: Correlation with Prevention of G1 Phase Arrest and Apoptosis. PLoS ONE 8 (2): e56381.
40. Massari ME, Murre C (2000) Helix-loop-helix proteins: regulators of transcription in eucaryotic organisms. Mol Cell Biol 20: 429–440.
41. Ruzinova MB, Benezra R (2003) Id proteins in development, cell cycle and cancer. Trends Cell Biol 13: 410–418.
42. Iavarone A, Lasorella A (2006) ID proteins as targets in cancer and tools in neurobiology. Trends Mol Med 12: 588–594.
43. Carey JP, Knowell AE, Chinaranagari S, Chaudhary J (2013) ID4 promotes senescence and sensitivity to doxorubicin-induced apoptosis in DU145 prostate cancer cells. Anticancer Res 33 (10): 4271–8.

12

Reprogramming Suppresses Premature Senescence Phenotypes of Werner Syndrome Cells and Maintains Chromosomal Stability over Long-Term Culture

Akira Shimamoto[1]*, **Harunobu Kagawa**[1], **Kazumasa Zensho**[1], **Yukihiro Sera**[1], **Yasuhiro Kazuki**[2], **Mitsuhiko Osaki**[2,3], **Mitsuo Oshimura**[2], **Yasuhito Ishigaki**[4], **Kanya Hamasaki**[5], **Yoshiaki Kodama**[5], **Shinsuke Yuasa**[6], **Keiichi Fukuda**[6], **Kyotaro Hirashima**[7], **Hiroyuki Seimiya**[7], **Hirofumi Koyama**[8], **Takahiko Shimizu**[8], **Minoru Takemoto**[9], **Koutaro Yokote**[9], **Makoto Goto**[10], **Hidetoshi Tahara**[1]*

1 Department of Cellular and Molecular Biology, Graduate School of Biomedical & Health Sciences, Hiroshima University, Hiroshima, Japan, 2 Department of Biomedical Science, Institute of Regenerative Medicine and Biofunction, Graduate School of Medical Science, Tottori University, Yonago, Japan, 3 Division of Pathological Biochemistry, Faculty of Medicine, Tottori University, Yonago, Japan, 4 Medical Research Institute, Kanazawa Medical University, Kahoku, Ishikawa, Japan, 5 Department of Genetics, Radiation Effects Research Foundation, Hiroshima, Japan, 6 Department of Cardiology, Keio University School of Medicine, Tokyo, Japan, 7 Division of Molecular Biotherapy, The Cancer Chemotherapy Center, Japanese Foundation For Cancer Research, Tokyo, Japan, 8 Department of Advanced Aging Medicine, Chiba University Graduate School of Medicine, Chiba, Japan, 9 Department of Clinical Cell Biology and Medicine, Chiba University Graduate School of Medicine, Chiba, Japan, 10 Division of Orthopedic Surgery & Rheumatology, Tokyo Women's Medical University Medical Center East, Tokyo, Japan

Abstract

Werner syndrome (WS) is a premature aging disorder characterized by chromosomal instability and cancer predisposition. Mutations in *WRN* are responsible for the disease and cause telomere dysfunction, resulting in accelerated aging. Recent studies have revealed that cells from WS patients can be successfully reprogrammed into induced pluripotent stem cells (iPSCs). In the present study, we describe the effects of long-term culture on WS iPSCs, which acquired and maintained infinite proliferative potential for self-renewal over 2 years. After long-term cultures, WS iPSCs exhibited stable undifferentiated states and differentiation capacity, and premature upregulation of senescence-associated genes in WS cells was completely suppressed in WS iPSCs despite *WRN* deficiency. WS iPSCs also showed recapitulation of the phenotypes during differentiation. Furthermore, karyotype analysis indicated that WS iPSCs were stable, and half of the descendant clones had chromosomal profiles that were similar to those of parental cells. These unexpected properties might be achieved by induced expression of endogenous telomerase gene during reprogramming, which trigger telomerase reactivation leading to suppression of both replicative senescence and telomere dysfunction in WS cells. These findings demonstrated that reprogramming suppressed premature senescence phenotypes in WS cells and WS iPSCs could lead to chromosomal stability over the long term. WS iPSCs will provide opportunities to identify affected lineages in WS and to develop a new strategy for the treatment of WS.

Editor: Zhongjun Zhou, The University of Hong Kong, Hong Kong

Funding: This work was supported by a Grant-in-Aid for Challenging Exploratory Research No. 25670030 (to A.S) and for Scientific Research No. 20014015 (to H.T) and No. 24590902 (to M.G) from the Ministry of Education, Culture, Sports, Science and Technology of Japan. This work was also supported by a Health and Labor Sciences Research Grant from the Ministry of Health Labor and Welfare of Japan (to A.S). The funders had no role in study design, data collection and analysis, decision to publish, or preparation of the manuscript.

Competing Interests: The authors have declared that no competing interests exist.

* Email: shim@hiroshima-u.ac.jp (AS); toshi@hiroshima-u.ac.jp (HT)

Introduction

Werner syndrome (WS) is a rare human autosomal recessive disorder characterized by early onset of aging-associated diseases, chromosomal instability, and cancer predisposition [1,2]. Fibroblasts from WS patients exhibit premature replicative senescence [3], and *WRN*, a gene responsible for the disease, encodes a RecQ-type DNA helicase [4–7], that is involved in maintenance of chromosome integrity during DNA replication, repair, and recombination [8,9]. WRN helicase is known to interact with a variety of proteins associated with DNA metabolism including

proteins of replication fork progression, base excision repair, and telomere maintenance [8,9]. The dysfunction of WRN helicase causes defects in telomeric lagging-strand synthesis and telomere loss during DNA replication [10]. Further, it is also reported that telomere loss caused by a defect in WRN helicase involves chromosome end fusions that are suppressed by telomerase [11]. These observations suggest that premature senescence in WS cells reflects defects in telomeric lagging-strand synthesis followed by accelerated telomere loss during DNA replication.

Somatic cell reprogramming follows the introduction of several pluripotency genes including Oct3/4, Sox2, Klf4, c-myc, Nanog and Lin-28 into differentiated cells such as dermal fibroblasts, blood cells, and other cell types [12–17]. During reprogramming, somatic cell-specific genes are suppressed, and embryonic stem cell (ESC)-specific pluripotency genes are induced, leading to the generation of iPSCs with undifferentiated states and pluripotency [18]. In addition, ESC-like infinite proliferative potential is directed by induction of the endogenous telomere reverse-transcriptase catalytic subunit (hTERT) gene and the reactivation of telomerase activity during reprogramming [13,18].

Recently, Cheung et al. demonstrated that cells from WS patients were successfully reprogrammed into iPSCs with restored telomere function, suggesting that the induction of hTERT during reprogramming suppresses telomere dysfunction in WS cells lacking *WRN* [19]. However, the effects of long-term culture on the undifferentiated states, self-renewal abilities, and differentiation potentials of WS iPSCs remain unknown. In a previous study, progressive telomere shortening and loss of self-renewal ability were observed in iPSCs from dyskeratosis congenita patient cells in a long-term culture [20], warranting the evaluation of the properties of patient cell-derived iPSCs with telomere dysfunctions over the long term.

In this study, we cultured WS iPSCs with self-renewal capacity and infinite proliferative potential for over 2 years and reported similar properties to those of normal iPSCs including undifferentiated states and differentiation ability. Notably, WS iPSCs maintained stable karyotypes and their potential to recapitulate premature senescence phenotypes during differentiation over the long term. The present data demonstrate that reprogramming suppresses premature senescence phenotypes in WS cells by reversing the aging process and restoring telomere maintenance over the long term.

Materials and Methods

Cell lines

WS patients were diagnosed on the basis of clinical symptoms and *WRN* gene mutations. A0031 WS patient fibroblasts from a 37-year-old male were obtained from Goto Collection of RIKEN Bioresource Center (https://www.brc.riken.jp/lab/cell/english/index_gmc.shtml) [21], and WSCU01 patient fibroblasts were isolated from a 63-year-old Japanese male who was diagnosed at Chiba University. Both fibroblast isolates had type 4/6 heterozygous mutations. TIG-3 human fetal lung-derived fibroblast cells and WS patient-derived fibroblasts were used to generate iPSC lines. PLAT-A cells (kindly provided from Dr. Toshio Kitamura) were used to produce retroviruses [22]. SNL 76/7 (SNL) cells (DS pharma biomedical) were used as feeder layers for reprogramming of fibroblasts and maintenance of iPSCs. The human fibroblast-derived iPSC line iPS-TIG114-4f1 was obtained from the National Institute of Biomedical Innovation [23].

PLAT-A cells, TIG-3 fibroblasts, TIG-114 fibroblasts from the 36-year-old male, and SNL cells were grown in the Dulbecco's modified Eagle's medium (DMEM; Sigma) supplemented with 10% fetal bovine serum (FBS; Hyclone) and antibiotics (Invitrogen). WS fibroblasts were maintained on collagen-coated dishes (Nitta Gelatin), SNL cells were maintained on gelatin-coated dishes (Nitta Gelatin), and iPSCs were maintained in the ES medium comprising Knockout DMEM (Invitrogen) supplemented with 20% Knockout Serum Replacement (Invitrogen), glutamine, non-essential amino acids, β-mercaptoethanol and 4-ng/ml basic FGF. All cells were maintained at 37°C under 5% CO_2 atmosphere.

Generation of iPSCs

The generation of iPSCs was performed as described previously [13]. Briefly, 2×10^6 PLAT-A cells were plated in T25 flasks (Biocoat, BD Falcon), and were transfected with 4 μg pMXs-OCT3/4, SOX2, KLF-4, and c-myc (Addgene) 1 day later. Twenty-four hours after transfection, the culture medium was replaced with a fresh medium and cells were incubated for 24 h prior to harvest of viral supernatants. Viral supernatants containing Yamanaka factors were combined in even ratios.

For reprogramming experiments, 3×10^5 fibroblasts were seeded on 60-mm dishes and were infected with viral supernatants containing Yamanaka factors in the presence of 8 μg/ml polybrene 1 day later. Four days after infection, fibroblasts were harvested, and 1×10^5 cells were reseeded onto mitomycin C-inactivated SNL feeder layers on 100-mm dishes. Twenty-four hours after reseeding, the medium was replaced with the ES medium, and cultures were maintained by replacing the medium every other day. Approximately 30 days after retroviral transduction, emerging iPSC colonies with ESC colony-like flat and round shapes were picked up by mechanical dissection and were plated onto fresh feeder layers on 4-well plates (Thermo Scientific Nunc). Subsequently, iPSC lines were established by successive passages onto fresh feeder layers with split ratios between 1:3 and 1:5 using dispase (Roche Applied Science).

Alkaline phosphatase activity

Undifferentiated states of emerging colonies were examined using alkaline phosphatase staining. After formalin fixation, colonies were stained with reaction buffer containing 100 mM Tris-Cl (pH 8.5), 0.25 mg/ml Naphthol AS-BI phosphate (Sigma) and 0.25 mg/ml fast red violet LB salt (Sigma).

Embryoid body formation and in vitro differentiation

Clumps of iPSCs were transferred to non-adherent polystyrene dishes containing the ES medium without basic FGF to form embryoid bodies (EBs). The medium was replaced every other day. After 8 days of floating culture, EBs were transferred onto gelatin-coated plates and were maintained in DMEM supplemented with 10% FBS, β-mercaptoethanol, and antibiotics for another 8 days. For detection of senescence phenotypes during differentiation, Y-27632-treated iPSCs were dissociated into single cell suspensions with Accutase (Innovative Cell Technologies) and 1×10^4 cells were transferred into 96-well V-shaped bottom plates (Greiner Bio-One) to form evenly sized EBs. After 12 days of EB formation in the ES medium without basic FGF, EBs were cultured in DMEM supplemented with 10% FBS, β-mercaptoethanol, and antibiotics.

Teratoma formation

After harvest, 1×10^6 iPSCs were injected into the testes of a severe combined immunodeficient (SCID) mice (CREA, Japan). Three months after injection, tumors were dissected and were fixed using 4% paraformaldehyde. Subsequently, dissected tumor tissues were embedded in paraffin and were sliced and stained with hematoxylin and eosin.

Western blot

Whole cell lysates were prepared in SDS sample buffer and subjected to electrophoresis on 8% SDS-polyacrylamide gels, and separated proteins were transferred onto PVDF membranes (FluoroTrans W, Pall Corporation). Membranes were blocked with TBS-T containing 5% skim milk and were then incubated with anti-WRN (1:500, 4H12, Abcom) or anti-β-actin (1:30000,

Ac-15, Sigma) monoclonal antibodies for 3 h at room temperature. Membranes were then washed with TBS-T and were incubated with horseradish peroxidase-conjugated anti-mouse IgG (1:5000, NA931V, GE) for 1 h at room temperature. Chemiluminescence reactions were performed using Western Lightning Plus-ECL (PerkinElmer) and were detected using exposure of x-ray films.

Mutation analysis

The DNA fragments mut.4 (c.3139-1G>C) and mut.6 (c.1105C>T) were amplified with the primer pairs WS_mut4_U, GGTAAACGGTGTAGGAGTCTGC and WS_mut4_L, CTTGTGAGAGGCCTATAAACTGG, and WS_mut6_U, TGAAGATTCAACTACTGGGGGAGTAC and WS_ mut6_L, ACGGGAATAAAGTCTGCCAGAACC, respectively, using genomic DNA as a template. Mutations were analyzed by direct sequencing using these PCR primers.

Short tandem repeat (STR) analysis

Genomic DNAs were purified from WS fibroblasts and their derivative iPSC clones using phenol/chloroform extraction and were then used for analysis using a Cell ID System (Promega). PCR products were analyzed using an Applied Biosystems 3130xl Genetic Analyzer and GeneMapper software.

Gene expression profiling

Cy3-labeled total RNAs were hybridized onto Human Genome U133 Plus 2.0 Arrays (GeneChip, Affymetrix). Arrays were then scanned using the GeneChip Scanner 3000 7G (Affymetrix), and the obtained data were analyzed by Affymetrix Expression Console Software. The microarray dataset has been deposited in the NCBI Gene Expression Omnibus database under Series Accession GSE62114.

Measurement of telomere length

Genomic DNAs were digested using $Hinf$I restriction enzyme (TakaraBio), and were subjected to electrophoresis on 1% agarose gels. Size-fractionated DNAs were transferred onto Hybond-N+ membranes (GE). Membranes were hybridized with a digoxigenin-labeled $(CCCTAA)_4$ probe, and TRFs were detected using TeloTAGGG Telomere Length Assays (Roche Applied Science) according to the manufacturer's instructions.

RT-PCR and real-time qRT-PCR analysis of mRNA expression

Total RNA was prepared using RNeasy spin columns (Qiagen) according to the manufacturer's instructions. RT-PCR was performed with 0.1 μg of total RNA using SuperScript One-Step RT-PCR (Invitrogen). Semi-quantitative analysis was performed after converting total RNA into cDNA using a High Capacity RNA-to-cDNA kit (Life Technologies), and real-time PCR was performed using a Rotor-Gene SYBR Green PCR kit (Qiagen). Relative gene expression levels were analyzed according to the ΔΔCt method using Ct values of GAPDH mRNA as an internal control. Primer sequences are listed in Tables S1 and S2.

Immunofluorescence cytochemistry

Following fixation of iPSCs and differentiated cells with 4% paraformaldehyde for 15 min at 4°C, cells were permeabilized with 0.1% Triton X-100, washed with PBS containing 2% BSA, and incubated with primary antibodies diluted in PBS containing 2% BSA.

Primary antibodies against Nanog (1:200, Cell Signaling, D73G4), SSEA-4 (1:200, Cell Signaling, MC813), Tra-1-60 (1:200, Cell Signaling, #4746), Tra-1-81 (1:200, Cell Signaling, #4745), βIII-tubulin (1:200, Millipore, TU-20), desmin (1:200, Neomarkers, RB-9014-P0), vimentin (1:200, Santa Cruz, V9), and α-fetoprotein (1:500, Sigma, HPA010607) were detected using the secondary antibodies Alexa 488-conjugated anti-goat IgG (1:500, Invitrogen, A11055), Alexa 488-conjugated anti-mouse IgG (1:500, Invitrogen, A11001), Alexa 488-conjugated anti-mouse IgM (1:500, Invitrogen, A21042), and Alexa 488-conjugated anti-rabbit IgG (1:500, Invitrogen, A11013). Cell nuclei were stained with 1- μg/ml 4',6-diamidino-2-phenylindole (DAPI).

Karyotype analysis

After culturing iPSCs in the ES medium containing 100-ng/ml colcemid for 5 h at 37°C, cells were harvested using trypsin and were treated with 0.075 M KCl for 15 min at 37°C. Cells were then fixed in Carnoy's fluid, and chromosome slides were prepared. G-banding analysis was conducted using a previously described method [24].

M-FISH was performed with the Multi-color probe kit "24XCyte" (MetaSystems, Altlussheim, Germany) according to the manufacturer's protocol with slight modifications. Briefly, probes were denatured at 75°C for 5 min and were hybridized to metaphase spreads, which were denatured in 0.07 N NaOH at room temperature for 1 min. Slides were then incubated at 37°C for 2 nights and were then washed in 0.4× SSC at 72°C for 2 min, in 2× SSC containing 0.05% Tween 20 at room temperature for 30 s, and in 2× SSC at room temperature for 1 min, and the mounting medium (DAPI, 125 ng/ml) and a cover slip were applied. Acquisition and analysis of M-FISH images were performed using a CytoVision ChromoFluor System (Applied Imaging, Newcastle upon Tyne, UK).

Transduction of hTERT gene

PT67 retrovirus packaging cells (Takara Bio USA, Madison, WI, USA) were transfected with pMSCV-hTERT-puro using GenePorter II according to the manufacturer's protocol. After 24 h, the culture medium was replaced, cells were incubated for a further 24 h period, and viral supernatants were harvested, A0031 and WSCU01 WS fibroblasts were infected with viral supernatant in the presence of 8 μg/ml polybrene. Confluent infected cells were then split into 2 new dishes, and puromycin selection of infected cells was initiated at the following passage. Confluent infected cells were then passaged in 4-fold dilutions, leading to an increase in 2 population doubling levels for each passage.

SA-β-gal assay

SA-β-gal staining was performed as described by Debacq-Chainiaux et al. [25].

Ethical statement

This study was approved by the Ethics Review Board of the Graduate School of Medicine, Chiba University and was conducted in accordance with the Declaration of Helsinki. Written informed consents were obtained from patients prior to tissue harvesting and iPSC generation, and patients were entitled to the protection of confidential information. Genome/gene analyses performed in this study were approved by the Ethics Committee for Human Genome/Gene Analysis Research at Hiroshima University. All animal experiments were performed in strict compliance with the protocol approved by the Institutional Animal Care and Use Committee of Tottori University (13-Y-

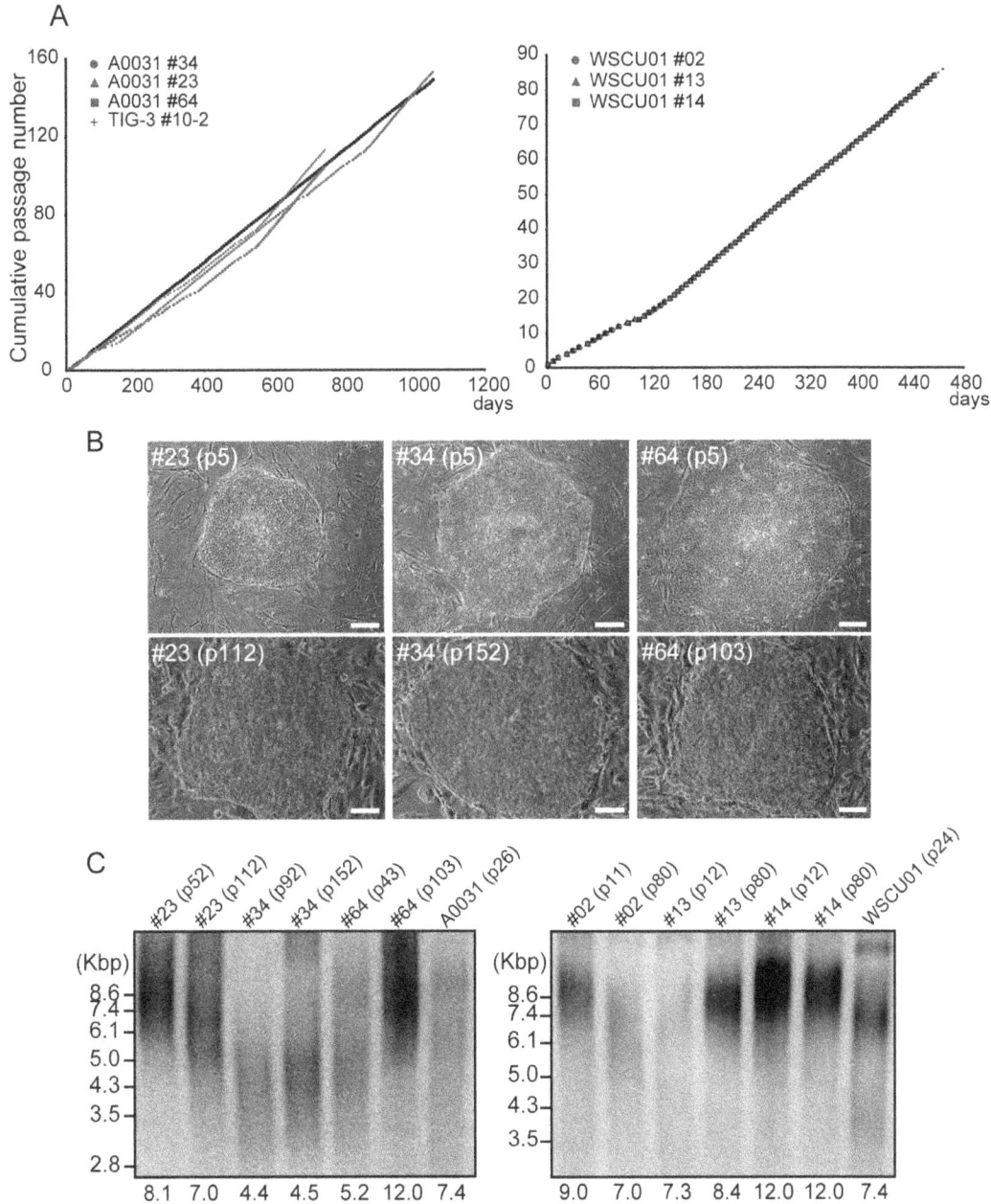

Figure 1. Infinite Proliferation of WS iPSCs after Long-Term Culture. (A) Cumulative passage number for WS iPSCs. (B) Colony morphologies of A0031-derived WS iPSC clones in early and late passages. Bars = 100 μm. (C) TRF length analysis of WS iPSC clones in early and late passages.

18), and the Animal Care and Use Committee of Chiba University (25–131). All recombinant DNA experiments were performed in strict conformance with the guidelines of the Institutional Recombinant DNA Experiment Safety Committee at Hiroshima University.

Results

Infinite proliferative potential of WS iPSCs after long-term culture

To determine whether reprogramming provides WS cells with infinite proliferative potential, we generated iPSCs from WS patient fibroblasts. Morphologically distinct colonies from parental cells emerged after transduction of Yamanaka factors using retroviruses and showed elevated alkaline phosphatase activity (Figures S1A and S1B). Colonies were picked up, and 6 WS iPSC lines were established using fibroblasts from 2 independent WS patients after several passages. In western blotting analysis using an anti-WRN antibody, WRN protein was not detected in WS iPSCs but was expressed in both normal fibroblasts and iPSCs (Figure S2A). Direct sequencing analysis of WS iPSCs identified compound heterozygous Mut4/Mut6 mutations in the *WRN* gene similar to those observed in parental cells, and the derivation of WS iPSCs from parental cells was confirmed by STR analysis (Figures S2B and S2C). Finally, the 6 WS iPSC lines #23, #34, and #64 from A0031 and #02, #13, and#14 from WSCU01 were successfully established.

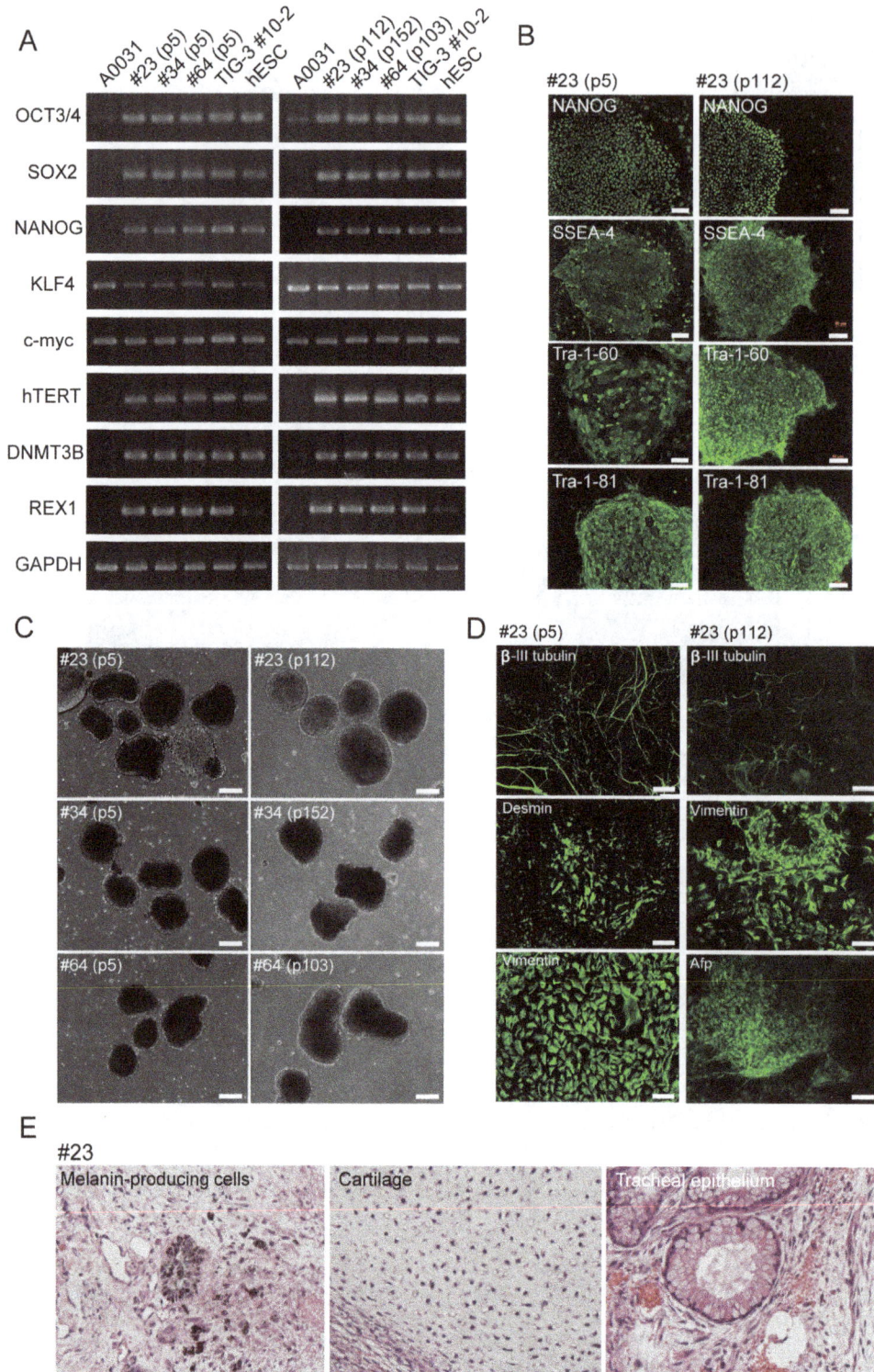

Figure 2. Sustained ESC-like characteristics of WS iPSCs after Long-Term Culture. (A) Expression of pluripotency genes in A0031-derived WS iPSC clones in early and late passages. (B) Expression of hESC markers in A0031-derived WS iPSC clone #23 in early and late passages. Bars = 100 μm. (C) EB formation in A0031-derived WS iPSC clones from early and late passages. Bars = 100 μm. (D) Immunocytochemical analysis of differentiation of EBs into 3 germ layers for A0031-derived iPSC clone #23 in early and late passages. β-III tubulin (ectoderm), desmin (mesoderm), vimentin (mesoderm and parietal endoderm), and α-fetoprotein (Afp, endoderm). Bars = 100 μm. (E) Hematoxylin and eosin histology of teratomas from A0031-derived iPSC clone #23. Formation of all 3 germ layers is shown including melanin-producing cells (ectoderm), cartilage (mesoderm), and tracheal epithelium (endoderm).

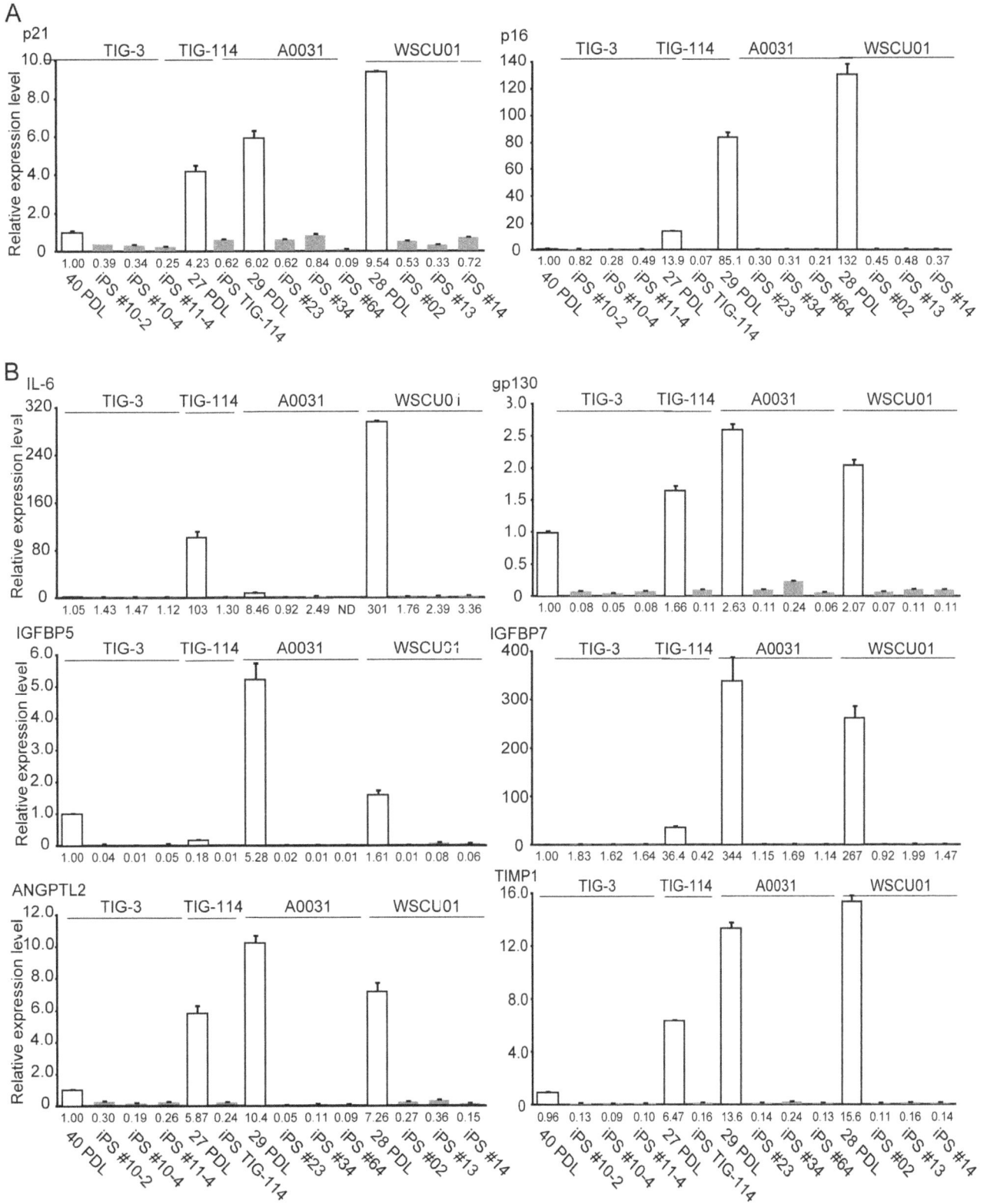

Figure 3. Suppression of Senescence-Associated Gene Expression in Reprogrammed WS iPSCs. (A) Expression of CDKI genes in parental fibroblasts and iPSCs. White columns show relative expression levels in the parental fibroblasts TIG-3, TIG-114, A0031, and WSCU01, and gray columns show those of their derived iPSC clones. Numbers under the horizontal axis in each graph show relative values in mRNA expression compared with that in TIG-3 fibroblasts. Values represent means of three technical replicates ± SD. (B) Expression of SASP genes in parental fibroblasts and iPSCs. Each graph is shown as in (A).

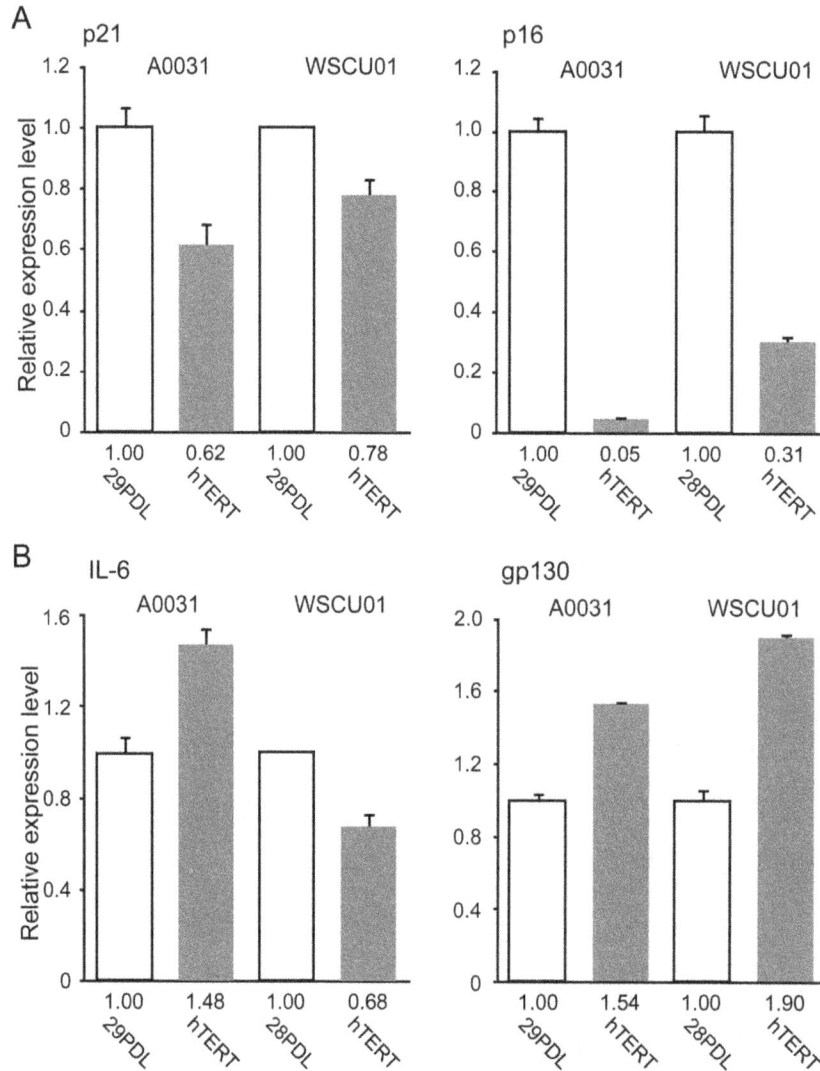

Figure 4. Reprogramming of the SASP gene loci is mediated by factors other than activated telomerase. (A) Expression of CDKI genes in WS fibroblasts and their hTERT-transduced derivatives. White columns show relative expression levels in A0031 and WSCU01 fibroblasts, and gray columns show those of their hTERT-transduced derivatives. Numbers under the horizontal axis in each graph show relative values in mRNA expression compared with that in parental fibroblasts. Values represent means of three technical replicates ± SD. (B) Expression levels of SASP genes in WS fibroblasts and their hTERT-transduced derivatives. Each graph is shown as in (C).

WS iPSC lines from A0031 were cultured for 120 continuous passages over 2 years without morphological changes or loss of growth capacity (Figures 1A and 1B). Moreover, iPSC lines from WSCU01 proliferated for a year (Figures 1A and S1C). Average terminal restriction fragment (TRF) lengths in clones #23, #34, and #64 (A0031) were decreased, invariable, and increased during long-term culture, respectively, and similar telomere dynamics were observed in WSCU01-derived iPSC clones (Figure 1C).

Sustained ESC-like characters of WS iPSCs after long-term culture

To determine the persistence of ESC-like characteristics in WS iPSCs, we compared undifferentiated states and differentiation potentials between WS iPSCs from early and late passages. WS iPSC lines expressed pluripotency genes and hESC-specific surface markers during early passages (around p10), and during late passages (around p100; Figures 2A, 2B, S3 and S4). These iPSC lines also showed sustained formation of embryoid bodies and differentiation into 3 germ layers (Figures 2C, 2D, and S5). Furthermore, at around p50, WS iPSC lines generated teratomas that contained tissue structures of all 3 germ layers. These were consistent with those shown in normal iPSC lines after transplantation into the testes of SCID mice (Figures 2E and S6). Thus, reprogrammed WS fibroblasts acquired infinite proliferative potential, and the ESC-like characteristics of the resulting iPSCs were maintained for more than 2 years.

Suppression of senescence-associated gene expression in WS iPSCs after long-term culture

Global gene expression analysis using DNA chips showed pronounced similarities among pluripotent stem cells including WS iPSCs. However, marked differences between WS iPSC and WS fibroblasts were observed (Figure S7). Heat map analysis also showed a high analogy of global gene expression profiles in these

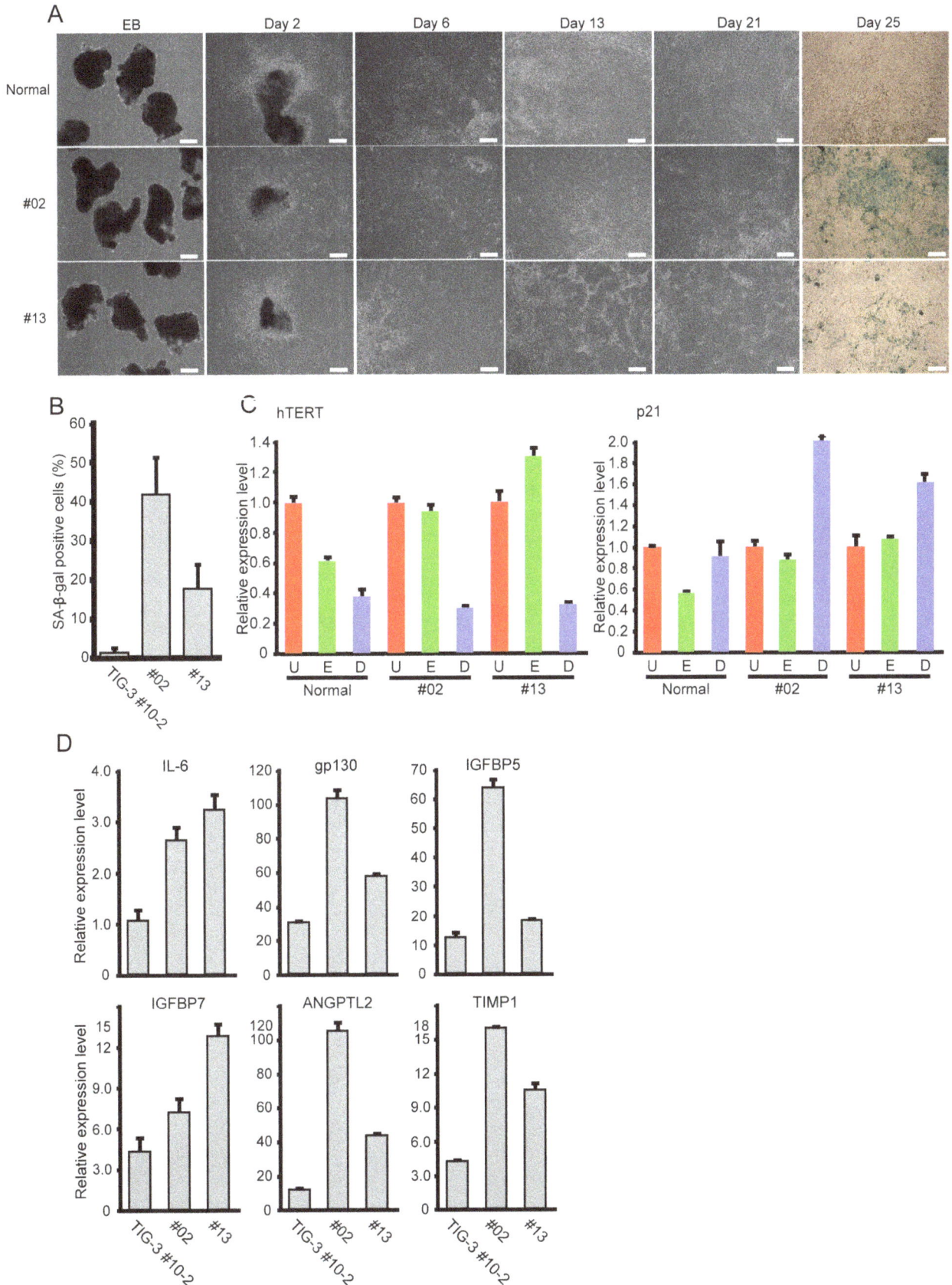

Figure 5. Recapitulation of Premature Senescence Phenotypes in Differentiated Cells from WS iPSCs. (A) Differentiation of EBs from normal (TIG-3) and WS (WSCU01 #02 and #13) iPSCs. Differentiated cells from WS iPSCs showed premature senescence. SA-β-gal staining was performed on day 25 of differentiation. Bars = 100 μm. (B) Percentage of senescent cells after 25 days of differentiation. SA-β-gal-positive cells were

counted in three randomly selected fields with 40× magnification. Values represent means of the three fields ± SD. (C) Expression of hTERT and p21 mRNAs in undifferentiated iPSCs ("U," red columns), EBs after 12 days of formation ("E," green columns), and differentiated cells after 25 days of differentiation ("D," blue columns). Values represent means of three technical replicates ± SD. (D) Expression of SASP genes in differentiated cells from normal (TIG-3) and WS (WSCU01 #02 and #13) iPSCs after 25 days of differentiation. Graphs shows fold changes relative to undifferentiated iPSCs. Values represent means of three technical replicates ± SD.

pluripotent stem cell lines, but distinctly different profiles from those of WS fibroblasts (Figures S8A). Recent studies of aging have identified senescence-induced inflammatory and secretory factors that are collectively referred to as the senescence-associated secretory phenotype (SASP) and are the hallmarks of aging. It is widely accepted that age-associated inflammatory responses contribute to human aging mechanisms [26]. Accordingly, we observed downregulation of SASP secretory factors, including inflammatory cytokines, growth factors and MMPs, in both normal and WS iPSCs compared with WS fibroblasts (Figures S8B). Subsequently, we performed real-time qRT-PCR analysis using PDL-matched normal and patient fibroblasts, and their iPSC derivatives which were maintained in long-term culture. Although relative expression levels of the senescence-associated cyclin-dependent kinase inhibitor (CDKI) genes *p21Waf1/Cip1* and *p16INK4a* in normal fibroblasts correlated with the donor age, the expression levels of these genes were higher in WS fibroblasts than in normal fibroblasts, indicating that replicative senescence was prematurely induced in WS cells (Figure 3A). However, expression levels of these genes were significantly reduced in all iPSC clones from normal and WS cells (Figure 3A), suggesting that these gene loci are reprogrammed to the same degree in normal and WS iPSCs. Thus, we examined the expression of the typical SASP genes *IL-6* and *gp130* [27] and found higher expression levels in WS fibroblasts than in normal fibroblasts (Figure 3B). Moreover, expression levels of these genes drastically decreased in both normal and WS iPSCs compared with parental fibroblasts. Similarly, expression levels of the SASP genes *IGFBP5*, *IGFBP7*, *ANGPTL2*, and *TIMP1* ([28–31] were significantly decreased in both normal and WS iPSCs compared with parental fibroblasts (Figures 3B).

Reprogramming of the SASP gene loci is mediated by factors other than activated telomerase

WS fibroblasts were previously shown to bypass premature senescence following introduction of the telomerase gene *hTERT*

[32], Similarly, the present WS cells bypassed premature replicative senescence, and hTERT allowed cell division for over 150 PDL in A0031 cells, and 40 PDL in WSCU01 cells compared with parental cells that became senescent at less than 30 PDL (Figures S9A and S9B). TRF length analysis showed that hTERT-expressing WS cells acquired longer telomeres during passages than parental cells (Figures S9C). To examine whether the expression of hTERT was sufficient to suppress the upregulation of aging-associated genes in WS cells, we compared expression levels of CDKI and SASP genes between WS fibroblasts and their hTERT-expressing derivatives. Whereas a decline in p21waf1/cip1 and p16INK4a mRNA expression was observed in hTERT-expressing cells (Figure 4A), IL-6 and gp130 expression was not suppressed following the introduction of hTERT, suggesting that reprogramming of the SASP gene loci is mediated by factors other than activated telomerase (Figure 4B). The present data show complete suppression of premature senescence phenotypes in WS cells using transcription factor-induced reprogramming and suggest that persistence of the undifferentiated state and pluripotency are crucial for reversing the aging process.

Recapitulation of premature senescence phenotypes in differentiated cells from WS iPSCs

To establish cell lineages that prematurely senesced, EBs consisting of equal numbers of iPSCs maintained in long-term culture were differentiated in serum-containing medium. Differentiated cells from WS iPSC-derived EBs were outgrown less rapidly than those from normal iPSC-derived EBs (Figure 5A, Day 2). These cells exhibited flat and enlarged morphology (Figure 5A, Day 6, 13, and 21) and became positive for SA-β-gal staining (Figure 5A, Day 25, and Figure 5B). Whereas expression levels of hTERT were downregulated equally in differentiated cells from normal and WS iPSCs, p21 mRNA was more highly induced in differentiated cells from WS iPSCs than those from normal iPSCs (Figure 5C). Expression levels of the SASP genes were also significantly increased in differentiated cells from WS iPSCs

Table 1. Results of chromosome analysis of WS iPSC clones and their parenral cells.

Cell lines	Numbers of cells analyzed by G-banding	Numbers of cells analyzed by M-FISH	Karyotypes
A0031	20 (13/7)	ND	46,XY,del(8)(q22q24)/46,XY,t(1;14)(p34.1;q13),t(4;7)(p15.2;q22),del(8)(q22q24)
iPS#23	20	10	46,XY,t(1;14)(p34.1;q13),t(4;7)(p15.2;q22),del(8)(q22q24),der(21)t(17;21)(?;q22.3)
iPS#34	20	10	46,XY,t(1;14)(p34.1;q13),t(4;7)(p15.2;q22),del(8)(q22q24)
iPS#64	20	10	46,XY,t(1;14)(p34.1;q13),t(4;7)(p15.2;q22),del(8)(q22q24),der(19)t(2;19)(?;p13.3)
WSCU01	20	ND	46,XY,normal
iPS#02	20	10	47,XY,+del(20)(p?)
iPS#13	20	10	46,XY,normal
iPS#14	20	10	46,XY,normal

Abbreviations: t, translocation; del, deletion; der, derivative chromosome; p, short arm; q, long arm.

A A0031
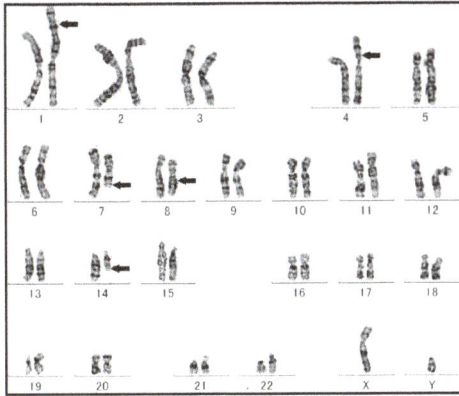

B #34
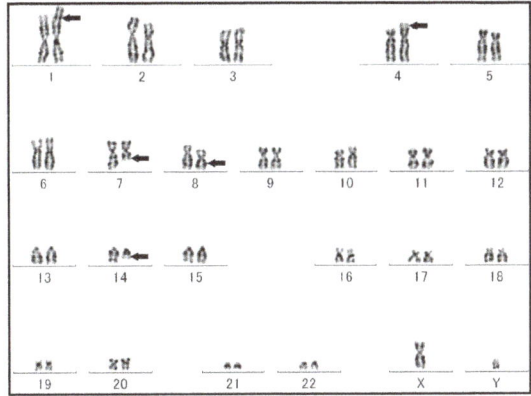

C #23
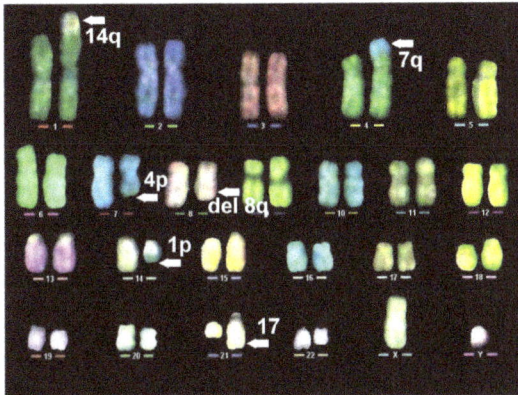

F #02
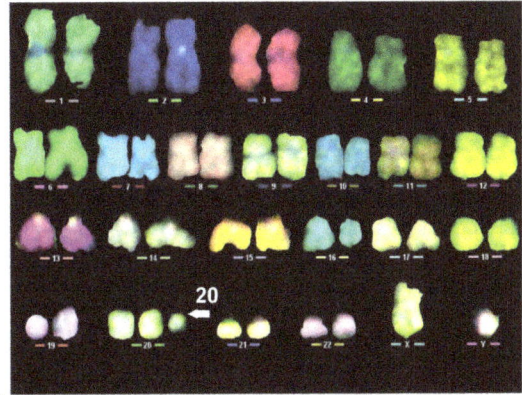

D #34
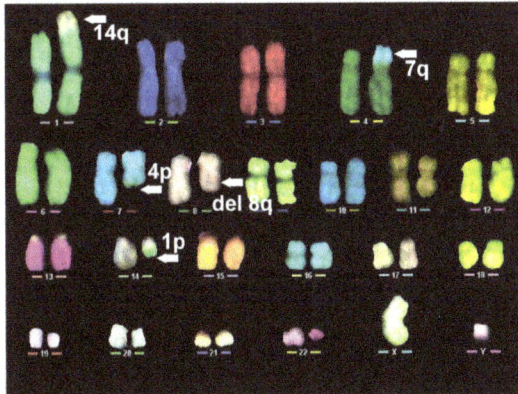

G #13
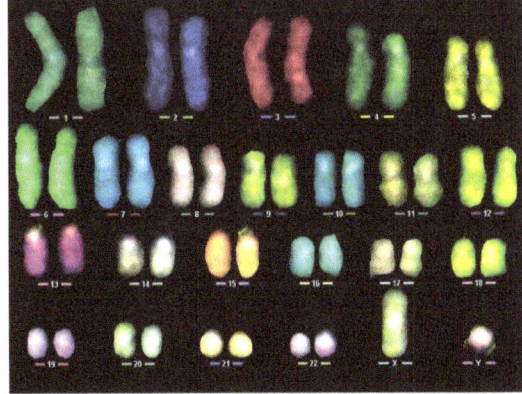

E #64
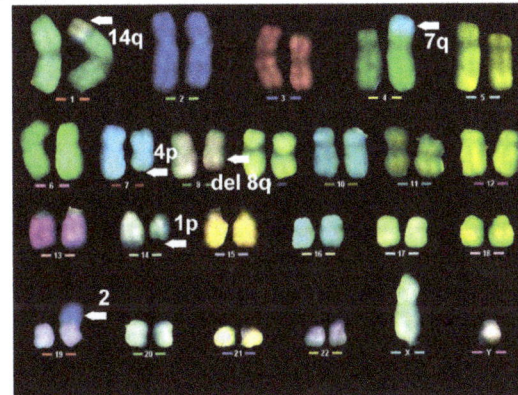

H #14
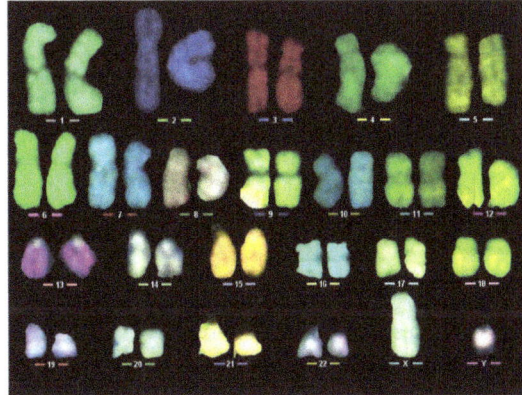

Figure 6. Karyotype Analysis of WS iPSCs. Chromosomal profiles of G-band analysis. (A) Parental A0031 fibroblast and (B) A0031-derived iPSC clone #34. Arrows indicate translocation breakpoints. Chromosomal profiles of M-FISH analysis. A0031-derived iPSC clones (C) #23, (D) #34, and (E) #64 and WSCU01-derived iPSC clones (F) #02, (G) #13, and (H) #14. Arrows indicate translocation breakpoints or an extra chromosome.

compared with those from normal iPSCs (Figure 5D). These results demonstrated recapitulation of premature senescence phenotypes with downregulation of hTERT in differentiated cells from WS iPSCs.

Karyotype analysis of WS iPSCs

WS is characterized by genomic instability, and gene translocation events have been observed during culture of patient-derived cells [33]. Because reprogramming of somatic cells and subsequent maintenance of iPSCs involves extensive cell division, WS iPSCs may acquire additional chromosomal abnormalities. Thus, we compared chromosomal profiles of long-term cultured WS iPSC clones with those of parental WS fibroblasts by karyotype analysis. The subsequent G-banding stain and multicolor fluorescence *in situ* hybridization (M-FISH) analysis are summarized in Table 1.

Chromosomal profiles of parental A0031 WS fibroblasts showed mosaicism with the following abnormal karyotypes: 46, XY with a deletion in 8q and 46, XY with a deletion in 8q along with reciprocal translocations between 1p and 14q, and 4p and 7q (Figure 6A). These karyotypes support previous observations of chromosomal instability in WS cells [33]. Whereas, 1 of the derived iPSC clones (#34) had the same chromosomal profile as its parent cells (Figures 6B and 6D), the other 2 A0031-derived iPSC clones (#23 and #64) had the translocations 21q and 19p, respectively, in addition to those of the parental karyotype (Table 1, Figures 6C and 6E). Moreover, whereas parental WSCU01 fibroblasts and 2 of their derived iPSC clones (#13 and #14) had normal karyotypes (Table 1, Figures 6G and 6H), the remaining iPSC clone #02 carried the abnormal karyotype 47 (XY with an additional aberrant chromosome derived from chromosome 20; Table 1, Figure 6F).

The observation that 3 of 6 WS iPSC clones had the same karyotypes as their parental cells after approximately 100 passages suggests that karyotypes of WS cells are stabilized following reprogramming.

Discussion

In this study, we demonstrated that WS fibroblasts could be reprogrammed into iPSCs using Yamanaka factors, and the resulting iPSCs showed unlimited proliferative capacity that was sufficient for self-renewal over a period of 2 years. WS iPSCs also exhibited undifferentiated states and differentiation potential after long-term culture. Subsequently, we showed that WS iPSCs maintain immortality and ESC-like characteristics that indicate corrected telomere dysfunction following reprogramming of WS cells. Although WRN was not essential for generation of iPSCs, WRN helicase may protect genome integrity by mechanism other than the maintenance of telomere in iPSCs.

TRF length analysis indicated that WS iPSC lines maintained telomere with size variation in each clone. It is known that human iPSCs derived from normal somatic cells showed varied telomere length, and variation of telomere length among human iPSC clones is thought to partly depend on acquired telomerase activity associated with their reprogrammed states [34,35]. Therefore, variation of telomere length observed among WS iPSC clones would be due to clonal variation in telomerase activity rather than telomere dysfunction associated with *WRN* deficiency.

Normal human iPSCs are known to acquire genomic instability with a high incidence of additions, deletions and translocations [36,37]. In contrast, chromosomal aberrations are frequently caused by telomere dysfunctions in WS fibroblasts following the induction of cell cycle progression [11]. Nonetheless, the present data show unexpected maintenance of chromosomal profiles in WS iPSC clones during long-term culture for more than 100 passages although half of these clones acquired additional chromosomal abnormalities. Previously, the introduction of hTERT reduced the chromosomal aberrations in cells from WS patients [11]. In agreement, the present data indicate endogenous hTERT expression in WS iPSCs, but not in parental fibroblasts, suggesting that reprogramming suppresses chromosomal instability in WS cells by reactivating telomerase.

Previous studies show that WS fibroblasts express inflammatory cytokines [38] and WS is associated with inflammatory conditions such as atherosclerosis, diabetes and osteoporosis [39–43]. The present data indicate that both CDKI and SASP genes are prematurely induced in WS fibroblasts compared with PDL-matched normal fibroblasts. However, expression levels of these genes were completely suppressed in WS iPSCs to the same degree observed in normal iPSCs. In contrast, hTERT did not suppress SASP genes in WS fibroblasts, as shown by previous study [44], although a decline in p21waf1/cip1 and p16INK4a mRNAs was observed. Taken together, these observations suggest that pluripotency-associated transcription factor-induced reprogramming reverses the aging process in both normal and WS cells. Furthermore, differentiated cells from EBs of long-term cultured WS iPSCs showed premature senescence phenotypes, thus demonstrating that WS iPSCs stably maintained their potential to recapitulate premature senescence phenotypes during differentiation over the long term. In addition, embryoid body-mediated iPSC differentiation recapitulated premature senescence phenotypes in WS iPSCs, suggesting that it would provide a simple and rapid way to identify cell lineages affected in WS.

In the present study, we demonstrated the potential of WS iPSCs to proliferate infinitely and differentiate into various cell types, which could be used to provide patient cells in large quantities over the long term. Because WS-specific iPSCs may be differentiated into multiple cell types, their experimental use may resolve the major pathogenic processes of WS for which cell types available from patients are usually limited to lymphocytes and/or fibroblasts. The present technologies may also be used to develop cell transplantation therapies for WS patients using gene-corrected patient cells. The present observations indicate that WS iPSCs may be a powerful tool for understanding normal aging and the pathogenesis of WS.

Supporting Information

Figure S1 Generation of WS iPSCs. (A) Generation of iPSCs. Normal (TIG-3) and Werner syndrome (A0031 and WSCU01) fibroblasts are shown in the left panels, and emergence of morphologically distinct ESC-like colonies from parental cells is shown in the right panels. (B) Alkaline phosphatase activity of ESC-like colonies derived from TIG-3 and A0031 fibroblasts. (C) Colony morphologies of WSCU01-derived WS iPSC clones in early and late passages. Bars = 100 μm.

Figure S2　Evidences that WS iPSCs were derived from patients. (A) Western blot analysis of WRN helicase protein in WS iPSCs. (B) Direct sequencing analysis identified compound heterozygous mut.4/mut.6 mutations in WS iPSCs. Mut.4 is a C to G substitution at the splice-donor site bordered by exon 26, as shown by an arrow in the illustration of the double-strand base sequence. Obtained pherograms show antisense peak shapes. A peak corresponding to mut.4 in normal TIG-3 fibroblast shows a single "C," whereas the WS iPSC clone #34 from A0031 fibroblasts gave double peaks showing "G" in addition to "C." Mut.6 is a T to C substitution in exon 9. A peak corresponding to mut.6 in normal cells showed a single "C," whereas WS iPSC gave double peaks showing "T" in addition to "C." C, blue; G, black; T, red; A, green. (C) STR analysis of A0031-derived iPSC clone #34, showing that iPSC clone #34 was derived from the parental A0031 fibroblasts.

Figure S3　Expression of pluripotency genes in WSCU01-derived WS iPSC clones in early and late passages.

Figure S4　Expression of hESC markers in WS iPSCs in early and late passages. A0031-derived clones #34, and #64, and WSCU01-derived clones #02, #13, and #14 are shown. Bars = 100 μm.

Figure S5　Immunocytochemistry for differentiation of embryoid bodies into 3 germ layers for WS iPSCs in early and late passages. A0031-derived clones #34, and #64, and WSCU01-derived clones #02, #13, and #14 are shown. Bars = 100 μm.

Figure S6　Hematoxylin and eosin histology of teratomas derived from iPSCs. Hematoxylin and eosin histology of teratomas derived from iPSCs. The normal TIG-3 fibroblast-derived clone #10-2, A0031-derived clones #34, and #64, and the WSCU01-derived clone #02 are shown. Formation of all 3 germ layers is shown with melanin-producing cells and glial tissue (ectoderm), cartilage (mesoderm) and intestinal epithelia. Glands are lined by columnar epithelia and tracheal epithelium (endoderm).

Figure S7　Figure Scatter plots comparing gene expression profiles.

Figure S8　Analysis of senescence-associated gene expression in iPSCs. (A) Heat map analysis of WS iPSC #34 and parental WS A0031 fibroblasts, normal TIG-3 fibroblast-derived iPSCs, and hESC; 3277 probes with >5-fold differences in expression between A0031 fibroblast and WS iPSC were included in the heat map. (B) Heat map analysis of the gene profiles of secreted protein probes with >2-fold differences in expression between A0031 fibroblasts and the 3 pluripotent stem cell lines WS iPSC, TIG-3 iPSC, and hESC.

Figure S9　hTERT bypassed premature replicative senescence of WS fibroblasts. (A) Morphologies of growing normal TIG-3 fibroblasts, and A0031 and WSCU01 WS fibroblasts. WS fibroblasts showed premature senescence. SA-β-gal staining was performed for WSCU01 (lower). Bars = 100 μm. (B) Cumulative population doubling levels for hTERT-expressing WS cells. (C) TRF lengths of A0031 fibroblasts and their TERT-transduced derivatives.

Table S1

Table S2

Acknowledgments

We are grateful to Miho Kusuda-Furue (National Institute of Biomedical Innovation), Hidenori Akutsu (National Center for Child Health and Development) and Haruhiko Koseki (RCAI RIKEN) for their help, encouragement and suggestions. We also thank M. K. F and Bunsyo Shiotani for the critical review of draft manuscripts, and the Analysis Center of Life Science, Natural Science Center for Basic Research and Development of Hiroshima University for processing microarray data.

Author Contributions

Conceived and designed the experiments: AS. Performed the experiments: AS HK KZ YS YK MO MO HK TS KH HS YI KH YK. Analyzed the data: AS YK MO MO TS KH HS YI KH YK. Contributed reagents/materials/analysis tools: MG MT KY SY KF HT. Wrote the paper: AS MG. Final approval of the version to be published: AS HT.

References

1. Goto M, Miller RW, Ishikawa Y, Sugano H (1996) Excess of rare cancers in Werner syndrome (adult progeria). Cancer Epidemiol Biomarkers Prev 5: 239–246.
2. Goto M (2000) Werner's syndrome: from clinics to genetics. Clin Exp Rheumatol 18: 760–766.
3. Salk D, Au K, Hoehn H, Martin GM (1981) Effects of radical-scavenging enzymes and reduced oxygen exposure on growth and chromosome abnormalities of Werner syndrome cultured skin fibroblasts. Hum Genet 57: 269–275.
4. Yu CE, Oshima J, Fu YH, Wijsman EM, Hisama F, et al. (1996) Positional cloning of the Werner's syndrome gene. Science 272: 258–262.
5. Oshima J, Yu CE, Piussan C, Klein G, Jabkowski J, et al. (1996) Homozygous and compound heterozygous mutations at the Werner syndrome locus. Hum Mol Genet 5: 1909–1913.
6. Goto M, Imamura O, Kuromitsu J, Matsumoto T, Yamabe Y, et al. (1997) Analysis of helicase gene mutations in Japanese Werner's syndrome patients. Hum Genet 99: 191–193.
7. Matsumoto T, Imamura O, Yamabe Y, Kuromitsu J, Tokutake Y, et al. (1997) Mutation and haplotype analyses of the Werner's syndrome gene based on its genomic structure: genetic epidemiology in the Japanese population. Hum Genet 100: 123–130.
8. Shimamoto A, Sugimoto M, Furuichi Y (2004) Molecular biology of Werner syndrome. Int J Clin Oncol 9: 288–298.
9. Rossi ML, Ghosh AK, Bohr VA (2010) Roles of Werner syndrome protein in protection of genome integrity. DNA Repair (Amst) 9: 331–344.
10. Crabbe L, Verdun RE, Haggblom CI, Karlseder J (2004) Defective telomere lagging strand synthesis in cells lacking WRN helicase activity. Science 306: 1951–1953.
11. Crabbe L, Jauch A, Naeger CM, Holtgreve-Grez H, Karlseder J (2007) Telomere dysfunction as a cause of genomic instability in Werner syndrome. Proc Natl Acad Sci U S A 104: 2205–2210.
12. Takahashi K, Yamanaka S (2006) Induction of pluripotent stem cells from mouse embryonic and adult fibroblast cultures by defined factors. Cell 126: 663–676.
13. Takahashi K, Tanabe K, Ohnuki M, Narita M, Ichisaka T, et al. (2007) Induction of pluripotent stem cells from adult human fibroblasts by defined factors. Cell 131: 861–872.
14. Yu J, Vodyanik MA, Smuga-Otto K, Antosiewicz-Bourget J, Frane JL, et al. (2007) Induced pluripotent stem cell lines derived from human somatic cells. Science 318: 1917–1920.
15. Aoi T, Yae K, Nakagawa M, Ichisaka T, Okita K, et al. (2008) Generation of pluripotent stem cells from adult mouse liver and stomach cells. Science 321: 699–702.
16. Stadtfeld M, Hochedlinger K (2010) Induced pluripotency: history, mechanisms, and applications. Genes Dev 24: 2239–2263.

17. Okita K, Yamanaka S (2011) Induced pluripotent stem cells: opportunities and challenges. Philos Trans R Soc Lond B Biol Sci 366: 2198–2207.

18. Stadtfeld M, Maherali N, Breault DT, Hochedlinger K (2008) Defining molecular cornerstones during fibroblast to iPS cell reprogramming in mouse. Cell Stem Cell 2: 230–240.

19. Cheung HH, Liu X, Canterel-Thouennon L, Li L, Edmonson C, et al. (2014) Telomerase protects werner syndrome lineage-specific stem cells from premature aging. Stem Cell Reports 2: 534–546.

20. Batista LF, Pech MF, Zhong FL, Nguyen HN, Xie KT, et al. (2011) Telomere shortening and loss of self-renewal in dyskeratosis congenita induced pluripotent stem cells. Nature 474: 399–402.

21. Goto M, Ishikawa Y, Sugimoto M, Furuichi Y (2013) Werner syndrome: A changing pattern of clinical manifestations in Japan (1917~2008). Biosci Trends 7: 13–22.

22. Morita S, Kojima T, Kitamura T (2000) Plat-E: an efficient and stable system for transient packaging of retroviruses. Gene Ther 7: 1063–1066.

23. Amps K, Andrews PW, Anyfantis G, Armstrong L, Avery S, et al. (2011) Screening ethnically diverse human embryonic stem cells identifies a chromosome 20 minimal amplicon conferring growth advantage. Nat Biotechnol 29: 1132–1144.

24. Ohtaki K, Sposto R, Kodama Y, Nakano M, Awa AA (1994) Aneuploidy in somatic cells of in utero exposed A-bomb survivors in Hiroshima. Mutat Res 316: 49–58.

25. Debacq-Chainiaux F, Erusalimsky JD, Campisi J, Toussaint O (2009) Protocols to detect senescence-associated beta-galactosidase (SA-betagal) activity, a biomarker of senescent cells in culture and in vivo. Nat Protoc 4: 1798–1806.

26. Goto M (2008) Inflammaging (inflammation + aging): A driving force for human aging based on an evolutionarily antagonistic pleiotropy theory? Biosci Trends 2: 218–230.

27. Salama R, Sadaie M, Hoare M, Narita M (2014) Cellular senescence and its effector programs. Genes Dev 28: 99–114.

28. Kojima H, Kunimoto H, Inoue T, Nakajima K (2012) The STAT3-IGFBP5 axis is critical for IL-6/gp130-induced premature senescence in human fibroblasts. Cell Cycle 11:

29. Wajapeyee N, Serra RW, Zhu X, Mahalingam M, Green MR (2008) Oncogenic BRAF induces senescence and apoptosis through pathways mediated by the secreted protein IGFBP7. Cell 132: 363–374.

30. Tabata M, Kadomatsu T, Fukuhara S, Miyata K, Ito Y, et al. (2009) Angiopoietin-like protein 2 promotes chronic adipose tissue inflammation and obesity-related systemic insulin resistance. Cell Metab 10: 178–188.

31. Gilbert LA, Hemann MT (2010) DNA damage-mediated induction of a chemoresistant niche. Cell 143: 355–366.

32. Wyllie FS, Jones CJ, Skinner JW, Haughton MF, Wallis C, et al. (2000) Telomerase prevents the accelerated cell ageing of Werner syndrome fibroblasts. Nat Genet 24: 16–17.

33. Salk D, Au K, Hoehn H, Stenchever MR, Martin GM (1981) Evidence of clonal attenuation, clonal succession, and clonal expansion in mass cultures of aging Werner's syndrome fibroblasts. Cytogenet Cell Genet 30: 108–117.

34. Mathew R, Jia W, Sharma A, Zhao Y, Clarke LE, et al. (2010) Robust activation of the human but not mouse telomerase gene during the induction of pluripotency. FASEB J 24: 2702–2715.

35. Vaziri H, Chapman K, Guigova A, Teichroeb J, Lacher M, et al. (2010) Spontaneous reversal of the developmental aging of normal human cells following transcriptional reprogramming. Regen Med 5: 345–363.

36. Taapken SM, Nisler BS, Newton MA, Sampsell-Barron TL, Leonhard KA, et al. (2011) Karotypic abnormalities in human induced pluripotent stem cells and embryonic stem cells. Nat Biotechnol 29: 313–314.

37. Martins-Taylor K, Nisler BS, Taapken SM, Compton T, Crandall L, et al. (2011) Recurrent copy number variations in human induced pluripotent stem cells. Nat Biotechnol 29: 488–491.

38. Kumar S, Vinci JM, Millis AJ, Baglioni C (1993) Expression of interleukin-1 alpha and beta in early passage fibroblasts from aging individuals. Exp Gerontol 28: 505–513.

39. Murano S, Nakazawa A, Saito I, Masuda M, Morisaki N, et al. (1997) Increased blood plasminogen activator inhibitor-1 and intercellular adhesion molecule-1 as possible risk factors of atherosclerosis in Werner syndrome. Gerontology 43 Suppl 1: 43–52.

40. Yokote K, Hara K, Mori S, Kadowaki T, Saito Y, et al. (2004) Dysadipocytokinemia in werner syndrome and its recovery by treatment with pioglitazone. Diabetes Care 27: 2562–2563.

41. Rubin CD, Zerwekh JE, Reed-Gitomer BY, Pak CY (1992) Characterization of osteoporosis in a patient with Werner's syndrome. J Am Geriatr Soc 40: 1161–1163.

42. Davis T, Kipling D (2006) Werner Syndrome as an example of inflamm-aging: possible therapeutic opportunities for a progeroid syndrome? Rejuvenation Res 9: 402–407.

43. Goto M, Sugimoto K, Hayashi S, Ogino T, Sugimoto M, et al. (2012) Aging-associated inflammation in healthy Japanese individuals and patients with Werner syndrome. Exp Gerontol 47: 936–939.

44. Choi D, Whittier PS, Oshima J, Funk WD (2001) Telomerase expression prevents replicative senescence but does not fully reset mRNA expression patterns in Werner syndrome cell strains. FASEB J 15: 1014–1020.

13

Amelioration of Reproduction-Associated Oxidative Stress in a Viviparous Insect Is Critical to Prevent Reproductive Senescence

Veronika Michalkova[1,2,9], **Joshua B. Benoit**[1*,9,¤], **Geoffrey M. Attardo**[1], **Jan Medlock**[3], **Serap Aksoy**[1]

1 Department of Epidemiology of Microbial Diseases, Yale School of Public Health, New Haven, Connecticut, United State of America, **2** Section of Molecular and Applied Zoology, Institute of Zoology, Slovak Academy of Sciences, Bratislava, Slovakia, **3** Department of Biomedical Sciences, Oregon State University, Corvallis, Oregon, United States of America

Abstract

Impact of reproductive processes upon female health has yielded conflicting results; particularly in relation to the role of reproduction-associated stress. We used the viviparous tsetse fly to determine if lactation, birth and involution lead to damage from oxidative stress (OS) that impairs subsequent reproductive cycles. Tsetse females carry an intrauterine larva to full term at each pregnancy cycle, and lactate to nourish them with milk secretions produced by the accessory gland (= milk gland) organ. Unlike most K-strategists, tsetse females lack an apparent period of reproductive senescence allowing the production of 8–10 progeny over their entire life span. In a lactating female, over 47% of the maternal transcriptome is associated with the generation of milk proteins. The resulting single larval offspring weighs as much as the mother at birth. In studying this process we noted an increase in specific antioxidant enzyme (AOE) transcripts and enzymatic activity at critical times during lactation, birth and involution in the milk gland/fat body organ and the uterus. Suppression of *superoxide dismutase* (*sod*) decreased fecundity in subsequent reproductive cycles in young mothers and nearly abolished fecundity in geriatric females. Loss of fecundity was in part due to the inability of the mother to produce adequate milk to support larval growth. Longevity was also impaired after *sod* knockdown. Generation of OS in virgin females through exogenous treatment with hydrogen peroxide at times corresponding to pregnancy intervals reduced survival, which was exacerbated by *sod* knockdown. AOE expression may prevent oxidative damage associated with the generation of nutrients by the milk gland, parturition and milk gland breakdown. Our results indicate that prevention of OS is essential for females to meet the growing nutritional demands of juveniles during pregnancy and to repair the damage that occurs at birth. This process is particularly important for females to remain fecund during the latter portion of their lifetime.

Editor: Kristin Michel, Kansas State University, United States of America

Funding: This study received support from the National Institutes of Health grant AI081774 and Ambrose Monell Foundation awarded to SA and from NIH F32AI093023 to JB. The funders had no role in study design, data collection and analysis, decision to publish, or preparation of the manuscript.

Competing Interests: The authors have declared that no competing interests exist.

* E-mail: joshua.benoit@uc.edu

¤ Current address: Department of Biological Sciences, McMicken College of Arts and Sciences, University of Cincinnati, Cincinnati, Ohio, United State of America

9 These authors contributed equally to this work.

Introduction

Reactive oxygen species (ROS) are produced by mitochondrial respiration, which can be exacerbated during metabolic dysfunction, or as part of an immune response to pathogens. These factors can negatively interact with other biological molecules leading to oxidative damage [1–6]. According to the free-radical theory of aging, an organism that is unable to prevent or repair oxidative stress (OS), accumulates damage which leads to organismal dysfunction, aging and death [7]. This theory hypothesizes that presence of antioxidant enzymes (AOEs) is associated with increased longevity [6,8–10]. However, recent studies have questioned the significance of the OS response on aging, and instead have suggested that other factors, such as dysregulation of nutrient signaling pathways, impaired proteolysis or reduced autophagy may be more important, with OS playing only a minor role in relation to aging [11–15]. In addition, the production of

low levels of ROS appears critical to longevity and metabolic health by acting on intracellular signaling molecules at times of stress [16]. An alternative hypothesis that encompasses both of these ideas is that under optimal conditions ROS plays a role in stress signaling and may even have a positive effect in the prevention of aging. However, under sub-optimal conditions, or periods of high stress, individuals may not be able to mount an adequate response to high levels of ROS [13,17,18], leading to cellular damage and accelerated senescence.

Reproductive processes (pregnancy, parturition, lactation, and involution) have been documented to cause oxidative damage in mammalian systems [19–24]. The prevention of OS by AOE expression is critical to fecundity. In *Drosophila*, mosquitoes and sand flies knockdown of AOEs leads to reduced egg production [8,9,25]. Tsetse flies undergo viviparous reproduction, which deviates from the norm of oviparity that occurs in most insects. Tsetse females develop a single oocyte per gonotrophic cycle, and nurture a single offspring in their uterus during embryonic and larval development [26]. Unlike other K-strategists however, tsetse females don't exhibit an apparent period of reproductive senescence. Instead, tsetse females remain fertile throughout their adult lifetime to allow production of 8–10 progeny. During pregnancy, a single larva is nourished in the uterus by the milk secretions from the modified female accessory gland (referred to as milk or uterine gland) [26]. The milk gland undergoes involution (regression and breakdown of milk gland cells to pre-lactation levels) at the completion of each pregnancy cycle [27]. Nearly 20–25 mg of nutrients, consisting of a lipid-protein emulsion within an aqueous base, are transferred to each progeny during the 5–6 day period of intrauterine larval development [27,28]. Over 50% of maternal lipid reserves are metabolized to provide the lipids and amino acids required for milk synthesis [29–32]. Larval progeny weigh as much as the mother at the time of birth. The fact that tsetse flies have such a heavy metabolic investment in their progeny makes the lack of reproductive senescence even more intriguing [33]. In addition, there is no observed difference in longevity between mated (reproductively active) and unmated tsetse females [33]. Other than a few specific examples, such as the naked mole rat [34], female fecundity typically declines or ceases with age. Furthermore, maternal investment in offspring development has other potential negative consequences on the mother, such as a reduction in longevity [35,36]. Little is known about the processes tsetse females utilize to prevent and repair damage that occurs during lactation and intrauterine larval development to maintain the ability to produce progeny late in life.

In this study, we investigated the role of the lactation, birth and involution processes upon reproductive senescence and longevity using the viviparous tsetse fly system. We particularly focused on interplay between OS generation and the AOE response in relation to fecundity and longevity as well as on how females compensate for reproduction-induced stress to maintain high progeny output late in life. Our results support the role of the antioxidant response as a critical mechanism to prevent the premature reproductive senescence that results from the induction of OS during tsetse reproduction/lactation/birth processes. We discuss the implications of our findings in light of the interactions between reproduction, OS and antioxidant dynamics, and senescence in organisms with heavy nutritional investment in their progeny, including mammals and birds.

Results

Milk Gland Protein Synthesis is High During Lactation and Declines Immediately After Birth

To provide a synopsis of the physiological changes that occur during the tsetse lactation and birth processes, we examined intrauterine larval size, maternal milk protein transcript abundance, and maternal lipid levels during pregnancy. Larval development occurs within the mother's uterus over a 5–6 day period. At the time of parturition the mature larva has a dry mass of over 10 mg (wet mass of 20–22 mg; Figure 1a), which is equivalent to the mass of the mother [27]. Predicted transcript levels for the twelve major milk proteins, which include Acid sphingomyelinase 1 (aSMase1 [37]), Transferrin (Trf [38]), a lipocalin (Milk Gland Protein 1; MGP1 [39]) and other milk proteins (MGP2-10 [40,41]) account for over 47% of the total number of predicted RNA-seq reads in a library generated from lactating females carrying a mature intrauterine larva (Figure 1b). Within 24–48 h post-parturition, expression levels for all twelve major milk proteins dramatically decline to dry (non-lactating) levels where the major milk protein transcripts account for only

2% of the total reads (Figure 1b). In addition, the lipid reserves of females decline by over 50% during the later stages of the lactation period at each pregnancy cycle (based on Attardo et al. [29] and Figure 1c). The lipid breakdown that occurs at each pregnancy cycle is critical for the generation of diacylglycerol and proline [26,42,43], which are the major circulating nutrients in tsetse hemolymph and required for milk generation [30,31,44]. During pregnancy tsetse females appear to devote almost half of their nutritional/transcriptional investment towards production of milk for larval development. This process is under tight transcriptional

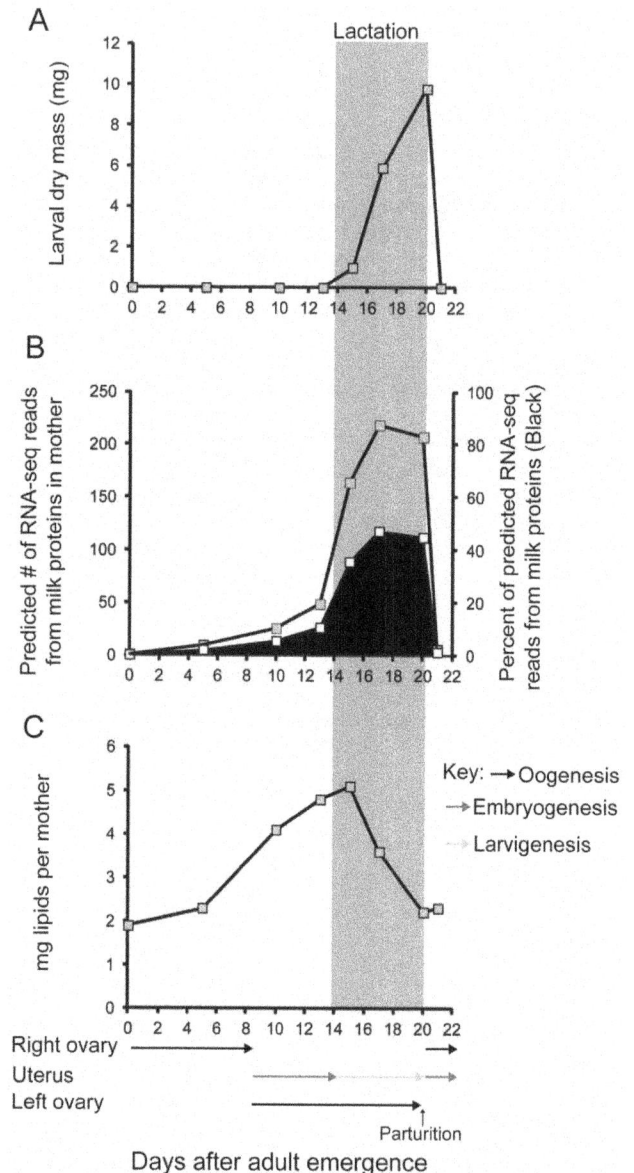

Figure 1. Tsetse fly investment in their progeny during lactation. A. Changes in dry mass of single intrauterine larva throughout development. B. Predicted read abundance for the 12 major milk protein genes (*milk gland protein 1–10, transferrin* and *acid sphingomyelinase 1*) throughout lactation based on fold changes in milk proteins in relation to transcriptome analysis measured at the peak of lactation (17–18 d) and 24–48 h after parturition according to Benoit et al. [40]. C. Total lipid content in females through pregnancy.

regulation, with milk synthesis shut down within 24–48 hour post parturition [1].

Lack of Increased OS Markers during Tsetse Lactation, Birth and Involution

To determine if there is an increased level of oxidative damage throughout the tsetse pregnancy and birth cycle, we measured levels of two types of oxidative damage, protein carbonyls (proteins damaged by OS) and malondialdehyde (MDA; marker of lipid peroxidation), throughout reproduction. We found no difference in lipid peroxidation or protein carbonyls levels between pregnant mothers harboring an (embryo, 1st, 2nd or 3rd instar larva) and mothers immediately after birth (Figure 2). Our results indicate that there is no significant oxidative damage that results from the substantial physiological changes associated with viviparous reproduction in tsetse.

Antioxidant (AOE) Gene Expression Increases during Lactation, Birth and Involution

We next measured transcript levels for nine genes that code for antioxidant enzymes throughout the first and the beginning of the second reproductive cycle to determine if lack of OS could result from increased AOE expression. Transcript levels for 6 of the 9

genes did not vary throughout pregnancy significantly (Table S2). However, there was a substantial increase in the expression of *Cu/Zn sod*, *Mn/Fe sod* and *catalase* genes during lactation, and this expression profile continued up to 24–48 h post parturition during milk gland involution (Figure 3a). The expression of all three AOE genes declined to their lowest level 48–72 h after parturition before increasing again during the second pregnancy cycle (Figure 3a). The AOE activity followed a similar pattern to that of the AOE gene expression with higher antioxidant activity detected during the latter periods of lactation continuing until 24–48 hours post parturition (Figure 3b).

Due to the drastic changes in transcript abundance during pregnancy, *Cu/Zn sod*, *Mn/Fe sod* and *catalase* expression levels were measured before and during lactation, as well as during the involution period post parturition in different tissues of the mother, including fat body/milk gland and uterus (Figure S1a–e). These analyses allowed us to determine that the substantial increase in the AOE response during the tsetse reproductive cycle is localized to the fat body/milk gland and uterine tissues. AOE transcripts

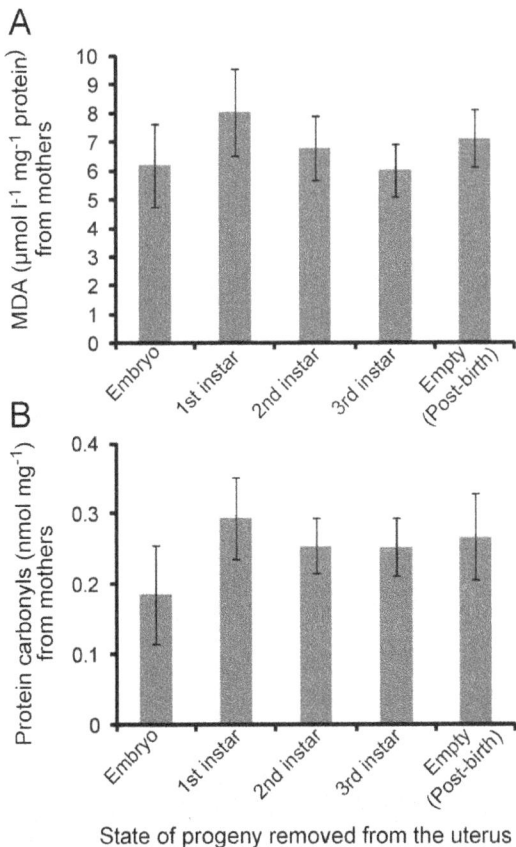

Figure 2. Levels of oxidative stress markers recovered from mothers through the 1st gonotrophic cycle. A. Lipid oxidation levels by measurement of lipid peroxidation. Samples were collected from female flies after progeny removal throughout reproduction. Mean ± SE of five groups of 3 flies. B. Protein oxidation by measurement of protein carbonyl levels. Mean ± SE of five groups of 3 flies.

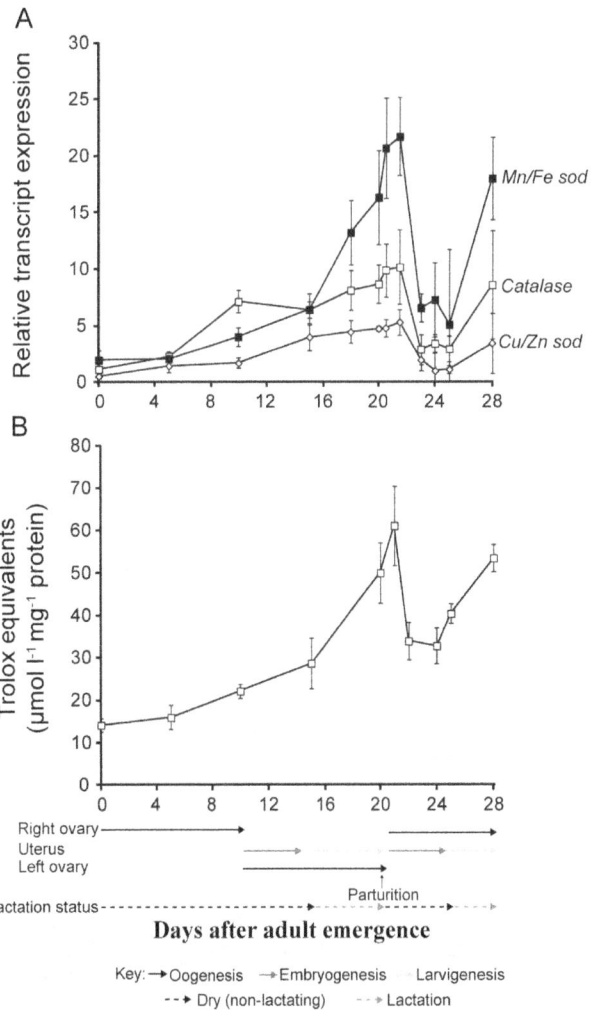

Figure 3. Antioxidant gene expression and activity levels throughout tsetse pregnancy. A. Transcript levels for *Mn/Fe superoxide dismutase* (*Mn/Fe sod*), *Cu/Zn sod* and *catalase* measured 24 h after the last blood meal. Each point represents the mean ± SE of four measurements. B. Antioxidant activity. Each sample represents the mean ± SE of four samples.

were found to increase in the fat body/milk gland and reproductive tract during lactation and involution (Figure S1a–c). A similar pattern was observed in regards to antioxidant activity with increased levels observed in the fat body/milk gland (Figure S1d). Separation of pure milk gland tissue is nearly impossible in tsetse females as it is intertwined with the fat body and trachea. Thus our dissections and measurements included both fat body and milk gland tissues. However, fluorescent in situ hybridization (FISH) analysis with gene specific primers indicates that the expression of both Mn/Fe sod and Cu/Zn sod occurs within the milk gland organ (Figure S2). These results show a substantial increase in AOE gene transcript levels and enzyme activity in response to lactation, birth and involution that is predominantly localized in tissues associated with larval growth and lactation.

Reduction of SOD Expression Impairs Lactation and Results in Loss of Fecundity

To determine the functional role of the AOE response during tsetse reproduction, we utilized RNA interference to suppress the transcript levels of sod genes. Injection of siRNA targeting Cu/Zn sod and Mn/Fe sod yielded a reduction in transcript abundance of over 65% for both genes, respectively (Figure S3a). Antioxidant enzymatic activity was also significantly reduced by 20–30% when individual genes were silenced, and was further suppressed by combined interference of both SOD genes by 60–70% (Figure S3b). We next evaluated the ability of pregnant females injected with both siCu/Zn sod and siMn/Fe sod to survive an exogenous H_2O_2 treatment, as an indication of their ability to respond to OS. We found that knockdown of SOD genes rendered reproductively active females over 50% less tolerant to H_2O_2 treatment as measured by survival in relation to control counterparts (Figure S3c). It appears that the two most abundant AOE gene products (Cu/Zn sod and Mn/Fe sod) likely enable flies to cope with pregnancy associated OS.

After demonstrating effective reduction of the antioxidant response by SOD gene knockdown, we assessed the effect of this phenotype on reproduction and lactation over the first three reproductive cycles in tsetse females by measuring progeny output. Knockdown of Cu/Zn or Mn/Fe sod individually during the first pregnancy cycle did not cause a significant reduction in pupal production during the next cycle relative to the control group that received siGFP treatments (Figure 4a). The combined knockdown of Cu/Zn and Mn/Fe sod in the first pregnancy cycle resulted in a slight reduction in progeny production in the second cycle (Figure 4a). However, the reduction of Cu/Zn sod alone during both the first and second cycles yielded nearly a 30% loss of fecundity during the third cycle (Figure 3a). Combined knockdown of both SOD genes during the first two cycles resulted in the lowest fecundity levels during the third cycle with a reduction of over 50% (Figure 4a). In addition to reduced progeny output, the length of the larval intrauterine development period was also extended by 15–20% following knockdown of a single SOD gene, and by over 30% when both SOD genes were suppressed in the earlier lactation cycles relative to the control treatment group (Figure 4b). The levels of protein carbonyl and markers of lipid peroxidation were also increased during subsequent pregnancy cycles following sod knockdown (Figure 5a and b). Collectively, our results indicate that SOD expression during periods of lactation and birth appears to be critical for the prevention of oxidative damage, and for the maintenance of tsetse's fecundity during subsequent reproductive cycles.

To determine the underlying aspects that lead to extended larval development period in SOD knockdown flies, we measured the transcript abundance of the three major milk proteins (MGP1,

MGP7 and aSMase1) during the third pregnancy cycle after siRNA injection in the previous two pregnancy cycles (either siGFP or siMn/Fe and siCu/Zn sod). We noted no significant differences in the expression levels of the milk protein genes between the two groups when analyzed early in the lactation period when a first instar larva was present in the uterus (Figure 4c). However, there was a 2–3 fold reduction in milk protein gene expression levels later in lactation when a second or third instar larva was present in the uterus and milk production is normally peaking (Figure 4d). Along with reduced transcript levels of three major milk proteins, we documented a 30–35% decrease in protein level for the major milk protein MGP1 after SOD knockdown (Figure S4). These results indicate that the reduced fecundity observed in the older females after SOD knockdown is likely due to the reduced levels of milk proteins generated by the milk gland, which is insufficient to support adequate larval development.

Reduction of Lactation-Associated AOEs Reduces Longevity and Development of Reproductive Senescence: Comparison with Reproductive Output in Other Animals

We compared data on reproductive rate relative to lifespan between tsetse and other organisms to examine how reproduction/aging dynamics of this fly relates to that of other organisms (Figure 6). In general, there is a period of time before an organism becomes reproductively active (Figure 6a). A decline in reproductive capacity usually occurs as organisms age. This typically happens gradually in insects such as med fly and Drosophila (Fig. 6a; [45–48]), but more rapidly after a critical age in the case of mammals, lions, and most other K-strategists. This rapid loss of fecundity represents declining reproductive fitness with age, or reproductive senescence (Figure 6a). Tsetse flies represent a drastic deviation from other animals in that they maintain their fecundity late in life (Figure 6a). Suppression of the two sod genes during lactation, birth and involution, however reduce tsetse's fecundity, making it more comparable with the fecundity parameters of other organisms. This is marked by a decline in the fecundity observed with age, and by a period of reproductive senescence late in life (Figure 6b). These results indicate that the increased expression of AOEs during lactation, birth and involution are critical for the prevention of reproductive decline and senescence.

Tsetse flies unique ability to maintain a high level of fecundity late in life is comparable to that of the naked mole rat, a rodent known for extreme longevity and high fecundity in old age [34]. Tsetse flies also live longer than other related insects and have no apparent decline in fecundity [34]. The lifespan (longevity) of both tsetse and the naked mole rat does not seem to be impacted by the act of reproduction. Our findings in tsetse implicate AOE expression at critical periods during each pregnancy cycle as a necessary mechanism that allows tsetse to maintain reproductive fitness and minimizes end of life reproductive senescence.

Pregnancy Stress can be Experimentally Induced by Exogenous H_2O_2 Treatment Followed by sod Knockdown

We noted a decrease in overall longevity upon sod knockdown, with the effect being more prominent in reproductively active flies (Figure 7a). Next we investigated whether increased lactation associated OS may also be responsible for the noted decrease in tsetse's longevity. We used exogenous H_2O_2 treatment to induce OS at critical times, mimicking the pregnancy-induced responses in age matched virgin females for comparison with pregnant but untreated counterparts. We injected virgin females with H_2O_2 at 10 day intervals, which correspond to the beginning of each

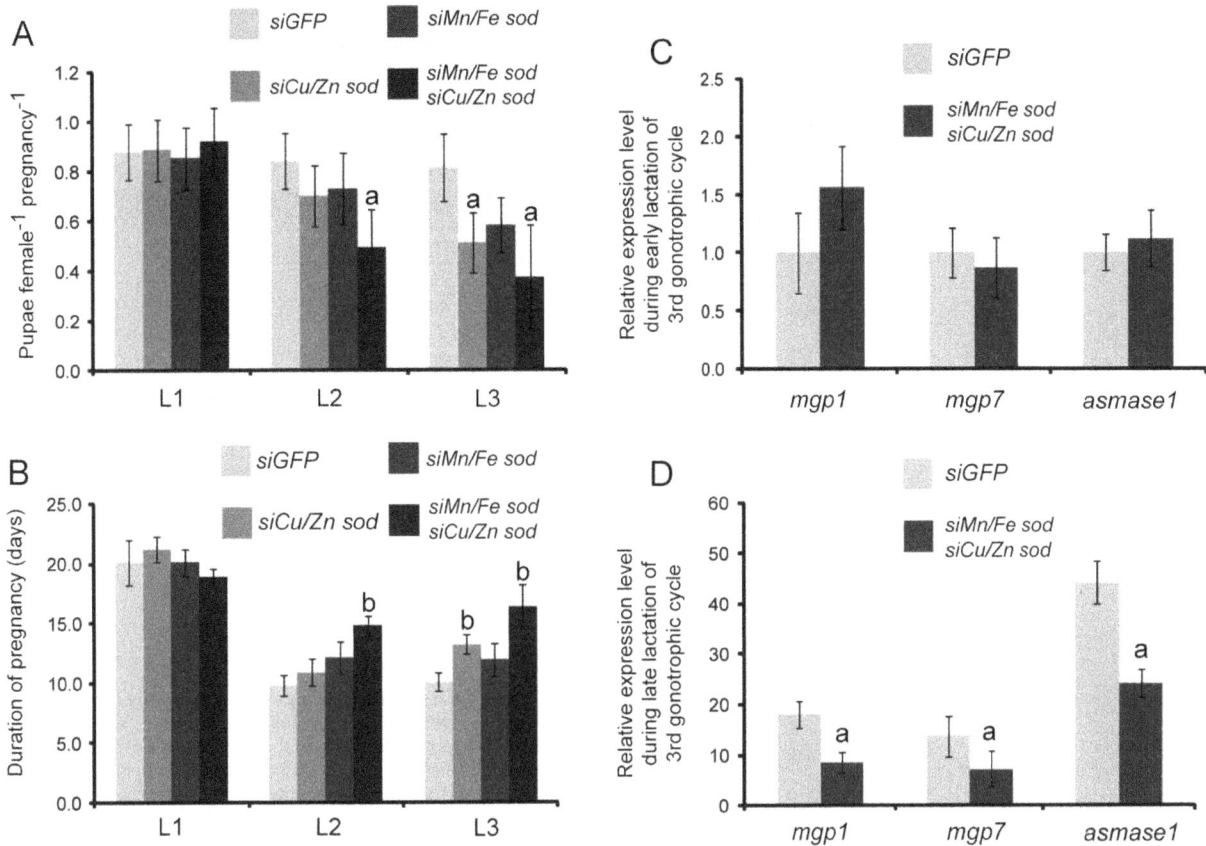

Figure 4. Effect of RNA interference of *Mn/Fe sod* and *Cu/Zn sod* on tsetse fecundity. A. Average number of pupae produced per female during generation of the 1st (L1), 2nd (L2) and 3rd (L3) pregnancy cycle after *sod* knockdown in the 14th day of the fly development and 5th day of subsequent pregnancy cycles. Mean ± SE of three groups of 15 flies. B. Length of the gonotrophic cycles analyzed under similar treatment as A. Mean ± SE of three groups of 15 flies are shown. Expression of *milk gland proteins* (*mgp1*, *mgp7* and *asmase1*) during the early (C, 1st instar larva present in uterus) and late stages (D, 3rd instar larva present in uterus) of lactation after *sod* knockdown during the first two pregnancy cycles.

pregnancy cycle starting on day 20 when females typically carry their first late stage third instar larva prior to parturition. These experiments were to specifically address if the bouts of oxidative stress associated with reproduction impact fly longevity without other physiological changes associated with lactation and birth, specifically after the reduction of the AOE response. We followed these flies for effects on longevity until death. Injection of virgin females with exogenous H_2O_2 resulted in a substantial decline in longevity with 50% mortality occurring nearly 50 days earlier than in the control virgin female group that received H_2O injections (Figure 7b). We next treated a group of virgin females with si*Mn/Fe* and si*Cu/Zn sod*, and found a small but significant reduction in their longevity when compared to control groups similarly injected with H_2O and siGFP, respectively (Figure 7b). However, injection with H_2O_2 after knockdown of *Mn/Fe* and *Cu/Zn sod* resulted in a drastic reduction in lifespan, which was not observed in either the siGFP or the H_2O_2 treatment groups (Figure 7b). These results indicate that OS, similar to that which occurs during lactation and parturition in tsetse, is particularly more detrimental to lifespan at times when SOD levels are low.

The SOD Response is Essential for Tsetse Population Sustainability

We performed population modeling to determine how suppression of the lactation-associated SOD response might alter

population growth dynamics using our data. Based on the modeling analysis, *siGFP* treated control flies had a probability of positive growth of 62.8% (Figure 8a). When flies were treated with *siMn/Fe sod* and *si Cu/Zn sod* double knockdown, we noted a negative impact on population growth, with only a 0.3% probability of a positive growth rate, the level necessary to support replacement of flies dying in the population (Figure 8a). Direct comparison of the growth rates between control and knockdown flies revealed an absolute difference in growth rate of 1.61 per year (95% CI = −0.214, 3.473, p-value for difference >0 = 4.06%; Figure 8b). The absolute values correspond to a decline in population size of 80.0% [95% confidence interval = −23.9%, 96.9%] after one year in the absence of an adequate SOD response during lactation. The modeling results indicate that the reproductive-associated antioxidant response is likely critical to maintain tsetse populations in the wild.

Discussion

In this study we used the viviparous tsetse fly to investigate the role of oxidative stress and antioxidant enzymes in reproductive senescence and female longevity. Tsetse females remain fertile for much of their adult-life, and once mated undergo multiple pregnancies (8–10) with no evidence of significant reproductive senescence. During this pregnancy period, they lactate to nurture their progeny to full term in their uterus by milk secretions

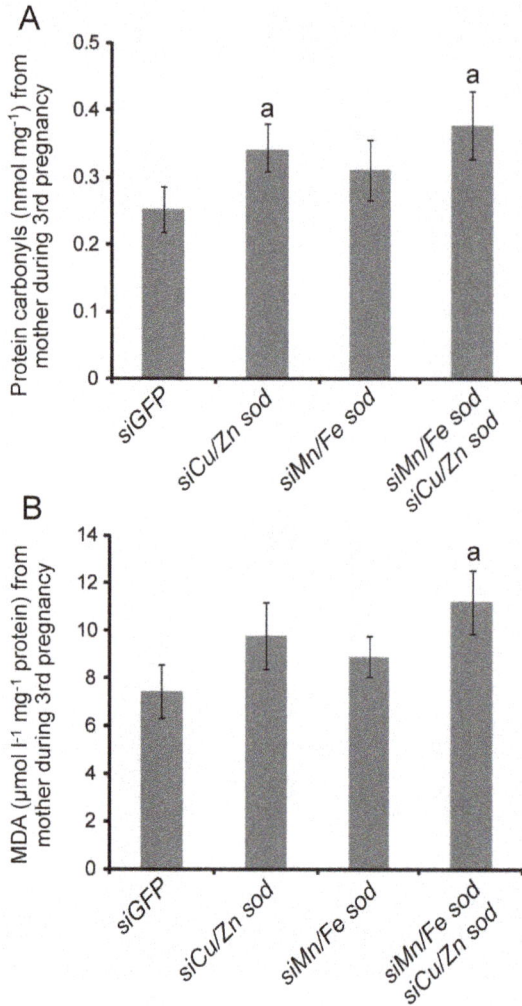

Figure 5. Oxidative stress markers recovered from females during their third pregnancy following *sod* knockdown during the first two reproductive cycles. A. Protein oxidation by measurement of protein carbonyl levels. Mean ± SE of five groups of 3 flies. B. Lipid oxidation levels measured by lipid peroxidation. Samples were collected from mothers carrying a 3rd instar larvae in their uterus. Mean ± SE of five groups of 3 flies.

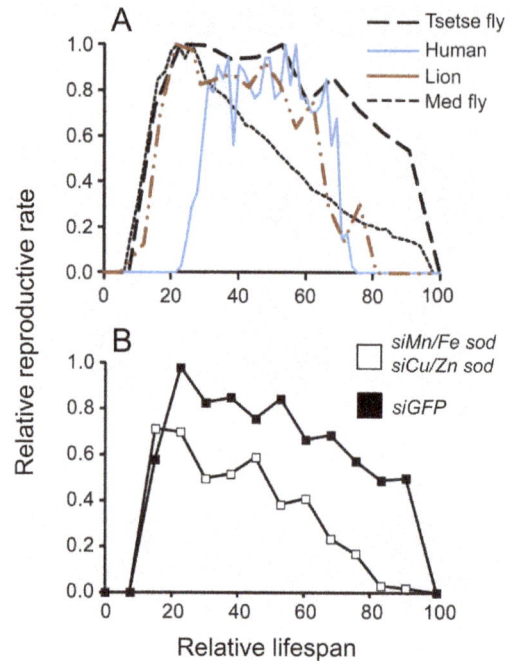

Figure 6. Age-related fecundity patterns in various species in comparison to tsetse flies. A. Medfly, (eggs/day) [46,47], human (traditional Ache population, progeny/year) [101], lions (progeny/year) [102], *Drosophila melanogaster* (eggs/day) [103] and tsetse fly (this study, [33]). B. Age-related fecundity patterns in tsetse fly after knockdown *Mn/Fe sod* and *Cu/Zn sod*. Mean ± SE for three groups of 15 flies.

produced from the milk gland organ. It appears that tsetse females can successfully manage reproduction-associated OS during the lactation, parturition and involution periods of the reproductive cycle. We found high levels of expression of the antioxidant pathway genes (*Cu/Zn sod*, *Mn/Fe sod* and *catalase*) late in pregnancy, and immediately after birth in reproduction associated tissues (milk gland/fat body and uterus). This increase in AOE appears to be important to maintain homeostasis with each subsequent pregnancy cycle, to prevent direct damage to the milk gland, and prevent interference with other underlying mechanisms necessary for lactation. Knockdown of the SOD response during lactation reduces milk protein generation in the subsequent reproductive cycles, results in reproductive senescence in older flies, and reduces longevity, particularly in reproductively active females. These results suggest that the spatially and temporally regulated AOE responses are a critical mechanism that protects the female reproductive system from OS over multiple cycles of lactation, parturition and involution. Population modeling predicts

that if tsetse females lack this lactation associated AOE response, natural population growth would decline by 80% within the year. We summarize the role of AOE expression during tsetse reproduction in Figure 9.

Similar to mammalian lactation, tsetse females nourish their progeny via secretion of milk from the milk gland organ [37,39,40]. Tsetse milk composition and production shares several similarities with mammalian systems. Mammalian systems have highly specialized lactating cells that cycle through periods of high activity during lactation to low/no activity following involution during the dry period [49,50]. The protein composition of tsetse and mammalian milk also show functional analogy between the two systems [51,52]. Comparable protein types include a lipocalin (MGP1 in tsetse versus β-lactoglobulin in mammals [39,53–56]), an iron-binding protein (Transferrin in tsetse versus Lactoferrin in mammals [38,57]), sphingomyelinase present either in milk or in the gut contents of nursing progeny [37,58–60] as well as immune proteins (peptidoglycan recognition protein PGRP-LB and UBA-SH3A in tsetse versus multiple mammalian immune proteins [40,51,54,61,62]). The lipid content of the milk secretions transferred to the developing offspring during lactation is also similar in both systems, both in composition and concentration [29,31,63]. In tsetse, the obligate symbiont *Wigglesworthia*, which provides critical nutrients for maintaining fecundity and for immune maturation, is transferred maternally in milk secretions [53,64,65]. Symbiotic bacteria in maternal milk secretions are also found in mammalian systems, and are thought to function as probiotics [64–65]. Lastly, tsetse and mammals have an expanded family of lactation-specific proteins (MGP 2–10 family in tsetse versus casein family in mammals [40,66,67]). The convergence between these disparate systems suggests that tsetse flies have

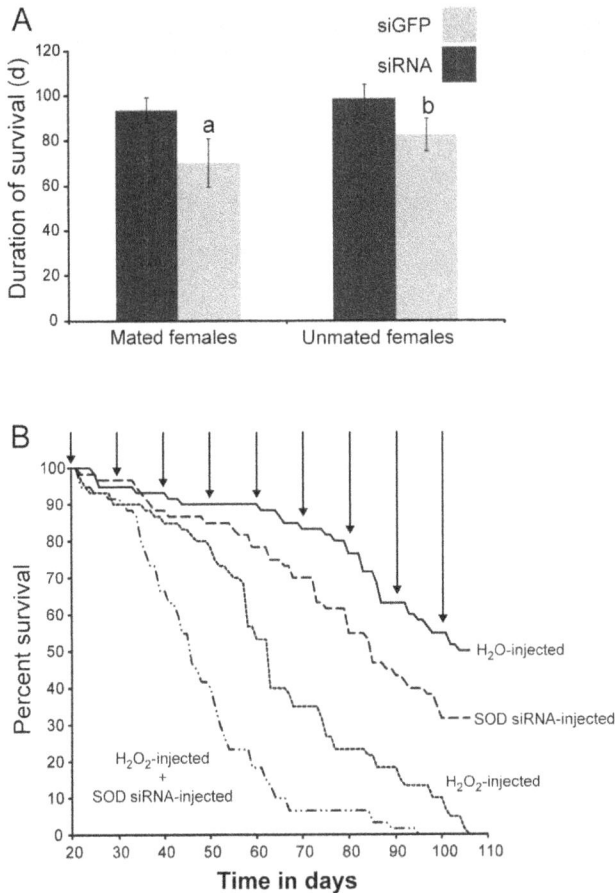

Figure 7. Survival of pregnant and virgin females following *sod* knockdown and exogenous treatment with H₂O₂. A. Longevity following *sod* knockdown in mated and unmated females. Mean ± SE of 15 flies. B. Survival of groups of virgin flies to mimic subjected to one of four treatments: H₂O or H₂O₂ injections at intervals during the peak of lactation that matched those of tsetse fly pregnancy, *Mn/Fe* and *Cu/Zn sod* during the first three pregnancy cycles and *Mn/Fe* and *Cu/Zn sod* during the first three pregnancy cycles along with H₂O₂ at intervals that match those of pregnancy. Survival data was measured using a Kaplan-Meier plot along with a log rank test. Arrows indicate treatment with H₂O or H₂O₂.

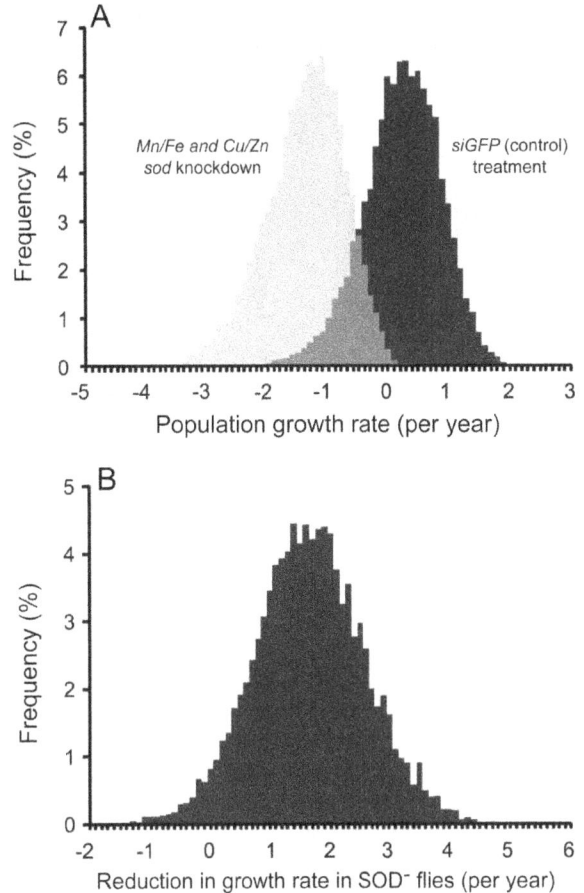

Figure 8. Population modeling following *sod* knockdown. A. Frequency of growth rate. B. Reduction in growth rate between *sod* knockdown and control (*siGFP*). Results represent 10,000 simulated replicates.

developed alternative yet functionally similar solutions to the problem of providing immature offspring with essential nutritional requirements.

The critical role of OS in relation to reproduction and progeny nourishment has been documented in many organisms, including *Drosophila* [68,69], birds [70,71], mammals [2,72,73] and blood feeding insects, such as sand flies and mosquitoes [8,9]. In terms of milk production, dairy cows express increased OS markers during lactation and in the subsequent period of involution [74]. However, increased OS during reproduction has not been documented for all organisms. Female house mice and bank voles do not show increased markers for OS during reproduction [75,76]. The lack of oxidative damage is not surprising as reproductive evolution has likely equipped animals with the ability to mitigate immediate and long-term damage associated with reproduction to maintain fecundity [77]. Similarly, in tsetse flies OS damage does not increase over the course of reproduction, and does not differ between fertile and infertile individuals. This is most likely due to increased AOE response mediated by the

expression of two SOD genes and a catalase gene late in intrauterine larval development, at parturition and during the subsequent period of involution that likely prevents excess ROS. Indeed, when RNA interference was utilized to reduce AOE genes during lactation, we observed a significant increase in oxidative damage during the subsequent periods of lactation and pregnancy. This damage resulted in impaired progeny output due to direct milk gland dysfunction or other mechanisms by which milk protein synthesis is impaired (i.e. reduction of available nutrients for milk protein synthesis). These results support the hypothesis that tsetse flies are adapted to mitigate the OS generated by the high energy demands of their intrauterine progeny by utilizing AOE pathways.

One of the most interesting findings from this study is there is no or minimal decline in fecundity as tsetse flies age. A few organisms, such as the naked mole rat [34], have high levels of progeny output during the later periods of life. For our studies, it is important to mention that our flies were held under laboratory conditions with regular access to meals throughout the course of the study. Although these conditions would seem to be optimal, flies do experience mechanical damage to their wings and bodies from housing within cages, suggesting that these flies likely experience stress throughout their lifetimes. However, colony conditions may be more stable than field conditions, thus OS is likely to be one of the many contributing factors involved in tsetse reproductive senescence. As an example, tsetse flies maintain tight control of

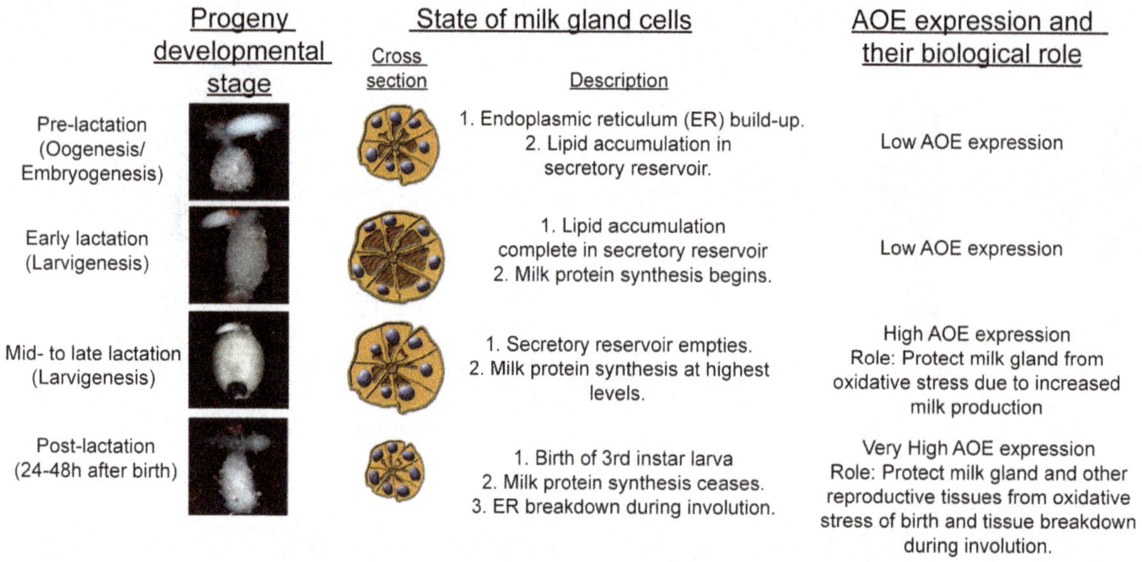

Figure 9. Summary for the role of oxidative stress and antioxidant enzyme expression during tsetse fly reproduction. Developmental images adapted from Benoit et al. [104]. Cross sections adapted from Ma and Denlinger [28], Hecker and Moloo [105] and Yang et al. [41].

lipid levels during the transition between lactation and dry periods [29,78]. These lipid reserves are critical for providing fat for incorporation into the milk and their breakdown generates amino acids necessary for milk protein generation [29–32]. If aging prevented lipid accumulation between periods of lactation,, potentially through dysregulation of insulin or juvenile hormone signaling that have been shown to regulate lipid homeostasis [78], flies may experience reproductive senescence due to the inability of older mothers to produce milk at adequate levels. Thus, there may be other factors beyond oxidative stress that could contribute to reproductive senescence in field flies. Even so, our study demonstrates that tsetse females lacking an oxidative stress response during lactation and birth have a discernible period of reproductive senescence and will be unable to maintain reproduction above replacement levels based on population modeling.

In relation to aging, mated and unmated tsetse females have the same lifespan (this study; [33]). This indicates that under laboratory conditions, there is no trade-off between fecundity and life span. This finding supports the discoveries reported in recent studies across multiple animal systems ranging from insects to mammals, which show that reproduction apparently has little to no effect on longevity [45,48,72,79]. Other studies have shown the fitness consequences due to reproduction such as impaired immunity and reduced resistance to environmental stress [25,72,80–82]. Our finding in tsetse shows that fecundity has a substantial cost on longevity when the AOE response is suppressed during reproduction. Recent studies have questioned the role of the OS response in relation to aging, since little to no change in lifespan was shown to occur after knockdown of *sod* genes [18,83], and overexpression of AOEs did not appear to extend lifespan in multiple model species [11,83]. Many of these studies however have utilized optimal rearing conditions, and it has been suggested that under suboptimal conditions OS could play a more important role in relation to aging [13]. It is possible that the observed impact on longevity in tsetse may not be due solely to oxidative damage, but may include other factors as well. A recent theory that has garnered support is the hyperfunction theory of aging, proposed by Williams [84] and Hamilton [85] with mechanisms focused on

by Blagosklonny [86–89]. This theory argues that unregulated processes associated with early-life fitness, such as growth and reproduction, can be damaging later in life. These uncontrolled processes can lead to negative-age related phenotypes and death. We have observed increased lipid levels in older flies, specifically in flies with a reduced ability to respond to OS during lactation. The inability to maintain lipid homeostasis suggests possible disruptions in the target of rapamycin (TOR), insulin signaling, or alternative nutrient sensing pathways, which is a major hallmark of aging [90]. Along with improper nutrient signaling, other hallmarks of aging, such as mitochondrial dysfunction and loss of proteostasis, may be altered in flies without their normal response to OS during lactation. Additional studies will be necessary to pinpoint the underlying pathologies that result from interference with the AOE response during tsetse lactation. Even so, our study suggests that reproductive-associated OS will lead to decreased longevity if the mechanisms for its suppression are impaired.

Summary

In this study, we show that the AOE response is critical for tsetse flies to manage OS generated during pregnancy and to maintain fecundity, particularly late in life. In the absence of the AOE response, there is a precipitous decline in fecundity, which is due, at least in part, to the inability of tsetse mothers to synthesize the milk nutrients required for progeny development. Population modeling reveals that in the absence of a well-regulated AOE response, the population growth rate will fall below replacement levels. These results suggest that the AOE response is likely a critical aspect that functions to compensate for the OS resulting from the massive metabolic demands generated by lactation in tsetse. In relation to organismal reproduction and senescence, it is likely that OS occurs during reproduction in most organisms, but females may have adapted to prevent the accumulation of oxidative damage during this period to allow for normal reproductive output as aging occurs.

Materials and Methods

Flies and antioxidant genes

Laboratory colonies of *Glossina morsitans morsitans*, established from a population collected in Zimbabwe, are utilized at Yale University for at least 20 years. Flies are maintained at 25°C and 50–60% RH using an artificial membrane feeding system [91]. Females were mated 3–5 d after emergence and collected according to developmental markers based on oocyte, embryo and larva presence [26,39]. Multiple antioxidant genes have been identified from tsetse flies based on previous studies (Table S1; [92]). Flies were stored in groups of 5 throughout our experiments for uniformity. We have provided a diagram of the experimental set-up to more easily interpret the results (Figure S5).

RNA and protein extraction

Temporal samples were acquired from pregnant flies with developing progeny removed so that transcript levels reflect only the changes occurring within the mother. Spatial samples were acquired from pregnant females with a 3rd instar larvae present within the uterus. Each sample was collected 24 h after blood feeding to remove effects of digestion. RNA and protein were extracted from whole flies and tissues using Trizol reagent according to the manufacturer's protocol (Invitrogen, Carlsbad, CA). cDNA was synthesized from 1 μg of total RNA using Superscript III reverse transcriptase kit (Invitrogen) based on the manufacturer's protocol, with the exception that cDNA synthesis was extended to 60 min. RNA and cDNA were stored at $-70°C$ until use. Protein was stored in protein pellet solubilization buffer (8M urea, 3M thiourea, 1% dithiothreitol and 4% CHAPS) at $-20°C$.

Transcript expression levels

The PCR amplification conditions were 95°C for 3 min, thirty cycles of 30 s at 95°C, 52 or 56°C for 1 min, and 1 min at 70°C in a Bio-Rad DNA Engine Peltier Thermocycler (Hercules, CA) with gene-specific primer sets. PCR products were purified and the amplified regions were validated by sequencing at the DNA Analysis Facility at Yale University. Levels of antioxidant and lactation-specific gene expression were determined by qPCR utilizing the iCycler iQ real-time PCR detection system (Bio-Rad, Hercules, CA) using gene specific primers (Table S1). The data were obtained in triplicate samples and were normalized to tsetse *tubulin* (*tub*, DQ377071.1) expression levels and analyzed with software version 3.1 (Bio-Rad). Transcript levels were assessed throughout the course of pregnancy for antioxidant genes, following knockdown of specific genes for validation and to determine if transcript levels of milk proteins were alters after perturbation of lactation-associated antioxidant responses (Figure S5).

RNA interference of antioxidant genes

Short interfering RNAs (siRNA) were synthesized commercially (IDT, Coralville, IA) and consist of two duplex sequences for *Cu/Zn sod* (CCGACGUGACGUAUCUCA and GUACUGAUGA-GAUACGUC) and *Mn/Fe sod* (AAUUGGAGCCAAAGCACC and CGACUAUGGUGCUUUGGC). Control siRNAs were designed against green fluorescent protein (GFP; GAUGCCAUU-CUUUGGUUUGUCUCCCAU and CUUGACUUCAGCAC-GUGUCUUGUAGUU). The concentration was determined by spectrophotometer and adjusted to 1 μg/μl. Each fly in the first treatment group was injected with 1.5 μl siRNA13d after emergence (single treatment) and flies in a second treatment group were injected again at 23 d (two treatments). This treatment procedure allowed for interference of the lactation-associated antioxidant response. For validation, transcript expression levels were determined by qPCR, antioxidant capacity and H_2O_2 tolerance was assessed 5–6 d after siRNA injections. Fecundity of the flies was measured over multiple gonotrophic cycles and displayed as the duration of pregnancy and the number of progeny generated per females during each gonotrophic cycle

Western blot analysis of tsetse milk proteins

Equal volumes of protein from three flies were combined for each time point, and analyzed by standard western blot protocol [39]. Antisera against Tubulin (Tub), Milk Gland Protein (MGP1) and Transferrin (Trf) were previously generated against recombinant tsetse proteins [38,39]. Analysis of Tubulin and MGP were performed utilizing the protein equivalent of 1/100th of a fly per well. Blots were blocked overnight in PBS, 3% BSA and 0.5% Tween 20 (blocking buffer). Tub and MGP1/Trf antisera were utilized at 1:5,000 and 1:20,000, respectively [38,39]. Signals were visualized with Supersignal West Pico Substrate (Pierce, Wobrun, MA) on an Image Station 2000R (Kodak, New Haven, CT). Western blot analysis was conducted for flies during the 3rd gonotrophic cycle after reduction of the AOE response in the previous two reproductive cycles (Figure S5).

In situ hybridization

Milk gland tubules together with fat body were collected from female flies carrying third instar larva and placed into Carnoy's fixative for a five day fixation period [53]. Digoxigenin-labeled RNA probes were generated using the MAXIscript T7 transcription kit following manufacturer's protocol (Ambion, Austin, TX) using a primer set with a T7 primer (Table S1) [52]. Antibody solutions were made featuring anti-Digoxigenin-rhodamine Fab fragments for FISH probe detection (1:200 dilution) (Roche) and rabbit anti-GmmMGP (1:2500) antibodies [39,53]. Alexa Fluor 488 goat anti-rabbit IgG (Invitrogen) at a dilution of 1:500 was added as a secondary antibody for immunohistochemistry [53]. Slides were mounted in VECTASHIELD Mounting Medium with DAPI (Vector laboratories Inc. Burlingame, CA). Samples were observed using a Zeiss Axioskop2 microscope (Zeiss, Thornwood, NY) equipped with a fluorescent filter. Samples were viewed and imaged at 400× magnification. Images were captured using an Infinity1 USB 2.0 camera and software (Lumenera Corporation, Ottawa, Ontario, Canada).

Trolox-equivalent antioxidant capacity (TEAC) assay

The TEAC assay was conducted according to Re et al [93], with modification by Lopez-Martinez et al. [88]. Female flies and dissected tissues were frozen in liquid nitrogen and stored at $-70°C$ until analysis. TEAC was measured using 2,2′-azino-bis-(3- ethylbenzothiazoline-6-sulfonic acid) (ABTS) radical cation decolorization assay. Samples were compared to a Trolox standard curve [0–150 μmol l^{-1} (ml^{-1}))] and results were expressed at Trolox equivalents per me soluble protein. Three pools of three samples were homogenized in PBS and centrifuged at 5000 g for 5 min at 4°C. The fly homogenate was diluted to a concentration of 2 mg protein ml^{-1}. The ABTS (7 mmol l^{-1} in 2.45 mmol l^{-1} potassium persulfate; Sigma-Aldrich, St Louis, MO, USA) was prepared before the assay and allowed to equilibrate in the dark at 25°C overnight. The protein samples and Trolox standard were combined with ABTS and incubated for 10 min at 25°C. Antioxidant capacity was measured at 734 nm on Synergy HT Multi-Mode Microplate Reader (BioTek). TEAC levels were assessed through the tsetse pregnancy cycle from females after removal of an embryo, 1st instar, 2nd instar and 3rd

instar larva from the uterus along with those immediately birth (no progeny in the uterus). In addition, TEAC levels were assessed following knockdown of *Cu/Zn sod* and *Mn/Fe sod* to determine if their knockdown impaired antioxidant levels.

Lipid peroxidation assay

Lipid peroxidation was measured by the amount of malondialdehyde (MDA), the main aldehyde product of lipid peroxidation, utilizing the thiobarbituric acid reactive substances test (TBARS). This assay was adapted from those previously described [94–97]. Individual flies, or tissues dissected from three individuals were pooled and homogenized in RIPA buffer with EDTA, respectively. The samples were split into two aliquots: one was used to determine the protein concentration as standardization and the second was treated with 10% trichloroacetic acid (TCA) then incubated in ice to precipitate proteins. Following TCA treatment, the sample was centrifuged for 2200 g for 15 min at 4°C. The supernatant was combined with 0.6% (w/v) thiobarbituric acid solution and heated at 95°C for 1 h. The samples were then allowed to cool to 25°C on ice and centrifuged (2200 g for 5 min) prior to absorbance measurement at 532 nm. MDA quantification was determined using an eight point MDA standard curve [0– 50 µmol l^{-1}] standardized in relation to total protein. MDA levels were assessed through the tsetse pregnancy cycle from females after removal of an embryo, 1st instar, 2nd instar and 3rd instar larva from the uterus along with those immediately birth (no progeny in the uterus; Figure S5). In addition, MDA levels were assessed in the third reproductive cycle following knockdown of *Cu/Zn sod* and *Mn/Fe sod* in the first two gonotrophic cycles to determine if their knockdown resulted in increased MDA levels.

Protein carbonyl assay

Protein oxidation was measured according to Levine et al. [98] with modifications by Lopez-Martinez et al. [95]. Whole flies and tissues were homogenized in a 5% sulfosalicylic acid. Excess amount of 2,4-dinitrophenylhydrazine (DNPH, Sigma) was utilized to extract carbonyls, the carbonyls were precipitated with TCA and multiple washes with ethanol:ethyl acetate solutions was utilized to remove excess DNPH. The resulting proteins were diluted in 6M guanidine hydrochloride. Sample absorbance was measured at 370 nm and compared to a BSA standard (nine points, 0.2 mg/ml) curve. Data are presented as nmol mg^{-1} soluble protein. Protein carbonyl levels were assessed through the tsetse pregnancy cycle from females after removal of an embryo, 1st instar, 2nd instar and 3rd instar larva from the uterus along with those immediately birth (no progeny in the uterus; Figure S5). In addition, protein carbonyl levels were assessed in the third reproductive cycle following knockdown of *Cu/Zn sod* and *Mn/Fe sod* in the first two gonotrophic cycles to determine if their knockdown resulted in increased protein carbonyl levels.

Effect of exogenous OS on nonreproductive (virgin) flies

For testing the periodic OS, unmated female flies were utilized under four separate treatment groups (Figure S5). The first treatment group was injected with 2 µl of 0.5% H_2O_2 at intervals of pregnancy (20, 30 and 40 d) during the first three reproductive cycles. The second treatment group was injected with water control, *Mn/Fe sod* and *Cu/Zn sod* siRNA (200 ng/µl) to determine the effect of SOD knockdown on survival, respectively. The third treatment group received *Mn/Fe sod* and *Cu/Zn sod* siRNA (200 ng/µl) along with 0.5% H_2O_2 to determine the effect of

increased OS after SOD knockout, respectively. Flies were held under standard colony rearing protocols and monitored until 100% mortality was reached. An outline of the experimental design is provided in Figure S5.

Population modeling following reduction of SOD response

To estimate the impact of reproductive-associated antioxidant response at the population scale, we built a simple mathematical model of a tsetse population growth. The model population for impaired reproductive-associated antioxidant response was parametrized with data from the si*Mn/FE* and si*Cu/Zn sod* treatments, while the non-impaired model population was parametrized with data from the control treatment, siGFP treatment (Table S3). For both model populations, we assumed normal, non-antioxidant-impaired mortality. We calculated the mean and standard deviation of fecundity and gonotrophic-cycle length for the control group and for the combined si*Mn/FE* and si*Cu/Zn sod* treatment group for 12 gonotrophic cycles (Table S3). For each gonotrophic cycle and each treatment group, we modeled fecundity F_{jk} as a beta random variable with parameters chosen to match the mean and standard deviation of the data. Similarly, we modeled gonotrophic-cycle length t_{jk} as a log normal random variable with parameters chosen to match the mean and standard deviation of the data for each gonotrophic cycle and each treatment group.

Given values of fecundity and gonotrophic cycle length, number of female offspring produced by a single female tsetse over its lifetime is $R_j = p \sum F_{jk} S_{jk}$ where p is the probability than a deposited pupa is female, which we took to be 55% [99] and S_{jk} is the survival, the probability of surviving to gonotrophic cycle k. We modeled survival as $S_{jk} = S_{pupa} s^{T_{jk}}$, where S_{pupa} is the probability that a deposited pupa survives to emerge as an adult, which we took to be a conservative number at 85% [99,100]; s is the probability of surviving each adult day, which we took to be 98% [99,100], and $T_{jk} = \sum t_{jk}$ is the number of days from emergence until the end of gonotrophic cycle k. The population growth rate is then $r_j = R_j D$, with the generation time defined to be $D = D_{pupa} + D_{adult}$ is the mean duration of the pupal stage, which we took to be 31.4 days [100]; and $D_{adult} = -(\log s)^{-1}$ is the mean adult lifespan. We calculated the population growth rate r_j for each treatment group and the difference in growth rate between the two treatment groups, $r_1 - r_2$, for 10,000 samples of our model.

Statistical analysis

Results were compared utilizing JMP or SAS statistical software programs (Cary, North Carolina, USA). Mean differences utilized between treatments were compared with one-way or two-way ANOVA with a Bonferroni correction followed by Tukey's post-hoc test. A Kaplan-Meier analysis was utilized to measure survival differences following treatment with H_2O_2.

Supporting Information

Figure S1 Antioxidant gene and activity levels in specific tissues before, during and after lactation. A, B and C. Transcript levels for *Mn/Fe superoxide dismutase* (*Mn/Fe sod*), *Cu/Zn sod* and *catalase*, respectively Each point represents the mean ± SE of four measurements. D. Antioxidant activity determined as Trolox-equivalent assay (µmol l^{-1} mg^{-1} protein). Each sample represents the mean ± SE of three samples.

Figure S2 Fluorescent *in situ* hybridization (FISH) analysis. Red for *Mn/FE sod* (A) and *Cu/Zn sod* (B) green for milk gland protein (MGP) immunohistochemistry. DAPI staining of nuclei in blue, is shown in a cross section of milk gland tubules. 1 = milk gland lumen; 2 = nuclei; 3 = secretory reservoir. Negative controls not treated with Digoxigenin-labeled antisense RNA probes displayed no signal.

Figure S3 RNA interference of *Mn/Fe sod* and *Cu/Zn sod*. A. Transcript levels. Mean ± SE of three samples. B. Antioxidant activity. Mean ± SE of four samples. C. Resistance to H_2O_2 injection. Mean ± SE of 15 flies.

Figure S4 Reduction in milk gland protein levels after SOD gene knockdown. Tubulin was utilized as an internal control. Relative protein levels were determined with densitometry through the utilization of ImageJ. Mean ± SE of three blots.

Figure S5 Diagram outlining experimental design.

Table S1 Quantitative PCR primer information utilized in this study.

Table S2 qPCR expression of multiple oxidative stress genes through tsetse pregnancy.

Table S3 Gonotrophic cycle length and fecundity by cycle number for control and si*Mn/Fe* and si*Cu/Zn sod* treatment groups. Cycle length is the duration of the gonotrophic cycle in days. Fecundity is probability that pupa was deposited during the cycle.

Acknowledgments

We thank Oleg Kruglov and Yineng Wu for their technical expertise.

Author Contributions

Conceived and designed the experiments: VM JBB GMA JM SA. Performed the experiments: VM JBB. Analyzed the data: VM JBB GMA JM SA. Contributed reagents/materials/analysis tools: VM JBB GMA JM SA. Wrote the paper: VM JBB GMA JM SA.

References

1. Attardo GM, Benoit JB, Michalkova V, Patrick KR, Krause TB, et al. (2013) The homeodomain protein Ladybird Late regulates milk protein gene expression during pregnancy in the tsetse fly (*Glossina morsitans*). PLoS Neg Trop Dis. DOI 10.1371/journal.pntd.0002645
2. Agarwal A, Gupta S, Sharma RK (2005) Role of oxidative stress in female reproduction. Reprod Biol Endocrinol 3: 28.
3. Murphy MP, Holmgren A, Larsson NG, Halliwell B, Chang CJ, et al. (2011) Unraveling the biological roles of reactive oxygen species. Cell Metab 13: 361–366.
4. Pamplona R, Costantini D (2011) Molecular and structural antioxidant defenses against oxidative stress in animals. Am J Physiol Regul Integr Comp Physiol 301: 843–863.
5. Lushchak VI (2011) Adaptive response to oxidative stress: Bacteria, fungi, plants and animals. Comp Biochem Physiol C Toxicol Pharmacol 153: 175–190.
6. Halliwell B, Gutteridge JMC (2007) Free Radicals in Biology and Medicine. United Kingdom: Oxford University Press. 704 p.
7. Harman D (1956) Aging - a theory based on free-radical and radiation-chemistry. J Gerontol 11: 298–300.
8. DeJong RJ, Miller LM, Molina-Cruz A, Gupta L, Kumar S, et al. (2007) Reactive oxygen species detoxification by catalase is a major determinant of fecundity in the mosquito *Anopheles gambiae*. Proc Natl Acad Sci USA 104: 2121–2126.
9. Diaz-Albiter H, Mitford R, Genta FA, Sant'Anna MRV, Dillon RJ (2011) Reactive oxygen species scavenging by catalase is important for female *Lutzomyia longipalpis* fecundity and mortality. PLoS One 6: e17486
10. Le Bourg E (2001) Oxidative stress, aging and longevity in *Drosophila melanogaster*. FEBS Lett 498: 183–186.
11. Cabreiro F, Ackerman D, Doonan R, Araiz C, Back P, et al. (2011) Increased life span from overexpression of superoxide dismutase in *Caenorhabditis elegans* is not caused by decreased oxidative damage. Free Radic Biol Med 51: 1575–1582.
12. Lewis KN, Andziak B, Yang T, Buffenstein R (2012) The naked mole-rat response to oxidative stress: Just deal with it. Antioxid Redox Signal doi:10.1089/ars.2012.4911.
13. Salmon AB, Richardson A, Perez VI (2010) Update on the oxidative stress theory of aging: does oxidative stress play a role in aging or healthy aging? Free Radic Biol Med 48: 642–655.
14. Speakman JR, Selman C (2011) The free-radical damage theory: Accumulating evidence against a simple link of oxidative stress to ageing and lifespan. Bioessays 33: 255–259.
15. Back P, Braeckman BP, Matthijssens F (2012) ROS in aging *Caenorhabditis elegans*: damage or signaling. Oxid Med Cell Longev 2012: 1–14.
16. Ristow M, Zarse K (2010) How increased oxidative stress promotes longevity and metabolic health: The concept of mitochondrial hormesis (mitohormesis). Exp Gerontol 45: 410–418.
17. Hekimi S, Lapointe J, Wen Y (2011) Taking a "good" look at free radicals in the aging process. Trends Cell Biol 21: 569–576.
18. Van Raamsdonk JM, Hekimi S (2012) Superoxide dismutase is dispensable for normal animal lifespan. Proc Natl Acad Sci USA 109: 5785–5790.
19. Piccione G, Alberghina D, Marafioti S, Giannetto C, Casella S, et al. (2012) Electrophoretic serum protein fraction profile during the different physiological phases in *Comisana* ewes. Reprod Domest Anim 47: 591–595.
20. Gillespie MJ, Haring VR, McColl KA, Monaghan P, Donald JA, et al. (2011) Histological and global gene expression analysis of the 'lactating' pigeon crop. BMC Genomics 12: 452.
21. Piccione G, Borruso M, Giannetto C, Morgante M, Giudice E (2007) Assessment of oxidative stress in dry and lactating cows. Acta Agriculturae Scand, Section A 19: 1–11.
22. Singh K, Davies SR, Dobson JM, Molenaar AJ, Wheeler TT, et al. (2008) cDNA microarray analysis reveals that antioxidant and immune genes are upregulatd during involution of the bovine mammary gland. J Dairy Sci 91: 2236–2246.
23. Castillo C, Hernandez J, Valverde I, Pereira V, Sotillo J, et al. (2006) Plasma malonaldehyde (MDA) and total antioxidant status (TAS) during lactation in dairy cows. Res Vet Sci 80: 133–139.
24. Castillo C, Hernandez J, Bravo A, Lopez-Alonso M, Pereira V, et al. (2005) Oxidative status during late pregnancy and early lactation in dairy cows. Vet J 169: 286–292.
25. Williams TD (2005) Mechanisms underlying the costs of egg production. Bioscience 55: 39–48.
26. Tobe SS, Langley PA (1978) Reproductive Physiology of *Glossina*. Annu Rev Entomol 23: 283–307.
27. Denlinger DL, Ma W-C (1974) Dynamics of the pregnancy cycle in the tsetse *Glossina morsitans*. J Insect Physiol 20: 1015–1026.
28. Ma WC, Denlinger DL, Jarlfors U, Smith DS (1975) Structural modulations in the tsetse fly milk gland during a pregnancy cycle. Tiss Cell 7: 319–330.
29. Attardo GM, Benoit JB, Michalkova V, Yang G, Roller L, et al. (2011) Analysis of lipolysis underlying lactation in the tsetse fly, *Glossina morsitans*. Insect Biochem Mol Biol 42: 360–370.
30. Langley PA, Bursell E (1980) Role of fat body and uterine gland in milk synthesis by adult female *Glossina morsitans*. Insect Biochem 10: 11–17.
31. Langley PA, Bursell E, Kabayo J, Pimley RW, Trewen MA, et al. (1981) Haemolymph lipid transport from fat body to uterine gland in pregnant females of *Glossina morsitans*. Insect Biochem 11: 225–231.
32. Pimley RW, Langley PA (1981) Hormonal control of lipid synthesis in the fat body of the adult female tsetse fly, *Glossina morsitans*. J Insect Physiol 27: 839–847.
33. Langley PA, Clutton-Brock TH (1998) Does reproductive investment change with age in tsetse flies, *Glossina morsitans morsitans* (Diptera: Glossinidae)? Funct Ecol 12: 866–870.
34. Buffenstein R (2008) Negligible senescence in the longest living rodent, the naked mole-rat: insights from a successfully aging species. J Comp Physiol B 178: 439–445.
35. Jasienska G (2009) Reproduction and lifespan: Trade-offs, overall energy budgets, intergenerational costs, and costs neglected by research. Am J Hum Biol 21: 524–532.
36. Dao A, Kassogue Y, Adamou A, Diallo M, Yaro AS, et al. (2010) Reproduction-longevity trade-off in *Anopheles gambiae* (Diptera: Culicidae). J Med Entomol 47: 769–777.

37. Benoit JB, Attardo GM, Michalkova V, Takac P, Bohova J, et al. (2012) Sphingomyelinase activity in mother's milk is essential for juvenile development: a case from lactating tsetse flies. Biol Reprod 87: 17, 1–10.

38. Guz N, Attardo GM, Wu Y, Aksoy S (2007) Molecular aspects of transferrin expression in the tsetse fly (Glossina morsitans morsitans). J Insect Physiol 53: 715–723.

39. Attardo GM, Guz N, Strickler-Dinglasan P, Aksoy S (2006) Molecular aspects of viviparous reproductive biology of the tsetse fly (Glossina morsitans morsitans): Regulation of yolk and milk gland protein synthesis. J Insect Physiol 52: 1128–1136.

40. Benoit JB, Attardo GM, Michalkova V, Bohova J, Zhang Q, et al. (2013) A novel highly divergent protein family from a viviparous insect identified by RNA-seq analysis: a potential target for tsetse fly-specific abortifacients. PLoS Genetics. DOI 10.1371/journal.pgen.1003874.

41. Yang G, Attardo GM, Lohs C, Aksoy S (2010) Molecular characterization of two novel milk proteins in the tsetse fly (Glossina morsitans morsitans). Insect Mol Biol 19: 253–262.

42. Bursell E (1977) Synthesis of proline by the fat body of the tsetse fly (Glossina morsitans): metabolic pathways. Insect Biochem 7: 427–434.

43. Pimley RW, Langley PA (1982) Hormone stimulated lipolysis and proline synthesis in the fat body of the adult tsetse fly, Glossina morsitans. J Insect Physiol 28: 781–789.

44. Tobe SS (1978) Changes in free amino acids and peptides in haemolymph of Glossina austeni during reproductive cycle. Experientia 34: 1462–1463.

45. Wit J, Sarup P, Lupsa N, Malte H, Frydenberg J, et al. (2013) Longevity for free? Increased reproduction with limited trade-offs in Drosophila melanogaster selected for increased life span. Exp Gerontol 48: 349–357.

46. Carey JR, Liedo P, Muller HG, Wang JL, Chiou JM (1998) Relationship of age patterns of fecundity to mortality, longevity, and lifetime reproduction in a large cohort of Mediterranean fruit fly females. J Gerontol A Biol Sci Med Sci 53: B245–251.

47. Carey JR, Liedo P, Muller HG, Wang JL, Vaupel JW (1998) Dual modes of aging in Mediterranean fruit fly females. Science 281: 996–998.

48. Khazaeli AA, Curtsinger JW (2013) Pleiotropy and life history evolution in Drosophila melanogaster: uncoupling life span and early fecundity. J Gerontol A Biol Sci Med Sci 68: 546–553.

49. McManaman JL, Neville MC (2003) Mammary physiology and milk secretion. Advanced Drug Deliv Rev 55: 629–641.

50. Neville MC, Picciano MF (1997) Regulation of milk lipid secretion and composition. Annu Rev Nutr 17: 159–183.

51. Lemay DG, Lynn DJ, Martin WF, Neville MC, Casey TM, et al. (2009) The bovine lactation genome: insights into the evolution of mammalian milk. Genome Biol 10: R43.

52. O'Donnell R, Holland JW, Deeth HC, Alewood P (2004) Milk proteomics. Int Dairy J 14: 1013–1023.

53. Attardo GM, Lohs C, Heddi A, Alam UH, Yildirim S, et al. (2008) Analysis of milk gland structure and function in Glossina morsitans: milk protein production, symbiont populations and fecundity. J Insect Physiol 54: 1236–1242.

54. Wickramasinghe S, Rincon G, Islas-Trejo A, Medrano JF (2012) Transcriptional profiling of bovine milk using RNA sequencing. BMC Genomics 13: 45.

55. Kontopidis G, Holt C, Sawyer L (2004) Invited review: beta-lactoglobulin: binding properties, structure, and function. J Dairy Sci 87: 785–796.

56. Lefevre CM, Digby MR, Whitley JC, Strahm Y, Nicholas KR (2007) Lactation transcriptomics in the Australian marsupial, Macropus eugenii: transcript sequencing and quantification. BMC Genomics 8: 417.

57. Strickler-Dinglasan PM, Guz N, Attardo G, Aksoy S (2006) Molecular characterization of iron binding proteins from Glossina morsitans morsitans (Diptera : Glossinidae). Insect Biochem Mol Biol 36: 921–933.

58. Nyberg L, Farooqi A, Blackberg L, Duan RD, Nilsson A, et al. (1998) Digestion of ceramide by human milk bile salt-stimulated lipase. J Pediatr Gastroenterol Nutr 27: 560–567.

59. Duan RD (2011) Physiological functions and clinical implications of sphingolipids in the gut. J Dig Dis 12: 60–70

60. Duan RD (2007) Sphingomyelinase and ceramidase in the intestinal tract. Eur J Lipid Sci Technol 109: 987–993.

61. Clarkson RW, Wayland MT, Lee J, Freeman T, Watson CJ (2004) Gene expression profiling of mammary gland development reveals putative roles for death receptors and immune mediators in post-lactational regression. Breast Cancer Res 6: R92–109.

62. Hettinga K, van Valenberg H, de Vries S, Boeren S, van Hooijdonk T, et al. (2011) The host defense proteome of human and bovine milk. PLoS One 6: e19433.

63. Cmelik SHW, Bursell E, Slack E (1969) Composition of the gut contents of thrid-instar tsetse larvae (Glossina morsitans Westwood). Comp Biochem Physiol 29: 447–453.

64. Pais R, Lohs C, Wu Y, Wang J, Aksoy S (2008) The obligate mutualist Wigglesworthia glossinidia influences reproduction, digestion, and immunity processes of its host, the tsetse fly. Appl Environ Microbiol 74: 5965–5974.

65. Weiss BL, Wang J, Aksoy S (2011) Tsetse immune system maturation requires the presence of obligate symbionts in larvae. PLoS Biol 9: e1000619.

66. Rijnkels M (2002) Multispecies comparison of the casein gene loci and evolution of casein gene family. J Mammary Gland Biol Neoplasia 7: 327–345.

67. Ginger MR, Grigor MR (1999) Comparative aspects of milk caseins. Comp Biochem Physiol B Biochem Mol Biol 124: 133–145.

68. Salmon AB, Marx DB, Harshman LG (2001) A cost of reproduction in Drosophila melanogaster: stress susceptibility. Evolution 55: 1600–1608.

69. Wang Y, Salmon AB, Harshman LG (2001) A cost of reproduction: oxidative stress susceptibility is associated with increased egg production in Drosophila melanogaster. Exp Gerontol 36: 1349–1359.

70. Alonso-Alvarez C, Perez-Rodriguez L, Garcia JT, Vinuela J, Mateo R (2010) Age and breeding effort as sources of individual variability in oxidative stress markers in a bird species. Physiol Biochem Zool 83: 110–118.

71. Heiss RS, Schoech SJ (2012) Oxidative cost of reproduction is sex specific and correlated with reproductive effort in a cooperatively breeding bird, the Florida scrub jay. Physiol Biochem Zool 85: 499–503.

72. Harshman LG, Zera AJ (2007) The cost of reproduction: the devil in the details. Trends Ecol Evol 22: 80–86.

73. Agarwal A, Gupta S, Sharma R (2005) Oxidative stress and its implications in female infertility - a clinician's perspective. Reprod Biomed Online 11: 641–650.

74. Sharma N, Singh NK, Singh OP, Pandey V, Verma PK (2011) Oxidative stress and antioxidant status during transition period in dairy cows. Asian-Aust J Anim Sci 24: 479–484.

75. Garratt M, Vasilaki A, Stockley P, McArdle F, Jackson M, et al. (2011) Is oxidative stress a physiological cost of reproduction? An experimental test in house mice. Proc Biol Sci 278: 1098–1106.

76. Oldakowski L, Piotrowska Z, Chrzaacik KM, Sadowska ET, Koteja P, et al. (2012) Is reproduction costly? No increase of oxidative damage in breeding bank voles. J Exp Biol 215: 1799–1805.

77. Metcalfe NB, Monaghan P (2013) Does reproduction cause oxidative stress? An open question. Trends Ecol Evol 28: 347–350.

78. Baumann AA, Benoit JB, Michalkova V, Mireji P, Attardo GM, et al. (2013) Juvenile hormone and insulin signaling pathways regulate lipid levels during lactation and dry periods of tsetse fly pregnancy. Mol Cell Endocrinol 372: 30–41.79.

79. De Loof A (2011) Longevity and aging in insects: Is reproduction costly; cheap; beneficial or irrelevant? A critical evaluation of the "trade-off" concept. J Insect Physiol 57: 1–11.

80. Norris K, Evans MR (2000) Ecological immunology: life history trade-offs and immune defense in birds. Behav Ecol 11: 19–26.

81. Owens IPF, Wilson K (1999) Immunocompetence: a neglected life history trait ot conspicuous red herring. Trends Ecol Evol 14: 170–172.

82. Fedorka KM, Zuk M, Mousseau TA (2004) Immune suppression and the cost of reproduction in the ground cricket, Allonemobius socius. Evolution 58: 2478–2485.

83. Van Remmen H, Ikeno Y, Hamilton M, Pahlavani M, Wolf N, et al. (2003) Life-long reduction in MnSOD activity results in increased DNA damage and higher incidence of cancer but does not accelerate aging. Physiol Genomics 16: 29–37.

84. Williams GC (1957) Pleiotropy, natural selection and the evolution of senescence. Evolution 11: 398–411.

85. Hamilton WD (1966) The moulding of senescence by natural selection. J Theor Biol 12: 12–45.

86. Blagosklonny MV (2012) Answering the ultimate question "what is the proximal cause of aging?". Aging 4: 861–877.

87. Gems D, Partridge L (2013) Genetics of longevity in model organisms: debates and paradigm shifts. Annu Rev Physiol 75: 621–644.

88. Blagosklonny MV (2007) Paradoxes of aging. Cell Cycle 6: 2997–3003.

89. Blagosklonny MV (2006) Aging and immortality: quasi-programmed senescence and its pharmacologic inhibition. Cell Cycle 5: 2087–2102.

90. Lopez-Otin C, Blasco MA, Partridge L, Serrano M, Kroemer G (2013) The hallmarks of aging. Cell 153: 1194–1217.

91. Moloo SK (1971) An artificial feeding technique for Glossina. Parasitology 63: 507–512.

92. Munks RJ, Sant'Anna MR, Grail W, Gibson W, Igglesden T, et al. (2005) Antioxidant gene expression in the blood-feeding fly Glossina morsitans morsitans. Insect Mol Biol 14: 483–491.

93. Re R, Pellegrini N, Proteggente A, Pannala A, Yang M, et al. (1999) Antioxidant activity applying an improved ABTS radical cation decolorization assay. Free Radic Biol Med 26: 1231–1237.

94. Lopez-Martinez G, Elnitsky MA, Benoit JB, Lee RE, Denlinger DL (2008) High resistance to oxidative damage in the Antarctic midge Belgica antarctica, and developmentally linked expression of genes encoding superoxide dismutase, catalase and heat shock proteins. Insect Biochem Mol Biol 38: 796–804.

95. Lopez-Martinez G, Hahn DA (2012) Short-term anoxic conditioning hormesis boosts antioxidant defenses, lowers oxidative damage following irradiation and enhances male sexual performance in the Caribbean fruit fly, Anastrepha suspensa. J Exp Biol 215: 2150–2161.

96. Uchiyama M, Mihara M (1978) Determination of malonaldehyde precursor in tissues by thiobarituric acid test. Anal Biochem 86: 271–278.

97. Ohkawa H, Ohishi N, Yagi K (1979) Assay for lipid peroxides in animal tissues by thiobarbituric acid reaction. Anal Biochem 95: 351–358.

98. Levine RL, Garland D, Oliver CN, Amici A, Climent I, et al. (1990) Determination of carbonyl content in oxidatively modified proteins. Methods Enzymol 186: 464–478.

99. Madubunyi LC (1989) Survival and productivity of the tsetse, Glossina morsitans morsitans Westwood (Diptera: Glossinidae) maintained under different feeding

regimens through four successive reproductive cycles in Zambia. Insect Sci Applic 10: 75–80.

100. Jarry M, Khaladi M, Gouteaux JP (1996) A matrix model for studying tsetse fly population. Entomol Exp Appl 78: 51–60.

101. Hill K, Hurtado M (1996) Aché life history: The ecology and demography of a foraging people. New York: Aldine de Gruyter. 570 p.

102. Packer C, Tatar M, Collins A (1998) Reproductive cessation in female mammals. Nature 392: 807–811.

103. Novoseltsev VN, Novoseltseva JA, Boyko SI, Yashin AI (2003) What fecundity patterns indicate about aging and longevity: insights from *Drosophila* studies. J Gerontol A Biol Sci Med Sci 58: 484–494.

104. Benoit JB, Yang G, Krause TB, Patrick KR, Aksoy S, et al. (2011) Lipophorin acts as a shuttle of lipids to the milk gland during tsetse fly pregnancy. J Insect Physiol 57: 1553–1561.

105. Hecker H, Moloo SK (1983) Quantitative morphological changes of the uterine gland cells in relation to physiological events during a pregnancy cycle in *Glossina morsitans morsitans*. J Insect Physiol 29: 651–658.

14

RPLP1, a Crucial Ribosomal Protein for Embryonic Development of the Nervous System

Laura Perucho[1], Ana Artero-Castro[2], Sergi Guerrero[2], Santiago Ramón y Cajal[2], Matilde E. LLeonart[2*], Zhao-Qi Wang[1,3]

1 Leibniz Institute for Age Research - Fritz Lipmann Institute (FLI), Jena, Germany, 2 Oncology and Pathology Group, Institut de Recerca Hospital Vall d'Hebron, Barcelona, Spain, 3 Faculty of Biology and Pharmacy, Friedrich Schiller University of Jena, Jena, Germany

Abstract

Ribosomal proteins are pivotal to development and tissue homeostasis. RP Large P1 (*Rplp1*) overexpression is associated with tumorigenesis. However, the physiological function of *Rplp1* in mammalian development remains unknown. In this study, we disrupted *Rplp1* in the mouse germline and central nervous system (*Rplp1$^{CNS\Delta}$*). *Rplp1* heterozygosity caused body size reductions, male infertility, systemic abnormalities in various tissues and a high frequency of early postnatal death. *Rplp1$^{CNS\Delta}$* newborn mice exhibited perinatal lethality and brain atrophy with size reductions of the neocortex, midbrain and ganglionic eminence. The Rplp1 knockout neocortex exhibited progenitor cell proliferation arrest and apoptosis due to the dysregulation of key cell cycle and apoptosis regulators (cyclin A, cyclin E, p21^{CIP1}, p27^{KIP1}, p53). Similarly, *Rplp1* deletion in pMEFs led to proliferation arrest and premature senescence. Importantly, *Rplp1* deletion in primary mouse embryonic fibroblasts did not alter global protein synthesis, but did change the expression patterns of specific protein subsets involved in protein folding and the unfolded protein response, cell death, protein transport and signal transduction, among others. Altogether, we demonstrated that the translation "fine-tuning" exerted by Rplp1 is essential for embryonic and brain development and for proper cell proliferation.

Editor: Gilbert Bernier, University of Montréal and Hôpital Maisonneuve-Rosemont, Canada

Funding: This work was supported by the Marató project TV3/052130 and the FIS project PI12/01104. MELL is a FIS investigator (Miguel Servet stabilized contract CP03/00101). Laura Perucho was supported by a fellowship from La Caixa and the Deutscher Akademischer Austauschdienst. The funders had no role in study design, data collection and analysis, decision to publish, or preparation of the manuscript.

Competing Interests: The authors have declared that no competing interests exist.

* Email: melleona@ir.vhebron.net

Introduction

The assurance of proper ribosome functionality is essential for the development of all multicellular organisms. Dysfunctions in most RPs induce developmental defects ranging from general translation impairment-related defects to tissue-specific phenotypes [1,2]. More than 50 ribosomal protein (RP)-encoding loci were found to be mutated in a group of developmental abnormalities in *Drosophila* termed "minutes" [3–6]. "Minutes" are characterized by general developmental retardation, a reduced body size, short, thin bristles and diminished fertility, all of which are likely caused by a reduction in protein synthesis. In mammals, RP genes mutations are associated with tissue-specific abnormalities such as the mouse Tail-short (Ts), Tail-short shionogi (Tss) and Rabotorcido (Rbt) mutants, which present with skeletal abnormalities, short, kinky tails and neural tube defects such as exencephaly, spina bifida and cleft palate [7,8]. Recent studies have shown that the developmental defects in Ts mutants are caused by mutations in *Rpl38*, thus affecting the production of RPL38 [1], which regulates axial-skeletal patterning by modulating the translation of a subset of Hox mRNAs [1]. Similarly, *Rpl24* hypomorphism causes Belly spot and tail (Bst) mutants, which present with white hind feet, kinky tails and ventral midline spots. *Rpl24* mutations impair *Rpl24* mRNA splicing and RPL24 production, thus affecting ribosome biogenesis, protein synthesis and the cell cycle [9].

The ribosomal stalk is a flexible lateral protuberance in the large ribosomal subunit that constitutes the specific elongation factor recognition motif [10–12]. In high eukaryotes, this stalk comprises RP Large P0 (P0) and two heterodimers formed by RP Large P1 (P1) and RP Large P2 (P2). This structure is known as the P complex or P proteins. P0 is connected to the rest of the ribosome through the ribosomal protein L12 and the 28S ribosomal RNA [13]. In contrast to other ribosomal proteins, P1 and P2 are not imported into the nucleus for their assembly, and constantly shuttle between the ribosome and the cytoplasm [14,15]. Interestingly, P1 and P2 stabilize each other in the cytoplasm [16,17]. Of importance is that ribosomal stalk protein alterations have been found in human tumors. For example, *Rplp1* mRNA levels are increased by five-fold in colorectal cancer tissues [18]. Similarly, human lymphoid cell lines containing mutant P53 were shown to overexpress P1 [19]. We previously found that the RNA and protein levels of P0, P1 and P2 (P proteins) were significantly increased in gynecologic tumors [20]. From a therapeutic point of view, gonadotropin-releasing hormone (GnRH) analogues, which are used to treat breast, prostate and ovarian cancers, have been found to exert their anti-proliferative effects through the down-regulation of P1 and P2 [21], suggesting the potential clinical implications of targeting ribosomal stalk proteins. Interestingly, previous work from our laboratory showed that P1 overexpression allows cells to bypass replicative senescence, likely due to cyclin E overexpression consequent to increased E2F1 promoter activity [22]. Moreover, P1 was found to cooperate with Ras^{Val12} in the transformation of murine NIH3T3 cells [22].

The requirement of ribosomal stalk proteins in proliferating cells differs vastly among species. *S. cerevisiae* homologs of P1 and P2 are dispensable for viability [23]. In contrast, the depletion of P2 in human cells does not affect viability, but rather impairs proliferation, likely by affecting the efficiency of eukaryotic translation initiation factor 5B (IF-2)-mediated ribosome assembly [16,24].

To date, the physiological function of *Rplp1* has remained elusive. This study explored the role of *Rplp1* in development and proliferation using *Rplp1*-deficient mouse models and derived cells. As proteins from the P complex are highly expressed in the fetal brain [25], we decided to explore the role of the P1 protein in brain development. We found that *Rplp1* was essential for embryonic and brain development. Rplp1 deletion induced proliferation defects and apoptosis *in vivo*. Moreover, Rplp1 deletion caused a senescence-associated proliferation arrest in primary mouse embryonic fibroblasts (pMEFs). Overall, we propose that *Rplp1* absence provokes a stress response associated with misfolded proteins that induces a different translation pattern, rather than a general disturbance of ribosomal function and/or protein synthesis.

Materials and Methods

Cell culture

Mouse embryonic fibroblasts (MEFs) were cultured in Dulbecco's Modified Eagle Medium (DMEM; Invitrogen Life Technologies, Carlsbad, CA, USA) supplemented with 10% fetal calf serum (FCS; Lonza, Basel, Switzerland), 2 mM L-glutamine (Invitrogen), 1 mM sodium pyruvate (Invitrogen, 11360-039), 100 units/mL of penicillin, 100 μg/mL of streptomycin (Pen/Strep; Invitrogen) and 0.5 mM β-mercaptoethanol (Invitrogen). Mouse embryonic stem (ES) cells (blastocysts derived from mouse strain 129/Sv) were cultured in Dulbecco's Modified Eagle Medium (DMEM) (Invitrogen) supplemented with 15% fetal calf serum (FCS) (Lonza), 2 mM L-glutamine (Invitrogen), 1 mM sodium pyruvate (Invitrogen), 1 mM MEM non-essential amino acids (Invitrogen), 100 units/mL of penicillin, 100 μg/mL of streptomycin (Pen/Strep; Invitrogen), 0.5 mM β-mercaptoethanol (Invitrogen) and 1000 U/mL LIF (Chemicon, Billerica, MA, USA). The culture medium was changed daily. Fresh medium was prepared every 2 to 3 days. All animal procedures followed Association for Assessment and Accreditation of Laboratory Animal Care guidelines and were approved by institutional Animal Care and Use Committee. Stable transfection was performed with 30 μg of retroviral vectors LMP^{shRNA} (control) LMP^{shp53}, and LMP^{shp16INK4A} into Phoenix cells. Phoenix cells were maintained in a Minimum Essential Media (Gibco) supplemented with 50 μg/mL penicillin-streptomycin and 10% FBS. After 48 hours, the Phoenix supernatant was added into MEF cells, which were selected with 1 μg/mL puromycin and further treated with OHT during 4 days in order to induce the Rplp1 knock-down. For the transient transfection 2×10^5 MEF cells were seeded per well in 6-well plates. After 24 h they were transfected with Lipofectamine 2000 with the p16^{INK4AsiRNA}, p53^{siRNA} and Cy3 dye-labeled negative control (AM17010). Then, the cells were treated with OHT during four days in order to induce the Rplp1 knock-down. Stable cell lines were done according.

Primary MEF (pMEF) immortalization

Early passage pMEFs (P2) were immortalized by p19^{ARF} knockdown. A plasmid encoding p19^{ARF} shRNA was transfected into the Phoenix E retroviral packaging cell line (based on HEK293 cells). After 15 hours, the medium was changed and the cells were incubated at 32°C to facilitate virus production. Forty-eight hours later, the viral supernatant was collected, filtered through a 0.45-μm filter and mixed 1:1 with MEF medium and polybrene to a final concentration of 8 μg/ml. The mixture was incubated at RT for 5 minutes and then added to 30% confluent primary MEFs. The pMEFs were incubated at 32°C with 5% CO$_2$. Twenty-four hours later, the medium was changed and the cells were transferred to a 37°C incubator. The cells were selected for 4 days post-infection with 2 μg/ml of puromycin.

Growth curve

The growth curves were performed with freshly isolated pMEFs. Briefly, 1.5×10^5 cells per clone were seeded in triplicates into 6-well plates. The triplicates were treated with 1 μM 4-hydroxytamoxifen (4-OHT) (Sigma-Aldrich, St. Louis, MO, USA) for 4 days, and the other triplicates were used as an untreated control. Every three days, the cells were trypsinized, counted and re-plated similarly. The growth curves were constructed by plotting the cumulative cell number versus the passage number.

Proliferation assay

pMEFs were treated with 1 μM 4-OHT for 4 days. Three days later, the cells were incubated for 2 hours with 10 μM bromodeoxyuridine (BrdU). After incubation, the cells were washed with PBS 1X, harvested and fixed with ice-cold ethanol. Next, the cells were centrifuged at 1000×g for 10 minutes. The supernatants were aspirated and the pellets resuspended in 3 mL of 0.08% pepsin in 0.1 M HCl, followed by an incubation at 37°C for 20 minutes with occasional mixing. The cells were then centrifuged as described above, and the pellets were resuspended in 1.5 mL of 2 M HCl. The mixtures were incubated at 37°C for 20 min. Next, 3 mL of 0.1 M sodium borate were added, and the samples were centrifuged. The pellets were resuspended in 2 mL of IFA/Tween20 (0.5% Tween 20 in IFA) and centrifuged. The cells were subsequently stained with 75 μL of a FITC-conjugated anti-BrdU antibody (Becton Dickinson, Franklin Lakes, NJ, USA) at a 1:5 dilution in IFA (10 mM HEPES, pH 7.4; 150 mM NaCl; 4% fetal bovine serum; 0.1% sodium azide) for 30 minutes on ice. Next, 2 mL of IFA/Tween 20 were added, and the cells were centrifuged and resuspended in 0.25 mL of IFA. Finally, 0.25 mL of a 20 μg/mL propidium iodide solution (PI) were added. The percentages of BrdU-positive cells were determined on a flow cytometer (FACSCanto, BD Biosciences; software FACS Diva, San Jose, CA, USA).

Cell cycle

Confluent primary or immortalized MEFs were trypsinized and resuspended in 1 mL of PBS 1X and subsequently fixed with ice-cold absolute ethanol for at least one hour. The cells were then incubated with DNase-free RNaseA (100 μg/mL; Sigma-Aldrich) at 37°C for 30 minutes, after which 100 μL of 1 mg/mL propidium iodide (PI) (Sigma) were added. Finally, the cell cycle profiles were collected using a flow cytometer (FACSCanto, BD Biosciences; software, FACS Diva) (BD Biosciences).

Apoptosis assay

Primary or immortalized MEFs were trypsinized and washed twice with PBS 1X. The supernatant was also collected to include the late apoptotic cells. The cells were resuspended in 0.1 mL of binding buffer (10 mM HEPES, pH 7.4; 140 mM NaCl; 2.5 mM CaCl$_2$) containing Annexin V-FITC (1:100 dilution; BD Biosciences). The mixture was incubated for 15 minutes at RT in the dark. Next, 400 μL of DAPI-containing binding buffer (final concentration, 0.2 μg/mL) were added. The samples were kept on ice for 15 minutes and then analyzed by flow cytometry.

Senescence assay

Primary or immortalized MEFs growing in culture dishes or on coverslips were washed once with PBS 1X and fixed with 2% formaldehyde and 0.2% glutaraldehyde for 10 minutes at RT. Next, the cells were washed twice with PBS 1X and stained with a β-galactosidase staining solution (40 mM citric acid/sodium phosphate pH 6.0, 0.15 M NaCl, 2 mM MgCl$_2$, 5 nM potassium ferrocyanide, 5 nM potassium ferricyanide, 1 mg/mL of X-Gal). The cells were incubated at 37°C in a dry incubator overnight. The reagents are included with the Senescence β-galactosidase staining kit (Cell Signaling, Danvers, MA, USA).

Protein synthesis

To measure protein synthesis, we used a system based on the azide-alkyne reaction (Click-it Protein synthesis kit) (Invitrogen). Briefly, newly synthetized proteins are labeled with an azide (or alkyne)-coupled methionine analog. A fluorophore or HRP-conjugated alkyne (or azide) is then used for detection. In our study, we used a biotin-conjugated alkyne to perform western blotting. Rplp1$^{F/F}$; Cre-ER^{T2}+ and Rplp1$^{+/F}$; Cre-ER^{T2}+ immortalized MEFs were treated with 1 μM 4-OHT for 4 days or left untreated (control). Three days later, the cells were washed once with warm PBS and incubated for 1 hour with methionine-free DMEM (Invitrogen) to deplete the methionine reserves of the cells. Next, the medium was removed, and the cells were incubated for 3 hours in methionine-free DMEM with the methionine analog azide-homoalanine (AHA; Invitrogen). The cells were then washed once with PBS, followed by the addition of lysis buffer (1% SDS, 50 mM Tris-HCl pH 8, 1 mM Na$_3$VO$_4$, 10 mM NaF, 0.1 mM PMSF, 1X Roche Complete Protease Inhibitor Cocktail; Roche, Basel Switzerland). The cells were collected with a cell scraper and incubated for 30 minutes in lysis buffer. Next, the cell lysates were sonicated (5 30-second on/off cycles; BioruptorPlus; Diagenode, Seraing, Belgium) and centrifuged at 15,700×g for 15 minutes at 4°C. The supernatant was transferred to a fresh Eppendorf tube. A Bradford assay was used to measure the protein concentration as follows: 1 μL of protein extract was mixed with 999 μL of a 1:5 dilution of Bradford solution (Bio-Rad) in water. The absorbance at 595 nm was determined with a spectrophotometer (Eppendorf BioPhotometer; Hamburg, Germany). Subsequently, 50 μg of protein were transferred to a new tube, to which were added 100 μL of biotin-alkyne in 2x reaction buffer (Invitrogen) and water to a final volume of 160 μL. The following reagents were then added sequentially: 10 μL of reagent C (CuSO$_4$) (Invitrogen), 10 μL of reagent D (buffer additive 1) and 20 μL of reagent E (buffer additive 2). The mixture was shaken for 20 minutes, and then 600 μL of methanol, 150 μL of chloroform and 400 μL of water were added. The mixture was vortexed and centrifuged for 5 minutes at 13,200×g. The upper aqueous phase was discarded, and 450 μL of methanol were added. The protein solution was centrifuged as described above, and the methanol was discarded. The remaining protein pellet was washed again with methanol as described above, after which the pellet was air-dried. The pellet was resuspended in SDS-sample buffer 1X (see 2.6.2), vortexed for 10 minutes and then heated for 10 minutes at 70°C. A quarter of the mixture was separated by SDS-polyacrylamide gel electro-

phoresis and then transferred to a PVDF membrane (Bio-Rad). The membrane was blocked for 30 minutes with 5% BSA in TBS-T and then for 30 minutes with an ABC peroxidase reagent (Vectastain Burlingame, CA, USA), which reagent contains a biotinylated horseradish peroxidase (HRP) that had been pre-incubated with avidin at a specific ratio to form large complexes. The membrane was washed 3 times for 5 minutes each at RT. Finally, the membrane was developed with an ECL kit (Pierce, Appleton, WI, USA). Cells that had been treated with 1 μg/mL of cycloheximide (Sigma), which inhibits the elongation step of protein synthesis, were used as a negative control.

Neurosphere formation assay

For this assay, freshly isolated neural stem cells were plated at a density of 8×10^5 cells/T-25 flask in DMEM/F12 (Invitrogen) supplemented with 20 ng/mL of EGF (Peprotech, Rocky Hill, NJ, USA), 20 ng/mL of bFGF (Peprotech), 1X B-27 (Invitrogen), 100 units/mL of penicillin and 100 μg/mL of streptomycin (Pen/Strep; Invitrogen). The cells were incubated at 37°C with 5%CO$_2$. Seven days later, the neurospheres were counted via microscopy to determine the number of neurospheres per mL.

PCR

DNA was isolated from mouse tails or cells. For Rplp1 PCR-genotyping, the following primers were used:
R1-1 5′-CGT GGT CTC CTA CTT CTG TG-3′
R1-2 5′-GAA AAG TGC CAG GAA ATC CAG T-3′
R1-15 5′-ATG CTG TGT CCA TTA TCC T-3′
The primers R1-1 and 2 yield bands of 145 bp for wild-type Rplp1 and 201 bp for floxed Rplp1. If Rplp1 is deleted, primers R1-1 and 15 yield a band of 411 bp. To detect the Rplp1 targeted allele, the following primers were used:
R1-3 5′-CTT CAT GTA GAA AGT TTA GGA CTT G-3′
R1-4 5′-CTA GTG AGA CGT GCT ACT TC-3′
R1-5 5′-ATG TTT TGT AGT TCA GGC TGG-3′
Primers R1-3 and 4 yield a band of 444 bp for targeted Rplp1 is targeted, whereas primers R1-3 and 5 yield a band of 158 bp for wild-type Rplp1.
For Cre PCR-genotyping, the following primers were used:
Cre1 5′-CGGTCGATGCAACGAGTGATG-3′
Cre2 5′-CCAGAGACGGAAATCCATCGC-3′
Actin-B2-1 5′-CACCGGAGAATGGGAAGCCGAA-3′
Actin-B2-2 5′-TCCACACAGATGGAGCGTCCAG-3′
The Cre1 and Cre2 primers detect the Cre transgene to yield a band of 643 bp. The Actin-B2-1 and Actin-B2-2 primers detect the Actin gene to yield a band of 294 bp and are used as a control. The PCR reaction conditions were as follows: For Rplp1, an initial denaturation step was performed for 3 minutes at 94°C, followed by 35 cycles of denaturation for 15 seconds at 94°C, primer annealing for 1 minute at 57°C and elongation for 2 minutes at 72°C and a final elongation step for 7 minutes at 72°C. For Cre, an initial denaturation step was performed for 3 minutes at 94°C, followed by 35 cycles of denaturation for 30 seconds at 94°C, primer annealing for 1 minute at 58.5°C and elongation for 2 minutes 30 seconds at 65°C and a final elongation step for 7 minutes at 65°C.

Southern Blot

Genomic DNA from cells or mouse tissues was digested either with AseI for the short arm and PflFI for the long arm or HindIII. The digested samples were separated on a 0.8% agarose gel in TAE buffer (40 mM Tris Base, 20 mM acetic acid, 1 mM EDTA). The DNA was fragmented by depurination in 250 nM HCl for 20 minutes and denatured in 500 mM NaOH, 1.5 M NaCl for 30 minutes. The DNA was then transferred to a Hybond XL membrane (GE Healthcare Life Sciences, Cleveland, Ohio). Next, the membrane was incubated for 20 minutes in 40 mM NaPi and baked for 1 hour at 80°C, followed by DNA crosslinking (UV Stratalinker; Stratagene, La Jolla, CA, USA). The membrane was then prehybridized in Church's buffer (500 mM NaPi pH 8, 7% SDS, 1 mM EDTA) for one hour at 65°C. Subsequently, the membrane was hybridized overnight with a dCTP α-^{32}P radio labeled probe in Church's buffer at 65°C. The sequences of the genomic probes were as follows:

P3LA (for long arm):

tcatttggctaggtggcaaggactgtgcctgcagattctccgtcactatcagtttttataaattg gagatgctcgcagttgctcatgctactatttcatatacatgaaaaaagatttgtttaaaaagtcg aatgtgctatttaacttggtacagctggcatttgactggaaaacaggtagtttttattataggat acaagctgatttcatagtgtagtcttcgattcttggagcgtttaagaaaagtttggagaaaaaca ttgctggtatatttgtggaaatgtgttttgaaatatagaaatctttactgcaagtgctcagaggtg ctttcactgttgaggcacggtacatgtgaagtacctgttcctgtgttctacagggttctcctctacc agagtttcaacagcttgtactttttgatatggctgtatatgaagaatgttttctatttagatgcctca gacacacttaagcgttatattgatcctgctgatactttaacagacctgctatttattacttcacaa agcagccataataattgggtttgatcaagaatgcgaaatggattatttgtcctgagctagccat aaacaggaagacctagagtcacgacaactgtaccctttgcccttgttgcaatggaagctccc aaacagactatctctctcatgctgttgtccaaagatgcctgttggttgttgactaagaagaga acgttgaatgattttcatgtttagtgtgggcaggtttgatttcggtgaacttgcattgtaaactgct gcacttctaatggaacctcaaagtaatcctgggttgtgcttgtttcccaat.

P1RA (for short arm):

aggcctgttatcagtgatgggtgtccgtagtcttgattttgaagggtcttgcattaaggaaac tgttcttttttgtaaattgagatgtgccaattttcattaagcaccaagacagggacaggaccaata tctaaaccagaaataatggtcccatttgtgctgggtggtggggtgagaaacagtatcctggggt tttatgggtgataacctgcactctgccggtcctgtctattcctgcatcttggatgttctaacatctt ccgttgcagaaggctattgcccagagaaaacagaagatgctttaaattttttattttttaaatt tttgaatcagggtgttcttctctatcccaagctggcctgaaactcactatgtagcctagagtgga ctggaaccttccagaaaccttcctgcctcagacttccaggtggctggtgtgacagctatactcc acatgactgctttgtggaactttaggttctatgtccagctaagatattaaagctattaaaagcaa aggggcaaaaagaataaaactattttgcagcttcctaggccctccacagtgcattgaccttctc agagggtgcagacagtctccataccacctacatgcagggtccctgtttgaagagcaaactca gttccctatgtactggagccataggcctgatttggagggtcccaacaagtagagtctggccac tttcctc.

Probe G (for HindIII digestion):

cagtgatagtattgtgaacctgggcttataatcttgtaacctgccacccacgtgtaggataa tggacacagcatgcctggccataggctgttatttagctcaaatagttctgggcctccaggttctg ctcaatttgacgtctacacttctgacatggaatgctaaggattgtattgcccaatgaaaatggat gttctggtccttgaggctcacctccttgatggggcattgtcttcccaaggtaacctttgtggagt tgggtgggggttagagttaaggaaaggtcttactgtgtagccttggctagtctggaaatcacc tgccttttggaaatttaacgaggggactggtaccctggttaattattgca.

The following day, the membrane was washed twice in washing buffer (1% SDS, 30 mM NaPi) for 5 minutes at 55°C, once for 15 minutes at 65°C and once for 30–45 minutes at 65°C. Finally, the membrane was exposed to a phosphoimager overnight and subsequently to X-Ray film for several days.

Protein isolation

For protein isolation, the cells were trypsinized and washed twice with ice-cold PBS. After centrifugation at $240 \times g$ and supernatant removal, the cell pellet was resuspended in 50 L of RIPA buffer (50 mM Tris-HCl, 150 mM NaCl, 1 mM EDTA, 0.25% sodium deoxycholate, 1 mM Na$_3$VO$_4$, 10 mM NaF, 0.1 mM PMSF, 1% NP-40, 1X Roche Complete Protease Inhibitor Cocktail; Roche) and incubated for 30 minutes on ice. The lysate was then sonicated (30-second on/off cycles; Bioruptor Plus; Diagenode) and centrifuged at $15,700 \times g$ for 15 minutes at 4°C, followed by transfer to a fresh Eppendorf tube and storage at −80°C. A Bradford assay was used to measure the protein concentration as follows: 1 µL of protein extract was mixed with 999 µL of a 1:5 dilution of Bradford solution (Bio-Rad) in water.

The absorbance at 595 nm was determined with a spectrophotometer (Eppendorf BioPhotometer; Eppendorf). For protein isolation from mouse tissues, the tissues were previously snap-frozen in liquid nitrogen and stored at −80°C. A single tissue piece was minced with a sharp scalpel, followed by the addition of RIPA buffer. The tissue was subsequently homogenized with a tissue homogenizer (Polytron PT 2500E). The tissue lysate was incubated for 30 minutes on ice, followed by the above-described procedure.

Western blot

For western blot analysis, the protein samples were separated by SDS-polyacrylamide gel electrophoresis (SDS-PAGE). After separation, the proteins were transferred to a PVDF membrane (Bio-Rad) that was subsequently blocked with 5% non-fat dried milk (NFDM) in TBS-T or in 5% BSA in TBS-T if antibodies against phosphorylated proteins were to be used. After blocking, the membrane was incubated overnight at 4°C with the primary antibody diluted in blocking solution. The membrane was then washed and incubated for 30 minutes to 2 hours at RT with the HRP-conjugated secondary antibody diluted in 5% NFDM in TBS-T. Finally, the membrane was washed and developed with an ECL kit (Pierce).

Two-dimensional gel electrophoresis

Protein extracts from three different $Rplp1^{i\Delta}$ pMEFs that had been treated with 4-OHT for four days or not (control) were separated by two-dimensional gel electrophoresis. The dysregulated proteins (p<0.01) in the $Rplp1^{i\Delta}$ pMEFs were selected and identified by ESI-MS as described in [26].

ROS assay

Control and inducible pMEFs were treated with OHT for 4 days. DCF-DA was then added to the cells for a 30 minutes incubation. The amount of DCF (the oxidized, fluorescent form of DCF-DA; Invitrogen) was then analyzed by flow cytometry.

Isolation, fixation and embedding of mouse tissues

To isolate mouse or mouse embryonic tissues, the mouse was first sacrificed by cervical dislocation. After cleaning with 70% ethanol, the abdominal wall and peritoneum were opened to expose the organs or embryos, which were removed with forceps and sharp scissors, washed in PBS and fixed ON in 4% PFA at 4°C or in Roti-Histofix (4% formaldehyde, Roth) at RT. To isolate the brains from E18.5 embryos, the heads were removed and immersed in PBS in a Petri dish. The skulls were carefully removed with fine forceps. This procedure was performed under a stereomicroscope (Zeiss Stemi 2000; Zeiss, Oberkochen, Germany). After fixation, the tissues were washed in PBS and incubated for 30 minutes at 4°C in 30% ethanol, followed by a transfer to 50% ethanol, processing and paraffin embedding. The paraffin-embedded tissues were then cut into 5-µm-thick slices with a microtome (Microm, Cavriago, Italy). The slices were mounted on glass slides and dried overnight at 55°C. Hematoxylin and eosin (H&E) staining or immunohistochemistry (IHC) were then performed. All of the procedures performed in this study were approved by the Ethical Committee of Animal Research at the Leibniz Institute for Age Research.

IHC and microscopy

To perform IHC analyses of the mouse embryonic brains, the paraffin sections were first deparaffinized. For antigen retrieval, the sections were incubated in 10 mM sodium citrate, pH 6.0 for

A

B

C

D

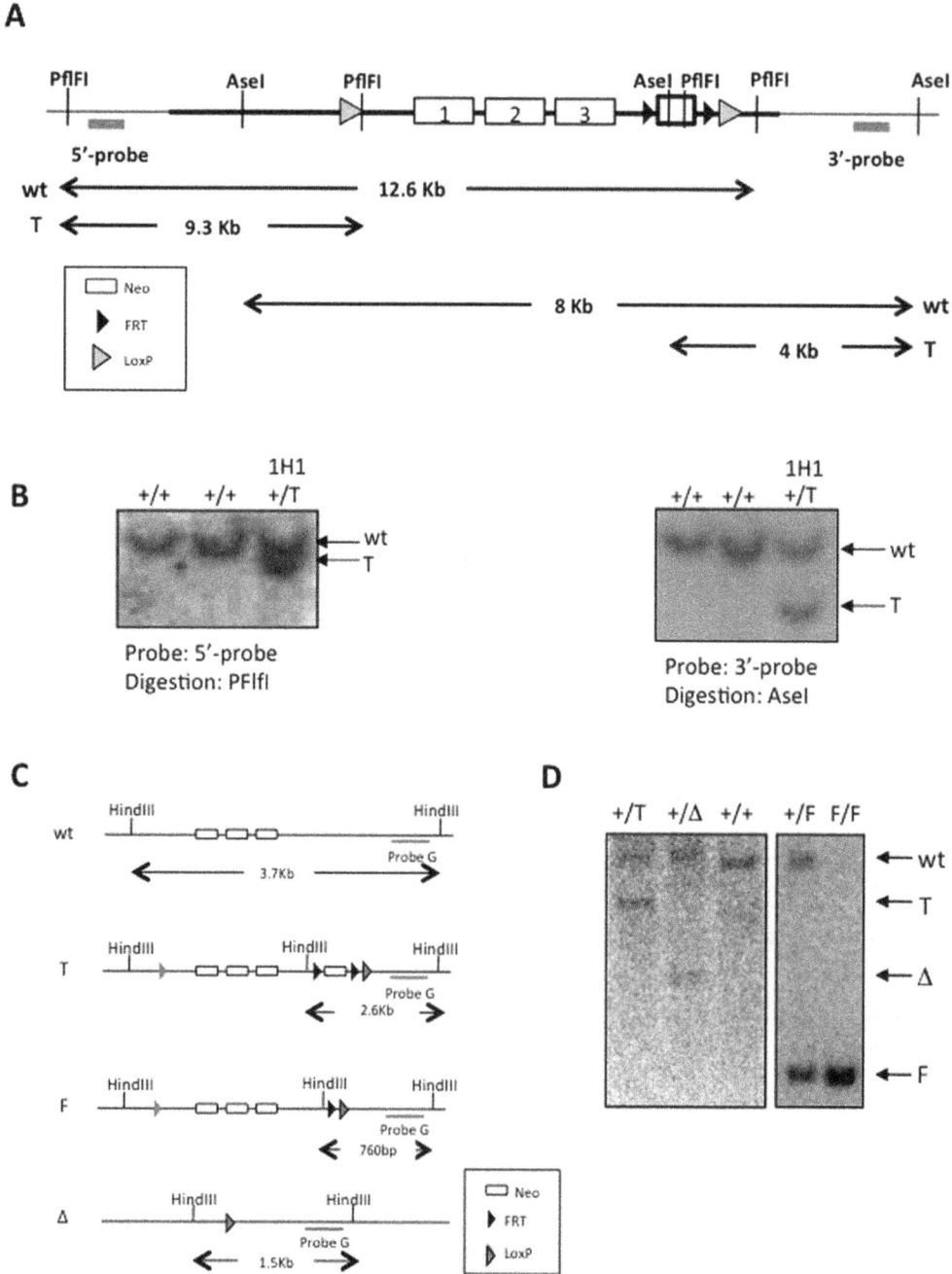

Figure 1. Generation of *Rplp1* knockout mice. (A) Gene targeting in ES cells. A Southern blotting strategy was used to screen the mutant alleles in ES cells. 5′- and 3′- external probes were hybridized to the Southern blots after genomic DNA digestion with *PflFI* and *AseI*, respectively. **(B)** Southern blot analysis of gene-targeted *Rplp1* ES cells. Two strategies were used to confirm the correct integration of the gene-targeting vector, using the 5′- and 3′- probes indicated in (A). A *Rplp1*$^{+/T}$ clone (1H1) is shown. **(C)** Southern blotting strategy for *Rplp1* mutant alleles. **(D)** Southern blot of mouse tails, showing *Rplp1*$^{+/+}$, *Rplp1*$^{+/T}$, *Rplp1*$^{+/F}$, *Rplp1*$^{F/F}$ and *Rplp1*$^{+/\Delta}$. Wt: wild-type allele. T: targeted allele. F: floxed allele. Δ: deleted allele.

10 minutes at a sub-boiling temperature in a microwave. The sections were allowed to cool at RT for 30 minutes and were then washed three times with PBS for 5 minutes each at RT. Next, the sections were incubated in blocking solution (1% BSA, 5% goat serum, 0.4% Triton X-100 in PBS) to avoid non-specific antibody binding for 1 hour at RT in a humidified chamber. The blocking solution was then removed, and a primary antibody dilution in blocking solution was added. The sections were incubated overnight at 4°C in a humidified chamber with the primary antibody. Next, the sections were washed three times in PBS at RT and incubated with a fluorochrome-conjugated secondary antibody diluted in blocking solution. The sections were then washed three times in PBS for 5 minutes each and finally mounted with coverslips using a DAPI-containing mounting medium (ProLong gold; Invitrogen). The mounted sections were air-dried for several hours and stored temporarily at 4°C and long-term at -20°C. IHC images were acquired with a fluorescence microscope (Zeiss Axio Imager ApoTome or Zeiss Axio Imager M1; Zeiss)

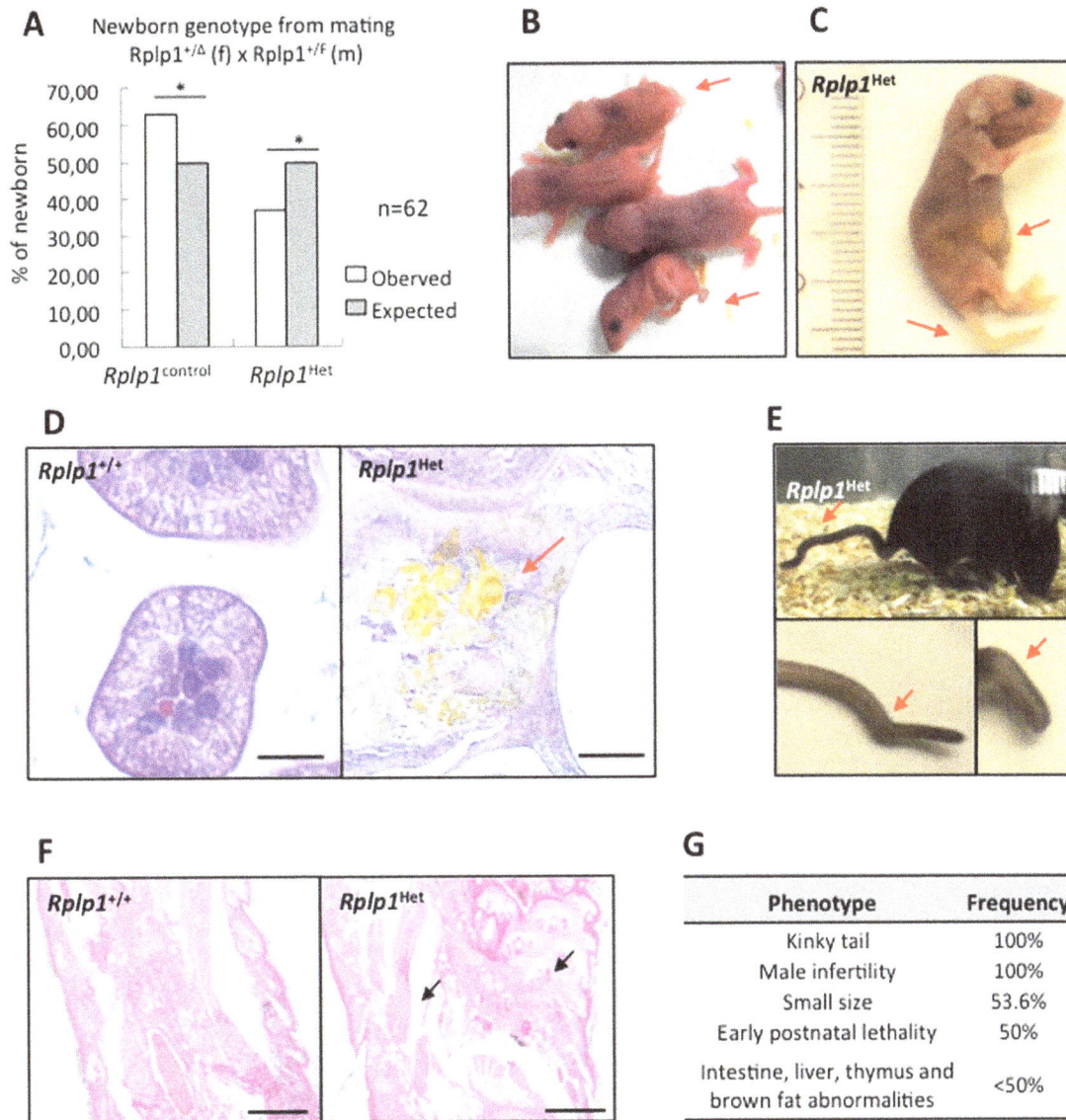

Figure 2. *Rplp1*^Het^ mice exhibit developmental defects. (A) Offspring genotype distribution from matings between *Rplp1*^+/Δ^ and *Rplp1*^+/F^ mice. Pearson's chi-squared test was used for the statistical analysis. X² = 0.04 (B) *Rplp1*^Het^ mice (red arrows) are smaller than their littermates. (C) Detail of a *Rplp1*^Het^ mouse with an abnormal, yellow-colored abdomen and a kinky tail. (D) H&E staining of *Rplp1*^+/+^ and *Rplp1*^Het^ mouse intestines from postnatal day 0. The intestines were perforated at different locations and meconium ileus (yellow) was present. Scale bar: 20 μm. (E) Kinky tails in *Rplp1*^Het^ mice. (F) H&E staining of *Rplp1*^Het^ and *Rplp1*^+/+^ mouse tails. Scale bar: 500 μm. (G) Overview of the phenotypes observed in *Rplp1*^Het^ mice.

coupled to a charge-coupled device (CCD)-camera (Zeiss AxioCamMRm) and AxioVision software (Carl Zeiss). Bright-field images were obtained with a Zeiss Axio Imager M1 microscope fitted with a CCD-camera (Zeiss AxioCam MRc5). The number of cells positive for a certain marker was determined with the ImageJ software program.

Terminal deoxynucleotidyl transferase dUTP nick-end labeling (TUNEL) of mouse brain sections

Paraffin sections of different embryonic brain stages were deparaffinized and incubated in 10 mM sodium citrate, pH 6.0 for 10 minutes at a sub-boiling temperature. The sections were cooled at RT for 30 minutes and washed three times for 5 minutes each at RT with PBS. The sections were incubated with a TUNEL reaction mixture (1x buffer, Amersham; 0.3 units/μL of terminal deoxynucleotidyltransferase, Amersham; 6.66 μM biotin-linked dUTP, Roche Diagnostics; water; Amersham, GE Healthcare Life Sciences) for 1 hour at 37°C in a humidified chamber. The sections were then washed three times for 5 minutes each in PBS at RT and incubated with a 1:500 dilution of streptavidin-Cy3 (Sigma-Aldrich) in PBS with 1% BSA for one hour at RT. The sections were washed three times for five minutes each with PBS and mounted with coverslips, using a DAPI-containing mounting medium (ProLong gold; Invitrogen). The mounted sections were air-dried for several hours and stored temporarily at 4°C and long-term at −20°C.

A

Newborn genotype from mating between
Rplp1+/F;NesCre+ mice

□ Oberved
■ Expected

n=176

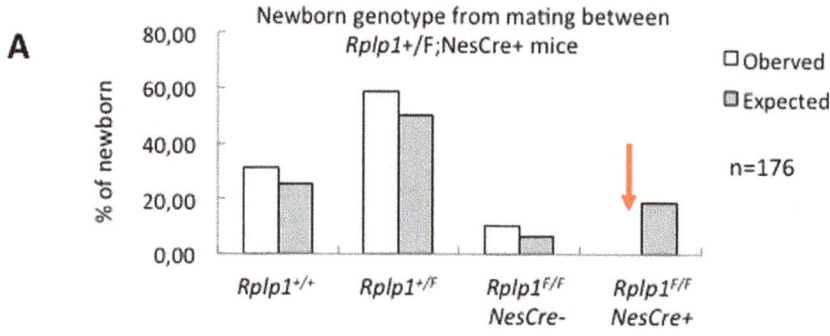

B

Control   *Rplp1^CNSΔ*

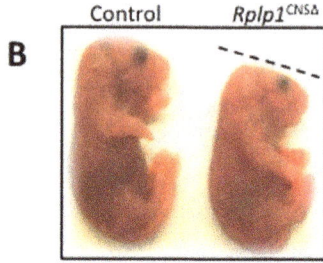

C

Control   *Rplp1^CNSΔ*

Cb

1 mm

Ctx

Ob

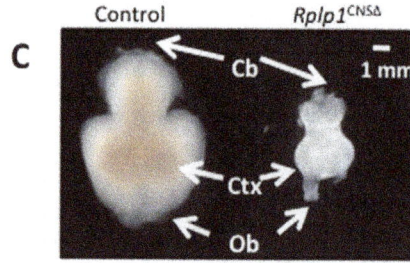

D

E12.5   E13.5   E15.5

Control

Rplp1^CNSΔ

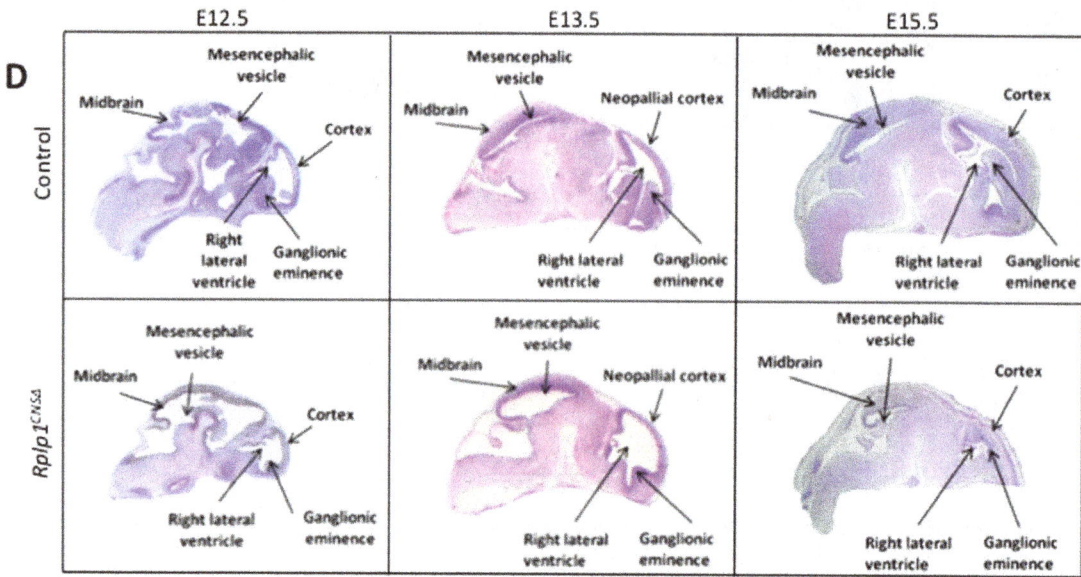

E

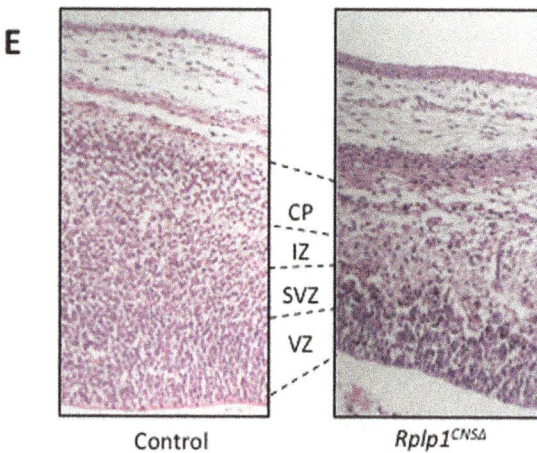

CP
IZ
SVZ
VZ

Control   *Rplp1^CNSΔ*

F

Control   *Rplp1^CNSΔ*

Rplp1 →
Rplp2 →

β-Actin

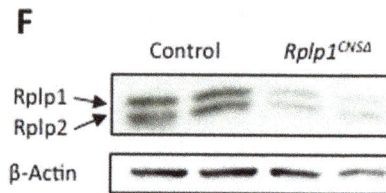

Figure 3. *Rplp1*^CNSΔ mice die perinatally and have reduced brain sizes and morphological defects. (**A**) Table showing the genotypes of the mice obtained from matings between *Rplp1+/F; NesCre+* mice. No *Rplp1*^CNSΔ mice were obtained. (**B**) *Rplp1*^CNSΔ and control E18.5 embryos. *Rplp1*^CNSΔ E18.5 embryos exhibited abnormal head morphology. (**C**) Pictures of *Rplp1*^CNSΔ and control E18.5 embryonic brains. The embryonic brain size is extremely reduced in *Rplp1*^CNSΔ embryos. (**D**) H&E staining images of control and *Rplp1*^CNSΔ embryonic brains at different stages. (**E**) Magnification of H&E stained control and *Rplp1*^CNSΔ E15.5 neocortexes. (**F**) Western blot showing efficient *Rplp1* deletion in *Rplp1*^CNSΔ mouse embryonic brains. RPLP2 expression was also downregulated in these mice. VZ: ventricular zone. SVZ: subventricular zone. IZ: intermediate zone. CP: cortical plate.

In vivo bromodeoxyuridine (BrdU)-proliferation assay

Pregnant females at E13.5 were injected intraperitoneally with a single 50-µg/g mouse body weight dose of BrdU (Sigma). After 30 minutes, the females were sacrificed by cervical dislocation and the embryos were collected. The embryonic heads were removed and fixed in 4% PFA at 4°C overnight. Portions of the embryos were used for DNA isolation and further analysis by PCR. The embryonic heads were processed as described in the IHC section. After deparaffination, the sections were incubated in 10 mM sodium citrate, pH 6.0 for 10 minutes at a sub-boiling temperature, cooled at RT for 30 minutes and washed three times for 5 minutes each with PBS at RT. Next, the sections were incubated in 2 M HCl at 37°C for 30 minutes to denature the DNA. The sections were washed three times in PBS for 5 minutes each, followed by a trypsin incubation (Zytomed, ZUCO43-15) for 20 minutes at 37°C. The sections were then washed three times for 5 minutes each in PBS and incubated for one hour at RT in a humidified chamber with blocking solution (1% BSA, 5% goat serum, 0.4% Triton X-100 in PBS). Finally, immunostaining was performed with an anti-BrdU antibody (Abcam, Cambridge, UK). The antibodies used are described in Table S1.

Results

Generation of *Rplp1* knockout mice

To dissect the role of *Rplp1 in vivo*, we generated *Rplp1* constitutive and conditional knockout mice. Briefly, the two homologous regions of the Rplp1 gene were amplified by PCR from Sv129/J background mouse genomic DNA. These PCR fragments were subcloned into the DTA vector, which contains a neomycin (neo) resistance gene to ampicillin and the DTA (Diphtheria Toxin A) gene. A single LoxP site and anFRT-Neo-FRT-LoxP cassette were inserted by homologous recombination upstream of exon 1 and downstream of exon 3, respectively (Figure 1A). After gene targeting in embryonic stem (ES) cells, a southern blot analysis with 5′- and 3′-external probes confirmed the correct gene targeting event in the ES cells (Figure 1A and 1B). The targeted ES clone (1H1) was injected into blastocysts of C57BL/6N mice to generate chimeras that gave rise to germline offspring carrying the *Rplp1* targeted (T) allele. The germline offspring (*Rplp1*^+/T) was confirmed by southern blotting (Figure 1C and 1D). The intercrossing of *Rplp1*^+/T mice with mice expressing Flp-recombinase (FLP) or Nestin-cre (NesCre) generated *Rplp1*

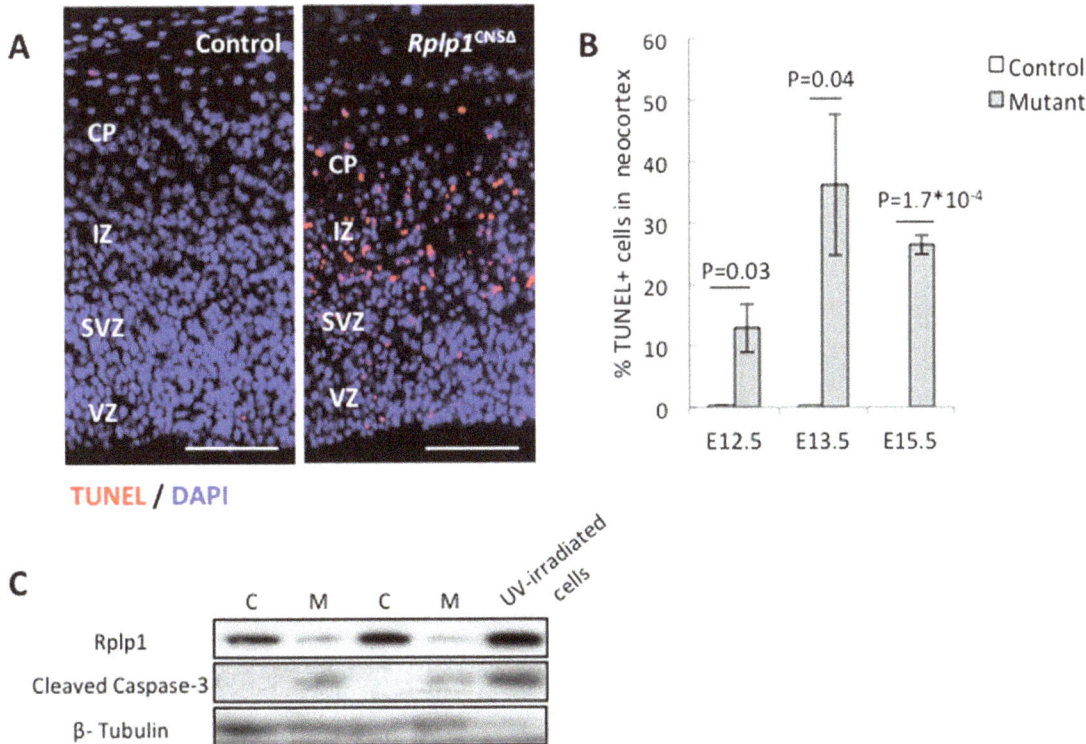

Figure 4. Increased apoptosis in the *Rplp1*^CNS neocortex. (**A**) TUNEL staining of sagittal control and *Rplp1*^CNSΔ embryonic brain sections. (**B**) Quantification of control and *Rplp1*^CNSΔ embryonic brain TUNEL staining at E12.5, E13.5 and E15.5. (**C**) Western blot analysis of cleaved caspase-3 in E13.5 embryonic brain protein extracts. C: control. M: mutant. VZ: ventricular zone. SVZ: subventricular zone. IZ: intermediate zone. CP: cortical plate. Scale bars: 50 µm. N = 3. Error bars: SEM.

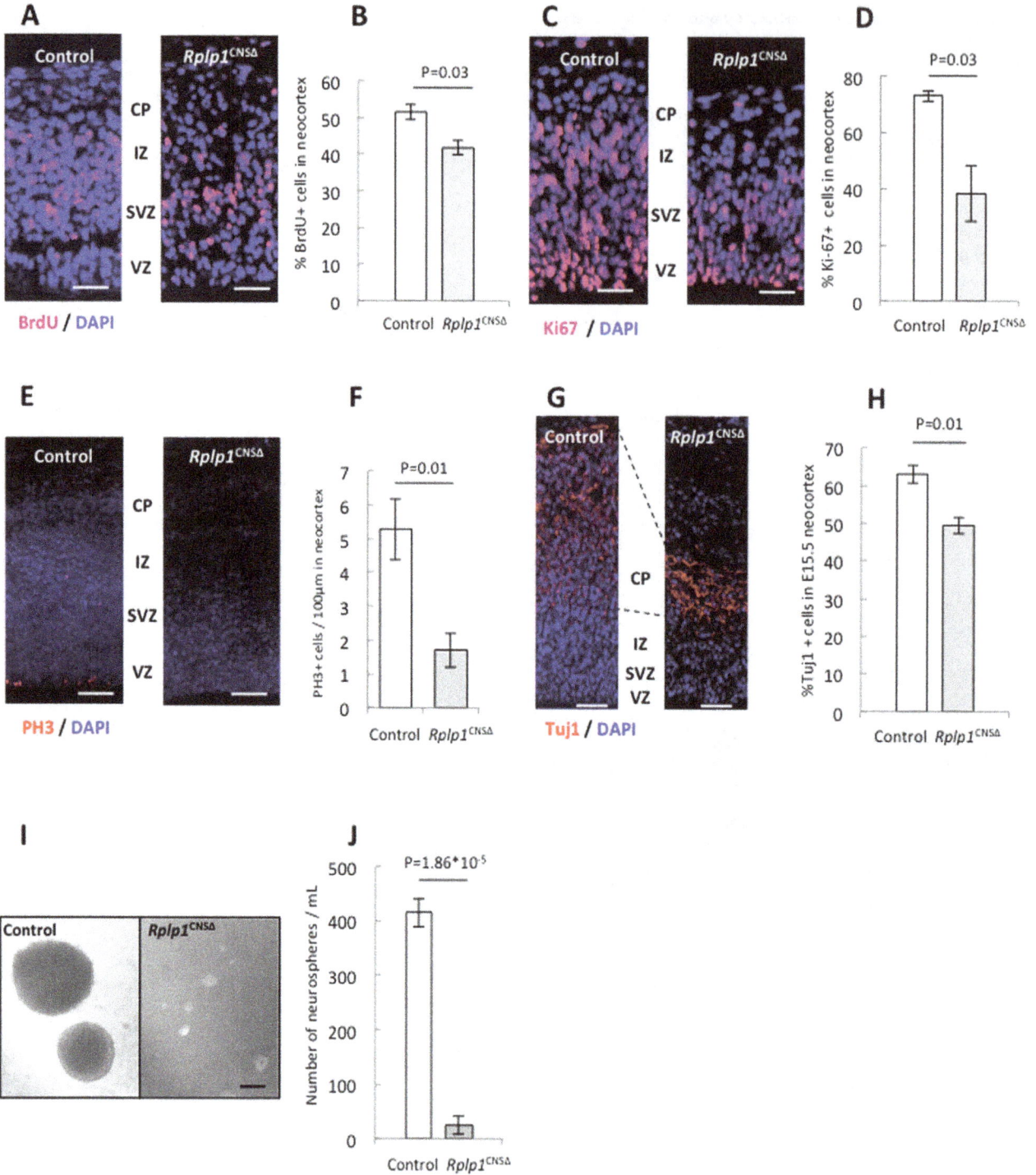

Figure 5. Proliferation defect in *Rplp1*^CNSΔ mouse embryonic brains. (**A**) BrdU staining of control and *Rplp1*^CNSΔ E13.5 embryonic brain paraffin sections after BrdU pulse-labeling for 1 h. Scale bars: 50 μm. N = 3. (**B**) Quantification of BrdU+ cells in the neocortex. (**C**) Ki67 staining in control and *Rplp1*^CNSΔ E13.5 embryonic brain paraffin sections. Scale bars: 50 μm. N = 3. (**D**) Quantification of Ki67+ cells in the neocortex. (**E**) Paraffin sections of control and *Rplp1*^CNSΔ E13.5 embryonic brains were stained for PH 3. Scale bars: 100 μm. N = 4. (**F**) Quantification of PH 3+ cells in the neocortex. (**G**) Paraffin sections of control and *Rplp1*^CNSΔ E15.5 embryonic brains were stained for Tuj1. Scale bars: 50 μm. N = 3. (**H**) Quantification of Tuj1+ cells in the neocortex. (**I**) Control and *Rplp1*^CNSΔ neurospheres formed *in vitro* after 7 days in culture. (**J**) Quantification of neurospheres per mL. Scale bars: 50 μm. N = 3. VZ: ventricular zone. SVZ: subventricular zone. IZ: intermediate zone. CP: cortical plate. Error bars: SEM.

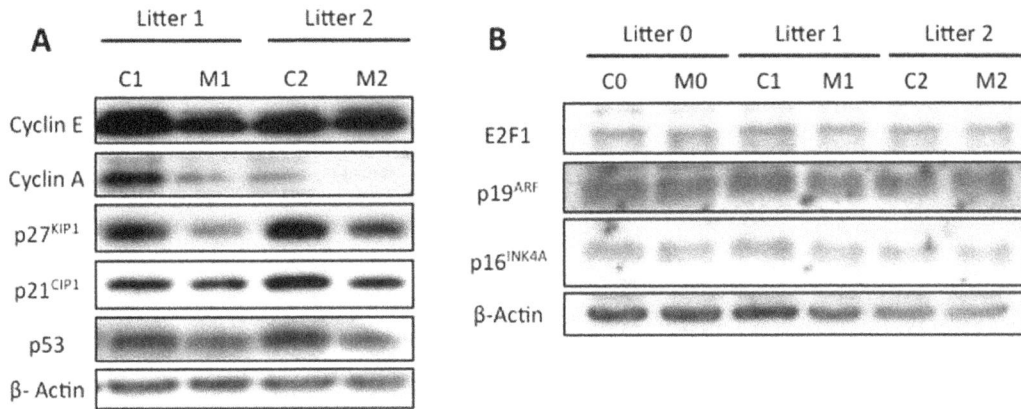

Figure 6. Cyclin A, cyclin E, P21^{CIP1}, P27^{KIP1} and P53 expression are downregulated in Rplp1$^{CNS\Delta}$ E13.5 embryonic brains. Western blot analysis of E13.5 embryonic brain samples was performed.

floxed (Rplp1$^{F/F}$) mice or deleted Rplp1 (Rplp1$^{+/\Delta}$) mice, respectively (Figure 1C and 1D).

Rplp1 heterozygous mice exhibit severe developmental defects

We obtained Rplp1$^{+/\Delta}$ and Rplp1$^{F/\Delta}$ mice (Rplp1 heterozygous mice, Rplp1^{Het}), which carry only one functional allele of Rplp1, from matings between Rplp1$^{+/F}$; NesCre$^+$ mice and between Rplp1$^{+/F}$; NesCre$^+$ mice. Rplp1^{Het} mice were born at a significantly reduced frequency (Figure 2A). Moreover, approximately 50% of the Rplp1^{Het} mice died during the early postnatal period. Rplp1^{Het} newborn mice were smaller than the control littermates (Figure 2B) and exhibited a yellow abdominal coloration (Figure 2C). A histological analysis of the intestinal sections revealed perforations in the small and large bowel. Yellow-colored meconium ileus was present in the lesions. The epithelial structure was destroyed and inflammatory cells were present around these lesions (Figure 2D). Additional abnormalities were observed in the liver, where there was very little hematopoiesis and erythroblasts and granular cells were lacking (Figure S1). The thymuses in Rplp1^{Het} mice were much smaller and exhibited abnormal organization. The brown fat adipoblasts were poorly differentiated (Figure S1). Rplp1^{Het} mice exhibited rigid, shorter, kinky tails (Figure 2E); a histological analysis of Rplp1^{Het} tail sections further revealed that the serial cartilage was disorganized and the long bones were abnormally enlarged (Figure 2F). Furthermore, Rplp1^{Het} male mice were infertile, making the generation of Rplp1 knockout mice impossible. However, the histological analyses of Rplp1^{Het} testes sections revealed no differences between the Rplp1^{Het} and control mice (Figure S1). The Rplp1^{Het} mouse phenotype is summarized in Figure 2G.

Rplp1 conditional deletion in the CNS causes perinatal lethality and reduced brain size

To study the role of Rplp1 in the CNS, Rplp1 conditional knockout mice (Rplp1$^{CNS\Delta}$) were generated by crossing Rplp1 floxed mice (Rplp1$^{F/F}$) with Nestin-Cre transgenic mice. Intercrossing between Rplp1$^{+/F}$; NesCre$^+$ mice did not yield any Rplp1$^{F/F}$; NesCre$^+$ (Rplp1$^{CNS\Delta}$) offspring, indicating that Rplp1$^{CNS\Delta}$ mice died during development or the early postnatal period (Figure 3A). We further analyzed the developmental stage at which the Rplp1$^{CNS\Delta}$ mice died. We found viable Rplp1$^{CNS\Delta}$ embryos at embryonic day (E) E12.5, E13.5, E15.5 and E17.5.

Furthermore, a cesarean procedure at E18.5 allowed us to recover viable Rplp1$^{CNS\Delta}$ embryos. However, these were small, featured flat heads (Figure 3B) and had dramatically reduced brain sizes (Figure 3C). Overall, the mutant mice were unable to survive.

Because the brain defects at developmental stage E18.5 were dramatic, we analyzed the structure of the Rplp1$^{CNS\Delta}$ embryonic brain at earlier stages. An histological examination revealed that at E12.5, compared with wild-type embryos, Rplp1$^{CNS\Delta}$ embryos showed a reduced ganglionic eminence, a thinner neocortex and an enlarged right lateral ventricle (Figure 3D). At E13.5, the mutant embryos exhibited enlarged ventricles, atrophy of the neopallial cortex and roof of the midbrain, a reduced ganglionic eminence and reduced cellularity in the thalamus. At E15.5 the cortex and the midbrain were very small and atrophic, suggesting that brain growth was arrested at E13.5 (Figure 3D). The brain atrophy and arrested development explained the flattened shape of the head observed at later stages (e.g., E18.5; Figure 3B). At E15.5, the mutant embryos had a thinner cortex, which was associated with an abnormal cortical layer structure (Figure 3E). Histological analysis showed that the mutant cortex had a thinner ventricular zone (VZ) and was devoid of subventricular zone (SVZ) and cortical plate (CP). Overall, the cellularity was greatly reduced. The efficient deletion of Rplp1 in Rplp1$^{CNS\Delta}$ embryonic brains was already evident at E13.5 (Figure 3F). Notably, we found that P2 was also knocked-out in the Rplp1$^{CNS\Delta}$ brains, possibly because P1 and P2 stabilize each other in the cytoplasm [17].

Taken together, our data show that Rplp1 deletion in the CNS affected brain size and development, thus causing perinatal lethality (Figure 3D).

Rplp1 deletion in the CNS causes increased apoptosis and proliferation arrest in progenitor cells

To study the causes of the decreased cellularity in the Rplp1$^{CNS\Delta}$ neocortex, we evaluated apoptosis. Terminal deoxynucleotidyl transferase UTP nick-end labeling (TUNEL) staining revealed increased apoptosis in the neocortexes of the E12.5, E13.5 and E15.5 brain sections (Figure 4A and 4B). Concurrently, western blot analysis showed that caspase-3 activation was greatly increased in the E13.5 Rplp1$^{CNS\Delta}$ brains, as determined by its cleavage (Figure 4C).

Next, we examined whether Rplp1 deletion caused a proliferation defect in the mouse embryonic brain. First, we performed an in vivo BrdU labeling assay by pulse-labeling the E13.5 embryos with BrdU for 30 minutes. We found that the number of BrdU$^+$

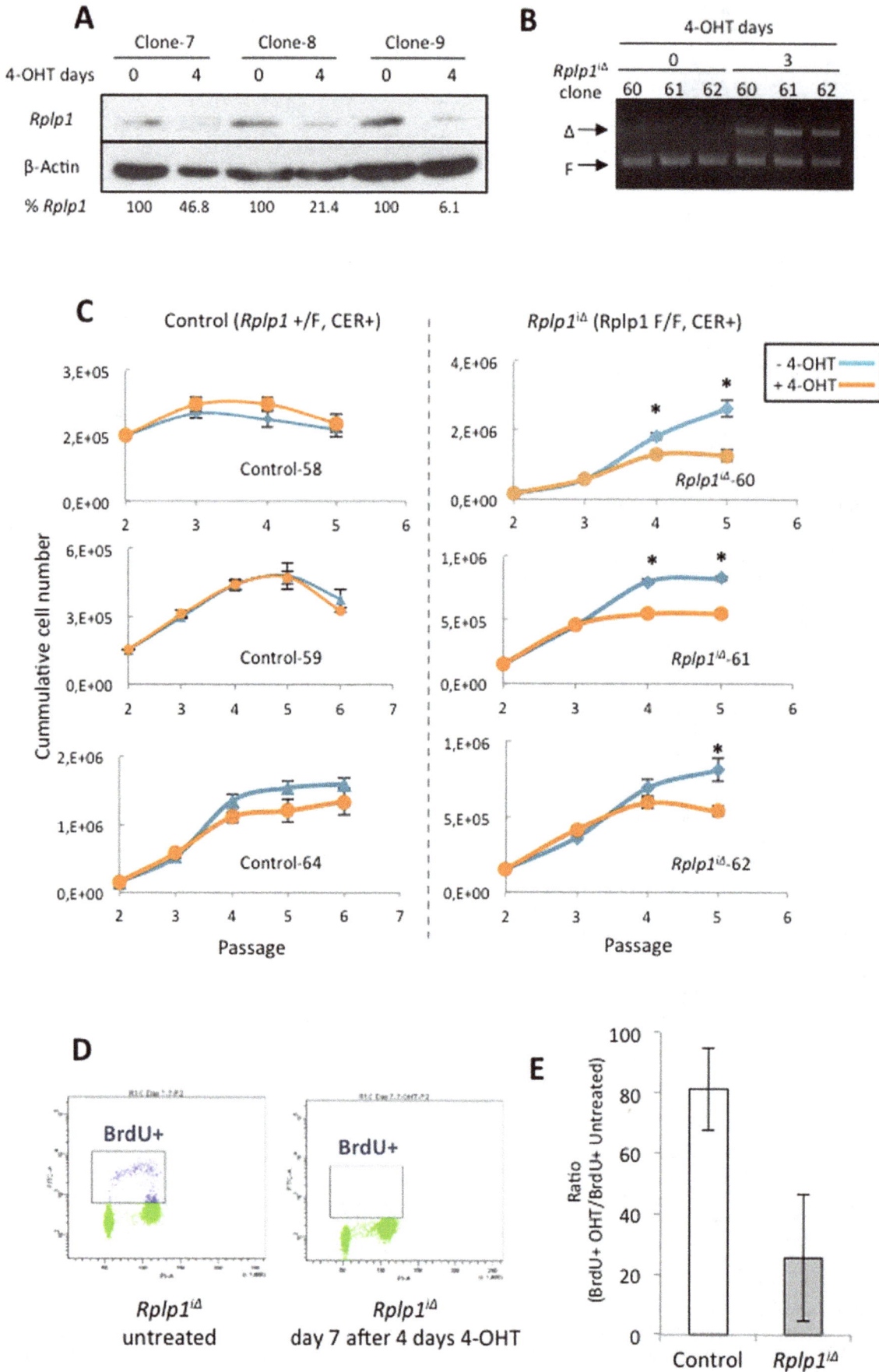

A

Clone-7   Clone-8   Clone-9

4-OHT days   0   4   0   4   0   4

Rplp1

β-Actin

% Rplp1   100   46.8   100   21.4   100   6.1

B

4-OHT days

Rplp1^iΔ clone   0   3

60   61   62   60   61   62

Δ→

F→

C

Control (Rplp1 +/F, CER+)   Rplp1^iΔ (Rplp1 F/F, CER+)

- 4-OHT
+ 4-OHT

Control-58   Rplp1^iΔ-60

Control-59   Rplp1^iΔ-61

Control-64   Rplp1^iΔ-62

Cummulative cell number

Passage   Passage

D

BrdU+   BrdU+

Rplp1^iΔ   Rplp1^iΔ
untreated   day 7 after 4 days 4-OHT

E

Ratio (BrdU+ OHT/BrdU+ Untreated)

Control   Rplp1^iΔ

Figure 7. *Rplp1*-deleted primary MEF exhibit a proliferation defect. (A) Western blot analysis of *Rplp1*$^{i\Delta}$ pMEFs that were untreated or treated for 4 days with 1 μM 4-OHT. **(B)** PCR, showing *Rplp1* deletion in the inducible MEF cell lines used in (c). **(C)** Growth curves of control (*Rplp1*$^{+/F}$ CER$^+$) and *Rplp1*-inducible pMEF (*Rplp1*$^{i\Delta}$), that were untreated or treated with 1 μM 4-OHT for 4 days. Student's t-test was used to perform the statistical analysis. *: P<0.05. **(D)** *Rplp1*$^{i\Delta}$ and control pMEFs were treated with 1 μM 4-OHT for 4 days or left untreated. After 3 days, they were labeled with 10 μM BrdU for 2 hours, fixed and stained with an anti-BrdU antibody and PI. The cells were analyzed by flow cytometry. **(E)** BrdU$^+$ cells were quantified, and the ratio of BrdU$^+$ cells (treated/untreated) was plotted. Error bars: SEM.

cells was significantly reduced in the *Rplp1*$^{CNS\Delta}$ embryonic brain, thus indicating a proliferation defect (Figure 5A and 5B).

Next, immunostaining of the E13.5 brain sections with an anti-Ki67 antibody revealed that the number of Ki67$^+$ cells was significantly reduced in the *Rplp1*$^{CNS\Delta}$ embryonic brain, compared with the controls (Figure 5C and 5D), suggesting the presence of fewer cycling cells. Staining of the *Rplp1*$^{CNS\Delta}$ embryonic brain sections with an antibody against phosphorylated histone-3 (PH 3) consistently revealed reduced mitosis in the *Rplp1*$^{CNS\Delta}$ neocortex (Figure 5E and 5F). To further analyze the proliferation and apoptosis of *Rplp1*$^{CNS\Delta}$ neural progenitors, we performed a primary neurosphere formation assay and found that the *Rplp1*$^{CNS\Delta}$ neural progenitors formed very few neurospheres and the sizes of the formed neurospheres were dramatically reduced (Figure 5I and 5J), indicating compromised proliferation and enhanced apoptosis.

Consequent to the reduced proliferation and increased apoptosis, postmitotic neurons (Tuj1+) were found to be greatly reduced in the mutant neocortex (Figure 5G and 5H). These observations well explain the absence of the CP and intermediate zone (IZ) layers (Figure 3E) and contribute to an explanation of the brain atrophy of *Rplp1*$^{CNS\Delta}$ mice.

To further understand the proliferation defects observed in the *Rplp1*$^{CNS\Delta}$ embryonic brains, the key cell cycle regulators in the *Rplp1*$^{CNS\Delta}$ E13.5 brain were analyzed. The cyclin A and cyclin E protein levels were reduced in the mutant brain (Figure 6). Moreover, the protein levels of the CDK inhibitors p21^{CIP1} and p27^{KIP1} were reduced in the mutant brain (Figure 6). Similarly, p53 expression was slightly downregulated in the *Rplp1*-deleted embryonic brain (Figure 6) suggesting that p21^{CIP1} and p27^{KIP1} inhibition can be responsible for the apoptosis observed in the brain [27,28]. We conclude that *Rplp1* deletion in the developing CNS caused perinatal lethality, reduced brain size and morphological brain defects consequent to greatly increased apoptosis in association with a proliferation defect.

Rplp1 deletion in MEFs causes a p16^{INK4A}/pRb pathway-mediated proliferation defect and increased senescence

To further understand the role of *Rplp1* in cell proliferation and apoptosis, we generated *Rplp1*$^{F/F}$ mice after crossing *Rplp1*+/F mice with Cre-ER^{T2} transgenic mice [29], and subsequently isolated the *Rplp1*$^{F/F}$CER$^+$ (*Rplp1*$^{i\Delta}$) and *Rplp1*$^{+/F}$CER$^+$ (control) pMEFs. *Rplp1* was efficiently deleted in the *Rplp1*$^{i\Delta}$ pMEFs upon the addition of 1 μM 4-OHT for four days (Figure 7A and 7B). First, we assessed proliferation in *Rplp1*$^{i\Delta}$ and control pMEFs that had been treated with 1 μM 4-OHT for four days. *Rplp1*$^{i\Delta}$ pMEFs showed a proliferation defect, with reduced cell numbers (Figure 7C). Furthermore, BrdU labeling of *Rplp1*$^{i\Delta}$ and control pMEFs after four days of 1 μM 4-OHT revealed a considerable reduction of BrdU+ cells among the *Rplp1*$^{i\Delta}$cells, compared with the controls (Figure 7D and 7E). However, when we analyzed the cell cycle profiles, we found no obvious differences in the cell cycle distribution between the control cells and those with a single *Rplp1* allele deletion (Figure 8A). Next, we investigated whether increased apoptosis contributed to the reduced numbers of *Rplp1*$^{i\Delta}$ pMEFs. Fluorescence-activated cell sorting (FACS) analysis

revealed no obvious differences in the Annexin V+ cell populations of mutant and control cells that had been stained with Annexin V/DAPI (Figure 8B).

From the growth curve (Figure 7C), we noticed a premature cessation of proliferation in *Rplp1*$^{i\Delta}$ pMEFs after passage 4. To follow the fates of these cells, we performed β-galactosidase (β-gal) staining and found that the frequency of β-gal$^+$ cells was higher among *Rplp1*$^{i\Delta}$ pMEFs than among the controls (Figure 8C and 8D), indicating that *Rplp1* deletion caused early senescence in the pMEFs. To investigate the cause of this senescence, we analyzed the levels of important cell cycle regulatory proteins and found higher levels of the CDK inhibitor p16^{INK4A}, a marker of senescence associated with the downregulation of pRb activity (Figure 8E). However, the protein levels of p21^{CIP1} and p27^{KIP1} did not differ between the control and *Rplp1*$^{i\Delta}$ pMEFs (Figure 8F). Because senescence can be caused by the accumulation of reactive oxygen species (ROS) [30,31] and the non-essential ribosomal proteins RPL1, RPL32 and RPL36 can prevent intracellular ROS generation [32], we measured the intracellular ROS levels. No differences were observed between the deleted and control cells (Figure S2), suggesting that ROS was not the cause of senescence in *Rplp1*$^{i\Delta}$ pMEFs. Finally we expressed lentiviral vectors expressing p16^{INK4A}-shRNA and p53^{shRNA} in *Rplp1*$^{i\Delta}$ pMEFs which were further depleted for Rplp1 (see materials and methods). The inhibition of p16^{INK4A} in this context rescues, at least partially, the senescent phenotype while p53 inhibition does not seen to have any effect (data not shown). Moreover transient transfection strategy using siRNAs showed similar results (Figure S3). Taken together, these experiments showed that *Rplp1* deletion in pMEFs induced a p16^{INK4A}/pRb pathway-mediated proliferation defect and led to increased senescence.

Rplp1 deletion in MEFs does not affect global protein synthesis but alters the translation pattern

Rplp1 is important for proper ribosomal interactions with elongation factors, especially eEF-2 [33,34]. To assess whether Rplp1 deletion affected protein synthesis, *Rplp1*$^{i\Delta}$ and control immortalized MEFs were treated with 4-OHT for four days. Three days after the end of the treatment, the cells were labeled with a methionine analog (azide-homoalanine), and the de novo synthesized proteins were detected by western blotting (Figure 9A) and quantified by densitometry (Figure 9B). Proper *Rplp1* deletion was assessed by western blotting (Figure 9A). The experiment was performed with two pairs of control and *Rplp1*$^{i\Delta}$ immortalized MEFs. The protein synthesis level was unchanged when *Rplp1* was deleted. Therefore, *Rplp1* deletion in MEFs did not affect general protein synthesis.

Two-dimensional gel electrophoresis was performed to examine the protein translation pattern in *Rplp1*-deficient pMEFs. The proteins that were more strongly dysregulated in *Rplp1*$^{i\Delta}$ pMEFs were selected and identified by mass spectrometry. We identified fourteen proteins that were significantly dysregulated in *Rplp1*$^{i\Delta}$ pMEFs (p<0.01); these were associated with different cellular functions such as protein folding (70%), cell death (40%), gene expression (20%) and metabolism (20%) (Figure 9C and Table S2). In agreement with the finding that protein folding was the most

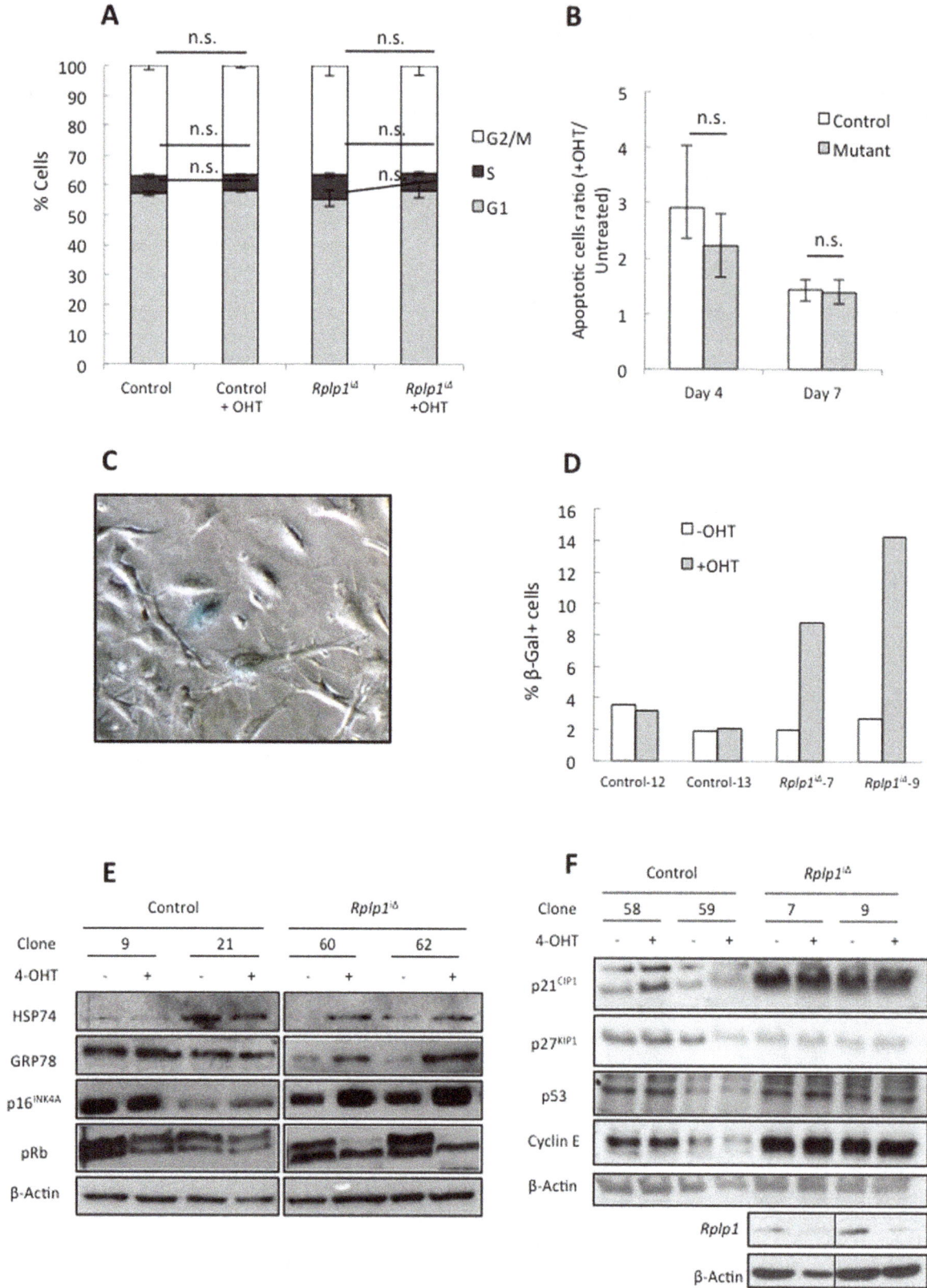

Figure 8. Increased senescence in *Rplp1*-deleted primary MEFs is mediated by the p16^INK4A/pRb pathway. (**A**) Quantification of the cell cycle profiles of control and *Rplp1^iΔ* pMEFs that were untreated or treated for 4 days with 4-OHT. Student's t-test was applied for the statistical analysis. n.s.: not significant. Error bars: SEM. N = 3. (**B**) *Rplp1^iΔ* and control pMEFs were treated with 1 μM 4-OHT for 4 days or left untreated. The cells were harvested, stained with Annexin V/DAPI and analyzed by flow cytometry on day 4 after the treatment (Day 4), or 3 days later (Day 7). Error bars: SEM. (**C**) β-galactosidase staining was performed in *Rplp1^iΔ* and control pMEFs that were treated with 1 μM 4-OHT for 4 days or left untreated. (**D**)

Quantification of the amount of β-gal+ cells for each analyzed clone analyzed. (**E and F**). Western blot analysis of protein extracts from $Rplp1^{i\Delta}$ and control pMEFs that were treated with 1 μM 4-OHT for 4 days or left untreated.

affected group, the upregulation of stress-related proteins such as the endoplasmic reticulum (ER) chaperones HSP74 and GRP78 was confirmed by western blot analysis (Figure 8E).

Discussion

To study the function of P1 *in vivo*, we generated *Rplp1* knockout mouse models. *Rplp1* null mice could not be generated due to the infertility of $Rplp1^{Het}$ mice. Surprisingly, $Rplp1^{et}$ mice, which carry only one *Rplp1* allele, presented with a severe phenotype that led to early postnatal death in approximately 50% of the offspring. $Rplp1^{Het}$ mice exhibited rigid, kinky, short tails. This phenotype is consistent with the general notion that RP mutational haploinsufficiency is often associated with severe defects in mammals. For example, the phenotype of $Rplp1^{Het}$ mice is reminiscent of that of Ts (Ts/+) mutant mice, which possess a spontaneous, dominant mutation in *Rpl38*. [1]. While homozygous Ts mutants die before implantation, the heterozygous mice present with a short, kinky tail and skeletal patterning defects [5]. *Rpl38* regulates 80S-mRNA complex formation for specific Hox mRNAs [1]. *Rpl24* heterozygosity in *Bst/+* mice was also shown to cause kinked tails [9]. RPL24 regulates ribosomal subunit association and protein translation [2]. These observations suggest that defects in ribosomal subunit joining or assembly might induce skeletal defects. For other RPs, single-allele deletion leads to lethality during gastrulation, a period during which cell division and differentiation increase drastically, due to an error in ribosomal biogenesis (i. e.: *RpS6* mutations) [2]. In contrast, heterozygous mutations in other RPs such as *Rps19* [35], *Rpl29* [36] and *Rpl24* [9] are compatible with embryonic development. Moreover, some human patients who carry *RPS19* mutations present with skeletal malformations [37].

Our results show that the specific knockout of *Rplp1* in the CNS provoked perinatal lethality and morphological brain defects. The observed brain atrophy was caused by the impaired proliferation and increased apoptosis of neuroprogenitors. $Rplp1^{CNS\Delta}$ mice exhibited neocortical apoptosis, which also contributed to brain atrophy. Consistently, deficiencies in other RPs such as *Rpl22* were shown to selectively arrest the development of α/β-T cells in a p53 activation and apoptosis-mediated manner [38]. RPL11 silencing was shown to induce p53-dependent apoptosis [39], and *Rps19* deficiency impaired ribosomal biogenesis and activated p53 in zebrafish [40]. Upon the silencing of other RPs such as RPL23 [41], RPS9 [42] or RPS6 [43], p53 becomes activated and induces apoptosis. In contrast, *Rplp1* deletion led to apoptosis independently of P53. This proliferation defect was accompanied by the downregulation of cyclin E, but appeared to be independent of p16^{INK4A} and p19^{ARF}. Surprisingly, the CDK inhibitors p21^{CIP1} and p27^{KIP1} were also downregulated. Although p21^{CIP1} and p27^{KIP1} exert direct cell cycle control at a nuclear level, these proteins can also exert other independent functions when cytoplasmically localized which could contribute to the observed abnormalities of the IZ and CP layers in the $Rplp1^{CNS\Delta}$ embryonic brain [44–46]. Moreover, the detrimental effect of a single-allele deficiency of *Rplp1* on neurosphere formation might be associated with the downregulation of p21^{CIP1} and p27^{KIP1}, as they have previously been associated with cell differentiation and apoptosis [27,28,44].

In agreement with our *in vivo* observations, the proliferation defects were also observed in $Rplp1^{i\Delta}$ pMEFs. Interestingly, the proliferation defect in $Rplp1^{i\Delta}$ pMEFs induced p16^{INK4A}/pRb pathway-mediated premature senescence, which was also p53-independent. Importantly p16^{INK4A} inhibition is able to bypass, at least partially, the senescence phenotype indicating that this pathway is crucial for Rplp1-deficiency-mediated senescence. This finding was consistent with finding that *Rplp1* overexpression could bypass senescence in pMEFs [22]. A similar proliferative defect was also previously observed in P1–P2 knocked-down human cells [47]. In contrast to the $Rplp1^{CNS\Delta}$ embryonic brain, the p27^{KIP1}, p21^{CIP1} and cyclin E protein levels were unaltered in $Rplp1^{i\Delta}$ pMEFs, indicating that *Rplp1* deletion has different consequences in specific tissues or cell types. This finding was also supported by the fact that, in strong contrast to proliferating cells, *Rplp1* deletion in post-mitotic mature B cells and follicular dendritic cells in $Rplp1^{B\Delta}$ mice did not result in an obvious phenotype (Perucho et al., unpublished observations). Given that embryonic stem (ES) cells contain high levels of P1 ([22] and data not shown), our results suggest that *Rplp1* is crucial in embryonic stem cells and progenitor cells (e.g., neural system), but dispensable in certain differentiated cells such as mature B cells. Consistent with this assumption, *Rplp1* expression was downregulated upon the differentiation of mouse ES cells to embryonic bodies [48]. It is also possible that in different cell types, the ability of the ribosomal subunits to compensate for losses in P1/P2 loss differs. For example, P0, P1 and P2 contain a common C-terminal domain that is responsible for the ribosomal interaction with EF-2 [33]. However, the C-terminal domain of P0 is not required for ribosomal activity when P1 and P2 are bound to the ribosome [49]. In other words, the C-terminal domain of P0 might be sufficient for ribosomal-translation factor interactions in some cell types or conditions, whereas in other cell types that require proliferation, P1 and P2 act as rate-limiting factors. For example, the proportions of ribosomal stalk proteins in the cytoplasm have been reported to vary from less than 1% [50] to 75% [51], possibly reflecting the different requirements among organisms and metabolic cell conditions [52].

On the other hand, *Rplp1* deletion (and concurrently *Rplp2* deletion) in the $Rplp1^{i\Delta}$ pMEFs did not affect global protein translation. This is in agreement with previous observations in human cells [47]. In contrast, the depletion of other RPs (i.e. *Rps9*) was shown to reduce the protein synthesis rate [42]. Interestingly, we identified 14 specific proteins that were dysregulated in $Rplp1^{i\Delta}$ pMEFs, most of which were ER chaperones. For example, most of the upregulated proteins in $Rplp1^{i\Delta}$ pMEFs are so in reaction with the ribosomal stress response (i.e.: GRP75, GRP78, SYAC and HSP74). In addition, some of the alterations observed in proliferation and apoptosis could be due to the reduced levels of Rab1b given its role in the control of cell growth [53–55]. The ER is home to an array of interlinked chaperone proteins upon which secreted proteins depend for correct folding, partner chain assimilation and final multimer assembly. The ER stress response constitutes a cellular process that is triggered by various conditions that disturb protein folding. Eukaryotic cells have developed an adaptive mechanism, the unfolded protein response (UPR), that acts to remove unfolded proteins and restore ER homeostasis [56]. In mammalian cells, imbalanced RP levels or the absence or malfunction of any RP has been shown to induce ribosomal stress, with severe consequences for cell survival [57]. Although this response has been linked to p53 [58], p53-independent mechanisms are also involved [59,60]. Interestingly, RP knockdown or

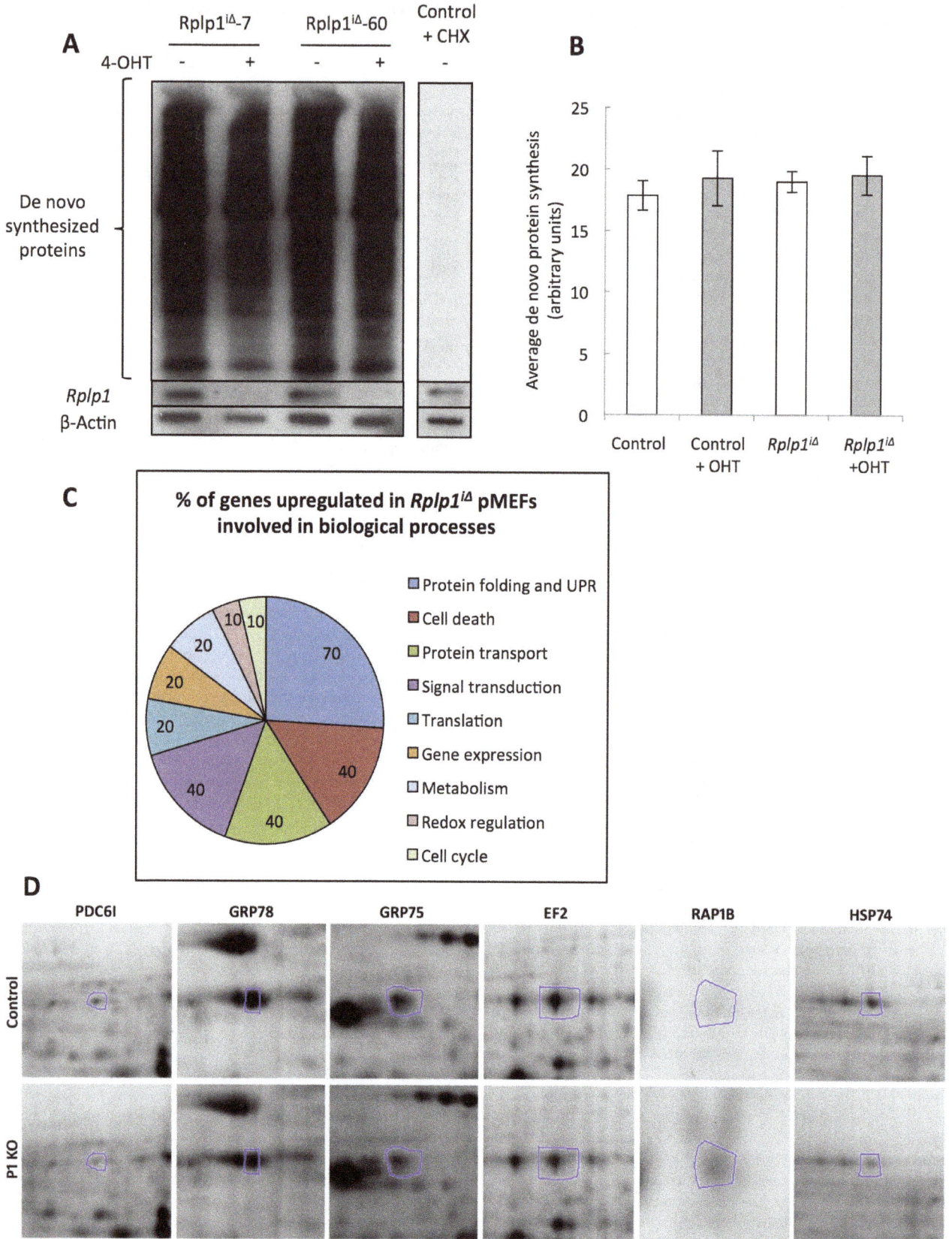

Figure 9. De novo protein synthesis is normal in *Rplp1*^{i∆} MEFs, but the protein expression pattern is altered. (**A**) Western blot analysis of newly synthesized proteins in *Rplp1*^{i∆} MEFs. Cycloheximide (CHX)-treated MEFs were used as a negative control. (**B**) Densitometric quantification of the newly synthesized proteins in *Rplp1*^{i∆} MEFs. Two control and 2 *Rplp1*^{i∆} MEF cell lines were used. Error bars: SEM. (**C**) Percentages of upregulated

and downregulated proteins involved in different biological processes in *Rplp1*[iΔ]pMEFs. The classification was performed according to gene ontology (www.geneontology.org). (**D**) Associated alterations in the levels of proteins that are dysregulated by a factor of 1.5 or more in ***Rplp1*[iΔ]pMEFs** cells. Representative photographs of the 2D gel are shown. Only portions of the 2D gel images corresponding to the indicated proteins are shown.

haploinsufficiency can provoke a ribosomal stress response that can be associated with senescence, UPR or other mechanisms [61,62]. The data presented herein link the ER-UPR with the senescence response in a single effector pathway downstream of ribosomal stress. Moreover, because protein folding is coupled with elongation, the absence of P1 and P2 might affect translation elongation by disrupting protein folding. EF-2 upregulation might reflect an attempt by the cell to compensate for the impaired stalk recognition, as P0, P1 and P2 comprise the EF-2 recognition motif [34]. For example, we cannot rule out the possibility that *Rplp1* has additional extra-ribosomal functions, as P2 [63], at replication forks [64]. The relationship between the dysregulated proteins in *Rplp1*[iΔ] pMEFs and the observed phenotype in the mutant mice remains to be fully characterized. Although the global protein level is unchanged, the absence of P1 might cause an increased translation error rate that would generate unfolded proteins.

Our results suggest that P1 has potential extraribosomal functions related to protein folding, a process that occurs outside the ribosome but within the ER compartment.

On the other hand, it has been hypothesized that *Rplp1* might be involved in internal ribosomal entry site (IRES)-dependent translation [16]. Interestingly, both the p27[KIP1] and p53 mRNAs contain IRES [65]. This alternative hypothesis should be explored in future studies. Importantly, the P1 disturbance particularly affected proliferating cells (neuroprecursors), strongly suggesting the following: that P1 plays specific roles in the ribosome by "fine-tuning" translation accordingly to the cellular requirements and/or that proliferating cells are equipped with an extra-sensitive ER stress response to preserve their stemness properties. Our work also suggests that *Rplp1* impairment-mediated activation of the ER stress pathway translates into different response mechanisms (senescence *in vitro* and apoptosis *in vivo*) that are incompatible with cell survival and normal development. Overall, our work shows that Rplp1 is crucial for development and proliferation and proposes P1 as a novel factor of protein proper folding and translational "fine-tuning".

Supporting Information

Figure S1 H&E staining of *Rplp1*[Het] and *Rplp1*[+/+] mice tissues. Scale bar: 50 μm. Liver, thymus and brown fat staining were

performed at postnatal day 1 (P1). Testis staining was performed at P30.

Figure S2 Senescence is not caused by increased ROS in *Rplp1*[iΔ]pMEFs. An intracellular ROS assay was performed in *Rplp1*[iΔ]and control pMEFs that were treated with 1 μM 4-OHT for 4 days or left untreated.

Figure S3 Senescence is bypassed at least partially by p16[INK4] inhibition. (**A**) Western-Blot of p16[NK4A] antibody indicating the efficiency of the p16[INK4AsiRNA]. (**B**) Quantification of senescent cells upon transient transfection with the indicated siRNAs (*p< 0.05). (**C**) Photographs of *Rplp1*[iΔ] and control pMEFs transfected with the p16[INK4AsiRNA] and further treated during 4 days with 1 M 4-OHT.

Table S1 List of antibodies used.

Table S2 Dysregulated proteins identified in *Rplp1*[iΔ] pMEFs by two-dimensional gel electrophoresis and classification according to gene ontology (www.geneontology.org) in the different biological processes in which they are involved. Green indicates protein involvement in a biological process and red indicates non-involvement.

Acknowledgments

We are grateful to all animal care technicians from the Leibniz Institute for Age Research. We are very gratefull with Dr. Manuel Serrano from the CNIO for providing the retroviral vectors LMP[shRNAs].

Author Contributions

Conceived and designed the experiments: LP AA SG MLL ZW. Performed the experiments: LP AA SG. Analyzed the data: LP AA SG SR MLL ZW. Contributed reagents/materials/analysis tools: MLL ZW. Wrote the paper: LP MLL ZW. Reviewed and evaluated the article: LP AA SR MLL ZW. Approved the final manuscript: LP AA SG SR MLL ZW.

References

1. Kondrashov N, Pusic A, Stumpf CR, Shimizu K, Hsieh AC, et al. (2011) Ribosome-mediated specificity in Hox mRNA translation and vertebrate tissue patterning. Cell 145: 383–397.
2. Panic L, Tamarut S, Sticker-Jantscheff M, Barkic M, Solter D, et al. (2006) Ribosomal protein S6 gene haploinsufficiency is associated with activation of a p53-dependent checkpoint during gastrulation. Molecular and cellular biology 26: 8880–8891.
3. Kongsuwan K, Yu Q, Vincent A, Frisardi MC, Rosbash M, et al. (1985) A Drosophila Minute gene encodes a ribosomal protein. Nature 317: 555–558.
4. Lambertsson A (1998) The minute genes in Drosophila and their molecular functions. Adv Genet 38: 69–134.
5. Marygold SJ, Roote J, Reuter G, Lambertsson A, Ashburner M, et al. (2007) The ribosomal protein genes and Minute loci of Drosophila melanogaster. Genome biology 8: R216.
6. Yoshihama M, Uechi T, Asakawa S, Kawasaki K, Kato S, et al. (2002) The human ribosomal protein genes: sequencing and comparative analysis of 73 genes. Genome Res 12: 379–390.
7. Hustert E, Scherer G, Olowson M, Guenet JL, Balling R (1996) Rbt (Rabo torcido), a new mouse skeletal mutation involved in anteroposterior patterning of the axial skeleton, maps close to the Ts (tail-short) locus and distal to the Sox9 locus on chromosome 11. Mamm Genome 7: 881–885.
8. Morgan WC (1950) A new tail-short mutation in the mouse whose lethal effects are conditioned by the residual genotypes. J Hered 41: 208–215.
9. Oliver ER, Saunders TL, Tarle SA, Glaser T (2004) Ribosomal protein L24 defect in belly spot and tail (Bst), a mouse Minute. Development 131: 3907–3920.
10. Moazed D, Robertson JM, Noller HF (1988) Interaction of elongation factors EF-G and EF-Tu with a conserved loop in 23S RNA. Nature 334: 362–364.
11. Uchiumi T, Honma S, Nomura T, Dabbs ER, Hachimori A (2002) Translation elongation by a hybrid ribosome in which proteins at the GTPase center of the Escherichia coli ribosome are replaced with rat counterparts. J Biol Chem 277: 3857–3862.
12. Uchiumi T, Traut RR, Kominami R (1990) Monoclonal antibodies against acidic phosphoproteins P0, P1, and P2 of eukaryotic ribosomes as functional probes. J Biol Chem 265: 89–95.
13. Egebjerg J, Douthwaite SR, Liljas A, Garrett RA (1990) Characterization of the binding sites of protein L11 and the L10.(L12)4 pentameric complex in the GTPase domain of 23 S ribosomal RNA from Escherichia coli. J Mol Biol 213: 275–288.
14. Tsurugi K, Ogata K (1985) Evidence for the exchangeability of acidic ribosomal proteins on cytoplasmic ribosomes in regenerating rat liver. J Biochem 98: 1427–1431.

15. Zinker S, Warner JR (1976) The ribosomal proteins of Saccharomyces cerevisiae. Phosphorylated and exchangeable proteins. J Biol Chem 251: 1799–1807.

16. Martinez-Azorin F, Remacha M, Martinez-Salas E, Ballesta JP (2008) Internal translation initiation on the foot-and-mouth disease virus IRES is affected by ribosomal stalk conformation. FEBS Lett 582: 3029–3032.

17. Nusspaumer G, Remacha M, Ballesta JP (2000) Phosphorylation and N-terminal region of yeast ribosomal protein P1 mediate its degradation, which is prevented by protein P2. EMBO J 19: 6075–6084.

18. Zhang L, Zhou W, Velculescu VE, Kern SE, Hruban RH, et al. (1997) Gene expression profiles in normal and cancer cells. Science 276: 1268–1272.

19. Loging WT, Reisman D (1999) Elevated expression of ribosomal protein genes L37, RPP-1, and S2 in the presence of mutant p53. Cancer Epidemiol Biomarkers Prev 8: 1011–1016.

20. Artero-Castro A, Castellvi J, Garcia A, Hernandez J, Ramon y Cajal S, et al. (2011) Expression of the ribosomal proteins Rplp0, Rplp1, and Rplp2 in gynecologic tumors. Human pathology 42: 194–203.

21. Chen A, Kaganovsky E, Rahimipour S, Ben-Aroya N, Okon E, et al. (2002) Two forms of gonadotropin-releasing hormone (GnRH) are expressed in human breast tissue and overexpressed in breast cancer: a putative mechanism for the antiproliferative effect of GnRH by down-regulation of acidic ribosomal phosphoproteins P1 and P2. Cancer Res 62: 1036–1044.

22. Artero-Castro A, Kondoh H, Fernandez-Marcos PJ, Serrano M, Ramon y Cajal S, et al. (2009) Rplp1 bypasses replicative senescence and contributes to transformation. Exp Cell Res 315: 1372–1383.

23. Remacha M, Jimenez-Diaz A, Bermejo B, Rodriguez-Gabriel MA, Guarinos E, et al. (1995) Ribosomal acidic phosphoproteins P1 and P2 are not required for cell viability but regulate the pattern of protein expression in Saccharomyces cerevisiae. Molecular and cellular biology 15: 4754–4762.

24. Huang C, Mandava CS, Sanyal S (2010) The ribosomal stalk plays a key role in IF2-mediated association of the ribosomal subunits. J Mol Biol 399: 145–153.

25. Ishii K, Washio T, Uechi T, Yoshihama M, Kenmochi N, et al. (2006) Characteristics and clustering of human ribosomal protein genes. BMC Genomics 7: 37.

26. Colome N, Collado J, Bech-Serra JJ, Liiv I, Anton LC, et al. (2010) Increased apoptosis after autoimmune regulator expression in epithelial cells revealed by a combined quantitative proteomics approach. Journal of proteome research 9: 2600–2609.

27. Eymin B, Haugg M, Droin N, Sordet O, Dimanche-Boitrel MT, et al. (1999) p27Kip1 induces drug resistance by preventing apoptosis upstream of cytochrome c release and procaspase-3 activation in leukemic cells. Oncogene 18: 1411–1418.

28. Suzuki A, Tsutomi Y, Yamamoto N, Shibutani T, Akahane K (1999) Mitochondrial regulation of cell death: mitochondria are essential for procaspase 3-p21 complex formation to resist Fas-mediated cell death. Molecular and cellular biology 19: 3842–3847.

29. Feil R, Wagner J, Metzger D, Chambon P (1997) Regulation of Cre recombinase activity by mutated estrogen receptor ligand-binding domains. Biochem Biophys Res Commun 237: 752–757.

30. Chen QM, Bartholomew JC, Campisi J, Acosta M, Reagan JD, et al. (1998) Molecular analysis of H2O2-induced senescent-like growth arrest in normal human fibroblasts: p53 and Rb control G1 arrest but not cell replication. The Biochemical journal 332 (Pt 1): 43–50.

31. Frippiat C, Chen QM, Remacle J, Toussaint O (2000) Cell cycle regulation in H(2)O(2)-induced premature senescence of human diploid fibroblasts and regulatory control exerted by the papilloma virus E6 and E7 proteins. Experimental gerontology 35: 733–745.

32. Nakayashiki T, Mori H (2013) Genome-wide screening with hydroxyurea reveals a link between nonessential ribosomal proteins and reactive oxygen species production. J Bacteriol 195: 1226–1235.

33. Bargis-Surgey P, Lavergne JP, Gonzalo P, Vard C, Filhol-Cochet O, et al. (1999) Interaction of elongation factor eEF-2 with ribosomal P proteins. Eur J Biochem 262: 606–611.

34. Gomez-Lorenzo MG, Spahn CM, Agrawal RK, Grassucci RA, Penczek P, et al. (2000) Three-dimensional cryo-electron microscopy localization of EF2 in the Saccharomyces cerevisiae 80S ribosome at 17.5 A resolution. EMBO J 19: 2710–2718.

35. Draptchinskaia N, Gustavsson P, Andersson B, Pettersson M, Willig TN, et al. (1999) The gene encoding ribosomal protein S19 is mutated in Diamond-Blackfan anaemia. Nat Genet 21: 169–175.

36. Kirn-Safran CB, Oristian DS, Focht RJ, Parker SG, Vivian JL, et al. (2007) Global growth deficiencies in mice lacking the ribosomal protein HIP/RPL29. Dev Dyn 236: 447–460.

37. Matsson H, Davey EJ, Draptchinskaia N, Hamaguchi I, Ooka A, et al. (2004) Targeted disruption of the ribosomal protein S19 gene is lethal prior to implantation. Molecular and cellular biology 24: 4032–4037.

38. Anderson SJ, Lauritsen JP, Hartman MG, Foushee AM, Lefebvre JM, et al. (2007) Ablation of ribosomal protein L22 selectively impairs alphabeta T cell development by activation of a p53-dependent checkpoint. Immunity 26: 759–772.

39. Chakraborty A, Uechi T, Higa S, Torihara H, Kenmochi N (2009) Loss of ribosomal protein L11 affects zebrafish embryonic development through a p53-dependent apoptotic response. PLoS One 4: e4152.

40. Danilova N, Sakamoto KM, Lin S (2008) Ribosomal protein S19 deficiency in zebrafish leads to developmental abnormalities and defective erythropoiesis through activation of p53 protein family. Blood 112: 5228–5237.

41. Jin A, Itahana K, O'Keefe K, Zhang Y (2004) Inhibition of HDM2 and activation of p53 by ribosomal protein L23. Mol Cell Biol 24: 7669–7680.

42. Lindstrom MS, Nister M (2010) Silencing of ribosomal protein S9 elicits a multitude of cellular responses inhibiting the growth of cancer cells subsequent to p53 activation. PloS one 5: e9578.

43. Sulic S, Panic L, Barkic M, Mercep M, Uzelac M, et al. (2005) Inactivation of S6 ribosomal protein gene in T lymphocytes activates a p53-dependent checkpoint response. Genes Dev 19: 3070–3082.

44. Marone M, Bonanno G, Rutella S, Leone G, Scambia G, et al. (2002) Survival and cell cycle control in early hematopoiesis: role of bcl-2, and the cyclin dependent kinase inhibitors P27 and P21. Leukemia & lymphoma 43: 51–57.

45. Nguyen L, Besson A, Heng JI, Schuurmans C, Teboul L, et al. (2006) p27kip1 independently promotes neuronal differentiation and migration in the cerebral cortex. Genes & development 20: 1511–1524.

46. McAllister SS, Becker-Hapak M, Pintucci G, Pagano M, Dowdy SF (2003) Novel p27(kip1) C-terminal scatter domain mediates Rac-dependent cell migration independent of cell cycle arrest functions. Molecular and cellular biology 23: 216–228.

47. Martinez-Azorin F, Remacha M, Ballesta JP (2008) Functional characterization of ribosomal P1/P2 proteins in human cells. The Biochemical journal 413: 527–534.

48. Mansergh FC, Daly CS, Hurley AL, Wride MA, Hunter SM, et al. (2009) Gene expression profiles during early differentiation of mouse embryonic stem cells. BMC Dev Biol 9: 5.

49. Santos C, Ballesta JP (1995) The highly conserved protein P0 carboxyl end is essential for ribosome activity only in the absence of proteins P1 and P2. J Biol Chem 270: 20608–20614.

50. Mitsui K, Nakagawa T, Tsurugi K (1988) On the size and the role of a free cytosolic pool of acidic ribosomal proteins in yeast Saccharomyces cerevisiae. J Biochem 104: 908–911.

51. van Agthoven A, Kriek J, Amons R, Moller W (1978) Isolation and characterization of the acidic phosphoproteins of 60-S ribosomes from Artemia salina and rat liver. Eur J Biochem 91: 553–565.

52. Saenz-Robles MT, Remacha M, Vilella MD, Zinker S, Ballesta JP (1990) The acidic ribosomal proteins as regulators of the eukaryotic ribosomal activity. Biochimica et biophysica acta 1050: 51–55.

53. Sun L, Xie P, Wada J, Kashihara N, Liu FY, et al. (2008) Rap1b GTPase ameliorates glucose-induced mitochondrial dysfunction. Journal of the American Society of Nephrology: JASN 19: 2293–2301.

54. Yoshida Y, Kawata M, Miura Y, Musha T, Sasaki T, et al. (1992) Microinjection of smg/rap1/Krev-1 p21 into Swiss 3T3 cells induces DNA synthesis and morphological changes. Molecular and cellular biology 12: 3407–3414.

55. Ribeiro-Neto F, Urbani J, Lemee N, Lou L, Altschuler DL (2002) On the mitogenic properties of Rap1b: cAMP-induced G(1)/S entry requires activated and phosphorylated Rap1b. Proceedings of the National Academy of Sciences of the United States of America 99: 5418–5423.

56. Sano R, Reed JC (2013) ER stress-induced cell death mechanisms. Biochimica et biophysica acta 1833: 3460–3470.

57. Robledo S, Idol RA, Crimmins DL, Ladenson JH, Mason PJ, et al. (2008) The role of human ribosomal proteins in the maturation of rRNA and ribosome production. RNA 14: 1918–1929.

58. Morgado-Palacin L, Llanos S, Serrano M (2012) Ribosomal stress induces L11- and p53-dependent apoptosis in mouse pluripotent stem cells. Cell Cycle 11: 503–510.

59. Iadevaia V, Caldarola S, Biondini L, Gismondi A, Karlsson S, et al. (2010) PIM1 kinase is destabilized by ribosomal stress causing inhibition of cell cycle progression. Oncogene 29: 5490–5499.

60. Challagundla KB, Sun XX, Zhang X, DeVine T, Zhang Q, et al. (2011) Ribosomal protein L11 recruits miR-24/miRISC to repress c-Myc expression in response to ribosomal stress. Molecular and cellular biology 31: 4007–4021.

61. de Las Heras-Rubio A, Perucho L, Paciucci R, Vilardell J, Lleonart ME (2013) Ribosomal proteins as novel players in tumorigenesis. Cancer metastasis reviews 10.1007/s10555-013-9460-6.

62. Denoyelle C, Abou-Rjaily G, Bezrookove V, Verhaegen M, Johnson TM, et al. (2006) Anti-oncogenic role of the endoplasmic reticulum differentially activated by mutations in the MAPK pathway. Nature cell biology 8: 1053–1063.

63. Furukawa T, Uchiumi T, Tokunaga R, Taketani S (1992) Ribosomal protein P2, a novel iron-binding protein. Arch Biochem Biophys 298: 182–186.

64. Lopez-Contreras AJ, Ruppen I, Nieto-Soler M, Murga M, Rodriguez-Acebes S, et al. (2013) A proteomic characterization of factors enriched at nascent DNA molecules. Cell Rep 3: 1105–1116.

65. Stoneley M, Willis AE (2004) Cellular internal ribosome entry segments: structures, trans-acting factors and regulation of gene expression. Oncogene 23: 3200–3207.

15

Hinokitiol Induces DNA Damage and Autophagy followed by Cell Cycle Arrest and Senescence in Gefitinib-Resistant Lung Adenocarcinoma Cells

Lan-Hui Li[1,2], Ping Wu[1], Jen-Yi Lee[1], Pei-Rong Li[1], Wan-Yu Hsieh[1], Chao-Chi Ho[3], Chen-Lung Ho[4], Wan-Jiun Chen[1,5], Chien-Chun Wang[6], Muh-Yong Yen[6,7], Shun-Min Yang[8], Huei-Wen Chen[1]*

1 Graduate Institute of Toxicology, College of Medicine, National Taiwan University, Taipei, Taiwan, 2 Department of Laboratory, Kunming Branch, Taipei City Hospital, Taipei, Taiwan, 3 Department of Internal Medicine, National Taiwan University Hospital and National Taiwan University Medical College, Taipei, Taiwan, 4 Division of Wood Cellulose, Taiwan Forestry Research Institute, Taipei, Taiwan, 5 Graduate Institute of Oncology, College of Medicine, National Taiwan University, Taipei, Taiwan, 6 Division of Infectious Diseases, Kunming Branch, Taipei City Hospital, Taipei, Taiwan, 7 Department of Medicine, National Yang-Ming University, Taipei, Taiwan, 8 Department of Pathology, Tri-Service General Hospital, National Defense Medical Center, Taipei, Taiwan

Abstract

Despite good initial responses, drug resistance and disease recurrence remain major issues for lung adenocarcinoma patients with epidermal growth factor receptor (EGFR) mutations taking EGFR-tyrosine kinase inhibitors (TKI). To discover new strategies to overcome this issue, we investigated 40 essential oils from plants indigenous to Taiwan as alternative treatments for a wide range of illnesses. Here, we found that hinokitiol, a natural monoterpenoid from the heartwood of *Calocedrus formosana*, exhibited potent anticancer effects. In this study, we demonstrated that hinokitiol inhibited the proliferation and colony formation ability of lung adenocarcinoma cells as well as the EGFR-TKI-resistant lines PC9-IR and H1975. Transcriptomic analysis and pathway prediction algorithms indicated that the main implicated pathways included DNA damage, autophagy, and cell cycle. Further investigations confirmed that in lung cancer cells, hinokitiol inhibited cell proliferation by inducing the p53-independent DNA damage response, autophagy (not apoptosis), S-phase cell cycle arrest, and senescence. Furthermore, hinokitiol inhibited the growth of xenograft tumors in association with DNA damage and autophagy but exhibited fewer effects on lung stromal fibroblasts. In summary, we demonstrated novel mechanisms by which hinokitiol, an essential oil extract, acted as a promising anticancer agent to overcome EGFR-TKI resistance in lung cancer cells via inducing DNA damage, autophagy, cell cycle arrest, and senescence in vitro and in vivo.

Editor: Arianna L. Kim, Columbia University Medical Center, United States of America

Funding: This work was supported by the grants from Ministry of Science and Technology (102-2325-B-002-046-) and National Taiwan University Cutting-Edge Steering Research Project (NTU CESRP-10R71602C2 and 100R705057). The funders had no role in study design, data collection and analysis, decision to publish, or preparation of the manuscript.

Competing Interests: The authors have declared that no competing interests exist.

* Email: shwchen@ntu.edu.tw

Introduction

Lung cancer, especially lung adenocarcinoma [1], is the leading cause of cancer mortality worldwide, with a five-year overall survival rate of only 15% [2,3]. Clinical and epidemiologic evidence has shown that more than 50% of lung adenocarcinoma cases in Asia express the epidermal growth factor receptor (EGFR) mutation. Accordingly, EGFR-tyrosine kinase inhibitors (TKIs) have been developed and have been shown to improve survival over standard treatments [4,5]. Despite good initial responses to EGFR-TKIs, most lung adenocarcinoma patients with EGFR mutations who are taking EGFR-TKIs develop resistance within 9 months. Resistance may be due to either intrinsic or acquired tumor cell resistance to both conventional and targeted cancer therapies and remains one of the largest clinical obstacles [6]. Therefore, there is an urgent need to identify new strategies for the treatment of lung cancer patients with drug resistance.

Herbal compounds have been suggested as an important and classical source for developing strategies to treat cancers. In folk medicine, essential oil constituents from plants are used as alternative treatments for a wide range of illnesses including cancer prevention and treatment [7–9]. Recently, studies have reported that essential oils, including the leaf of *Porcelia macrocarpa* [10] and *Pyrolae herba* [11], the heartwood of *Cunninghamia lanceolata* var. konishii [12], and the seed of *Litsea cubeba* [13], possess anticancer effects against different types of human tumors. Taiwan is located in the subtropics and has abundant plants with essential oil extracts that have been suggested as potential candidates for new therapeutic compounds. Many essential oils are volatile, which may represent an advantage for lung cancer treatment; this consideration prompted us to screen the potency of essential oils against lung adenocarcinomas [13].

In this study, we screened over 40 different essential oils from 31 different indigenous plants from Taiwan to identify new strategies for overcoming treatment failure. Among the investigated substances, we determined that hinokitiol, from the essential oil of *Calocedrus formosana* heartwood, had the most potent anticancer effects on EGFR-TKI-resistant lung cancer cell lines (H1975 and PC9-IR). Here, we reveal the novel mechanisms by which hinokitiol exerts its potent anticancer effects on several lung adenocarcinoma cell lines as well as EGFR-TKI-resistant cells. Specifically, hinokitiol induces DNA damage, autophagy, cell cycle arrest in S phase, and senescence. The potential anti-tumor effect and mechanisms of hinokitiol were confirmed in a xenograft model. Our findings suggest that hinokitiol could be a promising compound for treating EGFR-TKI-resistant lung adenocarcinomas.

Materials and Methods

Essential oils and chemicals

A total of 40 essential oils from 31 local plants in Taiwan were extracted using a standard hydrodistillation technique, and the constituents were analyzed through GC-MS. Hinokitiol (β-thujaplicin) was purchased from Sigma (St. Louis, MO, USA) and dissolved in DMSO as a stock stored at $-20°C$. 3-methyladenine (3-MA) was purchased from Sigma (M9281) and dissolved in RPMI complete medium (Gibco, Breda, The Netherlands). Chloroquine was purchased from Sigma (C6628) and dissolved in DMSO as a stock stored at $-20°C$. Acridine orange was purchased from Sigma (A6014).

Cell lines and culture conditions

The human lung adenocarcinoma cell lines, A549 (EGFR wild type), H1975 (EGFR L858R/T790M, gefitinib-resistant), H1299 (EGFR wild type, p53 null), and H3255 (EGFR L858R) were purchased from American Type Culture Collection (ATCC; Manassas, VA, USA). PC9 (EGFR exon 19 deletion) and PC9-IR (EGFR exon 19 deletion, gefitinib-resistant) were kind gifts from Dr. C. H. Yang (Graduate Institute of Oncology, Cancer Research Center, National Taiwan University). Human stromal fibroblast tissues were harvested from freshly resected lung tumor tissues from lung cancer patients who underwent surgical resection at the National Taiwan University Hospital and were sampled at least 5 cm away from neoplastic lesions by a pathologist within 30 min. The detail processes and protocols of isolating human stromal fibroblasts were described as our previous report [14]. This research project was approved by the institutional review board of National Taiwan University College of Medicine (Taipei, Taiwan) and written informed consent was obtained from all patients. The cell lines including stromal fibroblasts were cultured in RPMI-1640 medium supplemented with 10% fetal bovine albumin and 1% penicillin/streptomycin in a humidified atmosphere of 5% CO_2 in air at 37°C.

Cell proliferation assay

The effects of essential oils on A549 cells were evaluated using MTT (3-(4,5-dimethylthiazol-2-yl)-2,5-diphenyltetrazolium bromide) assay. The effects of hinokitiol on a series of lung adenocarcinoma cell lines were assayed through trypan blue staining. For the MTT assay, $5×10^3$ cells were cultured in 96-well plates overnight and then incubated with the essential oils under investigation (diluted 1:10,000 in medium) for 48 h. At the indicated times, the medium was removed, and 0.5 mg/ml MTT solution, which was dissolved in the culture medium, was added to the wells. After a further 1.5 h of incubation, the medium was removed, and DMSO was added to the plates. The color intensity was measured at 570 nm using a multi-label plate reader (Vector3; Perkin-Elmer, USA). For trypan blue staining, $2×10^4$ cells were cultured in 12-well plates overnight and then incubated with 0.3125–10 μM hinokitiol for 24, 48, and 72 h. At the indicated times, the cells were trypsinized and stained with trypan blue. The viable cells that excluded trypan blue were counted in a counting chamber. For the 3-MA treated experiment, $5.5×10^3$ cells were cultured in 96-well plates overnight and then incubated with 2.5 mM 3-MA for 1 hour prior to 5 μM hinokitiol treatment for 48 h. At the indicated times, the cells were trypsinized and stained with trypan blue. The viable cells were counted in a counting chamber.

Colony formation assay

H1975 and PC9-IR cells were cultured overnight in a 6-well plate at a density of 80 cells per well. Hinokitiol was freshly prepared at concentrations of 0.5, 1, or 5 μM and added to the wells. The cells were then incubated for 3 days. On the 4th day, the cells were incubated with drug-free complete medium and cultured for another 7–10 days. The colonies were fixed in 4% ice-cold paraformaldehyde for 15 minutes at 37°C, and each well was stained with 0.1% crystal violet overnight at room temperature. The colonies were then counted.

Gene expression profile by Affymetrix array analysis

The microarray experiments were performed using the Affymetrix Human Genome GeneChip expression by the Microarray Core Facility of National Taiwan University according to the manufacturer's protocols (Affymetrix, Santa Clara, CA, USA). All experiments were performed with complementary RNA probes prepared from H1975 or PC9-IR cells treated with or without 5 μM hinokitiol. All data were collected and analyzed according to the Affymetrix manual, and the raw microarray data were uploaded to the CRSD2 web server made in-house [15] and to GeneGo (http://www.genego.com/metacore) for pathway analysis.

DNA damage and autophagy gene expression profiling using real-time PCR arrays

Human DNA damage and autophagy signaling PCR arrays (SuperArray Bioscience), each of which assessed the expression of 84 genes, were used to assess the effect of hinokitiol on H1975 cells and stromal fibroblasts. The synthesis of complementary DNA, real-time PCR, and statistical analyses were performed according to the manufacturer's instructions, and the data shown represent the average of three replicates.

Cell cycle analysis

For propidium iodide (PI; Sigma) staining, H1975 cells and lung stromal fibroblasts ($5×10^5$) were cultured in 6-cm dishes overnight and then incubated with 5 μM hinokitiol for 72 h. At the indicated times, the cells were trypsinized and fixed in 70% ice-cold alcohol at $-20°C$ overnight. The fixed cells were washed twice in phosphate-buffered saline (PBS) and resuspended in a solution containing 0.1% Triton X-100, 200 μg/ml RNase A, and 20 μg/ml PI in PBS. The cells were incubated for 20 minutes at room temperature in the dark, and the stained nuclei were analyzed using a flow cytometer (FC500, Beckman Coulter). 5-Bromodeoxyuridine (BrdU)-labeled cells were measured using a BrdU flow kit (BD Pharmingen, USA) according to the manufacturer's instructions. Briefly, H1975 cells ($5×10^5$) were cultured in 6-cm dishes overnight and then incubated with 5 μM hinokitiol for 72 h. The cells were labeled with 10 μM BrdU for 12 h before harvesting. At the indicated times, the BrdU-labeled cells were

Table 1. The screening of essential oils on A549 cell proliferation as determined using MTT assay.

Essential oils	Proliferation rate (%)
Eucalyptus camaldulensis flower	93.2±13.2
Eucalyptus grandis leaf	95.8±8.7
Cinnamomum subavenium Miq.(Fu-Shan No. 4)	101.6±8.6
Cunninghamia konishii leaf	100.4±1.0
Eucalyptus camaldulensis leaf	97.8±4.6
Cinnamomum subavenium Miq. (Dasyue Mountain)	95.8±1.6
Cinnamomum subavenium Miq (Liouguei)	92.6±8.7
Eucalyptus urophylla leaf	100.1±2.5
Cinnamomum camphora (L.) Presl twig	101.3±2.8
Cinnamomum camphora (L.) Presl bark	99.7±0.1
Cinnamomum camphora (L.) Presl flower	102.1±4.1
Cinnamomum camphora (L.) Presl heartwood	97.8±2.7
Litsea cubeba stem	98.0±2.4
Litsea cubeba fruit	88.9±8.9
Litsea cubeba old twig	87.4±0.4
Litsea cubeba leaf	104.1±1.4
Litsea cubeba young twig	100.7±1.6
Cryptomeria japonica heartwood	88.8±2.6
Eucalyptus urophylla flower	107.8±3.5
Taiwania cryptomerioides Hayata leaf	87.4±0.7
Calocedrus Formosana heartwood	64.7±6.5*
Calocedrus formosana leaf	93.9±3.5
Taiwania cryptomerioides Hay. leaf	89.4±2.7
Houttuynia cordata Thunb	95.7±6.1
Machilus japonica Sieb. & Zucc (Chihtuan No. 1)[#]	69.9±1.8*
Machilus japonica Sieb. & Zucc (Chihtuan No. 2)[#]	100.1±9.3
Essential oils	**Proliferation rates (%)**
Eucalyptus camaldulensis leaf	67.1±6.7*
Nothaphoebe konishii (Hay.)	67.7±1.7*
Machilus japonica Siebold et Zucc[#]	101.1±0.8
Cunninghamia konishii heartwood	71.4±3.4*
Cinnamomum camphora (L.) Presl leaf	100.2±0.2
Chamaecyparis formosensis bark	98.2±1.9
Chamaecyparis formosensis sapwood	95.8±7.4
Machilus thunbergii	92.6±4.5
Beilschmiedia erythrophloia Hayata	97.9±0.6
Clausena excavata Burm. f.	100.0±1.7
Juniperus formosana Hayata leaf	98.8±3.9
Lavandula pinnata	100.5±2.7
Nepeta cataria L.	101.0±6.2

The proliferation rates (%) are represented as the mean ± SD (%) compared with the corresponding control (0.1% DMSO) at 48 h ($n=3$). * indicates the top 5 potent essential oils. [#] belongs to the same species but was collected in different geographic areas in Taiwan.

fixed, permeabilized, stained and analyzed using a flow cytometer (FC500, Beckman Coulter).

Annexin V staining

Apoptosis was measured using an annexin V apoptosis assay kit (BD Pharmingen, USA) according to the manufacturer's instructions. Briefly, H1975 cells and lung stromal fibroblasts (5×10^5 cells) were cultured in 6-cm dishes overnight and then incubated with 5 μM hinokitiol for 72 h. At the indicated times, both floating and attached cells were collected and stained with annexin V-conjugated with Alexa Fluor 488 dye and PI. The stained cells were analyzed using a flow cytometer (FC500, Beckman Coulter).

A

B

C

D

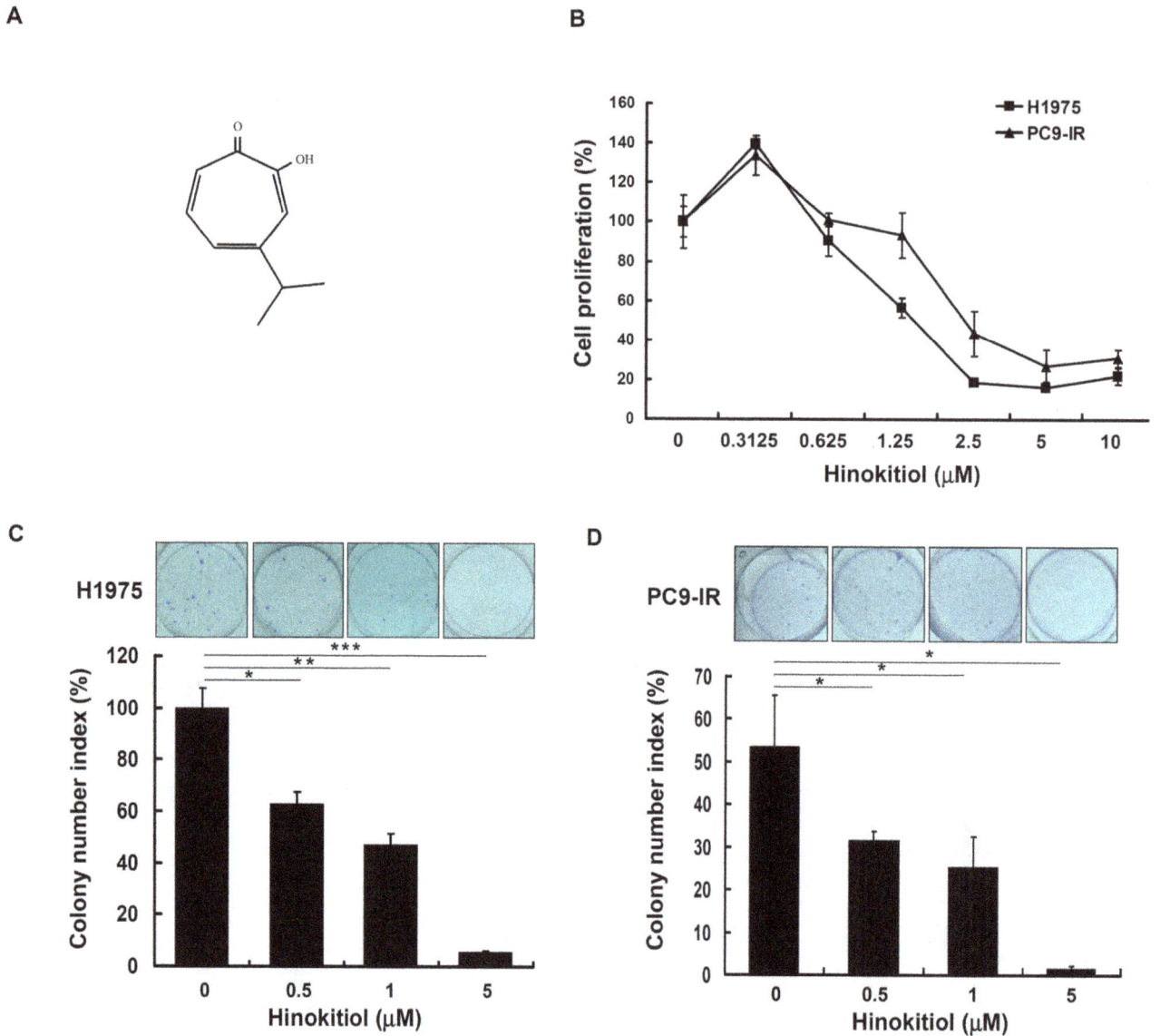

Figure 1. The effects of hinokitiol on cell proliferation. (A) The chemical structure of hinokitiol. (B) The effect of a 72-h hinokitiol treatment on H1975 and PC9-IR cell proliferation, as assayed through trypan blue staining. (C) The effect of hinokitiol on the colony formation ability of H1975 cells. (D) The effect of hinokitiol on the colony formation ability of PC9-IR cells. In (B), (C), and (D), the results are representative of three different experiments and are expressed as the mean ± SD and as % of control. *, **, and *** indicate a significant difference at the level of $p<0.05$, $p<0.01$, and $p<0.001$, respectively.

Table 2. The effect of hinokitiol on adenocarcinoma cell proliferation as determined through trypan blue staining.

Hinokitiol	48 h			72 h		
Conc. (µM)	0	5	10	0	5	10
A549	100±4.0	52.7±3.6	34.7±5.2	100±7.7	28.9±1.1	18.2±7.2
PC9	100±21.2	52.8±7.8	22.0±8.9	100±7.9	21.9±4.2	15.9±1.8
H1299	100±24.4	82.8±0	41.4±19.5	100±20.2	12.7±4.5	15.1±1.1
H3255	100±18.7	37.0±4.3	22.6±16.0	100±4.9	25.3±3.3	18.4±6.5
PC9-IR	100±12.5	73.5±12.5	36.8±6.2	100±1.1	37.4±3.2	8.4±3.2
H1975	100±9.4	55.3±3.4	40.3±10.8	100±8.1	38.9±12.5	16.8±6.5

The number of viable cells was determined through trypan blue staining, and the proliferation rates (%) are represented as the mean ± SD (%) compared with the corresponding control (0.1% DMSO) at the indicated times ($n = 3$).

A

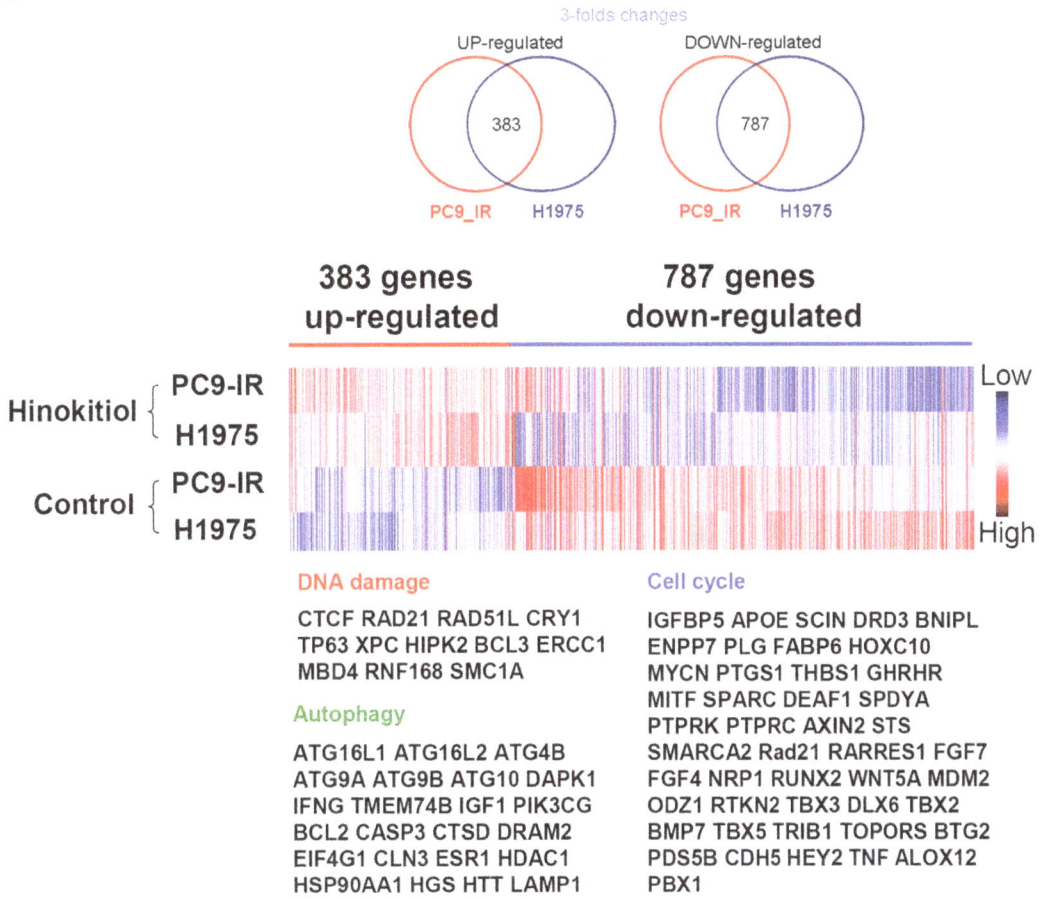

3-folds changes

UP-regulated   DOWN-regulated

383   787

PC9_IR H1975   PC9_IR H1975

383 genes up-regulated   **787 genes down-regulated**

Hinokitiol { PC9-IR / H1975

Control { PC9-IR / H1975

Low ... High

DNA damage

CTCF RAD21 RAD51L CRY1
TP63 XPC HIPK2 BCL3 ERCC1
MBD4 RNF168 SMC1A

Autophagy

ATG16L1 ATG16L2 ATG4B
ATG9A ATG9B ATG10 DAPK1
IFNG TMEM74B IGF1 PIK3CG
BCL2 CASP3 CTSD DRAM2
EIF4G1 CLN3 ESR1 HDAC1
HSP90AA1 HGS HTT LAMP1

Cell cycle

IGFBP5 APOE SCIN DRD3 BNIPL
ENPP7 PLG FABP6 HOXC10
MYCN PTGS1 THBS1 GHRHR
MITF SPARC DEAF1 SPDYA
PTPRK PTPRC AXIN2 STS
SMARCA2 Rad21 RARRES1 FGF7
FGF4 NRP1 RUNX2 WNT5A MDM2
ODZ1 RTKN2 TBX3 DLX6 TBX2
BMP7 TBX5 TRIB1 TOPORS BTG2
PDS5B CDH5 HEY2 TNF ALOX12
PBX1

B

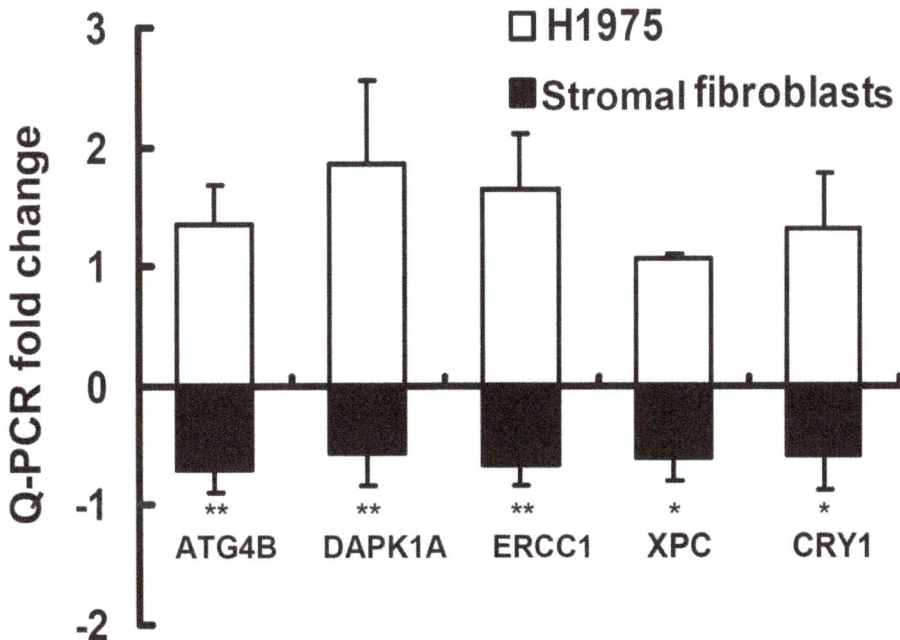

Figure 2. The effects of hinokitiol on gene expression. (A) Microarray profiling of H1975 cells and PC9-IR cells treated with 5 μM hinokitiol for 48 h. **(B)** Q-PCR array validation of the expression of genes related to DNA damage and autophagy in H1975 cells and lung stromal fibroblasts after 5 μM hinokitiol treatment for 24 h. The results are representative of those obtained in three different experiments and are expressed as the fold change compared with control. * and ** indicate a significant difference at the level of $p<0.05$ and $p<0.01$, respectively.

Acridine orange staining

To assess the formation of acidic vesicular organelles (AVOs), H1975 cells (5×10^5 cells) were seeded in 6-cm dishes with 5 μM hinokitiol for 8 h. At the indicated times, the cells were washed with PBS twice, followed by staining with 1 μg/ml acridine orange (Sigma, A 6014) in PBS containing 5% fetal bovine serum (FBS) at 37°C for 15 min. The stained cells were harvested and washed twice with PBS. The stained cells were then resuspended in PBS with 5% FBS and analyzed using a flow cytometer (FC500, Beckman Coulter).

Western blot analysis

H1975, H1299, and lung stromal fibroblasts (5×10^5) were cultured in 6-cm dishes overnight and then incubated with 5–25 μM hinokitiol for 4–72 h. Whole cell lysates were prepared using mammalian protein extraction reagent (Pierce, Rockford) containing protease inhibitors (Cytoskeleton, PICO2) and phosphatase inhibitors (Sigma). The lysates were clarified by centrifugation. Each sample, containing 40 μg protein, was separated on a 7.5–15% sodium dodecyl sulfate polyacrylamide gel (SDS–PAGE). The proteins were transferred by electroblotting to nitrocellulose membranes. The membranes were blocked for 60 min in 5% skim milk in TBST (Tris-buffered saline containing 20 mM NaF, 2 mM EDTA, and 0.2% Tween 20) at room temperature. Immunoblotting was performed using the following specific primary antibodies: total EGFR (Cell Signaling Technology, #2232S), phospho-EGFR (Y1068, Cell Signaling Technology, #2236S), and total ERK (Zymed Laboratories, 13-6200); phospho-ERK (T202/Y204, BD Transduction Laboratories, 612358); p21 (Santa Cruz C-19); cyclin D1 (Santa Cruz A-20); cyclin E2 (Cell Signaling Technology, #4132); cyclin A2 (GeneTex GTX103042); cyclin B1 (GeneTex GTX100911); γ-H2AX (Ser139, Millipore, #05-636); LC3 (Cell Signaling Technology, #3868); total ATM (GeneTex GTX70103); phospho-ATM (Ser1981, GeneTex, GTX61739); total SMC3 (Bethyl A302-068A); phospho-SMC3 (Ser1981, Bethyl, A300-480A); total p53 (Santa Cruz DO-1); phospho-p53 (Ser 15, GeneTex, GTX21431); p62 (Cell Signaling Technology, #5114S) and ATG5 (Cell Signaling Technology, #12994). The secondary antibodies were horseradish peroxidase-conjugated immunoglobulins. The antibodies were used according to the conditions recommended by the manufacturers. The bound antibodies were detected using the Enhanced Chemiluminescence System (Santa Cruz). Chemiluminescent signals were captured using the Fujifilm LAS 3000 system (Fujifilm, Tokyo, Japan). The expression level of each protein was quantified with the NIH ImageJ program using β-actin as a loading control.

Immunofluorescence γ-H2AX focus assay and confocal microscopy

H1975 cells were seeded on coverslips, allowed to attach overnight, and incubated with 5 μM hinokitiol for 48 h. After hinokitiol treatment, the cells were fixed with 4% paraformaldehyde for 10 min at room temperature and washed three times with PBS. After fixation, the cells were permeabilized with 0.5% Triton X-100 in PBS for 5 min and then blocked with 0.1% Tween 20 and 1% BSA in PBS for 5 min. The cells were incubated for 1 h with a mouse anti-γ-H2AX monoclonal antibody (Upstate, 1:800 dilution) and stained with DAPI (Sigma, D9542) and phalloidin dye (Alexa flour 647). The stained cells were examined using a

confocal laser scanning microscope (TCS SP5, Leica) at 400× magnification. All experiments were performed in triplicate.

β-Galactosidase staining for senescence

Senescence-associated-β-gal (SA-β-Gal) activity was measured using a β-gal staining kit (Cell Signaling Technology, #9860) at pH 6 according to the manufacturer's instructions. Briefly, 1×10^5 cells were incubated with 5 μM hinokitiol for 72 h, washed once with PBS, and fixed with 2% formaldehyde and 0.2% glutaraldehyde in PBS for 15 min. The cells were then washed twice with PBS and stained with a solution containing 5-bromo-4-chloro-3-indolyl-b-D-galactopyranoside (X-gal). Following incubation for 10–12 h at 37°C, senescent cells were identified by their blue staining using standard light microscopy (DMIRB, Leica).

siRNA transfection

Knockdown using specific RNA and scramble RNA interference was performed. Briefly, a mixture of 2 μg ATG5 siRNA plasmid (Invivogen, psirna42-hatg5) or scramble siRNA plasmid (Invivogen, ksirna42-lucgl3) and transfection reagent (Lipofectamine, Invitrogen) in serum-free culture medium was incubated with H1975 cells (2.5×10^5 cells) in 6-well dishes for 6 h. Then, complete culture medium and 5 μM hinokitiol were added, and the samples were incubated for 72 h. Corresponding protein down-regulation was confirmed using western blot analysis.

Ethics statement

All animal manipulations were performed in the Laboratory Animal Center of National Taiwan University College of Medicine (Taipei, Taiwan) in accordance with the protocols approved by the Institutional Animal Care and Use Committee of National Taiwan University College of Medicine (Taipei, Taiwan). All manipulations were performed humanely under isoflurane anesthesia, and all efforts were made to minimize suffering.

Animal model and experimental protocol

Six-week old NOD-SCID mice were purchased from LASCO Charles River Technology (Taiwan) and maintained in a specific pathogen-free environment. For subcutaneous xenografts, H1975 cells (1×10^6 cells in 100 μl of HBSS) were injected subcutaneously in the right flank of the animals. The hinokitiol treatment (2 or 10 mg/kg in PBS with 5% DMSO, i.p.) was initiated when the tumors reached 20 mm^3 and was administered daily until the animals were sacrificed at days 14 or 21. The tumors were measured every 4 days using a caliper, and the tumor volume was calculated according to the following formula: $V = 0.4\times a^2 b$, where a refers to the smaller diameter and b is the diameter perpendicular to a. At the end of the experiments, the mice were humanely euthanized through CO_2 inhalation to minimize suffering. Tumor xenografts were removed and weighed. A sample of tissue from each tumor was fixed in formalin and then embedded in paraffin.

Histological and immunohistochemical staining analysis

Paraffin sections were deparaffinized with xylene and then submitted to hematoxylin and eosin staining and immunohistochemical staining. Hematoxylin and eosin staining was carried out

A

Hinokitiol (h)

0	4	8	12	24	48	
						p53
1	0.8	0.5	0.5	0.5	0.7	
						γ-H2AX
1	0.8	0.9	1.1	3.0	6.4	
						β-actin

CDDP (h)

0	8	12	24	48	
					p53
1	0.5	0.9	4.4	8.9	
					γ-H2AX
1	0.9	1.1	1.6	3.4	
					β-actin

B

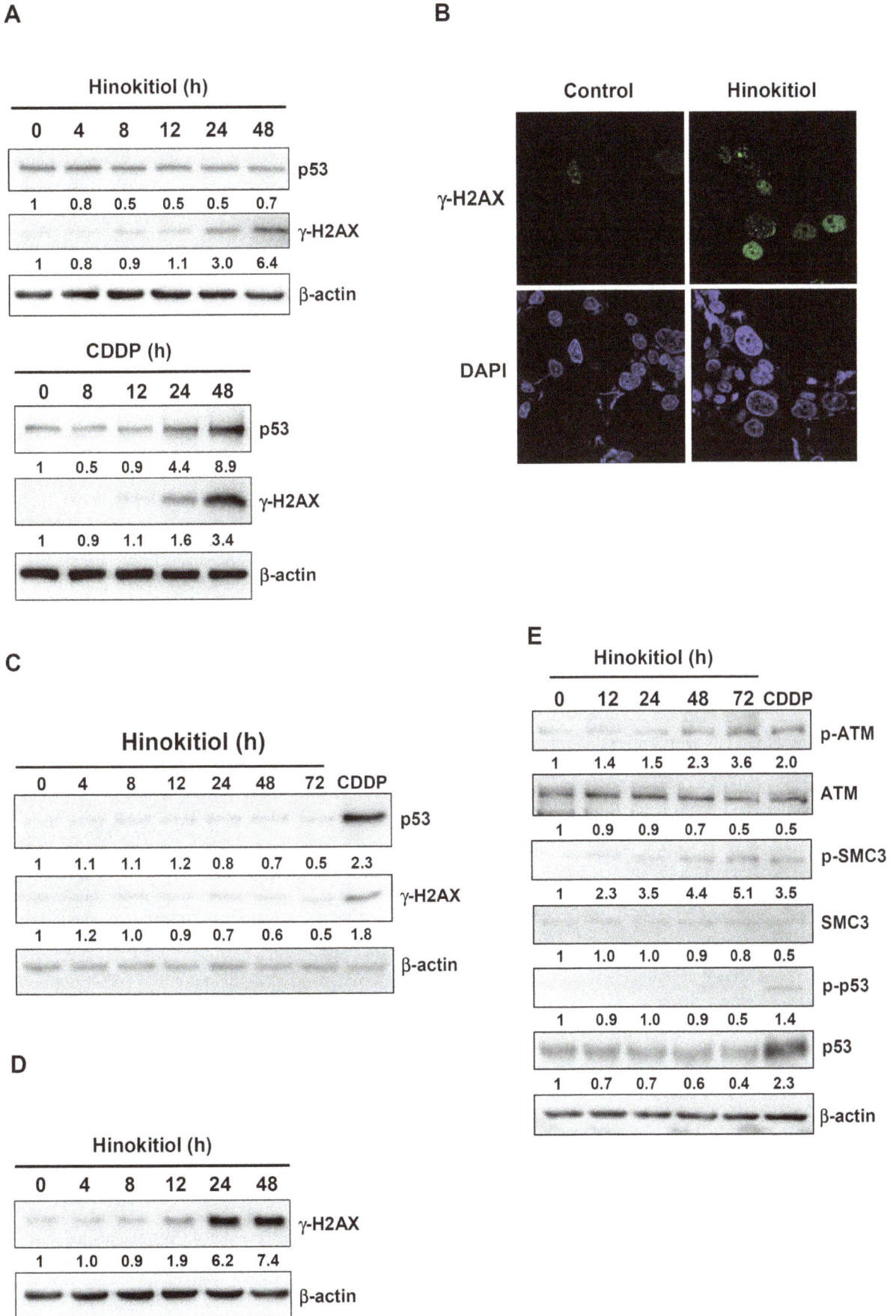

C

Hinokitiol (h)

0	4	8	12	24	48	72	CDDP	
								p53
1	1.1	1.1	1.2	0.8	0.7	0.5	2.3	
								γ-H2AX
1	1.2	1.0	0.9	0.7	0.6	0.5	1.8	
								β-actin

D

Hinokitiol (h)

0	4	8	12	24	48	
						γ-H2AX
1	1.0	0.9	1.9	6.2	7.4	
						β-actin

E

Hinokitiol (h)

0	12	24	48	72	CDDP	
						p-ATM
1	1.4	1.5	2.3	3.6	2.0	
						ATM
1	0.9	0.9	0.7	0.5	0.5	
						p-SMC3
1	2.3	3.5	4.4	5.1	3.5	
						SMC3
1	1.0	1.0	0.9	0.8	0.5	
						p-p53
1	0.9	1.0	0.9	0.5	1.4	
						p53
1	0.7	0.7	0.6	0.4	2.3	
						β-actin

Figure 3. The effects of hinokitiol on the expression of DNA damage regulatory proteins. (A) The effect of hinokitiol (5 μM) or cisplatin (25 μM) on the level of γ-H2AX phosphorylation and total p53 expression in H1975 cells, as assayed using western blots. **(B)** Assessment of hinokitiol-induced DNA damage in H1975 cells through an immunofluorescence γ-H2AX focus assay. **(C)** The effect of hinokitiol (5 μM) on the level of γ-H2AX phosphorylation and total p53 expression in lung stromal fibroblasts, as assayed using western blots. **(D)** The effect of hinokitiol (5 μM) on the level of γ-H2AX phosphorylation in H1299 cells. **(E)** The effect of hinokitiol (25 μM) or cisplatin (CDDP, 25 μM) on the phosphorylation and total level of ATM, SMC3, and p53 in H1975 cells. The expression level of each protein was quantified with the NIH ImageJ program using β-actin as a loading control.

using standard techniques. For the immunohistochemical staining, the paraffin sections were deparaffinized with xylene, and the antigens were retrieved by incubation in 0.01 M, pH 6.0 citrate buffer at 95°C for 20 min. The slides were then incubated in blocking buffer (3% BSA and 0.2% triton x-100 in PBS) for 1 h at room temperature. The primary antibodies (γ-H2AX, Ser139, Millipore, #MABE205; LC3, Cell Signaling Technology, #3868) were applied overnight at 4°C, and then washed three times with PBS for 5 min. These antibodies were detected using the IHC Select HRP/DAB kit (#DAB150, Millipore) according to the manufacturer's instructions. The slides were incubated for 1 h with biotinylated secondary antibody at room temperature, and then washed three times with PBS for 5 min. The slides were incubated for 30 min with streptavidin-HRP at room temperature, and then washed three times with PBS for 5 min. The substrate was developed using 4% DAB and the sections were counterstained with hematoxylin. The sections were dehydrated through graded alcohols, immersed in xyline, and mounted with coverslips. The tissue sections were observed under a standard light microscope (BX51, Olympus).

Statistical Analyses

All experiments were performed in triplicate and analyzed using the t-test (Excel; Microsoft) for significant differences. P values of <0.05 were considered significant.

Results

Screening for essential oils with anti-proliferative effects on lung adenocarcinoma cells

The essential oils isolated from 40 indigenous plants were evaluated for anti-proliferative effects in the human lung cancer cell line, A549, after 48 h of treatment. As shown in Table 1, five potent essential oils from *Calocedrus formosana* heartwood, *Machilus japonica* Sieb. and Zucc, *Eucalyptus camaldulensis* leaf, *Nothaphoebe konishii* (*Hay*.), and *Cunninghamia konishii* heartwood reduced cell proliferation to 64.7±6.5%, 69.9±1.8%, 67.1±6.7%, 67.7±1.7%, and 71.4±3.4% of control cells, respectively. The most potent essential oil, *Calocedrus formosana* heartwood extract, was selected for further evaluation.

Hinokitiol inhibits the proliferation of gefitinib-resistant human lung cancer cell lines

Hinokitiol is the major active compound in the essential oil of *Calocedrus formosana* heart wood [16], and its chemical structure is shown in Figure 1A. To investigate the potential anticancer activity of hinokitiol on human lung adenocarcinoma cells, six different human lung adenocarcinoma cell lines with different EGFR status, A549 (EGFR^{wt}), PC9 (EGFR^{del19}), H1299 (EGFR^{wt}), H3255 (EGFR^{L858R}), PC9-IR (EGFR^{del19}, with resistance to gefitinib) and H1975 (EGFR$^{L858R+T790M}$, with resistance to gefitinib) cells, were treated with hinokitiol (5 and 10 μM) for 48 and 72 h. Then, cell proliferation was evaluated by directly counting cells after trypan blue staining. As shown in Table 2, hinokitiol inhibited the proliferation of all cells in a time- and concentration-dependent manner. Interestingly, the gefitinib-

resistant cell lines, H1975 and PC9-IR, were inhibited by hinokitiol at a dose similar to that required for the gefitinib-sensitive cell lines PC9 and H3255. We further focused on the effects and underlying mechanisms of the action of hinokitiol on the gefitinib-resistant cells, H1975 and PC9-IR [17,18]. We found that hinokitiol had IC$_{50}$ values of 1.57 and 1.87 μM (72 h) in H1975 and PC9-IR cells, respectively (Fig. 1B). In addition, Figure 1C and 1D show that hinokitiol inhibited the colony formation ability of H1975 and PC9-IR cells in a concentration-dependent manner with an IC$_{50}$ <1 μM. These results indicated that hinokitiol potently reduced the proliferation and colony formation potential of H1975 and PC9-IR cells.

Transcriptomic and pathway analyses showing the potential molecular mechanisms of the effects of hinokitiol on H1975 and PC9-IR cells

To study the potential mechanisms of hinokitiol on gefitinib-resistant lung adenocarcinoma cells, we compared the gene expression profiles of H1975 and PC9-IR cells with or without hinokitiol using the Affymetrix human GeneChip. Here, we found that 383 genes were up-regulated over 3 fold, and 787 genes were down-regulated over 3 fold in both cell lines after 5 μM hinokitiol treatment for 48 h (Fig. 2A). The CRSD2 web server, Gene Ontology and Pathway Enrichment analysis, predicted that hinokitiol could affect certain key regulators/factors involved in DNA damage, autophagy, and cell cycle signaling in both cell lines. Furthermore, we examined DNA damage- and autophagy-related genes in H1975 cells and human lung stromal fibroblasts upon hinokitiol treatment using Q-PCR array (SuperArray Bioscience). We confirmed that two autophagy-related genes, *ATG4B* and *DAPK1A*, were up-regulated by hinokitiol treatment in H1975 cells but were down-regulated in stromal fibroblasts (> 1.5-fold change; Fig. 2B). In addition, three DNA damage-related genes, *ERCC1*, *XPC*, and *CRY1*, were up-regulated in hinokitiol-treated H1975 cells but down-regulated in stromal fibroblasts (> 1.5-fold change). These results indicated that hinokitiol induced the expression of certain DNA damage- and autophagy-related genes in cancer cells but not in human stromal fibroblasts.

Hinokitiol caused DNA damage in a p53-independent manner in lung adenocarcinoma cells but not in human lung stromal fibroblasts

According to our genome-wide transcriptomic analysis and Q-PCR validation, we found that the DNA damage-related genes *ERCC1*, *XPC*, and *CRY1* were up-regulated in hinokitiol-treated lung cancer cells. To further investigate whether hinokitiol can cause DNA damage, the levels of phosphorylated γ-H2AX and total and phosphorylated p53 were examined. Figure 3A shows that the levels of phosphorylated γ-H2AX were augmented after 48 h of hinokitiol treatment in H1975 cells, whereas total p53 was unchanged (Fig. 3A). The effect of hinokitiol on γ-H2AX phosphorylation was confirmed by immunostaining, which showed γ-H2AX protein accumulation in the nucleus of H1975 cells treated with hinokitiol (Fig. 3B), indicating that hinokitiol induced DNA damage in H1975 cells. Interestingly, hinokitiol did not induce DNA damage in human lung stromal fibroblasts

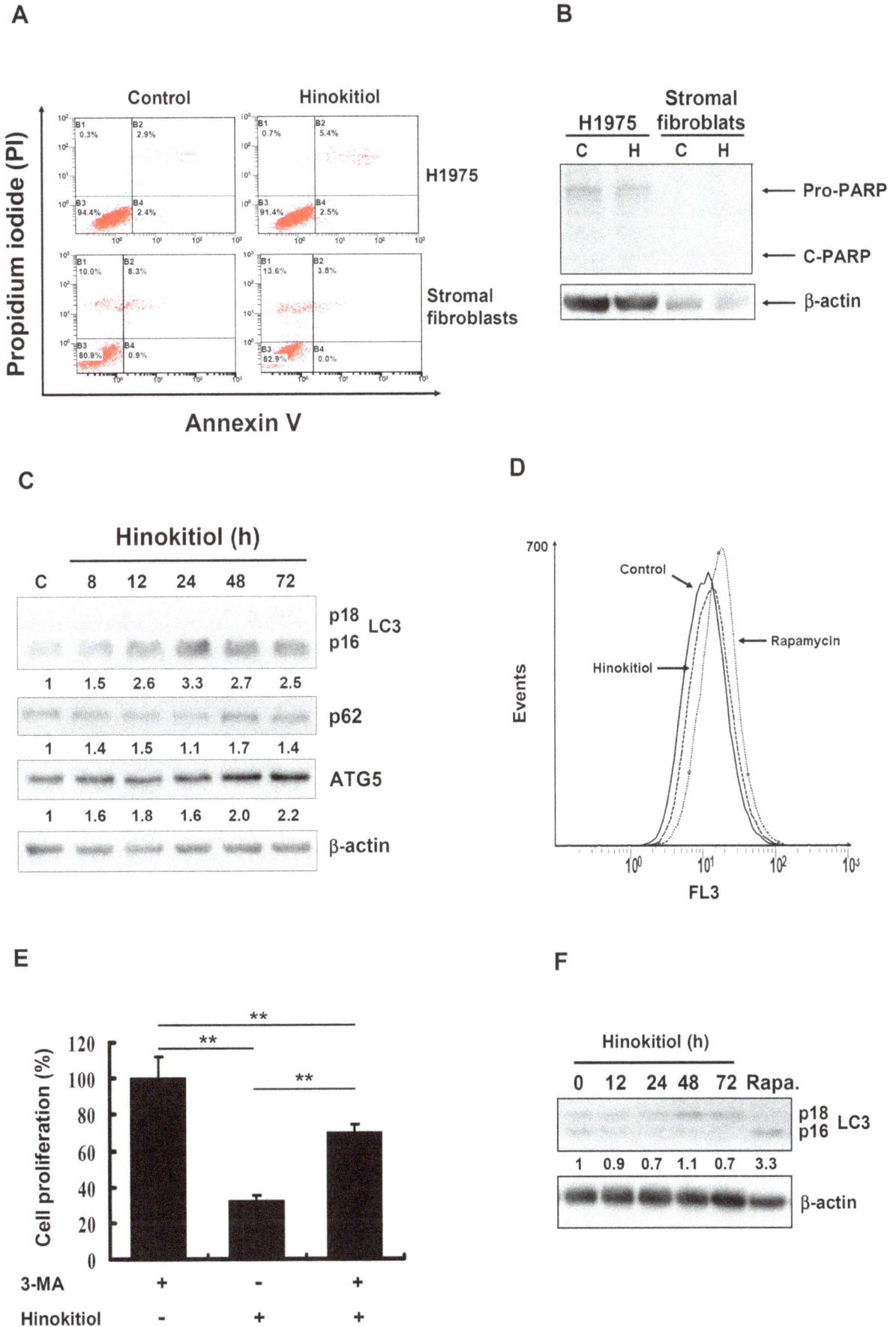

A

B

C

D

E

F

Figure 4. The effects of hinokitiol on apoptosis and autophagy. (**A**) Apoptosis was assessed using an annexin-V/PI binding assay in H1975 cells and lung stromal fibroblasts after 5 μM hinokitiol treatment. Western blot analysis of PARP in H1975 cells and lung stromal fibroblasts (**B**), LC3, p62 and ATG5 expression in (**C**) H1975 cells and (**F**) lung stromal fibroblasts. The treatment of 100 nM rapamycin for 48 h was used as a positive control for LC3 expression. The expression level of each protein was quantified with the NIH ImageJ program using β-actin as a loading control. (**D**) The formation of AVOs was quantified by flow-cytometry after acridine orange staining in H1975 cells treated with 5 μM hinokitiol for 8 h. (**E**) H1975 cells were pretreated with 2.5 mM of 3-MA for 1 h, followed by exposure to 5 μM hinokitiol for 48 h. Cell proliferation was analyzed through a trypan blue staining assay. The results are representative of three different experiments and are expressed as the mean ± SD. ** indicates a significant difference at the level of $p < 0.01$.

(Fig. 3C), and this result correlated with the expression of genes related to DNA damage shown in Figure 2. To confirm whether hinokitiol-induced DNA damage occurred independent of p53, we treated p53-null H1299 cells with hinokitiol and found that hinokitiol still induced DNA damage in these cells (Fig. 3D). Furthermore, we detected the major regulatory pathway of DNA damage response in the H1975 cells, such as the levels of phosphorylated and total ATM and SMC3. Additionally, we further detected the phosphorylated p53 to corroborate the DNA damage response is independent of p53 status evidenced by the phosphorylated or total p53 were unchanged by hinokitiol treatment (25 μM hinokitiol; Fig. 3E).

Hinokitiol induced autophagy in lung adenocarcinoma cells but not in human lung stromal fibroblasts

To gain further insight into the mode of action by which hinokitiol limited cancer cell proliferation, the effect of hinokitiol on apoptosis was examined by flow cytometry with annexin V-FITC/PI staining in H1975 cells. We found that hinokitiol treatment for 72 h did not significantly affect the percentage of cells in early or late apoptosis (Fig. 4A). Hinokitiol also did not induce apoptosis in human stromal fibroblasts (Fig. 4A). In addition, hinokitiol treatment did not induce detectable PARP cleavage in H1975 cells or human stromal fibroblasts (Fig. 4B). These results prompted us to investigate whether hinokitiol induced autophagy in H1975 cells. We found that the expression of LC3-II, p62 and ATG5 proteins, which are markers of autophagosome formation [19,20], increased after the hinokitiol treatment (Fig. 4C). Figure 4E provides additional evidence that hinokitiol induces cell autophagy, showing that 3-MA, an autophagy inhibitor, partially rescued the inhibition of cell growth induced by hinokitiol. In addition, we confirmed the autophagic response to hinokitiol by the analysis of the formation of AVOs. The flow cytometry analysis showed that the number of acidic vesicles in the H1975 cells slightly increased after hinokitiol exposure (Fig. 4D). Interestingly, hinokitiol did not induce significant levels of autophagy in human stromal fibroblasts (Fig. 4F), and this result correlated with the expression of genes related to autophagy shown in Figure 2.

Effects of hinokitiol on cell cycle arrest

We observed that hinokitiol reduced the proliferation of cancer cells, but this was not due to cytotoxicity (Fig. 4A & B). As such, we examined the effect of hinokitiol treatment on the cell cycle distribution of H1975 cells and found that the ratio of cells in S phase significantly increased after hinokitiol treatment. Concomitantly, the percentage of cells in the G1 phase was reduced compared with control cells. This result indicated that hinokitiol induced the accumulation of cancer cells in the S phase of the cell cycle (Fig. 5A). Interestingly, this effect on cell cycle distribution was not significantly observed in human lung stromal fibroblasts treated with hinokitiol (Fig. 5B). Furthermore, we used the BrdU flow assay to corroborate the S-phase arrest data in response to hinokitiol exposure in H1975 cells. In Fig. 5C, the percentage of

BrdU-negative cells in S-phase was higher in the hinokitiol exposure group; whereas the newly incorporated BrdU-labeled cells in S-phase were lower in H1975 cells. Moreover, both cancer and stromal fibroblasts in the sub-G1 phase were unaffected by the treatment with hinokitiol (Fig. 5A & B); these results were associated with the lack of apoptosis in H1975 cells, as shown in Fig. 4A & B. To investigate the underlying mechanism by which hinokitiol treatment induced cell-cycle arrest at S phase, we examined the key regulators during cell cycle progression. We found that the protein levels of cyclin D1, p21, cyclin A2, and cyclin B1 were down-regulated and that the levels of cyclin E2 were 1.9 times up-regulated in response to a 72-h treatment with hinokitiol compared with control (Fig. 5D). In addition, we found that the phosphorylation levels of EGFR and ERK, the up-stream signaling regulators of cyclin D1 [21], were significantly reduced after long-term treatment with hinokitiol (5 μM hinokitiol, 72 h; Fig. 5E). The nuclear staining in H1975 cells revealed that the proportion of abnormal mitosis was reduced after 5 μM hinokitiol exposure for 72 h (Fig. 5F).

Hinokitiol induced cellular senescence in both human lung cancer cells and lung stromal fibroblasts

Taken together, our results showed that hinokitiol inhibited cell proliferation by inducing DNA damage, autophagy, and cell cycle arrest in lung adenocarcinoma cells but not in human lung stromal fibroblasts. Because apoptosis and autophagy were not observed in hinokitiol-treated fibroblasts, we sought to evaluate whether cellular senescence could be triggered by hinokitiol treatment. The effect of hinokitiol on cellular senescence was assessed through SA-β-Gal staining, and we found that hinokitiol treatment (5 μM, 72 h) induced cellular senescence in H1975 cells and, more significantly, in human lung stromal fibroblasts (Fig. 6A). Next, we further clarify whether autophagy induced senescence in the H1975 cells after hinokitiol treatment. Thus, we used the autophagy inhibitors 3-MA and chloroquine and transfected the cells with siRNA against ATG5 to evaluate the hinokitiol-induced senescence. In Figure 6B & C, hinokitiol-induced senescence was attenuated by cotreatment with 3-MA (2.5 mM), chloroquine (10 μM), and transfected with ATG5 siRNA plasmid (2 μg). Accordingly, we conclude that hinokitiol inhibited cell proliferation in normal and tumor cells through different mechanisms, including modulating cell autophagy, cell cycle regulation, the p53-independent DNA damage response, and senescence.

Effects of hinokitiol on tumor growth of H1975 cell xenografts in SCID mice

The *in vivo* antitumor activity of hinokitiol was evaluated using H1975 cell xenografts in NOD-SCID mice. The intra-peritoneal administration of hinokitiol at low (2 mg/kg/day) and high (10 mg/kg/day) doses for 21 days significantly reduced the tumor volume (47.58% and 47.59%, respectively; Fig. 7A) compared with the control group. The size and weight of the excised tumors showed that hinokitiol effectively inhibited tumor growth *in vivo* (Fig. 7B). The histological examination of the tumor sections

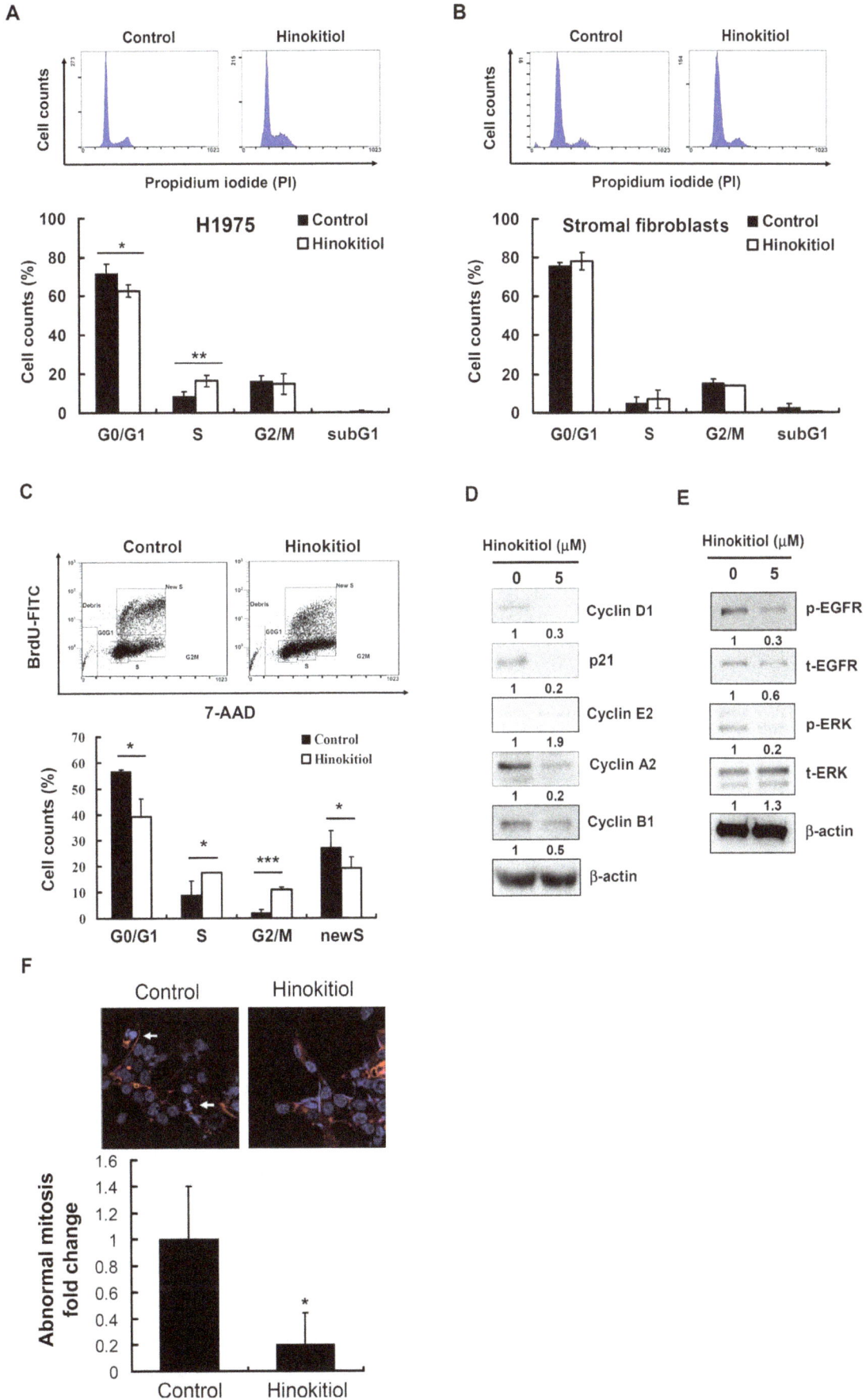

Figure 5. The effect of hinokitiol on cell cycle distribution. H1975 cells **(A)** and lung stromal fibroblasts **(B)** were treated with 5 µM hinokitiol for 72 h. The cell cycle distribution was determined by flow cytometry after the nuclei were stained with PI. **(C)** BrdU incorporation assay was applied in H1975 cells treated with 5 µM hinokitiol for 72 h. **(D)** Western blot analysis of cyclin D1, p21, cyclin E2, cyclin A2, and cyclin B1 expression in H1975 cells. **(E)** Western blot analysis of EGFR and ERK expression in H1975 cells. The expression level of each protein was quantified with the NIH ImageJ program using β-actin as a loading control. **(F)** Abnormal mitotic morphology stained with DAPI and phalloidin were quantified at 400× magnification under a confocal microscope (TCS SP5, Leica). In **(A)**, **(B)** and **(C)**, the results are representative of three different experiments, and the histogram shows the quantification expressed as the mean ± SD. *, ** and *** indicate a significant difference at the level of $p<0.05$, $p<0.01$ and < 0.001, respectively. In **(F)**, the histogram shows the quantification expressed as the mean ± SD of ratio in 5-10 fields per coverslip. * indicates significant differences at the level of $p<0.05$.

revealed that hinokitiol was able to reduce abnormal mitosis compared with the control group at days 14 and 21 (Fig. 7C). To further investigate whether the tumor growth inhibition was related to DNA damage and autophagy, we confirmed the presence of γ-H2AX and LC3 expression in the tumor tissue using immunohistochemical staining. The histological analysis revealed that hinokitiol induced γ-H2AX and LC3 at days 14 and 21 (Fig. 7D) compared with the control group levels. These *in vivo* data suggest that hinokitiol reduced tumor growth, potentially through the attenuation of tumorigenicity, and induced DNA damage and autophagy to suppress tumor progression.

Discussion

Natural herbs have been suggested as promising potential resources for the development of novel chemotherapeutics for cancer treatment. In this study, we assessed the effects of hinokitiol, which is also known as β-thujaplicin. Hinokitiol is the essential oil of a plant-derived, naturally occurring, aromatic, seven-membered tropolone compound found in cupressaceous plants such as the heartwood of *Chamaecyparis taiwanensis* and the leaves of *Calocedrus formosana* [22]. Hinokitiol has been reported to have applications in regulating several biological activities including anti-inflammation [23], anti-bacterial [24], anti-fungal [25], and anti-viral activities [26]. It has also been shown to have anti-proliferative effects in various cancer cell lines including melanoma [27], prostate carcinoma [28], oral cancer [22] and colon cancer cells [29]. However, the effects of hinokitiol on lung adenocarcinoma cells and the mechanisms underlying its effects have not been fully elucidated. In previous studies, the effective dose of hinokitiol against cancer cells ranged from 5 to 800 µM [27,30]. Considering the bioavailability and the anti-proliferation evidence in this study, we selected 5 µM as the dose in the beginning. In addition, we determined the IC_{50} of hinokitiol in H1975 and PC9-IR cells are less than 2 µM. In order to determine the effect of hinokitiol on cell proliferation in series of cell lines, we used a wide range of doses, including a higher dose of 10 µM. For these reasons, we selected doses of 5 and 10 µM hinokitiol in the trypan blue staining test (Table 2) and a dose of 5 µM for the following experiments. The data showed that 5 µM could induce significant phenotypic changes under our conditions.

In this study, we demonstrated that hinokitiol significantly inhibited cell proliferation in a series of lung adenocarcinoma cell lines, including EGFR-mutant and TKI-resistant cells, H1975 and PC9-IR, respectively. The mechanism of H1975 resistance to gefitinib is due to T790M mutation, whereas that of PC9-IR, which was selected from parental PC9 cells that had been continuously exposed to increasing concentrations of gefitinib, could be associated with persistent activation of ERK pathway [18,31]. In addition, the IC_{50} of gefitinib is more than 10 µM in H1975 [32] but more than 5 µM in PC9-IR, both of which contrast with 41 nM in the parental PC9 cells [18,31].

DNA damage induction is an effective mode of action of anticancer agents. Anticancer agents act by producing sufficient DNA strand breaks in cancer cells to evoke cell repair systems, cell cycle arrest, or cell death programs [33,34]. Many direct or indirect stresses lead to γ-H2AX expression, which is a sensitive central marker for DNA double-strand breaks (DSBs). These stresses including reactive oxygen species (ROS), DNA alkylation, topoisomerase poisons, repair deficiency, telomere shortening, meiosis breaks, and infection can activate ataxia telangiectasia, rad3-related (ATR), DNA-dependent protein kinase (DNA-PK) and ataxia telangiectasia mutated (ATM). ATM kinase is the major regulator of the recruitment of DNA damage response proteins to the DSB site and is considered a major mediator of γ-H2AX phosphorylation [35–37]. In addition to γ-H2AX, SMC3 is a substrate of ATM. SMC3 is a component of cohesin, which segregates the chromosome properly during S-phase, and its phosphorylation is required for DNA repair in response to DNA damage [37,38]. Cohesin recruitment continuously enhances ATM and γ-H2AX phosphorylation [39]. In this study, we demonstrated that in lung adenocarcinoma cells, hinokitiol caused DNA damage by inducing DSBs. This observation was further supported by the increase in the phosphorylation levels of ATM, γ-H2AX, and SMC3. The induction of γ-H2AX by hinokitiol was further confirmed in the xenografts model. Moreover, XPC, ERCC1, and CRY1, which are involved in the DNA damage repair system and correlate with S-phase arrest and senescence, were also activated by hinokitiol. In addition, the accumulation of DNA damage was considered to be the major trigger of the cell senescence phenotype [40]. Accordingly, we suggest that hinokitiol induced cell cycle arrest in S phase and triggered senescence to prevent cell replication and the transmission of damaged DNA to daughter cells.

Presently, the molecular mechanism of hinokitiol-induced DNA damage is not fully understood. Although oxidative stress can cause DNA damage, we found that hinokitiol did not induce ROS generation in lung adenocarcinoma cells (data not shown). Metals have been demonstrated to play an important role in cell proliferation and survival, and metal-chelating agents can cause DNA damage and cell death in cancer cells [41]. Hinokitiol has metal-chelating activity, and in prostate carcinoma cells, it is able to inhibit the Fe-containing enzyme ribonucleotide reductase and disrupt zinc finger motifs, thus interfering with DNA synthesis and cellular activities [28]. We suggest that hinokitiol-induced DNA damage might be associated with its metal-chelating activity. Anticancer agents can induce DSBs, cell cycle arrest, and cell death via p53-dependent and -independent pathways [42,43]. We demonstrated that DNA damage induced by hinokitiol was independent of p53, as demonstrated by the increased γ-H2AX expression without total or phosphorylated p53 activation in p53-wild-type H1975 cells and p53-null H1299 cells. Hinokitiol targeted cancer cells independent of their p53 status and can therefore be employed in a broad spectrum of tumors [43,44]. Recent studies have shown that DNA damage signaling cascades are important inducers of autophagy, which maintains the balance between synthesis, degradation, and the recycling of cellular components process [45,46]. In this study, hinokitiol induced

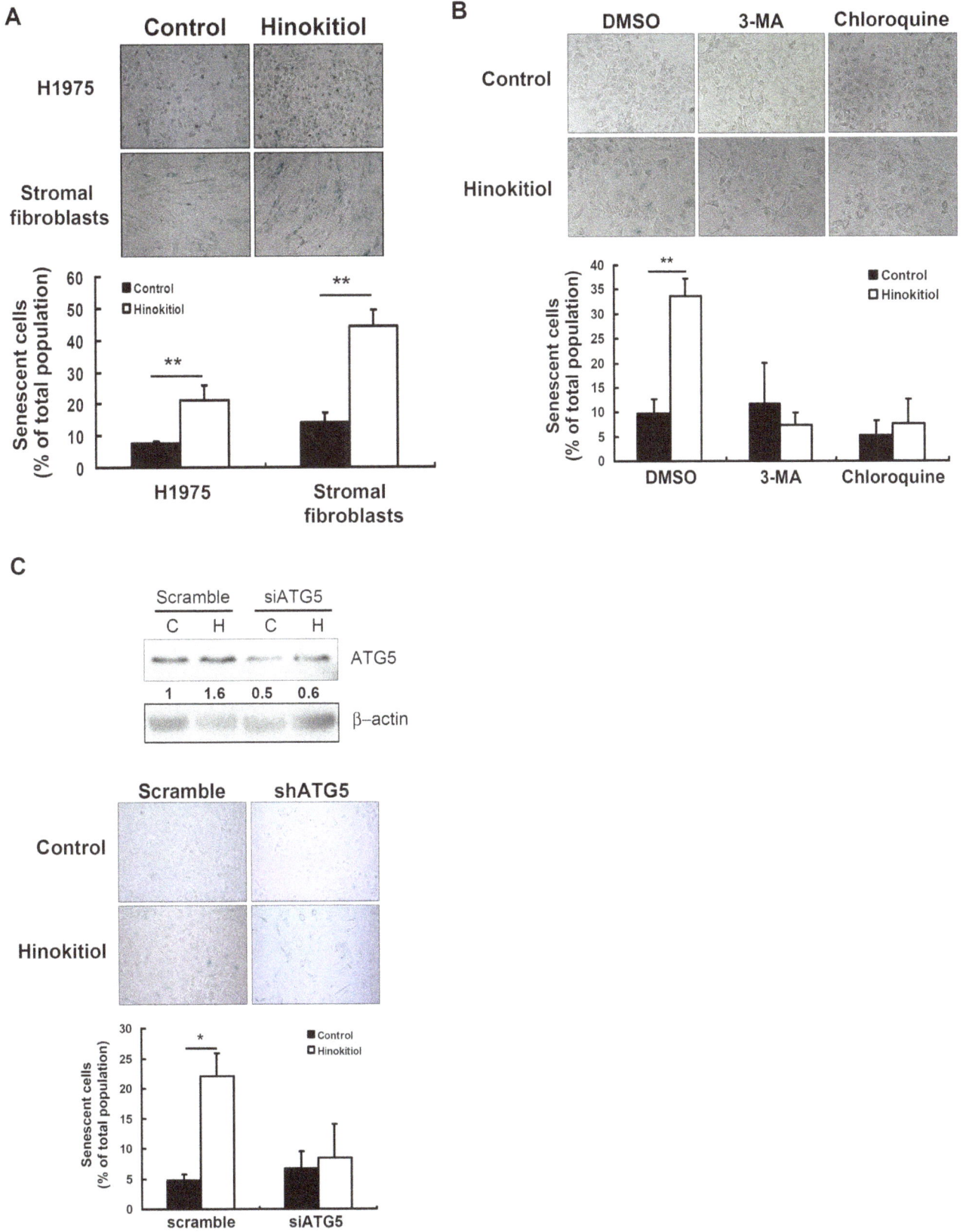

Figure 6. Hinokitiol induced cellular senescence in H1975 cells and lung stromal fibroblasts. (A) The senescent cells were quantified at 200× magnification under a standard light microscope. (B) Hinokitiol induced cellular senescence was attenuated by autophagy inhibitors in H1975 cells. (C) Hinokitiol induced cellular senescence was attenuated by transfection of siRNA against ATG5 in H1975 cells. Corresponding protein expression was detected by western blot. The expression level of each protein was quantified with the NIH ImageJ program using β-actin as a loading

control. In (A), (B) and (C), each value is the mean ± SD of 3-5 fields of three different experiments. * and ** indicate a significant difference at the level of $p<0.05$ and $p<0.01$, respectively.

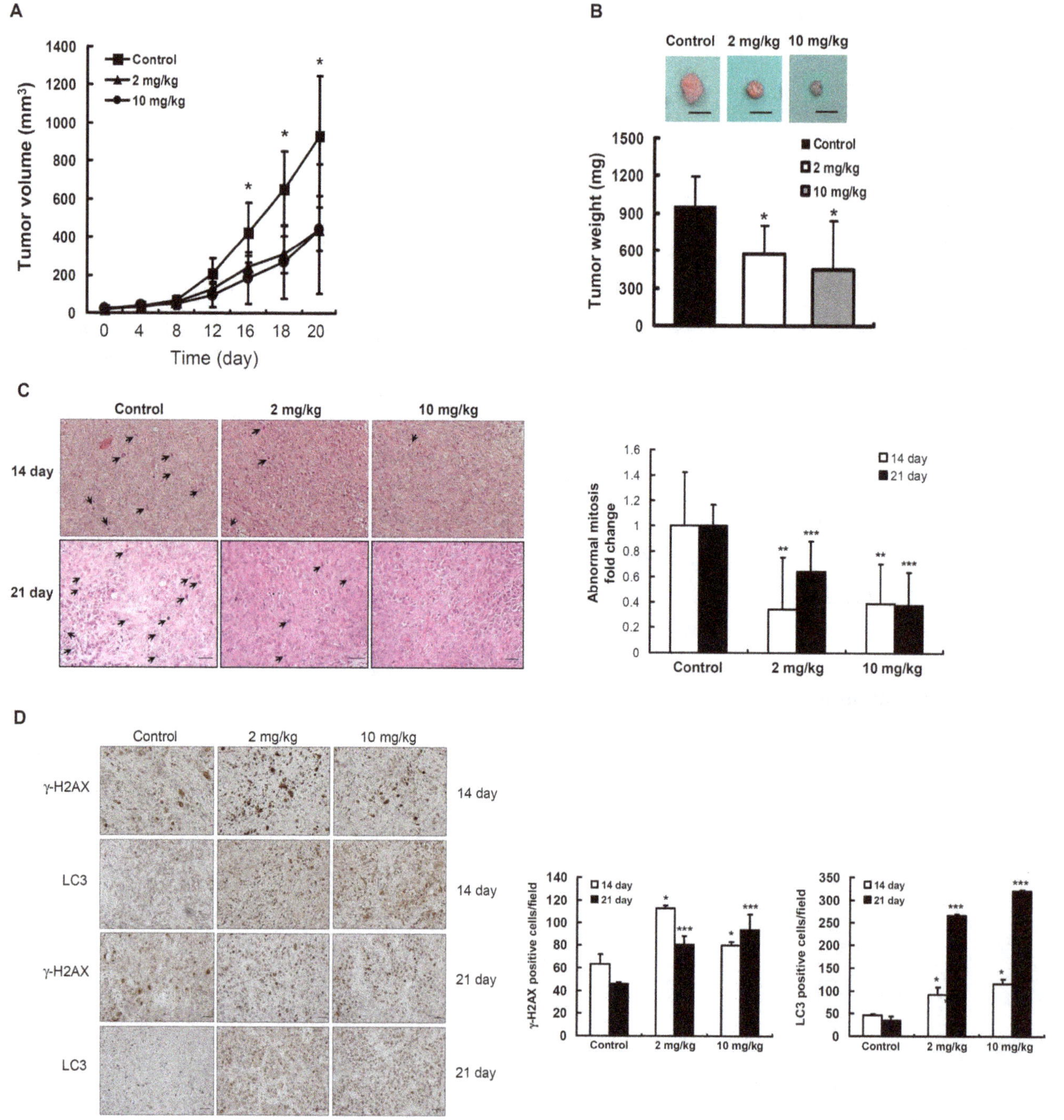

Figure 7. *In vivo* antitumor activity of hinokitiol. (A) The growth curves of subcutaneous xenografts of H1975 are shown. (B) The excised tumors were weighed and imaged. All results are given as the mean ± SD; n = 5 - 7 for each group. *indicates a significant difference at the level of $p<0.05$ compared with the control group. (C) Hematoxylin and eosin-stained tumor sections at days 14 or 21 from each group were analyzed. Arrow heads indicate the atypical nuclei or abnormal mitosis. Immunohistochemically stained tumor sections at days 14 or 21 from each group were analyzed to assess γ-H2AX and LC3 expression (D). The atypical nuclei, abnormal mitosis, and positive cells were quantified at 400× magnification under a standard light microscope (Olympus BX51, Japan). Each value is the mean ± SD of 5–10 fields of triplicate tumor sections. *, ** and *** indicate a significant difference compared with its' own control at the level of $p<0.05$, $p<0.01$, and $p<0.001$, respectively.

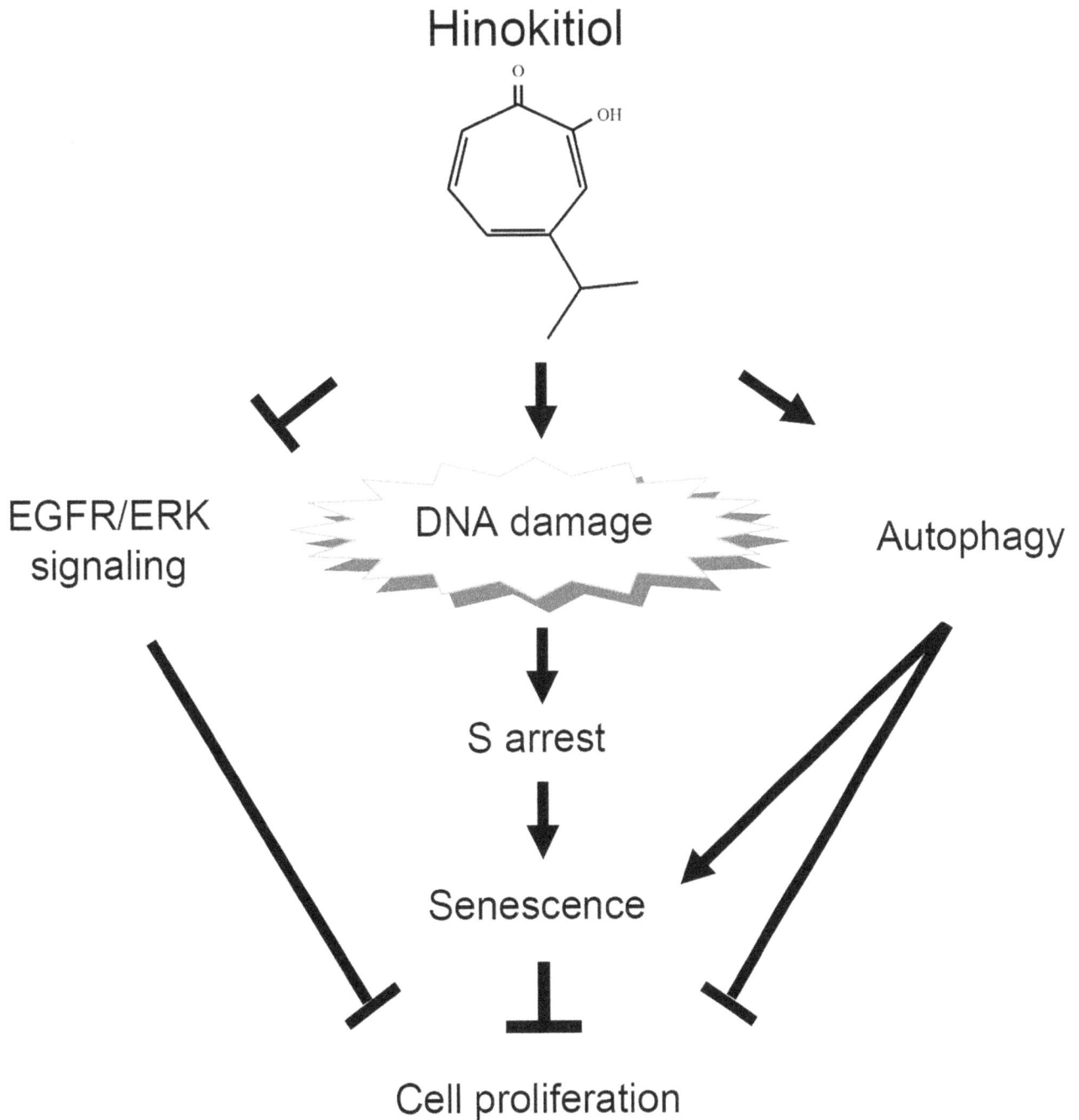

Figure 8. A schematic representation of the hypothetical mechanisms for the role of hinokitiol in suppressing lung adenocarcinomas.

autophagy, but not apoptosis or necrosis, in lung adenocarcinoma cells in vitro and in vivo, as demonstrated by LC3, ATG5, and p62 expression and AVO formation measurements. These data confirmed that hinokitiol treatment triggered autophagy and that autophagic flux was activated. Moreover, 3-MA pretreatment partially rescued the inhibition of cell growth induced by hinokitiol, implying that hinokitiol might induce autophagic cell death in lung adenocarcinomas. However, the precise mechanism by which DNA damage triggers autophagy in this context requires further study. In addition, autophagy was identified as an effector mechanism that regulates senescence [47,48]. In this study,

hinokitiol-triggered senescence was attenuated when autophagy was chemically or genetically down-regulated. These data provided new insight that autophagy might regulate senescence and consequently suppress cell progression and limit tumorigenesis. However, the detail mechanism of how hinokitiol triggered senescence without inducing DNA damage or autophagy response in lung stromal fibroblasts is unclear and further investigations are needed. In addition, previous studies have reported that sudden changes of culturing conditions are a stress to trigger senescence [49]. In this study, the stromal fibroblasts dissect from human lung have to adapt to artificial environments, as well as the absence of surrounding cell types and extracellular matrix components in culture dishes. This inadequate culture condition might offer a potential explanation of why stromal fibroblasts are more sensitive to hinokitiol induced senescence. The other possibility could be due to that unlike the tumor cell lines, the normal stromal fibroblasts are not immortalized.

The impairment of cell cycle progression is one of the mechanisms of anticancer agents [50]. The protein cyclin E2, which is essential for the transition from G1 to S phase [51], was slightly induced by hinokitiol even though other cell cycle check point regulators were down-regulated. The cell cycle analysis by PI staining and BrdU incorporation assays consistently suggested that hinokitiol inhibited the proliferation of cells by arresting the cell cycle in S phase. In addition, the down-regulation of EGFR expression and the inhibition of EGFR signaling cascades, such as the RAS/MAPK, PI(3)K/Akt, PLCc/PKC, and Jak/STAT pathways, offer potential therapeutic strategies for inhibiting cell proliferation [2,6]. We showed that hinokitiol inhibited EGFR phosphorylation and reduced ERK expression, which offers a possible mechanism by which hinokitiol suppressed proliferation in H1975 cells.

In this study, although the proliferation of stromal fibroblasts was also inhibited by hinokitiol treatment (data not shown), we found that hinokitiol induced DNA damage, autophagy, and cell cycle arrest to a greater extent in lung cancer cells than in stromal fibroblasts. The possible mechanisms of selectivity may be due to the following: 1) aneuploidy, which is a hallmark of cancer, increases the efficacy of anticancer agents [52]; 2) tumor cells are frequently more sensitive to Fe than normal cells and thus are more vulnerable to metal-chelating agents [28]; 3) the acidic environment in tumors enhances the growth inhibition and DNA fragmentation induced by metal-chelating agents [41]; 4) cancer cells with abundant topoisomerase 2α (Top2α) expression are more sensitive to DNA breaks induced by Top2α inhibitors [30]; 5) either the bioavailability or sensitivity of the drug towards certain biological targets in the cells may be altered [53]; 6) defects in the repair systems of tumor cells may increase their vulnerability [33]; or 7) in solid tumors, anticancer agents may enhance oxidative stress under hypoxic conditions [54].

In this study, we selected NOD-SCID mice as the xenograft model, based on previous studies [55,56]. Tumorigenesis studies revealed that the presence of atypical nuclei indicates higher tumorigenicity or malignancy [57,58]. The size and weight of

tumors were obviously lower, and the histological examination revealed fewer abnormal mitosis or atypical nuclei in treated mice. The IHC data indicated that the higher expression levels of γ-H2AX and LC3-II in hinokitiol-exposed mice might suppress tumor progression, resulting in the inhibition of tumor growth [59,60]. In addition, Shimizu et al. indicated that the acute oral LD_{50} for hinokitiol is as high as 469–504 mg/kg for mice [61]. Both 2-year chronic and carcinogenic toxicity studies have indicated that at dietary doses of 20.9–25.9 mg/kg/day in rats, hinokitiol does not have significant toxicity [62]. In this study, the mice in the hinokitiol group maintained a normal weight throughout treatment, and did not show any abnormalities with respect to food intake. Furthermore, hinokitiol treatment did not produce any severe adverse effects or life-threatening toxicities, as monitored by animal survival and behavior. Taken together, our data support the idea that hinokitiol might be used as a novel and safe strategy for the treatment of lung adenocarcinoma.

Conclusions

This study reports, for the first time, that hinokitiol, isolated from *Calocedrus formosana* heartwood, possesses potent anticancer effects against lung adenocarcinoma cells via the induction of DNA damage, autophagy, cell cycle arrest, and senescence, as depicted in Fig. 8. Its antitumor activity *in vivo* occurred without weight loss or other life-threatening toxicities to the animal, supporting the potential of this naturally occurring compound as a candidate therapeutic agent in lung cancer treatments.

Acknowledgments

We deeply appreciate the technical support and assistance from the Microarray Core Facility of National Taiwan University-Center of Genomic Medicine (NTUCGM), the imaging core at the First Core Labs, National Taiwan University College of Medicine, and the Department of Laboratory, Taipei City Hospital Kunming Branch.

Author Contributions

Conceived and designed the experiments: LHL PW CCH HWC. Performed the experiments: LHL PW JYL WYH WJC. Analyzed the data: LHL PW JYL WYH SMY. Contributed reagents/materials/analysis tools: PRL CLH CCW MYY. Contributed to the writing of the manuscript: LHL HWC.

References

1. Liu F, Yu G, Wang G, Liu H, Wu X, et al. (2012) An NQO1-initiated and p53-independent apoptotic pathway determines the anti-tumor effect of tanshinone IIA against non-small cell lung cancer. PLoS One 7(7): e42138.

2. Ma L, Wen ZS, Liu Z, Hu Z, Ma J, et al. (2011) Overexpression and small molecule-triggered downregulation of CIP2A in lung cancer. PLoS One 6(5): e20159.

3. Roberts PJ, Stinchcombe TE (2013) KRAS mutation: should we test for it, and does it matter? J Clin Oncol 31(8): 1112–1121.

4. Broet P, Dalmasso C, Tan EH, Alifano M, Zhang S, et al. (2011) Genomic profiles specific to patient ethnicity in lung adenocarcinoma. Clin Cancer Res 17(11): 3542–3550.

5. Lee H, Kim SJ, Jung KH, Son MK, Yan HH, et al. (2013) A novel imidazopyridine PI3K inhibitor with anticancer activity in non-small cell lung cancer cells. Oncol Rep 30(2): 863–869.

6. Brand TM, Iida M, Luthar N, Starr MM, Huppert EJ, et al. (2013) Nuclear EGFR as a molecular target in cancer. Radiother Oncol 108(3): 370–377.

7. Rogerio AP, Andrade EL, Leite DF, Figueiredo CP, Calixto JB (2009) Preventive and therapeutic anti-inflammatory properties of the sesquiterpene alpha-humulene in experimental airways allergic inflammation. Br J Pharmacol 158(4): 1074–1087.

8. Darmanin S, Wismayer PS, Camilleri Podesta MT, Micallef MJ, Buhagiar JA (2009) An extract from Ricinus communis L. leaves possesses cytotoxic properties and induces apoptosis in SK-MEL-28 human melanoma cells. Nat Prod Res 23(6): 561–571.

9. Bhalla Y, Gupta VK, Jaitak V (2013) Anticancer activity of essential oils: a review. J Sci Food Agric [Epub ahead of print]

10. da Silva EB, Matsuo AL, Figueiredo CR, Chaves MH, Sartorelli P, et al. (2013) Chemical constituents and cytotoxic evaluation of essential oils from leaves of Porcelia macrocarpa (Annonaceae). Nat Prod Commun 8(2): 277–279.

11. Cai L, Ye H, Li X, Lin Y, Yu F, et al. (2013) Chemical constituents of volatile oil from Pyrolae herba and antiproliferative activity against SW1353 human chondrosarcoma cells. Int J Oncol 42(4): 1452–1458.

12. Su YC, Hsu KP, Wang EI, Ho CL (2012) Composition, anticancer, and antimicrobial activities in vitro of the heartwood essential oil of Cunninghamia lanceolata var. konishii from Taiwan. Nat Prod Commun 7(9): 1245–1247.

13. Seal S, Chatterjee P, Bhattacharya S, Pal D, Dasgupta S, et al. (2012) Vapor of volatile oils from Litsea cubeba seed induces apoptosis and causes cell cycle arrest in lung cancer cells. PLoS One 7(10): e47014.

14. Chen WJ, Ho CC, Chang YL, Chen HY, Lin CA, et al. (2014) Cancer-associated fibroblasts regulate the plasticity of lung cancer stemness via paracrine signalling. Nat Commun 5: 3472.

15. Liu CC, Lin CC, Chen WS, Chen HY, Chang PC, et al. (2006) CRSD: a comprehensive web server for composite regulatory signature discovery. Nucleic Acids Res 34(Web Server issue): W571–577.

16. Yen TB, Chang HT, Hsieh CC, Chang ST (2008) Antifungal properties of ethanolic extract and its active compounds from Calocedrus macrolepis var. formosana (Florin) heartwood. Bioresour Technol 99(11): 4871–7.

17. Sudo M, Chin TM, Mori S, Doan NB, Said JW, et al. (2013) Inhibiting proliferation of gefitinib-resistant, non-small cell lung cancer. Cancer Chemother Pharmacol 71(5): 1325–1334.
18. Chang TH, Tsai MF, Su KY, Wu SG, Huang CP, et al. (2011) Slug confers resistance to the epidermal growth factor receptor tyrosine kinase inhibitor. Am J Respir Crit Care Med 183(8): 1071–1079.
19. Schnekenburger M, Grandjenette C, Ghelfi J, Karius T, Foliguet B, et al. (2011) Sustained exposure to the DNA demethylating agent, 2'-deoxy-5-azacytidine, leads to apoptotic cell death in chronic myeloid leukemia by promoting differentiation, senescence, and autophagy. Biochem Pharmacol 81(3): 364–378.
20. González-Rodríguez A, Mayoral R, Agra N, Valdecantos MP, Pardo V, et al. (2014) Impaired autophagic flux is associated with increased endoplasmic reticulum stress during the development of NAFLD. Cell Death Dis 17(5): e1179.
21. Lee J, Ryu SH, Kang SM, Chung WC, Gold KA, et al. (2011) Prevention of bronchial hyperplasia by EGFR pathway inhibitors in an organotypic culture model. Cancer Prev Res (Phila) 4(8): 1306–15.
22. Shih YH, Chang KW, Hsia SM, Yu CC, Fuh LJ, et al. (2013) In vitro antimicrobial and anticancer potential of hinokitiol against oral pathogens and oral cancer cell lines. Microbiol Res 168(5): 254–262.
23. Shih MF, Chen LY, Tsai PJ, Cherng JY (2012) In vitro and in vivo therapeutics of beta-thujaplicin on LPS-induced inflammation in macrophages and septic shock in mice. Int J Immunopathol Pharmacol 25(1): 39–48.
24. Morita Y, Matsumura E, Okabe T, Fukui T, Shibata M, et al. (2004) Biological activity of alpha-thujaplicin, the isomer of hinokitiol. Biol Pharm Bull 27(6): 899–902.
25. Komaki N, Watanabe T, Ogasawara A, Sato N, Mikami T, et al. (2008) Antifungal mechanism of hinokitiol against Candida albicans. Biol Pharm Bull 31(4): 735–737.
26. Budihas SR, Gorshkova I, Gaidamakov S, Wamiru A, Bona MK, et al. (2005) Selective inhibition of HIV-1 reverse transcriptase-associated ribonuclease H activity by hydroxylated tropolones. Nucleic Acids Res 33(4): 1249–1256.
27. Liu S, Yamauchi H (2009) p27-Associated G1 arrest induced by hinokitiol in human malignant melanoma cells is mediated via down-regulation of pRb, Skp2 ubiquitin ligase, and impairment of Cdk2 function. Cancer Lett 286(2): 240–249.
28. Liu S, Yamauchi H (2006) Hinokitiol, a metal chelator derived from natural plants, suppresses cell growth and disrupts androgen receptor signaling in prostate carcinoma cell lines. Biochem Biophys Res Commun 351(1): 26–32.
29. Lee YS, Choi KM, Kim W, Jeon YS, Lee YM, et al. (2013) Hinokitiol inhibits cell growth through induction of S-phase arrest and apoptosis in human colon cancer cells and suppresses tumor growth in a mouse xenograft experiment. J Nat Prod 76(12): 2195–202.
30. Shih YH, Chang KW, Hsia SM, Yu CC, Fuh LJ, et al. (2013) In vitro antimicrobial and anticancer potential of hinokitiol against oral pathogens and oral cancer cell lines. Microbiol Res 168(5): 254–62.
31. Huang MH, Lee JH, Chang YJ, Tsai HH, Lin YL, et al. (2013) MEK inhibitors reverse resistance in epidermal growth factor receptor mutation lung cancer cells with acquired resistance to gefitinib. Mol Oncol 7(1): 112–20.
32. La Monica S, Galetti M, Alfieri RR, Cavazzoni A, Ardizzoni A, et al. (2009) Everolimus restores gefitinib sensitivity in resistant non-small cell lung cancer cell lines. Biochem Pharmacol 78(5):460–8.
33. Calderon-Montano JM, Burgos-Moron E, Orta ML, Pastor N, Perez-Guerrero C, et al. (2012) Guanidine-reactive agent phenylglyoxal induces DNA damage and cancer cell death. Pharmacol Rep 64(6): 1515–1525.
34. Hisatomi T, Sueoka-Aragane N, Sato A, Tomimasu R, Ide M, et al. (2011) NK314 potentiates antitumor activity with adult T-cell leukemia-lymphoma cells by inhibition of dual targets on topoisomerase II{alpha} and DNA-dependent protein kinase. Blood 117(13): 3575–3584.
35. Bonner WM, Redon CE, Dickey JS, Nakamura AJ, Sedelnikova OA, et al. (2008) GammaH2AX and cancer. Nat Rev Cancer 8(12): 957–967.
36. Podhorecka M, Skladanowski A, Bozko P (2010) H2AX Phosphorylation: Its Role in DNA Damage Response and Cancer Therapy. J Nucleic Acids 2010: 9.
37. Watrin E, Peters JM (2009) The cohesin complex is required for the DNA damage-induced G2/M checkpoint in mammalian cells. EMBO J 28(17): 2625–35.
38. Caron P, Aymard F, Iacovoni JS, Briois S, Canitrot Y, et al. (2012) Cohesin Protects Genes against cH2AX Induced by DNA Double-Strand Breaks. PLoS Genetics 8(1): e1002460
39. Mah LJ, El-Osta A Karagiannis TC (2010) gammaH2AX: a sensitive molecular marker of DNA damage and repair. Leukemia 24(4): 679–686.
40. Wang C, Jurk D, Maddick M, Nelson G, Martin-Ruiz C, et al. (2009) DNA damage response and cellular senescence in tissues of aging mice. Aging Cell 8(3): 311–23.
41. Shamim U, Hanif S, Albanyan A, Beck FW, Bao B, et al. (2012) Resveratrol-induced apoptosis is enhanced in low pH environments associated with cancer. J Cell Physiol 227(4): 1493–1500.
42. Chiu SJ, Lee YJ, Hsu TS, Chen WS (2009) Oxaliplatin-induced gamma-H2AX activation via both p53-dependent and -independent pathways but is not associated with cell cycle arrest in human colorectal cancer cells. Chem Biol Interact 182(2–3): 173–182.
43. Hebar A, Rutgen BC, Selzer E (2012) NVX-412, a new oncology drug candidate, induces S-phase arrest and DNA damage in cancer cells in a p53-independent manner. PLoS One 7(9): e45015.
44. Lam M, Carmichael AR, Griffiths HR (2012) An aqueous extract of Fagonia cretica induces DNA damage, cell cycle arrest and apoptosis in breast cancer cells via FOXO3a and p53 expression. PLoS One 7(6): e40152.
45. Rodriguez-Rocha H, Garcia-Garcia A, Panayiotidis MI, Franco R (2011) DNA damage and autophagy. Mutat Res 711(1–2): 158–166.
46. Polewska J, Skwarska A, Augustin E, Konopa J (2013) DNA-damaging imidazoacridinone C-1311 induces autophagy followed by irreversible growth arrest and senescence in human lung cancer cells. J Pharmacol Exp Ther 346(3): 393–405.
47. Young AR, Narita M, Ferreira M, Kirschner K, Sadaie M, et al. (2009) Autophagy mediates the mitotic senescence transition. Genes Dev 23(7): 798–803.
48. Luo Y, Zou P, Zou J, Wang J, Zhou D, et al. (2011) Autophagy regulates ROS-induced cellular senescence via p21 in a p38 MAPKα dependent manner. Exp Gerontol 46(11): 860–7.
49. Kuilman T, Michaloglou C, Mooi WJ, Peeper DS (2010) The essence of senescence. Genes Dev 24(22): 2463–79.
50. Szmulewitz RZ, Clark R, Lotan T, Otto K, Taylor Veneris J, et al. (2012) MKK4 suppresses metastatic colonization by multiple highly metastatic prostate cancer cell lines through a transient impairment in cell cycle progression. Int J Cancer 130(3): 509–20.
51. Kitagawa M, Niisato N, Shiozaki A, Ohta-Fujimoto M, Hosogi S, et al. (2013) A regulatory role of K(+)-Cl(−) cotransporter in the cell cycle progression of breast cancer MDA-MB-231 cells. Arch Biochem Biophys 539(1): 92–8.
52. Tang YC, Williams BR, Siegel JJ, Amon A (2011) Identification of aneuploidy-selective antiproliferation compounds. Cell 144(4): 499–512.
53. Cho JY, Kim AR, Jung JH, Chun T, Rhee MH, et al. (2004) Cytotoxic and pro-apoptotic activities of cynaropicrin, a sesquiterpene lactone, on the viability of leukocyte cancer cell lines. Eur J Pharmacol 492(2–3): 85–94.
54. Chowdhury G, Junnotula V, Daniels JS, Greenberg MM, Gates KS (2007) DNA strand damage product analysis provides evidence that the tumor cell-specific cytotoxin tirapazamine produces hydroxyl radical and acts as a surrogate for O(2). J Am Chem Soc 129(42): 12870–12877.
55. Weeks LD, Fu P, Gerson SL (2013) Uracil-DNA glycosylase expression determines human lung cancer cell sensitivity to pemetrexed. Mol Cancer Ther 12(10): 2248–60.
56. Chen HW, Lee JY, Huang JY, Wang CC, Chen WJ, et al. (2008) Curcumin inhibits lung cancer cell invasion and metastasis through the tumor suppressor HLJ1. Cancer Res 68(18): 7428–38.
57. Sugiyama A, Miyagi Y, Komiya Y, Kurabe N, Kitanaka C, et al. (2003) Forced expression of antisense 14-3-3beta RNA suppresses tumor cell growth in vitro and in vivo. Carcinogenesis 24(9): 1549–59.
58. Patanè S, Avnet S, Coltella N, Costa B, Sponza S, et al. (2006) MET overexpression turns human primary osteoblasts into osteosarcomas. Cancer Res 66(9): 4750–7.
59. White E, Lowe SW (2009) Eating to exit: autophagy-enabled senescence revealed. Genes Dev 23(7): 784–7.
60. Hiyoshi H, Abdelhady S, Segerström L, Sveinbjörnsson B, Nuriya M, et al. (2012) Quiescence and γH2AX in neuroblastoma are regulated by ouabain/Na,K-ATPase. Br J Cancer 106(11): 1807–15.
61. Shimizu M, Noda T, Yamano T, Yamada A, Morita S (1993) Acute Oral Toxicity of Natural Food Additives in Mice and Rats. Seikatsu Eisei 37: 215–220. (Japanese)
62. Imai N, Doi Y, Nabae K, Tamano S, Hagiwara A, et al. (2006) Lack of hinokitiol (beta-thujaplicin) carcinogenicity in F344/DuCrj rats. J Toxicol Sci 31(4): 357–370.

16

Ginsenoside Rg1 Prevents Cognitive Impairment and Hippocampus Senescence in a Rat Model of D-Galactose-Induced Aging

Jiahong Zhu[1]⑨¶, Xinyi Mu[1]⑨¶, Jin Zeng[2], Chunyan Xu[1], Jun Liu[1], Mengsi Zhang[1], Chengpeng Li[1], Jie Chen[3], Tinyu Li[3], Yaping Wang[1]*

1 Department of Histology and Embryology, Laboratory of Stem Cells and Tissue Engineering, Chongqing Medical University, Chongqing, China, **2** The Land Force Lintong Sanatorium, Xi'an, Shanxi, China, **3** Chongqing Stem Cell Therapy Engineering Technical Center, Chongqing, China

Abstract

Neurogenesis continues throughout the lifetime in the hippocampus, while the rate declines with brain aging. It has been hypothesized that reduced neurogenesis may contribute to age-related cognitive impairment. Ginsenoside Rg1 is an active ingredient of *Panax ginseng* in traditional Chinese medicine, which exerts anti-oxidative and anti-aging effects. This study explores the neuroprotective effect of ginsenoside Rg1 on the hippocampus of the D-gal (D-galactose) induced aging rat model. Sub-acute aging was induced in male SD rats by subcutaneous injection of D-gal (120 mg/kg·d) for 42 days, and the rats were treated with ginsenoside Rg1 (20 mg/kg·d, intraperitoneally) or normal saline for 28 days after 14 days of D-gal injection. In another group, normal male SD rats were treated with ginsenoside Rg1 alone (20 mg/kg·d, intraperitoneally) for 28 days. It showed that administration of ginsenoside Rg1 significantly attenuated all the D-gal-induced changes in the hippocampus, including cognitive capacity, senescence-related markers and hippocampal neurogenesis, compared with the D-gal-treated rats. Further investigation showed that ginsenoside Rg1 protected NSCs/NPCs (neural stem cells/progenitor cells) shown by increased level of SOX-2 expression; reduced astrocytes activation shown by decrease level of *Aeg-1* expression; increased the hippocampal cell proliferation; enhanced the activity of the antioxidant enzymes GSH-Px (glutathione peroxidase) and SOD (Superoxide Dismutase); decreased the levels of IL-1β, IL-6 and TNF-α, which are the proinflammatory cytokines; increased the telomere lengths and telomerase activity; and down-regulated the mRNA expression of cellular senescence associated genes $p53$, $p21^{Cip1/Waf1}$ and $p19^{Arf}$ in the hippocampus of aged rats. Our data provides evidence that ginsenoside Rg1 can improve cognitive ability, protect NSCs/NPCs and promote neurogenesis by enhancing the antioxidant and anti-inflammatory capacity in the hippocampus.

Editor: Alexandra Kavushansky, Technion - Israel Institute of Technology, Israel

Funding: The work was supported by National Natural Science Foundation of China (No 30973818), and the Science Foundation of Ministry of Education of China (No 20125503110006). The funders had no role in study design, data collection and analysis, decision to publish, or preparation of the manuscript.

Competing Interests: The authors have declared that no competing interests exist.

* Email: ypwangcq@aliyun.com

⑨ These authors contributed equally to this work.

¶ These authors should be considered co-first authors.

Introduction

With the growing population and extended lifespan, brain aging becomes a worldwide problem due to its substantial associated disability. For example, one of the strongest risk factors for the Alzheimer's disease is brain aging. The brain is particularly vulnerable to oxidative stress because of its high oxygen metabolic rate and its relative deficiency in both free-radical scavenging enzymes and antioxidant molecules compared with other organs [1,2]. During aging, the accumulation of free radicals progressively damages the brain structure and function. Hippocampus is closely related to learning and memory abilities, and as an area where NSCs/NPCs (neural stem cells/progenitor cells) exist in the adult brain, it is of a particular interest in the age-associated neurodegeneration.

Panax ginseng has been used as a tonic drug in traditional Chinese medicine for over 2000 years. Ginsenoside Rg1 is one of the most active ingredients of *Panax ginseng*, and has been proven to have various pharmacological actions in anti-oxidation, anti-aging and particularly in memory deterioration [3,4]. Our previous work has showed a protective anti-aging function of Ginsenoside Rg1 in the neuron system that delays senescence of NSCs/NPCs *in vitro* [5].

To elucidate the function and the underlying mechanism of Ginsenoside Rg1 in age-associated neurodegeneration, we employed the D-gal (D-galactose) induced aging rat model. Chronic systemic exposure of rodents to D-gal induces accelerated aging including deterioration of cognitive and motor skills that are similar to symptoms in natural aging. Therefore, it is regarded and widely used as an ideal model to study the mechanisms and screen drugs for brain aging [6–9]. We investigated the effect of Rg1 on spatial memory and hippocampal histopathological damages in the D-gal induced aging rat model. Senescence-associated biomarker, neurogenesis, oxidative stress biomarkers, neuroinflammation biomarkers, telomere shortening and senescence-associated genes expression in the hippocampus were examined. We propose that ginsenoside Rg1 is able to improve cognitive ability, protect NSCs/NPCs and promote neurogenesis by its anti-oxidative and anti-inflammation capacity.

Materials and Methods

Ethics Statement

All experiments were performed in accordance with institutional and national guidelines and regulations and were approved by the Chongqing Medical University Animal Care and Use Committee.

Animal treatment

Three months old male Sprague-Dawley rats were purchased from the Medical and Laboratory Animal Center of Chongqing and housed in a temperature and light-controlled room with free access to water and food. All surgeries were performed under sodium pentobarbital anesthesia, and all the efforts were made to minimize suffering.

Sixty animals were randomly divided into 4 groups (control, D-gal-administration, Rg1 treatment, and D-gal-administration plus Rg1 treatment). In the D-gal-administration group, D-gal (120 mg/kg·d) was injected subcutaneously daily into rats for 42 days. In the D-gal-administration plus Rg1 treatment group, ginsenoside Rg1 (20 mg/kg·d) was injected peritoneally daily concomitantly for 28 days from day 15 of D-gal injection. All control animals were given saline in the same volume subcutaneously and peritoneally, respectively. In the Rg1 treatment group, saline at the same volumn with D-gal injection was injected subcutaneously for 42 days, and Rg1 (20 mg/kg·d) was injected peritoneally for 28 days from day 15 of saline injection. The body weights were measured every 3 days,there were no significant differences between the groups. The body weight data are provided in the supporting information (Figure S1 in File S1).

Reagents

Ginsenoside Rg1 (RSZD-121106, Purity = 98.3%) was purchased from Xi'an Haoxuan Biological Technology Co., Ltd (Xi'an, China), dissolved in ddH$_2$O at the concentration of 20 mg/ml, and sterilized by ultrafiltration. GSH/GSH-px kit, SOD kit and MDA kit were purchased from Nanjing Jiancheng Bioengineering Institute (Nanjing, China). IL-1β kit, IL-6 kit and goat anti-rabbit secondary antibody were purchased from Wuhan Boster Bio-engineering Co., Ltd. (Wuhan, China). TNF-α Kit was obtained from Uscn Life Science Inc. (Wuhan, China). BCA kit and SA-β-gal Staining kit were purchased from Beyotime Institute of Biotechnology (Shanghai, China). Anti-β-tubulin III antibody was obtained from Sigma Co. LLC. Anti-GFAP antibody was purchased from Wuhan Sanying Biotechnology Inc. (Wuhan, China).

Morris Water Maze Performances

After the 42-day treatment, spatial memory of the rats was assayed by Morris water maze task. The maze was a tank (80 cm in radius and 45 cm high) filled with water at approximately 24°C. The tank was divided into 4 quadrants, one of which contained a circular escape platform (8 cm in diameter) placed at a fixed position, 2.5 cm below the surface of the water. There were visual cues around the water maze. Oriented navigation trials were performed 4 times per day, for 7 consecutive days with a constant interval of 1 h. In each trial, the animals were gently placed in water in one of the four quadrants, and the starting quadrant was varied randomly over the trials. Rats were allowed a maximum of 90 sec to find the escape platform, where it remained for 30 sec.

For all training trials, the time that it took the rat to reach the submerged platform (escape latency) was recorded to assess spatial learning ability. On the eighth day, another set of tests consisting of a 120 sec trial with the platform removed was conducted. Besides escape latency before reaching the platform, time spent in the target quadrant and the number of target crossings over the previous location of the target platform were recorded to assess spatial memory ability. The target quadrant was defined as the quadrant that previously contained the platform, the radius of which was limited to 70 cm in this assessment.

Detection of oxidation-associated biomarkers

After the therapy, hippocampuses were collected and lysed in ice bath for 30 min. The supernatant was collected after centrifugation (12000 rpm, 4°C, 30 min). GSH-px activity and GSH content, SOD activity and MDA content were detected by chemical colorimetric analysis according to the manufacturer's instructions.

To detect GSH-Px activity, the enzymatic reaction in the tube, which contained NADPH, reduced GSH, sodium azide and glutathione reductase, was initiated by addition of H$_2$O$_2$. And the change in absorbance at 340 nm was monitored. Activity is expressed as U/mg protein. To detect reduced GSH content in each group, 1% trichloroacetic acid was added to the lysates. After centrifugation at 10 000×g for 15 min, protein free lysates were obtained. The reaction mixture for determination of GSH content consisted of lysates and 5, 5′-dithiobis-(2-nitrobenzoic acid) (DTNB) 6 mmol/L. The absorbance at 405 nm was monitored for 6 min using a microtiter plate reader (Bio-Rad Ltd, Japan). The content of GSH was calculated as 1 mg GSH/g protein from the change in the rate of absorbance on the basis of a standard curve.

The assay for total superoxide dismutases (SOD) is based on the ability to inhibit the oxidation of oxymine by the xanthine-xanthine oxidase system. One unit (U) of SOD activity was defined as the amount that reduced the absorbance at 550 nm by 50%, and data were expressed as units per microgram of hippocaumpus protein. Thiobarbituric acid reaction (TBAR) method was used to determine the MDA which can be measured at the wave length of 532 nm by reacting with thiobarbituric acid (TBA) to form a stable chromophore production. MDA content was expressed as nmol per milligram of hippocampal protein. Protein concentration was measured using the method of Bradford. Bovine serum albumin was used as a standard.

Detection of proinflammatory cytokines in the hippocampus by ELISA

The supernatant was collected as above, and the levels of proinflammatory cytokines IL-1β, IL-6 and TNF-α in the hippocampus in each group were measured by ELISA kit following the manufacture's instructions. The level of both cytokines was determined by the competitive binding of the cytokines in the samples with ^{125}I-radiolabled IL-1β and TNF-a standards respectively. Data were shown as the actual content of the lysates per mg tissue lysates.

Tissue processing and immunofluorescence

Animals were reanaesthetized and transcardially perfused with 4% buffered paraformaldehyde solution (pH 7.4), then the brains were separated and post-fixed for 4 hours, followed by dehydration in 20% sucrose at 4°C. Free floating sections of 20 μm were cut with a cryotome.

For immunofluorescence analysis, appropriate sections were recovered and washed with TBS with 0.3% Triton X-100 followed by blocking with 1.5% normal goat for 4 h at room temperature. Sections were then incubated with anti-β-tubulin III (a neuron marker), anti-GFAP (an astrocyte marker) and Gal-c (a mature oligodendrocyte marker) antibodies all diluted at 1:200 for 24 h at 4°C. Later, after TBS washes, sections were incubated with secondary antibodies for 1 h at 37°C. DAPI was used for nuclear staining. Finally, 20 μl of glycerole was applied to each slide and a cover slip was sealed in place. All slides were viewed directly under a fluorescence microscope (Eclipse, Nikon). Controls included omitting the primary and secondary antibodies. The total numbers of cells were estimated on three randomly selected sections taken through the central extent of the dentate gyrus area.

Senescence-associated β-galactosidase cytochemical staining

The SA-β-gal (senescence-associated β-galactosidase) staining was carried out according to the manufacturer's instructions. Frozen section preparation procedure described above was used for cytochemical staining. In brief, slides were washed twice by PBS, fixed by Fixative Solution for 15 min at room temperature, and stained by X-Gal Staining Solution (100 mM sodium phosphate, 2 mM MgCl2, 150 mM sodium chloride, 0.01% sodium deoxycholate, 0.02% NP-40, 5 mM potassium ferricyanide, 5 mM potassium ferrocyanide, and 1 mg/ml X-gal, pH 6) for 24 hours at 37°C in dark without CO_2. After the incubation, sections were washed in PBS and viewed under bright field at 400×magnification. Quantitative image analysis was performed by a blinded observer counting at least 3 random fields. The intensity of SA-β-gal-positive cells was evaluated by means of a ROD (relative optical density) value. ROD of SA-β-gal-positive cells in CA3 area of the hippocampus was obtained after transformation of mean gray values into ROD using the formula: ROD = log (256/mean gray). Images were collected from at least three different sections per structure and per animal by Image Pro Plus software.

Cell proliferation analyses

On the day 41 of treatment, BrdU (50 mg kg^{-1} in saline) was administered intraperitoneally three times with an interval of 4 hours. 12 hours after the final administration, the rats (5–6 animals per group) were reanaesthetized and perfused transcardially with 4% PFA in PBS. Hippocampuses were collected and postfixed. Frozen sections and immunofluorescence were performed as previously described. The primary antibody was the mouse monoclonal anti-BrdU (1:200; Sigma Co. LLC.). The total number of BrdU+ cells was estimated on three randomly selected sections taken through the central extent of the dentate gyrus area with a fluorescence microscope (Eclipse, Nikon).

Western blotting analysis

Hippocampuses in each group were collected after the therapy. Total protein was extracted, and the concentrations were measured by a BCA procedure. Samples containing 50 μg protein were separated on SDS-PAGE and transferred to PVDF membranes. Membranes were incubated overnight at 4°C with the anti-SOX2 antibody diluted at 1 : 500. The secondary antibody was diluted at 1 : 5,000 in TBST. The membranes were visualized using the enhanced chemiluminescence detection system (Pierce, USA). The level of β-actin was used as an internal control. Relative intensities were quantified using Quantity One (Bio Rad).

RNA extraction and realtime quantitative RT-PCR

Hippocampuses were collected after the therapy. Total mRNA was extracted using TRIZOL Reagent (TaKaRA, Japan), according to the manufacturer's protocol. OD260/OD280 of RNA: 1.8~2.0. First-strand cDNA was created by RT (TaKaRA, Japan). Real-time PCR was carried out using BIO-RAD sequence detection system (cfx96). DNA was amplified by an initial incubation at 94°C for 5 min followed by 40 cycles of 94°C denaturation for 15 sec, annealing at 60°C for 60 sec, 72°C extension for 1 min. mRNA expression levels were normalized against *Gapdh* mRNA level and analyzed by the comparative cycle threshold method. The PCR primers used are provided in the supporting information (Table S1 in File S1).

Measurement of telomere length by Southern blot

Telomere lengths were measured from the hippocampus according to the previously described method [10]. In brief, after extraction, DNA was inspected for integrity, digested, resolved by gel electrophoresis, transferred to a membrane, hybridized with labeled probes and exposed to X-ray film. The telomere lengths were measured by Western Biotechnology Corporation (Chongqing, China).

Detection activity of telomerase by silver staining TRAP-PCR

The supernatant was collected as above. The concentrations were measured by Coomassie brilliant blue. The PCR reaction mixture contained 5 μl 10× TRAP buffer, 1 μL dNTPs, 1 μl Taq polymerase,1 μl TS primer and 2 μl extract of telomerase, was incubated for 30 min at 23°C for telomerase-mediated extension of the TS primer. The reaction mixture was subjected to 35 cycles at 94°C for 30 sec, 50°C for 30 sec, and 72°C for 90 sec. TRAP reaction products were separated by 10% polyacrylamide gel electrophoresis and detected by SYBR green (Gene, Inc.) staining.

Statistical analysis

SPSS version 17.0 software was used for statistical analyses. One-way ANOVA was used for comparison of mean values across the groups and multiple comparisons were made by LSD test. Differences were considered significant at $P<0.05$.

Results

Ginsenoside Rg1 restored cognitive impairment caused by D-gal administration

The hidden-platform version of the Morris water maze, a hippocampus-dependent task, requires an animal to learn and remember the relationships between multiple distal cues and the platform location to escape the water [11]. As shown in Figure 1A, rats in the D-gal administration group had significant impairment in spatial learning ability during the seven-day place navigation training because of the longer escape latency compared to the control rats ($P<0.05$); while ginsenoside Rg1 treatment to D-gal administrated rats significantly shortened the escape latency to the similar levels of the control rats. Rats in the Rg1 treatment group showed similar spatial learning ability to that of the control rats during the navigation training.

To assess the spatial memory more directly, the rats were subjected to another trial in which the target platform was removed on the next day after the navigation training. As shown in Figure 1B, for the D-gal administered rats it took longer time to reach the location of the removed platform, and crossed the location fewer times compared to the control group. However, rats

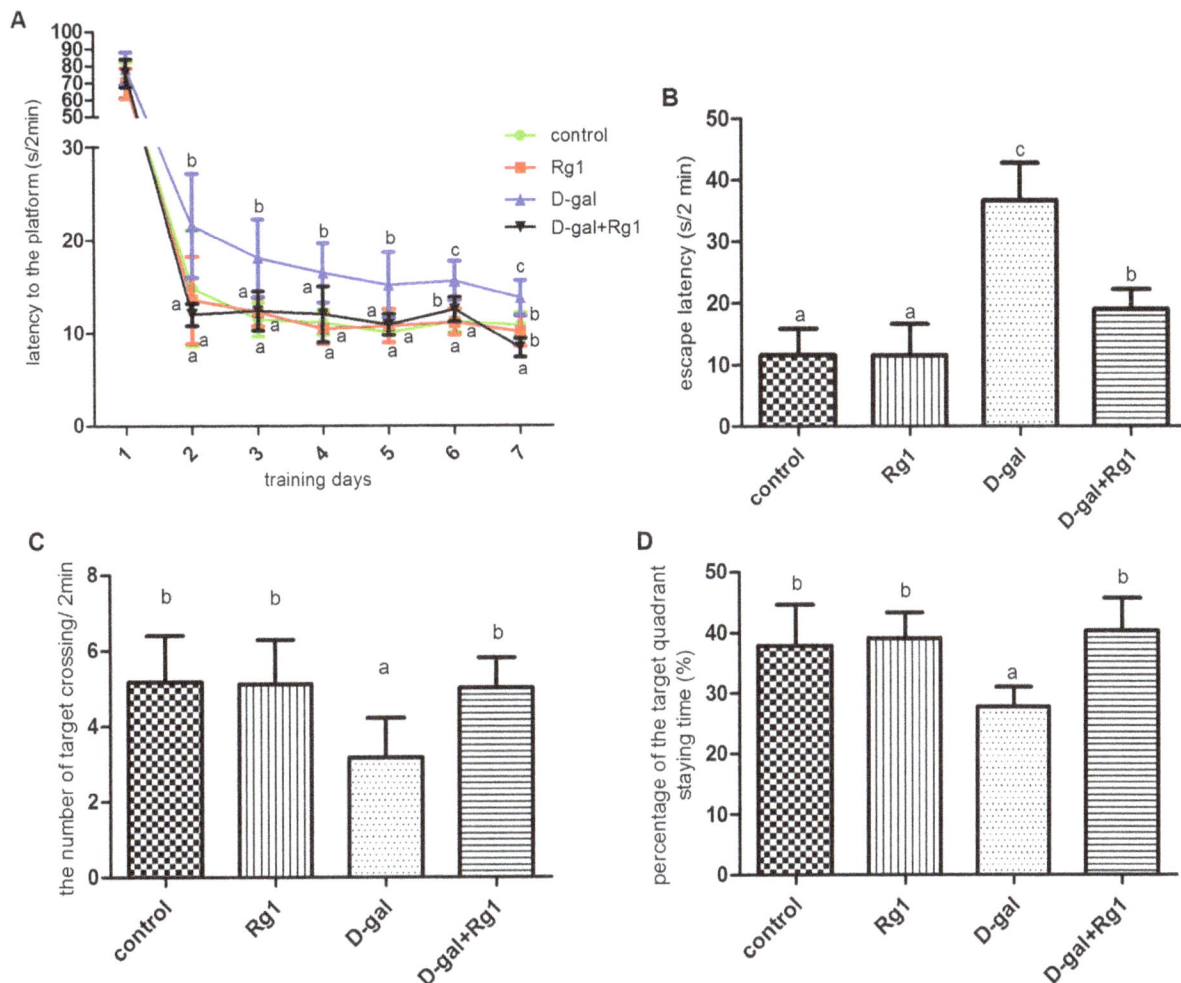

Figure 1. The effect of ginsenoside Rg1 on cognitive impairment caused by D-gal administration ($\bar{x} \pm s$, n = 5). The Morris water maze test was carried out to test the spatial learning and memory ability of rats. A. Latencies to find a hidden platform in the water maze during the seven days of place navigation training. On the eighth day, another set of tests was performed when the target platform was removed: B. The escape latency of the rats when the platform was removed. C. The times of rats' crossing the target quadrant. D. The percentage of time that the rats stayed in the quadrant where the platform was once placed. Different letters represent significantly different values as assessed by ANOVA and LSD tests with P<0.05.

in both Rg1 treatment group and D-gal administration plus Rg1 treatment group showed no remarkable differences in the escape latency and target crossing times compared to the control group. In addition, rats in the control group, Rg1 treated group and D-gal administration plus Rg1 treatment group spent more time in the target quadrant than the D-gal administrated rats.

These results indicated that aging model rats had impairments in spatial learning and memory, while the treatment of ginsenoside Rg1 could restore the age-related cognitive impairment caused by D-gal administration.

Ginsenoside Rg1 reduced the SA-β-Gal stainings in hippocampus of brain-aged rats

Aging is known to be associated with a slow decline in brain functions and be accompanied by progressive memory loss, dementia and cognitive dysfunctions. As the hippocampus is closely related to learning and memory ability, we have speculated that the loss of cognitive capacity of the rats in the D-gal administration group is related to the hippocampus aging.

SA-β-gal is one of the most widely used biomarkers for aging cells [12], and aged cells are stained in blue by it in the cytoplasm. As shown in Figure 2, barely any SA-β-gal positive cells were observed in DG area among all the groups, while aged cells were observed in the CA3 area. This pattern was consistent with a previous study [13]. The intensity of SA-β-gal staining was evaluated by means of a ROD (relative optical density) value. The ROD of the SA-β-gal stainingwas not statistically significant between the control group and the Rg1-treated group. Remarkably, D-gal administration induced a remarkable increase in the ROD of the SA-β-gal staining, compared to the control group (Figure 2, Table 1). However, in the D-gal administration plus Rg1 treatment group, the ROD was significantly reduced (Figure 2, Table 1). It demonstrates that Rg1 can protect the hippocampus against senescence.

Table 1. The effect of ginsenoside Rg1 on the senescence-associated SA-β-Gal stainings in area CA3 in the hippocampus of brain-aged rats ($\bar{x} \pm s$, $n = 5$).

Group	ROD of SA-β-Gal
control	11.8 ± 4.6^{a}
Rg1	12.4 ± 6.3^{a}
D-gal	67.8 ± 18.67^{c}
D-gal + Rg1	36.2 ± 12.46^{b}
	$P = 0.000$

The SA-β-gal (senescence-associated β-galactosidase) staining was carried out on the slides. ROD (relative optical density) of SA-β-gal-positive cells in CA3 area of the hippocampus was obtained after transformation of mean gray values into ROD using the formula: ROD = log (256/mean gray). Images were collected from at least three randomly selected sections per structure and per animal by Image Pro Plus software. Data are expressed as mean $\pm$ SD. Different letters represent significantly different values as assessed by ANOVA and LSD tests with $P < 0.01$.

The effect of ginsenoside Rg1 on the telomere lengths and telomerase activity in hippocampus of brain-aged rats

Telomeres become progressively shortened with each replication of cells and this feature is widely used to evaluate senescence. And the telomerase is responsible for telomere length maintenance. We detected both telomere lengths and telomerase activity in the hippocampus to evaluate the effect of ginsenoside Rg1 on brain senescence.

As we expected, both the telomere lengths and the telomerase activity were reduced in the D-gal-administration group, compared with the control, while ginsenoside Rg1 remarkably increased these two parameters in the D-gal administration plus Rg1 treatment group (Figure 3). Moreover, there were no differences between the control group and the Rg1 treatment group (Figure 3).

Ginsenoside Rg1 promoted neurogenesis in dentate gyrus of hippocampus of brain-aged rats

Although new neurons are generated in the adult hippocampus throughout life by NSCs/NPCs, the rate declines with the increasing age [14–17]. Here, we observed the NSCs/NPCs differentiation in hippocampus by immunofluorescence with anti-β-tubulin III (a neuron marker), anti-GFAP (glial fibrillary acid protein, an astrocyte marker) and Gal-c (galactocerebroside, a mature oligodendrocyte marker) antibodies. Though naïve NSCs/NPCs can be marked by GFAP as well, the astrocytes can be identified by the strong expression of GFAP and its morphological character of ramified branches.

Neurons positive for β-tubulin III had a large and irregularly shaped soma and an eccentrically-placed spherical nucleus in the dentate gyrus (DG) area of hippocampus, and oligodendrocytes positive for Gal-c had a few branches, while astrocytes showed activated characteristics by exhibiting hypertrophy, with very thick, highly ramified and intensely immunostained branches in the D-gal-administration group (Figure 4, panel 1). Furthermore, a remarkable decrease of the cells positive for β-tubulin III and a significant increase of the cells positive for Gal-c and GFAP were observed in the D-gal-administration group, compared with the control group and the Rg1 treated group (Figure 4, Table 2). However, in the D-gal-administration plus Rg1 treatment group, the number of cells positive for β-tubulin III increased remarkably, while the number of cells positive for Gal-c and GFAP decreased, compared with the D-gal-administration group (Figure 4, Table 2). This suggests that Rg1 promote NSCs/NPCs differentiation into neurons rather than glial cells in the aged hippocampus.

The effect of ginsenoside Rg1 on the expression of SOX2, Nestin and Aeg1 in hippocampus of brain-aged rats

A continuous decrease in the number of NSCs/NPCs underlies the age-related decline in hippocampal neurogenesis [18]. Commonly used markers for neural stem cells include SOX2 and Nestin. The transcription factor SOX2 is involved in the proliferation and/or maintenance of NSCs/NPCs and in neuro-

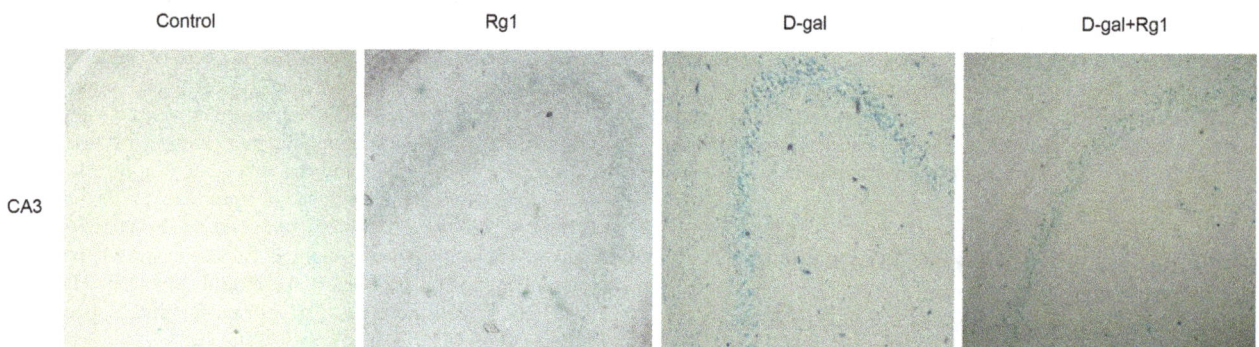

Figure 2. Ginsenoside Rg1 reduced the SA-β-Gal stainings in area CA3 in hippocampus of brain-aged rats ($\times$200). The hippocampuses were collected and fixed after the treatment. The SA-β-gal (senescence-associated β-galactosidase) staining was carried out on the slides to explore the aging of the hippocampus. The aged cells are stained in blue in the cytoplasm. The intensity of SA-β-gal-positive was evaluated by means of a ROD (relative optical density) value (Table 1).

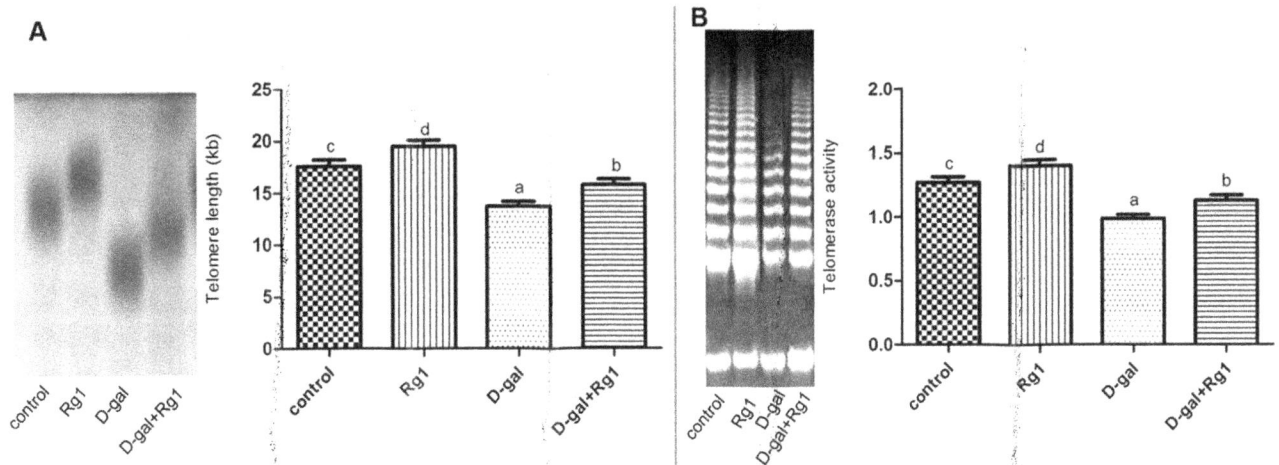

Figure 3. The effect of ginsenoside Rg1 on the telomere lengths and telomerase activity in hippocampus of brain-aged rats ($\bar{x}\pm s$, **n = 5).** A. The effect of ginsenoside Rg1 on the telomere lengths. The DNA of the hippocampus in each group was collected, and telomere lengths were evaluated by Southern Blot. B. The effect of ginsenoside Rg1 on the telomerase activity. The supernatant of the hippocampus in each group was collected and the telomerase activities were detected by silver staining TRAP-PCR. The bar graph indicates quantitative results of telomere lengths and telomerase activity. Different letters represent significantly different values as assessed by ANOVA and LSD tests with P<0.05.

genesis [19]. The intermediate filament protein, Nestin, is expressed predominantly in stem cells of the adult brain and is required for the proper self-renewal of NSCs [20]. We further detected the expression of SOX2 and Nestin to investigate the effect of Rg1 on NSCs/NPCs survival in aged hippocampus. In accordance with our expectation, the protein expression of SOX2 in the D-gal-administration group was significantly lower than that of the control group. Although Rg1 didn't increase SOX2 expression of the Rg1 treated group relatively to the controls, Rg1 treatment partially rescued the reduction of SOX2 expression in the D-gal-administration plus Rg1 treatment group (Figure 5A). It suggests that the ginsenoside Rg1 can protect NSCs/NPCs in the hippocampus of aged rats.

However, the expression of *Nestin* mRNA was increased violently in the D-gal administration group, and the treatment of Rg1 reversed this D-gal induced increase (Figure 5B). As re-expression of *Nestin* also associated with the astroglial activation during neurodegeneration [21], and the GFAP positive cells in the D-gal administration group showed activated astrocyte appearance (Figure 4), we suppose that the enhanced expression of *Nestin* is due to the activation of astroglials. Therefore, we further explored the expression of *Aeg1* (astrocyte elevated gene-1), a novel modulator of reactive astrogliosis. In accordance with the

expression of *Nestin*, the expression of *Aeg1* increased remarkably in the D-gal administration group, and decreased significantly in the D-gal-administration plus Rg1 treatment group (Figure 5C). Additionally, the expression levels of SOX2, *Nestin* and *Aeg1* of the Rg1 treatment group weren't significantly different from the control group. The results demonstrate that astrocytes are activated by D-gal administration as in early stage of neurodegenetive disease or brain damage; however, astrocytes activation is reduced by Rg1 treatment.

Ginsenoside Rg1 increases neurogenesis in brain aged rats by increasing new cell number

To explore whether ginsenoside Rg1 induced new cells production in the hippocampus, the total number of new cells was estimated in the dentate gyrus of all groups using immuno-fluorescence of BrdU (Figure 6). A student's t-test confirmed that the total number of BrdU$^+$ cells was lower in the dentate gyrus of D-gal administered rats relative to controls (Figure 6; Table 2). Although single treatment with Rg1 could not increase the total new cell number compared with the control, BrdU$^+$ cells increased notably in the D-gal-administration plus Rg1 treatment group relatively to the D-gal administered rats (Figure 6; Table 2). It

Table 2. The effect of ginsenoside Rg1 on the cell distributions in DG area of hippocampus in brain-aged rats.

Group	β-tubulin III	GFAP	Gal-c	Brdu
control	90.72±20.31^b	225.42±57.20^a	13.01±1.73^a	12.80±3.70^b
Rg1	98.2±20.0^b	212.4±36.57^a	12.54±2.06^a	14.20±5.54^b
D-gal	42.12±10.82^a	351.90±89.30^b	39.03±5.20^c	6.80±3.35^a
D-gal + Rg1	60.48±15.54^a	265.30±67.33^a	28.81±3.83^b	12.40±2.07^b
	p = 0.000	p = 0.016	p = 0.000	p = 0.039

The immunofluorescence of β-tubulin III (for neuron), GFAP (for astrocyte) Gal-C (for oligodendrocyte) and BrdU (for newly generated cell) was carried out on the slides. The numbers of marked cells were estimated on three randomly selected sections taken through the central extent of the dentate gyrus area. The experiments were performed three times with similar results. Data are expressed as mean ± SD. Different letters represent significantly different values as assessed by ANOVA and LSD tests with P<0.05.

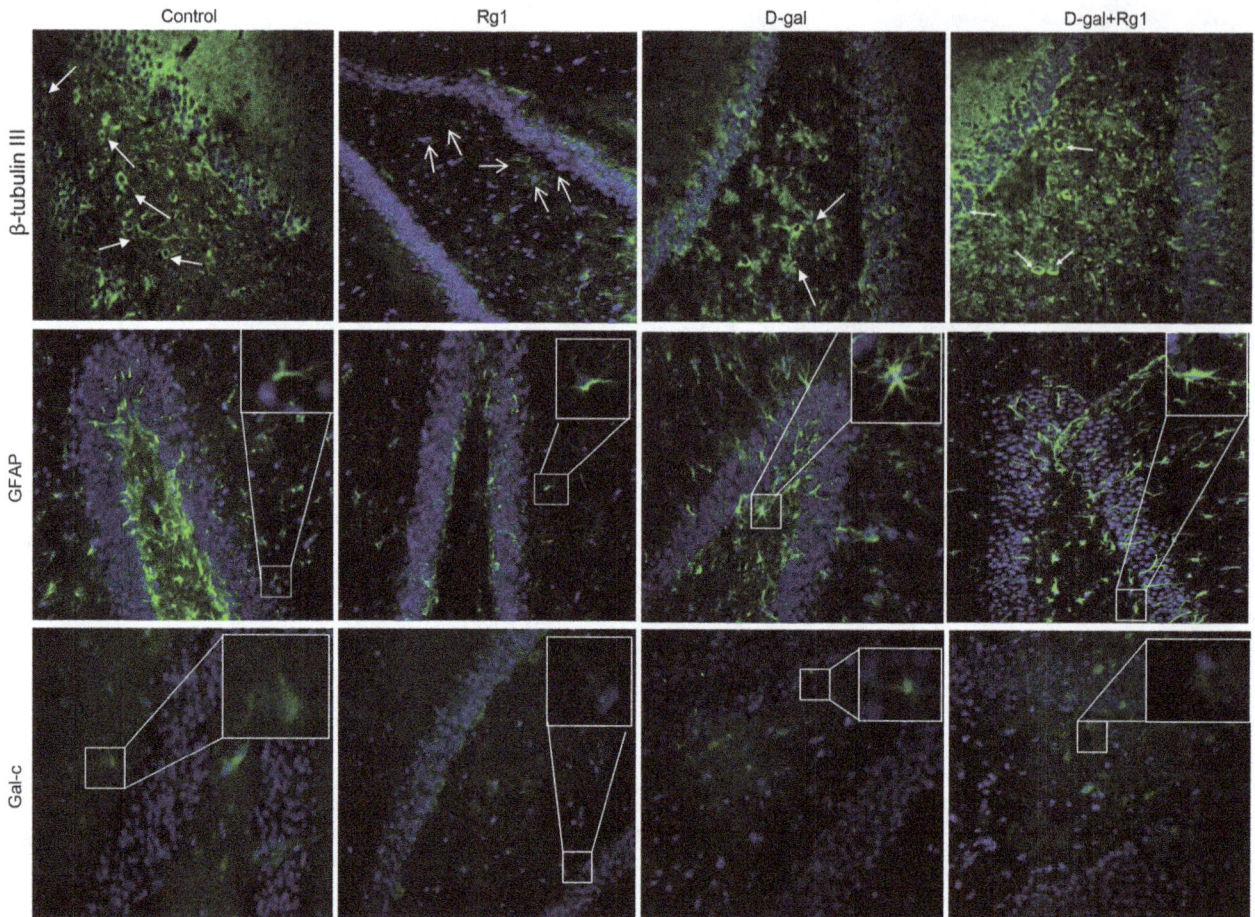

Figure 4. The effect of ginsenoside Rg1 on the NSCs/NPCs differentiation in DG area of hippocampus in brain-aged rats (×400). Hippocampuses in each group were collected and fixed after the treatment. Immunofluorescence was performed on the frozen sections of the hippocampus to visualize neurons, astrocytes and oligodendrocytes. Neurons were positive for β-tubulin III with relatively large and round cell body and less branches. Astrocytes were positive for GFAP with ramified branches. Astrocytes were activated by exhibiting hypertrophy, with very thick, highly ramified and intensely immunostained branches. Oligodendrocytes were positive for Gal-C with a few branches. DAPI was used for nuclear staining (blue). Numbers of the three types of cells in the DG area were analyzed under a fluorescence microscope (Table 2).

suggests that Rg1 promotes neurogenesis by increasing the number of new cells.

The anti-oxidative effect of ginsenoside Rg1 on the hippocampus in brain-aged rats

Oxidative stress of ROS (reactive oxygen species) is one of the main causes of cells' senescence. SOD (Superoxide Dismutase) and GSH-px (glutathione peroxidase) are two important enzymes that participate in the removal of ROS from the cellular environment. MDA (Malondialdehyde) is an end-product of ROS-induced peroxidation, and it is widely used as an oxidative stress biomarker; while GSH is the substrate of GSH-Px and its consumption decreases with age. We evaluated the SOD activity and MDA contents, GSH-Px activity and GSH reduced level in the hippocampus to figure out whether the anti-aging effect of ginsenoside Rg1 was mediated by alleviating oxidative stress.

Compared to the control group, SOD activity, GSH-Px activity and GSH consumption decreased significantly and the MDA content increased remarkably in the hippocampus in D-gal-administration group (Table 3). Meanwhile, Rg1 rescued the reduction of SOD activity, GSH-Px activity and GSH consumed level significantly, and partially rescued the increase of MDA in

the D-gal-administration plus Rg1 treatment group (Table 3). Interestingly, Rg1 single treatment also increased the activity of the two anti-oxidative enzymes and the reduced level of GSH, and reduced the MDA content. It shows that ginsenoside Rg1 exerts antioxidant effects against oxidative stress, by enhancing activity of endogenous anti-oxidative defense enzymes.

Ginsenoside Rg1 decreased the levels of proinflammatory cytokines of hippocampus in brain-aged rats

Chronic inflammation in the brain is associated with natural aging and neurodegeneration. Increased levels of proinflammatory cytokines as IL-1β, IL-6 and TNF-α have been found in inflammatory tissue and correlated well with aged brain.

The levels of IL-1β, IL-6 and TNF-α increased significantly in the hippocampus of the D-gal-administration group, compared with the control group. However, the levels of the proinflammatory cytokines were reduced notably in the D-gal-administration plus Rg1 treatment group, relatively to the D-gal-administration group (Table 4). Meanwhile, Rg1 single treatment didn't reduce the levels of IL-1β, IL-6 and TNF-α in the Rg1 treatment group, compared with the controls. It suggests that inflammation in D-gal

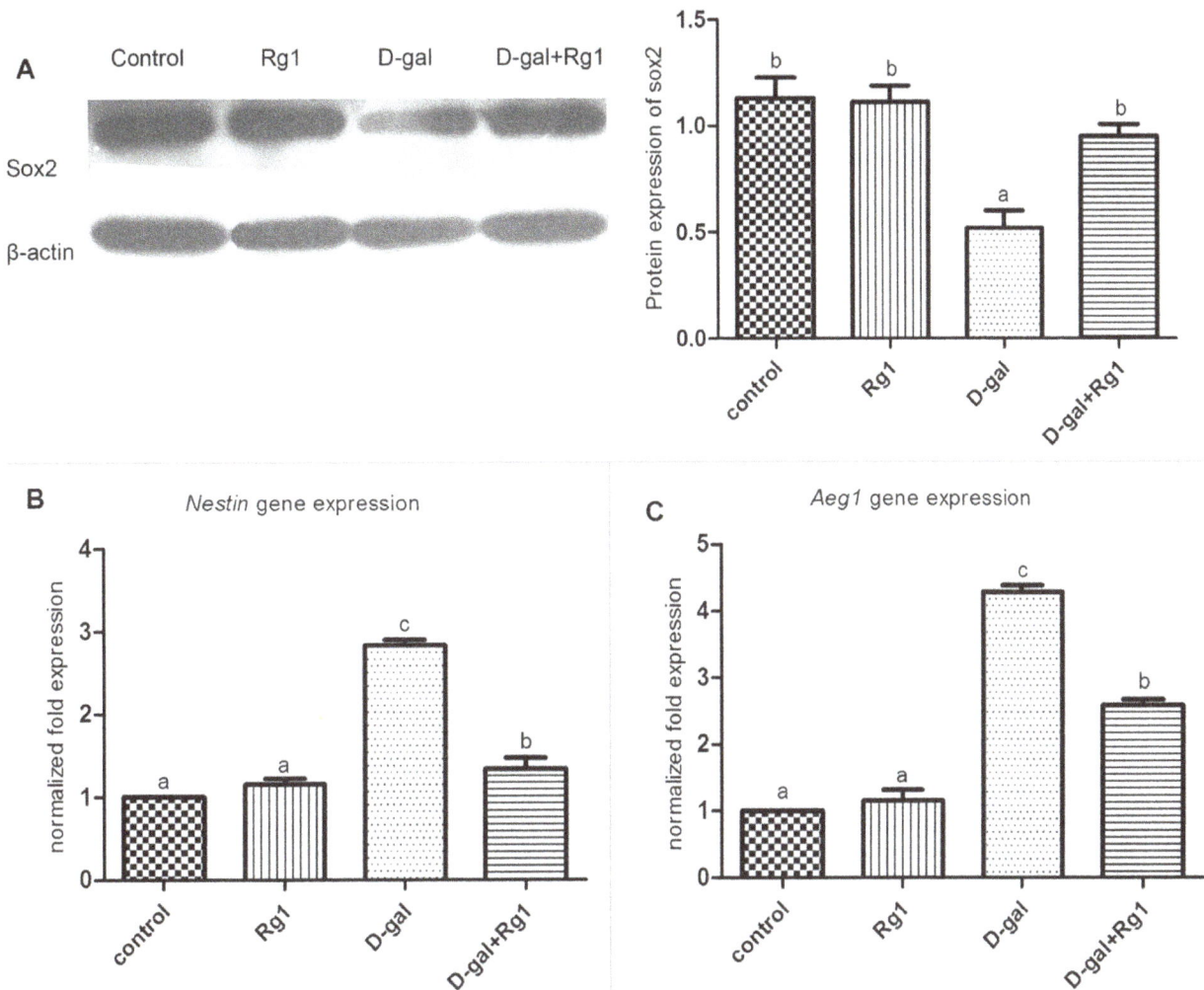

Figure 5. The effect of ginsenoside Rg1 on the expression of SOX2, *Nestin* and *Aeg1* in hippocampus of brain-aged rats. Hippocampuses in each group were collected. A. SOX2 protein expression was detected by western-blot, and β-actin was served as an internal standard. Relative intensities were quantified. B and C. *Nestin* and *Aeg1* mRNA expression was detected by realtime qRT-PCR. All values were normalized against *Gapdh* and expressed as a percentage of control. The experiments were performed three times with similar results. Data are expressed as mean ± SD. Different letters represent significantly different values as assessed by ANOVA and LSD tests with $P<0.05$.

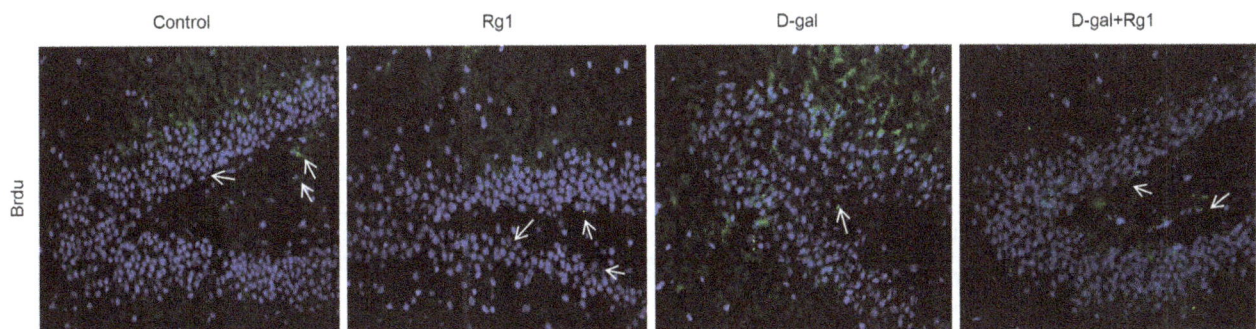

Figure 6. The effect of ginsenoside. Rg1 on cell proliferation in the DG area of the hippocampus of brain-aged rats. BrdU were administrated to the rats in each group three times on day 41 of the treatment to mark the newly generated cells. Hippocampuses were collected on the next day. Frozen slides were incubated with anti-BrdU antibodies. Arrows indicate newly generated cells which are stained by anti-BrdU antibody (green) around the nucleus (blue) during the final 24 hours of the treatment. Numbers of BrdU+ cells in the DG area were analyzed under a fluorescence microscope (Table 2).

Table 3. The effect of ginsenoside Rg1 on anti-oxidant ability in the hippocampus of brain-aged rats ($\bar{x}\pm s$, n = 5).

Group	SOD (U/mg prot)	MDA (nmol/mg prot)	GSH (mg/g prot)	GSH-px (U/mg prot)
control	4.52±0.57[c]	1.42±0.17[a]	1.83±0.16[b]	13.58±1.39[b]
Rg1	6.04±0.76[d]	1.12±0.11[d]	2.29±0.20[c]	15.54±1.15[c]
D-gal	2.95±0.37[a]	2.41±0.35[c]	0.55±0.05[a]	10.8±1.62[a]
D-gal + Rg1	3.64±0.46[b]	1.82±027[b]	2.11±0.19[c]	12.5±1.26[b]
	p = 0.000	p = 0.000	p = 0.000	p = 0.000

The supernatant of hippocampus in each group was collected. The anti-oxidative ability was determined by chemical colorimetric analysis of SOD activity and MDA content, and GSH-px activity and reduced GSH level. Data are expressed as mean ± SD. Different letters represent significantly different values as assessed by ANOVA and LSD tests with P<0.05.

induced aged hippocampus is alleviated by ginsenoside Rg1 treatment.

Ginsenoside Rg1 down-regulated the expression of senescence-associated genes in hippocampus of brain-aged rats

$P19^{Arf}$-Mdm2-p53-$p21^{Cip1/Waf1}$ pathway is a main signal transduction pathway involved in cell aging processes. Therefore, we performed qRT-PCR to explore the mRNA expressions of p53, $p19^{Arf}$ and $p21^{Cip1/Waf1}$, which are in the core position of the pathway. The expression of Gapdh was used as the inner control. As shown in Figure 7, the mRNA expression of p53, $p19^{Arf}$ and $p21^{Cip1/Waf1}$ in the D-gal-administration group was violently higher than that of the control group. However, in the D-gal-administration plus Rg1 treatment group, the expression of the genes was significantly lower than that of the D-gal-administration group (Figure 7). Meanwhile, there were no differences between the control group and the Rg1 treatment group. It indicates that ginsenoside Rg1 can down-regulate the expression of senescence-associated genes in the hippocampus of brain-aged rats.

Discussion

During natural aging, the brain undergoes progressive morphologic and functional changes resulting in the observed behavioral retrogression, such as declines in motor and cognitive performance. It will be of a great value to find out drugs against neurodegeneration to delay brain senescence. It has been reported that an increase of adult hippocampal neurogenesis may have therapeutic potential for reversing impairments in pattern separation and dentate gyrus dysfunction such as those seen during normal aging [22]. In the present study, we demonstrate

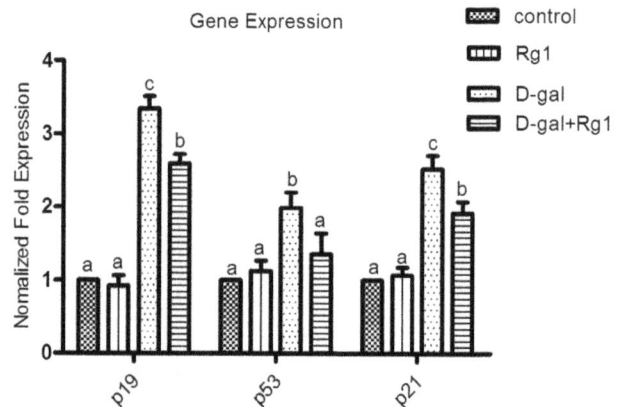

Figure 7. Ginsenoside Rg1 down-regulated the expression of $p19^{Arf}$, p53, $p21^{Cip1/Waf1}$ mRNA in hippocampus of brain-aged rats. The mRNA of hippocampus in each group was collected. Senescence-associated gene expressions were detected by qRT-PCR. All values were normalized against Gapdh and expressed as a percentage of control. The experiments were performed three times with similar results. Different letters represent significantly different values as assessed by ANOVA and LSD tests with P<0.05.

that ginsenoside Rg1 treatment protects hippocampus against abnormalities in a well-characterized aging rat model by D-gal administration. Rg1 treatment improved hippocampus-associated cognition, promoted NSCs/NPCs differentiation into neurons, and delayed cellular senescence in the hippocampus via antioxidant and anti-inflammation ability. D-gal administration model is a mimetic aging model related to free radical and the

Table 4. The effect of ginsenoside Rg1 on the levels of of IL-1β, IL-6 and TNF-α in the hippocampus of brain-aged rats ($\bar{x}\pm s$, n = 5, pg/mg).

Group	IL-1β	IL-6	TNF-α
control	0.456±0.019[b]	45.60±8.46[a]	3.885±0.321[a]
Rg1	0.409±0.020[a]	46.43±7.12[a]	3.445±0.286[a]
D-gal	0.620±0.030[c]	61.9±9.90[b]	6.005±0.945[c]
D-gal + Rg1	0.468±0.023[b]	57.96±9.57[b]	5.135±0.426[b]
	p = 0.000	p = 0.008	p = 0.000

The supernatant of hippocampus in each group was collected. The proinflammatory cytokines levels of IL-1β, IL-6 and TNF-α were measured by ELISA kit. Data are expressed as mean ± SD. Different letters represent significantly different values as assessed by ANOVA with P<0.05.

accumulation of waste substances in metabolism [23]. Similarly, the accumulation of free radicals progressively damages the brain function during natural aging, and D-gal-administrated rodents mimic many characteristics of the normal brain aging process. Therefore, D-gal-induced aging model is regarded as an ideal mimetic aging model to study the mechanism related to the brain aging and screen drugs for brain aging [24–26]. Furthermore, enhancing endogenous antioxidants is now widely regarded as an attractive therapy for conditions associated with mitochondrial oxidative stress, and ginsenoiside Rg1 is widely reported as having anti-oxidation effect [3–5]. Therefore, we employed D-gal administration model in this study as we established it previously [27]. In this study, we induced aging by D-gal administration and observed significant reduction in spatial memory, cell proliferation, and neurogenesis in the dentate gyrus. This result was supported by previous studies showing that proliferating progenitor cells were significantly decreased in the seventh week after D-gal administration [28,29]. In addition, D-gal can induce behavioral impairment in C57BL/6J mice [30] and decrease spatial preference for the target quadrant in the Morris water maze test [31].

We administered ginsenoiside Rg1 to control and D-gal mice and probed spatial memory and learning ability using a water maze test. The administration of ginsenoiside Rg1, a main active component of *Panax ginseng*, significantly reduced the escape latency in the D-gal group, while Rg1 administration to control mice did not significantly change the escape latency. In addition, the administration of Rg1 to D-gal-induced aging mice significantly improved the deficits in platform crossings in probe trial and spatial preference for the target quadrant. This result was coincided with a previous study that Rg1 has profound neuroprotective effects in an Alzheimer mouse model [32].

Rg1 administration to D-gal-induced aging mice significantly increased SA-β-gal expression and telomerase, and decrease telomere length in the hippocampus compared to that in the D-gal group. SA-β-gal, which reflects the function of the lysosomes, accumulates in aging cells as the lysosomes begin to malfunction. A telomere is a region of repetitive nucleotide sequences at the end of a chromatid. Telomere shortening can limit stem cell functions and regeneration during aging [33]. Both of the biomarkers are widely used to evaluate senescence. It indicates that ginsenoside Rg1 is able to protect against the senescence of the hippocampus, which is coincident with our previous study of the effect of ginsenoside Rg1 on NSCs/NPCs senescence *in vitro* [5].

Aging is associated with a continuous decline in the neurogenesis in the DG area of the normal hippocampus, because of the age-driven disappearance of NSCs/NPCs via their conversion into mature hippocampal astrocytes [18]. Therefore, we propose that the anti-aging effects produced by Rg1 also correlate with increased neurogenesis. Our data in this study supported this hypothesis. Four weeks of Rg1 treatment promoted NSCs/NPCs differentiation to neurons rather than glial cells, because the number of the cells positive for β-tubulin III increased and that of the cells positive for GFAP and Gal-C decreased, compared with the D-gal administration group. β-tubulin III is widely regarded as a neuronal marker in developmental neurobiology and stem cell research [34]. Given the potential significance of new neurons for cognitive function, it has been hypothesized that reduced neurogenesis may contribute to age-related cognitive impairment [18]. The promoted neurogenesis of Rg1 treatment in this study supports the effect of ginsenoside Rg1 in improving cognitive ability (Figure 1) and the function of *Panax ginseng* in preventing memory deterioration. GFAP is highly expressed by astrocytes and is widely used as a marker for differentiated astrocytes, while

evidence also indicates that GFAP is expressed by developing NSCs/NPCs [35]. However, in the D-gal administration group of this study, GFAP-positive cells showed morphological characteristics of activated astrocytes. Considering that the activated astrocytes have been identified as a major brain-derived source of inflammatory cytokines [36], and elevated levels of IL-1β (Table 4) can lead to astrocytes activation in a positive feedback way [37], we believe that most GFAP positive cells represent astrocytes in this study. In addition, the treatment of Rg1 significantly decreased the GFAP-positvie and Gal-C –positive cells number. Our results suggest Rg1 can counteract the age-driven NSCs/NPCs deletion and excess astrogenesis and promote NSCs/NPCs differentiation into neurons.

We further examined whether Rg1 promoted neurogenesis by maintaining the NSCs/NPCs. We employed the wide-spreading NSCs/NPCs markers SOX2 and Nestin. The increase of SOX2 level in the Rg1 treatment plus D-gal administration group indicated that the Rg1 could protect NSCs/NPCs survival against D-gal induced aging (Figure 5A). The increase of newly generated cells indicated by BrdU in the Rg1 treatment plus D-gal administration group further revealed the NSCs/NPCs protective effect of Rg1 (Figure 6). Moreover, in NSCs/NPCs, telomeres shortened with age and that telomerase-deficient mice exhibited reduced neurogenesis [38]. In this study, the SOX2 expression was well correlated with the changes of lengths of telomeres and the activity of telomerase in each group. These results suggest that ginsenoiside Rg1 effectively protect NSCs/NPCs survival against D-gal induced aging.

Interestingly, *Nestin* expression increased in the D-gal administration group. Nevertheless, this observation was consistent with the bulk of studies suggesting that in pathological conditions adult glial cells are induced to revert to a more primitive glial form, so that earlier stages phenotypic features, including Nestin, were transiently re-expressed [20,39,40]. Another study also illustrated that Nestin was re-expressed in the activated astroglial in the damaged brains [21]. Altogether with the elevated levels of *Aeg1* (Figure 5C) which plays a novel role in mediating reactive astrogliosis and responses to pathogenic and aging factors, it indicates the astrocytes activation in the D-gal-induced aged brain. Moreover, for the increased levels of *Aeg1*, it was also consistent with the morphological characteristic of activated astrocytes in the D-gal-administration group (Figure 4). However, *Nestin* and *Aeg1* expression was down-regulated in the D-gal-administration plus Rg1 treatment group, indicating that the reactive astrogliosis induced by D-gal was alleviated by Rg1 treatment. This result further illustrated that Rg1 could protect the age-related NSCs/NPCs survival and reduce astrogenesis. Cognitive capacity was improved, neurogenesis was restored and reactive astrogliosis was attenuated by ginsenoside Rg1 treatment to D-gal administered rats. We did not elucidate the direct mechanism of Rg1 on these effects in the hippocampus. However, we assumed two possible mechanisms for these effects. One of these is the antioxidant function of Rg1 on the hippocampus, because the oxygen metabolism of D-gal produces many reactive oxygen species (ROS) and may impair learning and memory directly or indirectly [31]. In addition, ROS can potently inhibit neurogenesis and particularly NSCs/NPCs proliferation [41]. Oxidative damage can also affect glial cells, which are connected to neuronal death or decreases in neuronal proliferation [42]. In the present study, Rg1 treatment protected the hippocampus against oxidative stress by promoting the activities of SOD and GSH-Px, which are important anti-oxidative enzymes to remove the oxidative stress accumulated in aging. On the other hand, as the telomere is highly sensitive to the oxidative stress, the increased telomere length and telomerase activities in the D-gal-administration plus Rg1 treatment group may also be due to the effect of the anti-oxidant function of Rg1. These results suggest that ginsenoiside Rg1 effectively attenuates D-gal-induced oxidative damage in the hippocampus, possibly by eliminating free radicals through activating antioxidant enzymes. It should be noted that the activities of SOD and GSH-Px were remarkably increased in the Rg1 single-treated rats. It confirmed the anti-oxidative effect of ginsenoside Rg1, which was consistent with previous studies [43,44].

Oxidative stress has been implicated in proinflammation [33], and aging is also associated with inflammation [45]. When chronic inflammation occurs in the aged brain, a variety of neurotoxic products and proinflammatory cytokines such as IL-1β, IL-6, and TNF-α are released [45–48]. In the present study, Rg1 treatment significantly reduced the levels of IL-1β, IL-6, and TNF-α, compared with the D-gal administration group. It suggests that Rg1 can protect the hippocampus from age-induced chronic inflammation. Furthermore, the elevated levels of proinflammatory cytokines could also be a consequence of astrocytes activation. Sustained activation of astrocytes releases high amount of NO (nitric oxide) and proinflammatory cytokines which accumulate in aging process, to exacerbate neuronal impairments [49,50]. In this study, the attenuated activation status of astrocytes by the Rg1 therapy may be a combined outcome of the anti-inflammation and the neurogenesis-promoting capacity of ginsenoside Rg1.

Another possible mechanism is associated with $p19^{Arf}$/MDM2/ p53 signaling pathway because it is an important signaling pathway controlling senescence [51]. The accumulated P53 protein can transcriptionally activate $p21^{Waf1/Cip1}$[51,52] and other putative effectors [53] that inhibit various kinds of cdk-cyclin complexes. On the other hand, p53 has been shown to mediate all adverse effects of telomere attrition on cell cycle arrest and/or apoptosis in proliferative cells, including stem cell populations. These effects of telomere dysfunction on NSCs/ NPCs, including those on neuronal differentiation and neurogenesis, are mediated by activation of $p53$ [51]. In the present study, the reduced mRNA levels of $p53$, $p19^{Arf}$, $p21^{Cip1/Waf1}$ by Rg1 indicated that Rg1 regulates the expression of the genes to delay telomere shortening and hippocampus senescence.

Adult NSCs/NPCs exist in the hippocampus in mammals, and neurogenesis continues throughout the lifetime. Recent study suggests [54] that promoting neurogenesis in adult mammals might provide a therapeutic way to cure age-associated neurodegenerative diseases or to improve age-related cognitive impairment. In the present study, we provided evidence that ginsenoiside Rg1 treatment can prevent cognitive impairment and hippocampus senescence in a rat model of D-galactose-induced aging, suggesting Rg1 is involved in the anti-oxidation and anti-inflammation regulating telomere length, NSCs/NPCs survival and differentiation. These effects may serve as the elementary mechanism underlying nootropic and anti-aging actions of ginsenoside Rg1.

Supporting Information

File S1

Author Contributions

Conceived and designed the experiments: JHZ YPW. Performed the experiments: JHZ XYM JZ MSZ CPL CYX JL JC TYL. Analyzed the data: JZ JHZ. Contributed reagents/materials/analysis tools: ZJH XYM JZ. Wrote the paper: JHZ XYM.

References

1. Olanow CW (1992) An introduction to the free radical hypothesis in Parkinson's disease. Ann Neurol 32 Suppl: S2–9.
2. Jeong K, Shin YC, Park S, Park JS, Kim N, et al. (2011) Ethanol extract of Scutellaria baicalensis Georgi prevents oxidative damage and neuroinflammation and memorial impairments in artificial senescense mice. J Biomed Sci 18: 14.
3. Cheng Y, Shen LH, Zhang JT (2005) Anti-amnestic and anti-aging effects of ginsenoside Rg1 and Rb1 and its mechanism of action. Acta Pharmacol Sin 26: 143–149.
4. Chen X, Zhang J, Fang Y, Zhao C, Zhu Y (2008) Ginsenoside Rg1 delays tert-butyl hydroperoxide-induced premature senescence in human WI-38 diploid fibroblast cells. J Gerontol A Biol Sci Med Sci 63: 253–264.
5. Peng B, Wang CL, Feng L, Wang YP (2011) The effects and the underlying mechanisms of Ginsenoside Rg1 to regulate neural stem cell senescence. Chinese Journal of Cell Biology 33: 1116–1122.
6. Song X, Bao M, Li D, Li YM (1999) Advanced glycation in D-galactose induced mouse aging model. Mech Aging Dev 108: 239–251.
7. Yoo DY, Kim W, Kim IH, Nam SM, Chung JY, et al. (2012) Combination effects of sodium butyrate and pyridoxine treatment on cell proliferation and neuroblast differentiation in the dentate gyrus of D-galactose-induced aging model mice. Neurochem Res 37: 223–231.
8. Wei H, Li L, Song Q, Ai H, Chu J, et al. (2005) Behavioural study of the D-galactose induced aging model in C57BL/6J mice. Behav Brain Res 157: 245–251.
9. Wei H, Cai Y, Chu J, Li C, Li L (2008) Temporal gene expression profile in hippocampus of mice treated with D-galactose. Cell Mol Neurobiol 28: 781–794.
10. Zhang XP, Zhang GH, Wang YY, Liu J, Wei Q, et al. (2013) Oxidized low-density lipoprotein induces hematopoietic stem cell senescence. Cell Biol Int 37: 940–948.
11. Schenk F, Morris RG (1985) Dissociation between components of spatial memory in rats after recovery from the effects of retrohippocampal lesions. Exp Brain Res 58: 11–28.
12. Dimri GP, Lee X, Basile G, Acosta M, Scott G, et al. (1995) A biomarker that identifies senescent human cells in culture and in aging skin in vivo. Proc Natl Acad Sci U S A 92: 9363–9367.
13. Geng YQ, Guan JT, Xu XH, Fu YC (2010) Senescence-associated beta-galactosidase activity expression in aging hippocampal neurons. Biochem Biophys Res Commun 396: 866–869.
14. Seki T, Arai Y (1995) Age-related production of new granule cells in the adult dentate gyrus. Neuroreport 6: 2479–2482.
15. Kuhn HG, Dickinson-Anson H, Gage FH (1996) Neurogenesis in the dentate gyrus of the adult rat: age-related decrease of neuronal progenitor proliferation. J Neurosci 16: 2027–2033.
16. Kempermann G, Gast D, Gage FH (2002) Neuroplasticity in old age: sustained fivefold induction of hippocampal neurogenesis by long-term environmental enrichment. Ann Neurol 52: 135–143.
17. Gould E, Reeves AJ, Fallah M, Tanapat P, Gross CG, et al. (1999) Hippocampal neurogenesis in adult Old World primates. Proc Natl Acad Sci U S A 96: 5263–5267.
18. Encinas JM, Michurina TV, Peunova N, Park JH, Tordo J, et al. (2011) Division-coupled astrocytic differentiation and age-related depletion of neural stem cells in the adult hippocampus. Cell Stem Cell 8: 566–579.
19. Episkopou V (2005) SOX2 functions in adult neural stem cells. Trends Neurosci 28: 219–221.
20. Park D, Xiang AP, Mao FF, Zhang L, Di CG, et al. (2010) Nestin is required for the proper self-renewal of neural stem cells. Stem Cells 28: 2162–2171.
21. Geloso MC, Corvino V, Cavallo V, Toesca A, Guadagni E, et al. (2004) Expression of astrocytic nestin in the rat hippocampus during trimethyltin-induced neurodegeneration. Neurosci Lett 357: 103–106.
22. Sahay A, Scobie KN, Hill AS, O'Carroll CM, Kheirbek MA, et al. (2011) Increasing adult hippocampal neurogenesis is sufficient to improve pattern separation. Nature 472: 466–470.
23. Ho SC, Liu JH, Wu RY (2003) Establishment of the mimetic aging effect in mice caused by D-galactose. Biogerontology 4: 15–18.
24. Geng YQ, Guan JT, Xu XH, Fu YC (2010) Senescence-associated beta-galactosidase activity expression in aging hippocampal neurons. Biochem Biophys Res Commun 396: 866–869.
25. Zhang XL, An LJ, Bao YM, Wang JY, Jiang B (2008) d-galactose administration induces memory loss and energy metabolism disturbance in mice: protective effects of catalpol. Food Chem Toxicol 46: 2888–2894.
26. Prisila Dulcy C, Singh HK, Preethi J, Rajan KE (2012) Standardized extract of Bacopa monniera (BESEB CDRI-08) attenuates contextual associative learning deficits in the aging rat's brain induced by D-galactose. J Neurosci Res 90: 2053–2064.
27. Peng B, Chen MS, Pu Y, Wang YP (2011) Anti-aging effects of Ginsenoside Rg1 and it's mechanisms on brain aging rats induced by D-galactose. Journal of Chongqing Medical Vniversity 36: 419–422.

28. Cui X, Zuo P, Zhang Q, Li X, Hu Y, et al. (2006) Chronic systemic D-galactose exposure induces memory loss, neurodegeneration, and oxidative damage in mice: protective effects of R-alpha-lipoic acid. J Neurosci Res 84: 647–654.

29. Yoo DY, Kim W, Lee CH, Shin BN, Nam SM, et al. (2012) Melatonin improves D-galactose-induced aging effects on behavior, neurogenesis, and lipid peroxidation in the mouse dentate gyrus via increasing pCREB expression. J Pineal Res 52: 21–28.

30. Wei H, Li L, Song Q, Ai H, Chu J, et al. (2005) Behavioural study of the D-galactose induced aging model in C57BL/6J mice. Behav Brain Res 157: 245–251.

31. Lu J, Zheng YL, Luo L, Wu DM, Sun DX, et al. (2006) Quercetin reverses D-galactose induced neurotoxicity in mouse brain. Behav Brain Res 171: 251–260.

32. Fang F, Chen X, Huang T, Lue LF, Luddy JS, et al. (2012) Multi-faced neuroprotective effects of Ginsenoside Rg1 in an Alzheimer mouse model. Biochim Biophys Acta 1822: 286–292.

33. Jiang H, Ju Z, Rudolph KL (2007) Telomere shortening and ageing. Z Gerontol Geriatr 40: 314–224. Review.

34. Dráberová E, Del Valle L, Gordon J, Marková V, Smejkalová B, et al. (2008) Class III beta-tubulin is constitutively coexpressed with glial fibrillary acidic protein and nestin in midgestational human fetal astrocytes: implications for phenotypic identity. J Neuropathol Exp Neurol 67: 341–354.

35. Imura T, Nakano I, Kornblum HI, Sofroniew MV (2006) Phenotypic and functional heterogeneity of GFAP-expressing cells in vitro: differential expression of LeX/CD15 by GFAP-expressing multipotent neural stem cells and non-neurogenic astrocytes. Glia 53: 277–293.

36. Wang Z, Li DD, Liang YY, Wang DS, Cai NS (2002) Activation of astrocytes by advanced glycation end products: cytokines induction and nitric oxide release. Acta Pharmacol Sin 23: 974–980.

37. Sama MA, Mathis DM, Furman JL, Abdul HM, Artiushin IA, et al. (2008) Interleukin-1beta-dependent signaling between astrocytes and neurons depends critically on astrocytic calcineurin/NFAT activity. J Biol Chem 283: 21953–21964.

38. Ferrón SR, Marqués-Torrejón MA, Mira H, Flores I, Taylor K, et al. (2009) Telomere shortening in neural stem cells disrupts neuronal differentiation and neuritogenesis. J Neurosci 29: 14394–14407.

39. Clarke SR, Shetty AK, Bradley JL, Turner DA (1994) Reactive astrocytes express the embryonic intermediate neurofilament nestin. Neuroreport 5: 1885–1888.

40. Frisén J, Johansson CB, Török C, Risling M, Lendahl U (1995) Rapid, widespread, and longlasting induction of nestin contributes to the generation of glial scar tissue after CNS injury. J Cell Biol 131: 453–464.

41. Limoli CL, Giedzinski E, Baure J, Rola R, Fike JR (2006) Altered growth and radiosensitivity in neural precursor cells subjected to oxidative stress. Int J Radiat Biol 82: 640–647.

42. Kinsner A, Pilotto V, Deininger S, Brown GC, Coecke S, et al. (2005) Inflammatory neurodegeneration induced by lipoteichoic acid from Staphylococcus aureus is mediated by glia activation, nitrosative and oxidative stress, and caspase activation. J Neurochem 95: 1132–1143.

43. Kim JH (2012) Cardiovascular Diseases and *Panax ginseng*: A Review on Molecular Mechanisms and Medical Applications. J Ginseng Res 36: 16–26.

44. Chen C, Mu XY, Zhou Y, Shun K, Geng S, et al. (2014) Ginsenoside Rg1 enhances the resistance of hematopoietic stem/progenitor cells to radiation-induced aging in mice. Acta Pharmacol Sin 35: 143–150.

45. Gemma C, Bachstetter AD, Bickford PC (2010) Neuron-Microglia Dialogue and Hippocampal Neurogenesis in the Aged Brain. Aging Dis 1: 232–244.

46. Ershler WB, Keller ET (2000) Age-associated increased interleukin-6 gene expression, late-life diseases, and frailty. Annu Rev Med 51: 245–270.

47. Bonafè M, Olivieri F, Cavallone L, Giovagnetti S, Mayegiani F, et al. (2001) A gender-dependent genetic predisposition to produce high levels of IL-6 is detrimental for longevity. Eur J Immunol 31: 2357–2361.

48. Bruunsgaard H, Andersen-Ranberg K, Jeune B, Pedersen AN, Skinhøj P, et al. (1999) A high plasma concentration of TNF-alpha is associated with dementia in centenarians. J Gerontol A Biol Sci Med Sci 54: M357–364.

49. Lei M, Hua X, Xiao M, Ding J, Han Q, et al. (2008) Impairments of astrocytes are involved the d-galactose-induced brain aging. Biochem Biophys Res Commun 369: 1082–1087.

50. Mrak RE, Griffin WS (2000) Interleukin-1 and the immunogenetics of Alzheimer disease. J Neuropathol Exp Neurol 59: 471–476.

51. el-Deiry WS, Tokino T, Velculescu VE, Levy DB, Parsons R, et al. (1993) WAF1, a potential mediator of p53 tumor suppression. Cell 75: 817–825.

52. Harper JW, Adami GR, Wei N, Keyomarsi K, Elledge SJ (1993) The p21 Cdk-interacting protein Cip1 is a potent inhibitor of G1 cyclin-dependent kinases. Cell 75: 805–816.

53. Groth A, Weber JD, Willumsen BM, Sherr CJ, Roussel MF (2000) Oncogenic Ras induces p19ARF and growth arrest in mouse embryo fibroblasts lacking p21Cip1 and p27Kip1 without activating cyclin D-dependent kinases. J Biol Chem 275: 27473–27480.

54. Vivar C, van Praag H (2013) Functional circuits of new neurons in the dentate gyrus. Front Neural Circuits 7: 15.

Permissions

The contributors of this book come from diverse backgrounds, making this book a truly international effort. This book will bring forth new frontiers with its revolutionizing research information and detailed analysis of the nascent developments around the world.

We would like to thank all the contributing authors for lending their expertise to make the book truly unique. They have played a crucial role in the development of this book. Without their invaluable contributions this book wouldn't have been possible. They have made vital efforts to compile up to date information on the varied aspects of this subject to make this book a valuable addition to the collection of many professionals and students.

This book was conceptualized with the vision of imparting up-to-date information and advanced data in this field. To ensure the same, a matchless editorial board was set up. Every individual on the board went through rigorous rounds of assessment to prove their worth. After which they invested a large part of their time researching and compiling the most relevant data for our readers.

The editorial board has been involved in producing this book since its inception. They have spent rigorous hours researching and exploring the diverse topics which have resulted in the successful publishing of this book. They have passed on their knowledge of decades through this book. To expedite this challenging task, the publisher supported the team at every step. A small team of assistant editors was also appointed to further simplify the editing procedure and attain best results for the readers.

Apart from the editorial board, the designing team has also invested a significant amount of their time in understanding the subject and creating the most relevant covers. They scrutinized every image to scout for the most suitable representation of the subject and create an appropriate cover for the book.

The publishing team has been an ardent support to the editorial, designing and production team. Their endless efforts to recruit the best for this project, has resulted in the accomplishment of this book. They are a veteran in the field of academics and their pool of knowledge is as vast as their experience in printing. Their expertise and guidance has proved useful at every step. Their uncompromising quality standards have made this book an exceptional effort. Their encouragement from time to time has been an inspiration for everyone.

The publisher and the editorial board hope that this book will prove to be a valuable piece of knowledge for researchers, students, practitioners and scholars across the globe.

List of Contributors

Masashi Murakami, Misako Nakashima and Koichiro Iohara
Department of Dental Regenerative Medicine, Center of Advanced Medicine for Dental and Oral Diseases, National Center for Geriatrics and Gerontology, Research Institute, Morioka, Obu, Aichi, Japan

Kenichi Kurita
Department of Oral and Maxillofacial Surgery, School of Dentistry, Aichi-gakuin University, Nagoya, Aichi, Japan

Hiroshi Horibe
Department of Dental Regenerative Medicine, Center of Advanced Medicine for Dental and Oral Diseases, National Center for Geriatrics and Gerontology, Research Institute, Morioka, Obu, Aichi, Japan
Department of Oral and Maxillofacial Surgery, School of Dentistry, Aichi-gakuin University, Nagoya, Aichi, Japan

Yuki Hayashi
Department of Dental Regenerative Medicine, Center of Advanced Medicine for Dental and Oral Diseases, National Center for Geriatrics and Gerontology, Research Institute, Morioka, Obu, Aichi, Japan
Department of Pediatric Dentistry, School of Dentistry, Aichi-gakuin University, Nagoya, Aichi, Japan

Norio Takeuchi
Department of Dental Regenerative Medicine, Center of Advanced Medicine for Dental and Oral Diseases, National Center for Geriatrics and Gerontology, Research Institute, Morioka, Obu, Aichi, Japan
Department of Endodontics, School of Dentistry, Aichi-g akuin University, Nagoya, Aichi, Japan

Yoshifumi Takei
Department of Biochemistry and Division of Disease Models, Center for Neurological Diseases and Cancer, Nagoya University Graduate School of Medicine, Nagoya, Aichi, Japan

Megumi Sasatani, Daisuke Iizuka and Kenji Kamiya
Department of Experimental Oncology, Research Institute for Radiation Biology and Medicine, Hiroshima University, Hiroshima, Japan

Hidehiko Kawai and Fumio Suzuki
Department of Molecular Radiobiology, Research Institute for Radiation Biology and Medicine, Hiroshima University, Hiroshima, Japan

Lili Cao
Department of Experimental Oncology, Research Institute for Radiation Biology and Medicine, Hiroshima University, Hiroshima, Japan
Department of Molecular Radiobiology, Research Institute for Radiation Biology and Medicine, Hiroshima University, Hiroshima, Japan

Yuji Masuda
Departm ent of Experimental Oncology, Research Institute for Radiation Biology and Medicine, Hiroshima University, Hiroshima, Japan
Department of Genome Dynamics, Research Institute of Environmental Medicine, Nagoya University, Furo-cho, Chikusa-ku, Nagoya, Japan

Toshiya Inaba
Department of Molecular Oncology & Leukemia Program Project, Research Institute for Radiation Biology and Medicine, Hiroshima University, Hiroshima, Japan

Keiji Suzuki
Department of Radiation Medical Sciences, Atomic Bomb Disease Institute, Nagasaki University, Nagasaki, Japan

Akira Ootsuyama
Department of Radiation Biology and Health, School of Medicine, University of Occupational and Environmental Health, Kitakyushu, Japan

Toshiyuki Umata
Radioisotope Research Center, University of Occupational and Environmental Health, Kitakyushu, Japan

Yohko Yoshida, Yuka Hayashi, Masayoshi Suda and Ippei Shimizu
Department of Cardiovascular Biology and Medicine, Niigata University Graduate School of Medical and Dental Sciences, Niigata, Japan

Kaoru Tateno, Sho Okada, Junji Moriya, Masataka Yokoyama, Aika Nojima and Yoshio Kobayashi
Department of Cardiovascular Medicine, Chiba University Graduate School of Medicine, Chiba, Japan

Masakatsu Yamashita
Kazusa DNA Research Institute, Kisarazu, Chiba, Japan

Tohru Minamino
Department of Cardiovascular Biology and Medicine, Niigata University Graduate School of Medical and Dental Sciences, Niigata, Japan, PRESTO, Japan Science and Technology Agency, Kawaguchi, Saitama, Japan

Yuichi Katsuoka, Luna Izuhara and Hirotaka James Okano
Division of Regenerative Medicine, Department of Internal Medicine, The Jikei University School of Medicine, Tokyo, Japan

Shinya Yokote and Takashi Yokoo
Division of Nephrology and Hypertension, Department of Internal Medicine, The Jikei University School of Medicine, Tokyo, Japan

Shuichiro Yamanaka
Division of Regenerative Medicine, Department of Internal Medicine, The Jikei University School of Medicine, Tokyo, Japan
Division of Nephrology and Hypertension, Department of Internal Medicine, The Jikei University School of Medicine, Tokyo, Japan

Akifumi Yamada
Department of Pediatrics, The Jikei University School of Medicine, Tokyo, Japan

Yohta Shimada
Department of Gene Therapy, Institute of DNA Medicine, The Jikei University School of Medicine, Tokyo, Japan

Nobuo Omura and Takao Ohki
Department of Surgery, The Jikei University School of Medicine, Tokyo, Japan

Stefania Briganti, Enrica Flori, Barbara Bellei and Mauro Picardo
Laboratory of Cutaneous Physiopathology, San Gallicano Dermatologic Institute, Istituto di Ricovero e Cura a Carattere Scientifico, Rome, Italy

Jennifer P. Chou, Danielle M. Ryba and Megha P. Koduri
Department of Pathology & Laboratory Medicine, David Geffen School of Medicine, University of California Los Angeles, Los Angeles, California, United States of America

Rita B. Effros
Department of Pathology & Laboratory Medicine, David Geffen School of Medicine, University of California Los Angeles, Los Angeles, California, United States of America
UCLA AIDS Institute, David Geffen School of Medicine, University of California Los Angeles, Los Angeles, California, United States of America

Christina M. Ramirez
Department of Biostatistics, Fielding School of Public Health, University of California Los Angeles, Los Angeles, California, United States of America

Olga Alster, Anna Bielak-Zmijewska, Grazyna Mosieniak, Aleksandra Wojtala, Zbigniew Korwek and Ewa Sikora
Laboratory of the Molecular Bases of Aging, Nencki Institute of Experimental Biology, Polish Academy of Sciences, Warsaw, Poland
Maria Moreno-Villanueva and Alexander Burkle Molecular Toxicology Group, Department of Biology, University of Konstanz, Konstanz, Germany

Wioleta Dudka-Ruszkowska, Monika Kusio-Kobiałka and Katarzyna Piwocka
Laboratory of Cytometry, Nencki Institute of Experimental Biology, Polish Academy of Sciences, Warsaw, Poland

Jan K. Siwicki
Department of Immunology, Maria Sklodowska-Curie Memorial Cancer Center and Institute of Oncology, Warsaw, Poland

Keiko Fujimura, Shu Wakino, Hitoshi Minakuchi, Kazuhiro Hasegawa, Koji Hosoya, Motoaki Komatsu, Yuka Kaneko, Keisuke Shinozuka, Naoki Washida, Takeshi Kanda, Hirobumi Tokuyama, Koichi Hayashi and Hiroshi Itoh
Department of Internal Medicine, School of Medicine, Keio University, Tokyo, Japan

Sigrid Hatse, Barbara Brouwers, Patrick Schöffski and Hans Wildiers
Laboratory of Experimental Oncology (LEO), Department of Oncology, KU Leuven, and Department of General Medical Oncology, University Hospitals Leuven, Leuven Cancer Institute, Leuven, Belgium

Bruna Dalmasso
Laboratory of Experimental Oncology (LEO), Department of Oncology, KU Leuven, and Department of General Medical Oncology, University Hospitals Leuven, Leuven Cancer Institute, Leuven, Belgium
Department of Internal Medicine, Istituto di Ricerca a Carattere Clinico e Scientifico (IRCCS), Azienda Ospedaliera Universitaria (AOU) San Martino Istituto Nazionale Tumori (IST), Genoa, Italy

Annouschka Laenen
Interuniversity Centre for Biostatistics and Statistical Bioinformatics, Leuven, Belgium

Cindy Kenis
Laboratory of Experimental Oncology (LEO), Department of Oncology, KU Leuven, and Department of General Medical Oncology, University Hospitals Leuven, Leuven Cancer Institute, Leuven, Belgium
Department of Geriatric Medicine, University Hospitals Leuven, Leuven, Belgium

Laura Pintado-Berninches and Jaime Carrillo
Instituto de Investigaciones Biomédicas CSIC/UAM, Madrid, Spain

Cristina Manguan-Garcia, Rosario Machado-Pinilla, Leandro Sastre and Rosario Perona
Instituto de Investigaciones Biomédicas CSIC/UAM, Madrid, Spain
CIBER de Enfermedades Raras, Valencia, Spain

Carme Pérez-Quilis, Isabel Esmoris and Amparo Gimeno
Biomedical Research Institute INCLIVA, Valencia, Spain

Department of Physiology, Faculty of Medicine and Dentistry, University of Valencia, Valencia, Spain

Jose Luis García-Giménez and Federico V. Pallardó,
CIBER de Enfermedades Raras, Valencia, Spain
Biomedical Research Institute INCLIVA, Valencia, Spain
Department of Physiology, Faculty of Medicine and Dentistry, University of Valencia, Valencia, Spain

Marco Napolitano
IRCCS SDN Foundation, Naples, Italy

Filiberto Cimino
IRCCS SDN Foundation, Naples, Italy
Department of Molecular Medicine and Medical Biotechnologies, University of Naples Federico II, Naples, Italy
CEINGE – Advanced Biotechnologies, Naples, Italy

Marika Comegna, Mariangela Succoio, Lucio Pastore, Raffaella Faraonio and Fabiana Passaro
Department of Molecular Medicine and Medical Biotechnologies, University of Naples Federico II, Naples, Italy
CEINGE – Advanced Biotechnologies, Naples, Italy

Eleonora Leggiero
CEINGE – Advanced Biotechnologies, Naples, Italy

Akira Shimamoto, Harunobu Kagawa, Kazumasa Zensho, Yukihiro Sera and Hidetoshi Tahara
Department of Cellular and Molecular Biology, Graduate School of Biomedical & Health Sciences, Hiroshima University, Hiroshima, Japan

Yasuhiro Kazuki and Mitsuo Oshimura
Department of Biomedical Science, Institute of Regenerative Medicine and Biofunction, Graduate School of Medical Science, Tottori University, Yonago, Japan

Mitsuhiko Osaki
Department of Biomedical Science, Institute of Regenerative Medicine and Biofunction, Graduate School of Medical Science, Tottori University, Yonago, Japan
Division of Pathological Biochemistry, Faculty of Medicine, Tottori University, Yonago, Japan

Yasuhito Ishigaki
Medical Research Institute, Kanazawa Medical University, Kahoku, Ishikawa, Japan

Kanya Hamasaki and Yoshiaki Kodama
Department of Genetics, Radiation Effects Research
Foundation, Hiroshima, Japan

Shinsuke Yuasa and Keiichi Fukuda
Department of Cardiology, Keio University School
of Medicine, Tokyo, Japan

Kyotaro Hirashima and Hiroyuki Seimiya
Division of Molecular Biotherapy, The Cancer
Chemotherapy Center, Japanese Foundation For
Cancer Research, Tokyo, Japan
Hirofumi Koyama and Takahiko Shimizu
Department of Advanced Aging Medicine, Chiba
University Graduate School of Medicine, Chiba,
Japan

Minoru Takemoto and Koutaro Yokote,
Department of Clinical Cell Biology and Medicine,
Chiba University Graduate School of Medicine,
Chiba, Japan

Makoto Goto
Division of Orthopedic Surgery & Rheumatology,
Tokyo Women's Medical University Medical Center
East, Tokyo, Japan

Joshua B. Benoit, Geoffrey M. Attardo and Serap
Aksoy
Department of Epidemiology of Microbial Diseases,
Yale School of Public Health, New Haven,
Connecticut, United State of America

Veronika Michalkova
Department of Epidemiology of Microbial Diseases,
Yale School of Public Health, New Haven,
Connecticut, United State of America
Section of Molecular and Applied Zoology, Institute
of Zoology, Slovak Academy of Sciences, Bratislava,
Slovakia

Jan Medlock
Department of Biomedical Sciences, Oregon State
University, Corvallis, Oregon, United States of
America

Laura Perucho
Leibniz Institute for Age Research - Fritz Lipmann
Institute (FLI), Jena, Germany

Ana Artero-Castro, Sergi Guerrero, Santiago
Ramón y Cajal and Matilde E. LLeonart
Oncology and Pathology Group, Institut de Recerca
Hospital Vall d'Hebron, Barcelona, Spain

Zhao-Qi Wang
Leibniz Institute for Age Research - Fritz Lipmann
Institute (FLI), Jena, Germany
Faculty of Biology and Pharmacy, Friedrich Schiller
University of Jena, Jena, Germany

Ping Wu, Jen-Yi Lee, Pei-Rong Li, Wan-Yu Hsieh
and Huei-Wen Chen
Graduate Institute of Toxicology, College of Medicine,
National Taiwan University, Taipei, Taiwan

Lan-Hui Li
Graduate Institute of Toxicology, College of
Medicine, National Taiwan University, Taipei,
Taiwan
Department of Laboratory, Kunming Branch, Taipei
City Hospital, Taipei, Taiwan

Chao-Chi Ho
Department of Internal Medicine, National Taiwan
University Hospital and National Taiwan University
Medical College, Taipei, Taiwan

Chen-Lung Ho
Division of Wood Cellulose, Taiwan Forestry
Research Institute, Taipei, Taiwan

Wan-Jiun Chen
Graduate Institute of Toxicology, College of
Medicine, National Taiwan University, Taipei,
Taiwan
Graduate Institute of Oncology, College of Medicine,
National Taiwan University, Taipei, Taiwan

Chien-Chun Wang
Division of Infectious Diseases, Kunming Branch,
Taipei City Hospital, Taipei, Taiwan

Muh-Yong Yen
Division of Infectious Diseases, Kunming Branch,
Taipei City Hospital, Taipei, Taiwan
Department of Medicine, National Yang-Ming
University, Taipei, Taiwan

Shun-Min Yang
Department of Pathology, Tri-Service General
Hospital, National Defense Medical Center, Taipei,
Taiwan

Jiahong Zhu, Xinyi Mu, Chunyan Xu, Jun Liu,
Mengsi Zhang, Chengpeng Li and Yaping Wang
Department of Histology and Embryology,
Laboratory of Stem Cells and Tissue Engineering,
Chongqing Medical University, Chongqing, China

Jin Zeng
The Land Force Lintong Sanatorium, Xi'an, Shanxi, China

Jie Chen, Tinyu Li
Chongqing Stem Cell Therapy Engineering Technical Center, Chongqing, China

Index